Review of Surgery

Review of Surgery

Basic Science and Clinical Topics for ABSITE

Gamal Mostafa, MD
Lamont Cathey, MD
Frederick L. Greene, MD

Editors

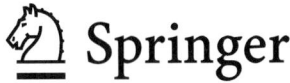 Springer

Gamal Mostafa, MD, Attending Surgeon, Department of General Surgery, Carolinas Medical Center, Charlotte, North Carolina, USA

Lamont Cathey, MD, Resident, Department of General Surgery, Carolinas Medical Center, Charlotte, North Carolina, USA

Frederick L. Greene, MD, Chairman, Department of General Surgery, Carolinas Medical Center, Charlotte, North Carolina, USA

Publisher's Note: Both the content of the In-Training Examination and the term "ABSITE" are protected by copyright held by the American Board of Surgery. The term "ABSITE" is used with the express permission of the American Board of Surgery.

Library of Congress Control Number: 2005939181

ISBN-10: 0-387-29080-X
ISBN-13: 978-0387-29080-5

Printed on acid-free paper.

Preface

One of the constants in the life of every young surgeon is the knowledge that one will be taking standardized examinations both during and after one's training in general surgery. As discussions continue regarding the best way to measure technical and professional competence, methods of testing will continue to take on new and more modern formats. It is obvious, however, that the knowledge base will continue to be a prime factor and that the volume of knowledge will continue to explode.

As we launched the development of a guide to facilitate the testing phase of surgical knowledge, the prime factors were to distill a large amount of information into a useable format and to provide the reader and future test taker with questions that would help during the study phase. As editors, we have had a number of years of training as well as participation in the training of others. We therefore appreciate the nuances and the types of material that are important, not only to answer test questions effectively, but also to have in our knowledge base in order to provide good clinical care. With these goals in mind, we developed this study guide.

The editors wish to thank our colleagues from Springer for their wonderful support, not only for agreeing to undertake this publishing venture, but also for their continued support and guidance throughout the development of this study guide. We are indebted to Cissy Moore-Swartz for her incredible technical support and for keeping the editors focused during the development phase. To have her as a member of our department in the capacity of editor, creator, and support person is an incredible resource.

Finally, the editors wish to dedicate this publication to all the surgical residents we have had the privilege to know and help train in the past and present and to those we hope will benefit from this labor as they face a variety of examinations in the future. We hope that this compendium is helpful in achieving success in the testing of their knowledge and surgical prowess.

Gamal Mostafa, MD
Lamont Cathey, MD
Frederick L. Greene, MD

Contents

Contributors

Heath Beckham, MD
Surgical Resident, Department of General Surgery, Carolinas Medical Center
Charlotte, North Carolina, USA

Justin M. Burns, MD
Surgical Resident, Department of General Surgery, Carolinas Medical Center
Charlotte, North Carolina, USA

Steven Camp, MD
Surgical Resident, Department of General Surgery, Carolinas Medical Center
Charlotte, North Carolina, USA

Jamie Cannon, MD
Surgical Resident, Department of General Surgery, Carolinas Medical Center
Charlotte, North Carolina, USA

Lamont Cathey, MD
Resident, Department of General Surgery, Carolinas Medical Center
Charlotte, North Carolina, USA

Alejandro Fernandez-Tatum, MD
Surgical Resident, Department of General Surgery, Carolinas Medical Center
Charlotte, North Carolina, USA

Frederick L. Greene, MD
Chairman, Department of General Surgery, Carolinas Medical Center
Charlotte, North Carolina, USA

Oliver Gunter, MD
Fellow, Trauma Department, Vanderbilt University, Nashville, Tennessee, USA

M. Daniel Isbell, MD
Surgical Resident, Department of General Surgery, Carolinas Medical Center
Charlotte, North Carolina, USA

Charles S. Joels, MD
Surgical Resident, Department of General Surgery, Carolinas Medical Center
Charlotte, North Carolina, USA

Philip D. Khan, MD
Surgical Resident, Department of General Surgery, Carolinas Medical Center
Charlotte, North Carolina, USA

Timothy Kuwada, MD
Attending Surgeon, Department of General Surgery, Carolinas Medical
Center, Charlotte, North Carolina, USA

Gamal Mostafa, MD
Attending Surgeon, Department of General Surgery, Carolinas Medical
Center, Charlotte, North Carolina, USA

James Norton, PhD
Statistician, Department of Statistics, Carolinas Medical Center
Charlotte, North Carolina, USA

Ankur R. Rana, MD
Surgical Resident, Department of General Surgery, Carolinas Medical Center
Charlotte, North Carolina, USA

Thomas M. Schmelzer, MD
Surgical Resident, Department of General Surgery, Carolinas Medical Center
Charlotte, North Carolina, USA

Part I
Physiology of the Cell

1
The Cell

Human cells express different shapes and functions. However, there are common structural and functional elements that allow cells to use energy, grow, and divide. All cells possess plasma membrane, and they contain specialized structures known as *organelles* that perform specific functions. Cell division, cell death, and cell signaling are complex cell biologic processes that are relevant in both health and disease.

The plasma membrane defines the boundary of the cell and is composed of phospholipids and proteins. The cell membrane is a continuous bilayer structure made of a sheet of phospholipid molecules with embedded proteins. The phospholipids are oriented in such a way that the hydrophilic phosphate portion is exposed to the aqueous surfaces and the insoluble hydrophobic portions are in the interior of the membrane. The animal eukaryotic cell membrane is distinguished from prokaryotic cells by its cholesterol content. The amount of membrane cholesterol determines the degree of its fluidity. Membrane proteins are globular units that can be attached to the inner or outer surface of the membrane or protrude through as transmembrane protein. Membrane proteins may function as carrier proteins, receptors, or enzymes.

The largest cellular organelle is the nucleus that contains all the chromosomal DNA in association with a specialized class of acidic proteins termed *histones*. DNA is the hereditary material that makes up genes. A gene is a segment of DNA that contains the code required for assembling one molecule, usually a protein. The genetic information is translated into RNA and then protein, leading to the expression of specific biologic characteristics of phenotypes.

Mitochondria are sausage-shaped organelles that are the major source of energy production. The mitochondrion is made up of two lipid bilayers. In the interior, the matrix space contains water-soluble enzymes that convert acetyl coenzyme A to carbon dioxide and water via the citric acid cycle. The respiratory enzyme chain involved in oxidative phosphorylation and the generation of adenosine triphosphate is attached to the inner membrane of the mitochondrion. The endoplasmic reticulum (ER) is a network of interconnected membranes that form closed vesicles, tubes, and saccules. The ER is involved in the synthesis of proteins and lipids. It is divided into rough ER, which is studded with ribosomes and involved in the synthesis of exportable proteins, and smooth ER, which lacks ribosomes and is involved in the synthesis of lipids. The rough ER is prominent in cells such as the pancreatic acini and plasma cells that secrete a large amount of proteins. Smooth ER is prominent in cells producing lipid derivatives, such as the adrenal cortex. Smooth ER also contains enzymes that detoxify endogenous metabolites and drugs. The Golgi complex is adjacent to the rough ER and is involved in sorting and packing of secreted proteins.

Cell signaling is the mechanism through which neighboring and distant cells influence the behavior of other cells. Cell signaling is important in both health and disease. Normal cell signaling is controlled by multiple signaling molecules. Signaling molecules include proteins, amino acids, steroids, and dissolved gases such as nitric oxide. These signaling molecules are also called *ligands*. Ligands bind to specific cell proteins called *receptors*. Receptors are located in the plasma membrane or the in the cytoplasm of the target cell. On ligand binding, the receptor is activated, and it generates intracellular signals that change the cell behavior. Ligands may act on the signaling cell itself (autocrine signaling) or on adjacent cells (paracrine signaling), or they may enter the circulation to act on distant cells (endocrine signaling). Most ligands are hydrophilic molecules. They bind to receptors on the cell surface of the target cells. Some ligands are hydrophilic molecules, such as steroid hormones, thyroid hormones, retinoids, and vitamin D. They diffuse across the cell membrane and bind to intracellular receptor proteins.

A cell division cycle is an organized sequence of complex biologic processes. Replication of DNA occurs in the synthesis (S) phase. Cell division occurs in the mitotic (M) phase. The intervals between these two phases are called gap 1 (G_1) and gap 2 (G_2) phases. When cells enter the G_1 phase, they receive signals that determine if they will proceed with DNA synthesis (i.e., enter the S phase) or exit the cycle. The control of the cell cycle is governed by the activation and inactivation of a family of regulatory proteins called *cyclin-dependent kinases*. Genes encode cell cycle regulatory proteins. These genes are often the target of mutations during neoplastic transformation. If the mutated gene is cancer causing, it is called an *oncogene*; its normal counterpart is called a *proto-oncogene*. Proto-oncogenes are typically involved in stimulatory signals, and mutation of a single copy is sufficient to cause increased cellular proliferation. Antiproliferative genes negatively control the cell division. These genes are referred to as *tumor suppressor genes* because they prevent excess and uncontrolled cell proliferation. Inactivation of these genes will cause the loss of proliferation control. Unlike proto-oncogenes, both copies of tumor suppressor genes must be deleted for malignant transformation to take place.

Apoptosis is physiologic cell death. It is implicated in various physiologic functions, including the remodeling of tissues during development and removal of senescent cells. As a physiologic process of cell elimination, it contrasts from the other form of cell death, necrosis. Necrosis is a passive energy-independent cell death. It requires an acute nonphysiologic injury, such as, ischemia, mechanical injury, or toxins. Necrosis will result in cell swelling and lysis. Cell lysis releases cytoplasmic contents into the extracellular milieu, resulting in inflammation. In contrast, apoptosis is a highly regulated energy-requiring form of cell death. Apoptotic cells undergo a sequence of morphological and biochemical changes. In the early phase of apoptosis, cells exhibit shrunken cytoplasm and detach from neighboring cells. Middle events include chromatin condensation with resultant crescent-shaped nuclei and then nuclear fragmentation. Late in apoptosis, the cells fragment into discrete plasma membrane-bound vesicles called *apoptotic bodies*. Apoptotic bodies are phagocytosed by surrounding cells and macrophages without inducing an inflammatory response.

Many stimuli activate the process of apoptosis. These include DNA damage through ionizing radiation, growth factor nutritional deprivation, activation of certain death receptors (Fas and tumor necrosis factor receptors), oxidative stress, and many chemotherapeutic agents. DNA damage activates *p53* functional activity, which results in cell cycle arrest in the G_1 phase in order to allow DNA repair. If the DNA damage is irreparable, death of the cell with apoptosis will occur. All signals of apoptosis converge to activate a common central process known as the *caspase cascade*. Caspases (cystine aspartate proteases) are proteolytic enzymes involved in the biochemical pathway that mediates apoptotic cell death. Tumor necrosis factor receptors (TNFRs) are a superfamily of transmembrane proteins that are present on all cells. Activation of these receptors may initiate apoptosis. During sepsis, down-regulation of macrophage and neutrophil TNFR is noted. This attenuation of TNFR activity may delay apoptosis of inflammatory cells and, therefore, prolong the inflammatory response. This prolonged survival of inflammatory cells augments the response to injury and infection and may precipitate multiple organ failure.

2
Cytokines

Cytokines are a diverse group of polypeptides and glycoproteins that are important mediators of inflammation. They are produced by various cell types, primarily by leukocytes. Cytokines are potent intercellular messengers, and they exert most of their actions on immune and inflammatory cells. Cytokines have certain distinctive features when compared with hormones. They are not stored intracellularly. When the cell is stimulated, cytokines are rapidly synthesized by messenger RNA transcription and quickly released. Cytokines exert their effects through very high-affinity binding to various receptors on target cells. Therefore, very small amounts of cytokines are required to produce their desired biologic effects. As a rule, cytokines mostly act on cells locally in an autocrine or paracrine fashion. However, when cytokines are produced in large amounts, they can enter the circulation and cause significant systemic effects.

Tumor Necrosis Factor and Interleukin-1

Tumor necrosis factor (TNF) and interleukin-1 (IL-1) are structurally dissimilar. However, their functions overlap considerably, and they act synergistically. Tumor necrosis factor was originally discovered as a substance causing ischemic necrosis of tumors in rabbits. It is produced mainly by monocytes and macrophages, and the most potent stimulus for its production is lipopolysaccharide (LPS) (endotoxin) from Gram-negative bacteria. However, other stimuli such as infection, trauma, ischemia, and toxins induce TNF release. Under normal physiologic circumstances, tissue TNF levels are not detectable, but TNF is the dominant cytokine secreted on activation of macrophages. Tumor necrosis factor is a proinflammatory cytokine, which directly depresses cardiac contractility, produces cachexia, and influences apoptosis. Tumor necrosis factor

results in an increased expression of endothelial E-selectin and leukocyte integrins. This promotes leukocyte adhesion to the endothelium. Several of the physiologic effects of "inflammation" can be attributed to the actions of TNF. Tumor necrosis factor acts on the hypothalamus via prostaglandin synthesis to cause fever, and it induces hepatocyte production of some of the acute-phase proteins, including C-reactive protein, fibrinogen, serum amyloid A, and α_1-antitrypsin. Large doses of TNF produce the classic symptoms of septic shock. Hypotension results from reduced vascular smooth muscle tone as well as myocardial depression, and disseminated intravascular coagulation results from endothelial expression of tissue factor and inhibition of thrombomodulin. Tumor necrosis factor is a potent regulator of cellular metabolism. It appears to be responsible for the syndrome of cachexia associated with chronic infection and malignancy. This effect may be related to the altered glucose and lipid metabolism.

Like TNF, IL-1 is produced primarily by macrophages. Interleukin-1 is also a pro-inflammatory cytokine, and its actions are similar to those of TNF. In contrast to TNF, IL-1 cannot induce apoptosis. Interleukin-1 induces fever when injected into experimental animals. It is likely that this pyrogenic action results from its interaction with the endothelial cells of the hypothalamic-pituitary portal venous system. This generates prostaglandins E. These prostaglandins act on the hypothalamus and alter the firing rate of thermosensitive neurons leading to fever. Therefore, antipyretic drugs such as aspirin are effective, because they inhibit the cyclooxygenase enzyme that converts arachidonic acid into prostaglandins.

Interferons

Interferon (IFN)-γ is produced by T cells and natural killer (NK) cells in response to antigens, an event greatly enhanced by IL-12. It activates macrophages, inducing them to kill microbes by activating enzymes that trigger synthesis of reactive oxygen metabolites and nitric oxide. IFN-α, and IFN-β are two functionally similar cytokines and are also called the *antiviral interferons*, because they are produced by antigen-stimulated T cells in response to viral infection. They inhibit viral replication by preventing infection of neighboring cells and putting cells into an antiviral state. They are frequently used in the clinical setting, and IFN-α seems to be an effective therapy for viral hepatitis.

Interleukin-6

Interleukin-6 is produced by mononuclear phagocytes, endothelial cells, and fibroblasts. The most prominent sources of IL-6 are LPS-stimulated macrophages and IL-1/TNF–stimulated stromal cells. Interleukin-6 was initially termed *hepatocyte-stimulating factor*. It acts as a potent stimulus for hepatocyte synthesis of acute-phase proteins. In contrast to other cytokines, IL-6 is more readily detected systemically. Interleukin-6 serves more of a classic endocrine function. This has an important clinical implication. Numerous studies have measured cytokine concentrations in the peripheral vasculature in an effort to identify markers of sepsis, predictors of mortality, and possible clinical interventions. The levels of the proinflammatory cytokines (TNF, IL-1) are not consistently correlated with either disease severity or mortality in patients with septic shock. The cytokine with which peripheral blood levels seem to correlate best with disease severity is IL-6.

Interleukin-2

Originally called *T-cell growth factor*, IL-2 acts in an autocrine manner on the T cells that produce it (i.e., T helper cells), up-regulating IL-2 receptors and thereby causing preferential proliferation of T cells specific for the stimulating antigen. It also promotes growth and differentiation of NK cells. Unlike other cytokines, which exert most of their effects via the innate immune system, IL-2 mediates acquired immunity, that is, the proliferation and differentiation of lymphocytes after antigen recognition.

Transforming Growth Factor-β

Transforming growth factor-β (TGF-β) is produced by a variety of cells, including activated T cells, phagocytes, and endothelial cells. It has potent anti-inflammatory effects. It inhibits T-cell differentiation and proliferation and macrophage activation. As an anti-inflammatory cytokine, it counteracts the effects of proinflammatory cytokines, causing down-regulation of endothelial adhesion molecules and down-regulation of TNF endothelial receptor expression. Transforming growth factor-β is one of the key cytokines involved in controlling tissue repair. Transforming growth factor-β is a potent inducer of extracellular matrix production and inhibitor of matrix degradation. The sustained production of this cytokine is implicated in the development of excessive tissue fibrosis. Overproduction of TGF-β is an important molecular event in inducing tissue fibrosis and may be an important mediator in a variety of disease states, such as liver cirrhosis, scleroderma, and keloid.

Certain Therapeutic Implications

Infliximab is a genetically engineered anti-TNF antibody that can bind to both cell-bound and -soluble TNF. It causes lysis of TNF-producing cells via complement- and antibody-dependent cytotoxicity. Infliximab is approved for use in patients with Crohn's disease, in whom it can induce and maintain remissions, result in endoscopically and histologically demonstrable mucosal healing, reduce the number of perianal fistulae, and decrease inflammation in ileoanal pouches. Infliximab is also used to treat other conditions such as rheumatoid arthritis, ankylosing spondylitis, and psoriatic arthritis.

It has long been recognized that the clotting system plays a major role in inflammation. This connection exists at several biologic levels. Disseminated intravascular coagulation is one of the cardinal signs of sepsis. Proinflammatory cytokines such as TNF, IL-1, and IL-6 are known to trigger activation of the clotting cascade by stimulating the release of tissue factor from monocytes and endothelium, leading to thrombin formation and a fibrin clot. These cytokines also inhibit endogenous fibrinolytic mechanisms by stimulating the release of plasminogen-activator inhibitor-1 from platelets and endothelium. Therefore, these proinflammatory cytokines can also be considered as procoagulants. Protein C is an endogenous anticoagulant that, when activated by thrombin bound to thrombomodulin, reduces the generation of thrombin by inactivating clotting factors Va and VIIIa. It also exerts an anti-inflammatory effect by inhibiting monocyte production of TNF, IL-1, and IL-6 and by limiting leukocyte adhesion to endothelium by binding selectins. Therefore, protein C clearly has an anti-inflammatory function. Decreased circulating levels of activated protein C are usually present in sepsis and are associated with increased mortality. These observations have led to the investigation of activated protein C as a potential treatment for severe sepsis. A multicenter, placebo-controlled phase III clinical trial documented a 6.1% reduction in total mortality in patients treated with drotrecogin alpha (the generic name for recombinant human activated protein C). The only major side effect with this agent was an increased risk of serious bleeding. Drotrecogin is thus the first therapy to have shown a real clinical benefit in sepsis trials. The U.S. Food and Drug Administration has approved this agent for treatment of sepsis. It is marketed under the brand name Xigris®.

3
Neutrophils

Neutrophils are the predominant inflammatory cell in a wound during the first 2 to 3 days after wounding; however, macrophages eventually become the predominant inflammatory cell in the wound. The normal immune action of the neutrophil is to phagocytose its target cell. This process results in the creation of a microenvironment inside the neutrophil known as a *phagosome*, which contains the targets for destruction. When the phagosome has been established, the neutrophil releases large quantities of reactive oxygen metabolites and proteases into it. Reactive oxygen metabolites and proteases act in synergy to digest phagocytosed matter. In cases of strong neutrophil activation, the cells may release their toxic products in concentrations that overwhelm the body's regulatory defenses, causing substantial damage to surrounding tissues through excess vascular permeability and parenchymal injury. After neutrophils phagocytose damaged material, they cease to function and often release lysosomal contents, which can contribute to tissue damage and a prolonged inflammatory response. Inflammatory cells and liquefied tissue are the constituents of pus, which may or may not be sterile, depending on whether bacteria are present. Unlike neutrophils, macrophages survive after phagocytosing bacteria or damaged material. The shift from neutrophils to macrophages as the predominant inflammatory cell type within the wound is at least in part due to macrophages' extended lifespan. Host defense systems require molecular oxygen to enable the humoral and cellular immune systems to function optimally. Normally, after opsonization a microorganism is phagocytosed by a neutrophil. The phagosome containing the bacteria then fuses with lysosomal granules within the neutrophils. In the presence of molecular oxygen, toxic oxygen radicals, such as hydrogen peroxide or superoxide, are generated, which result in lysis of bacteria. In the presence of devitalized tissue and in many shock states, delivery of oxygen to the neutrophils is inadequate. In these instances, even though phagocytosis may occur, bacteria may not be destroyed, and infection develops or persists.

To patrol the body effectively for infectious organisms and to repair injuries in disparate regions of the body, neutrophils must be able to circulate as nonadherent particles in blood and lymph and to adhere to and migrate through specific tissue sites where they are needed. Inflammatory events trigger release of circulating mediators such as cytokines, which produce generalized activation of endothelial cells and leukocytes, thereby rendering one or both cell types more adhesive. Circulating phagocytes then adhere to endothelium, they undergo diapedesis between the junctions of endothelial cells, migrate through the subendothelial matrix, and participate in the parenchymal inflammatory reaction. This phagocyte adherence, although essential to the immune response and to the repair of injury, may induce pathologic consequences. The importance of leukocyte adhesion to the endothelium in maintaining host defenses against infection is illustrated by a condition called *leukocyte adhesion deficiency I* (LAD I), which produces a profound defect in phagocyte accumulation because the leukocytes, although stimulated, cannot adhere and migrate to extravascular sites. Patients with LAD I have little or no pus at bacterial infection sites and suffer recurrent life-threatening bacterial infections. On the other hand, unmoderated leukocyte adhesion to the endothelium can also have pathologic consequences, such as lung failure (acute respiratory distress syndrome).

It has long been debated whether alterations in neutrophils or endothelial cells were responsible for the critical adhesive interaction. It is now clear that both cell types are involved. Several proteins, called *adherence molecules* (cell adhesion molecules), are currently identified. These molecules are classified into three categories, selectins, integrins, and immunoglobulins (Ig). L-selectin is expressed only on leukocytes, E-selectin is localized to endothelial cells, and P-selectin is found on platelets as well as endothelial cells. E-selectin is found exclusively on the surface of endothelial cells. Although not expressed on resting endothelium, E-selectin is markedly up-regulated in response to the cytokines interleukin-1 and tumor necrosis factor-α as well as to lipopolysaccharide. The integrin family comprises a vast number of adhesion molecules that mediate intercellular recognition and cellular binding to the extracellular matrix. These molecules are transmembrane receptors as opposed to selectins, which are surface molecules.

The selectins are expressed only on cells within the vasculature or the lymphatic system. Three selectins have been identified: L-selectin, P-selectin, and E-selectin. The selectins are responsible for the earliest interaction of circulating cells, setting the stage for integrin-mediated firm adherence. Without selectins, leukocytes interact poorly with endothelium. The selectin-mediated adhesion involves rapid on–off interaction and is observed under conditions of flow. On the other hand, integrin-dependent adhesion is sensitive to shear and is optimal under static conditions. Therefore, selectin receptors are responsible for the initial transient adhesion of neutrophils that occurs at sites of inflammation, known as *rolling*. The leukocyte integrin receptors interact with ligands on the endothelial cells, including members of the third major class of adhesion molecules, Ig. The integrin–Ig ligand interaction mediates firm adhesion of the neutrophils to endothelial cells at sites of inflammation as well as subsequent diapedesis and emigration. Together, these distinct adhesion systems create a process whereby neutrophils in flowing blood are initially "slowed" and "tethered" to endothelium by selectins. Then, once tethered, firm integrin–Ig adhesion results in diapedesis and neutrophil-mediated injury.

4
Macrophages

Monocytes are large cells with kidney-bean-shaped nuclei and abundant cytoplasm containing lysosomes. Monocytes are produced in the bone marrow and are found in the peripheral circulation (1% to 6% of all cells). The cells stay in the circulation for approximately 2 days until finding a permanent home in a particular body tissue. Once they transition into tissue, they are called *macrophages* (histiocytes).

Macrophages are phagocytizing cells and are present in most body tissues. The lifespan of a macrophage ranges from 2 to 4 months. The cells surveil the tissue through cell surface receptors or through pinocytosis. Macrophages migrate throughout the tissue via pseudopodal movement or can remain stationary. Macrophages are activated when they come in contact with inflammatory mediators (i.e., bacterial lipopolysaccharides [LPS], complement, bacterial DNA, inert microorganism particles, and interferon-γ). In contrast to inactivated macrophages, activated macrophages are more active, have more cytoplasm, and produce nitric oxide synthase. Macrophages phagocytize cellular debris and foreign particles. Specialized cell surface receptors help choose the targets for phagocytosis. Specific receptors include LPS receptors (i.e., CD14), mannose receptors, and scavenger receptors. More specifically, Toll-like receptors, which are expressed on macrophage surfaces, have a key role in their activation.

Phagocytosis ensues with several key steps. First, target particles are opsonized by immunoglobulins or complement proteins. Surface receptors on the macrophages interact with the opsonins and cause phagocytosis to begin. A specialized vacuole, called a *phagosome*, engulfs the particle. Next, lysosomes fuse with the phagosome,

emptying their enzymatic contents into it. The phagocytized particles are broken down by enzymatic digestion or by reactive oxygen species. However, some materials are resistant to breakdown, such as carbon from cigarette smoke and certain bacteria (i.e., mycobacteria). Resistant materials are surrounded by large numbers of macrophages forming a structure called a *granuloma*. Granulomas are composed of collections of mast cells, lymphocytes, and fibroblasts. The macrophages in granulomas resemble epithelial cells due to their close association and microvilli. Thus they are termed *epithelioid cells*. Multinucleate giant cells form from the fusion of monocytes at the lesion.

Activated macrophages contribute to the immune reaction and wound healing in various ways. The phagocytic actions help to eliminate cellular debris in fresh wounds before healing begins. Materials such as elastases, collagenases, lysozyme, hydrogen peroxide, and complement are released into the local area after macrophage activation. These substances have antimicrobial functions and help to refashion the extracellular matrix. Macrophages also secrete cytokines that affect the behavior of other cells as well (granulocyte-macrophage colony-stimulating factor, interleukin-6, fibroblast growth factors, and prostaglandins). Nitric oxide is released from activated macrophages and in turn causes histamine and vasoactive mediator release from mast cells and platelets. This provides a stimulus for the vascular response during inflammation. Interferon-α and interleukin-12 secreted by macrophages stimulate the proliferation and differentiation of lymphocytes. Macrophages also play an important role in processing antigens and presenting them to lymphocytes.

5
Lymphocytes

Lymphocytes are the major players in acquired immunity. Their role is to recognize antigens through a complex system of membrane surface receptors. Lymphocytes come in contact with antigens through direct contact or after they have been processed by antigen-presenting cells. T cells and B cells are the two major types of lymphocytes. T-cell lymphocytes are named as such because they are matured in the thymus. B cells are produced from the bone marrow. Together they account for about 95% of the circulating volume of lymphocytes. The ability to recognize an infinite number of antigens is the key to their immune activity. A variable family of genetic information imparts this ability to these unique cells. T and B cells are organized into subgroups according to membrane receptors, their location in the body, and their function.

T lymphocytes are subdivided according to their surface receptors (TCR-$\alpha\beta$ or TCR-$\gamma\delta$ plus CD3). Of the TCR-$\alpha\beta$ subset, up to 65% express CD4, and up to 35% express CD8. Immature thymocytes express both CD4 and CD8; however, only one receptor is expressed on mature cells. CD4 T lymphocytes recognize antigens that are associated with major histocompatibility complex (MHC) class II molecules, and CD8 T lymphocytes recognize those antigens associated with MHC class I molecules. T-helper cells (CD4 cells) produce cytokines that function in cell-mediated immunity. T_{H1} cells secrete interleukin-2 (IL-2) and interferon-γ. T_{H2} cells produce IL-4, IL-5, IL-6, IL-10, and IL-13, which stimulate antibody production.

B lymphocytes are the forerunners of plasma cells, which are cells that produce and secrete antibodies. B cells can be identified by the presence of immunoglobulins (IgM and IgD) on their cell surfaces. B cells also have receptors for complement and can be identified by another common surface marker, CD19. B cells differentiate into plasma cells after stimulation by T cells. Plasma cells have distinct histologic characteristics, which include a round eccentric nucleus with a cartwheel arrangement of heterochromatin. Their cytoplasm is filled with dense granular structures that contain antibodies. The cytoplasm also has a basophilic staining pattern and an extensive network of endoplasmic reticulum. Plasma cells, unlike B cells lack the immunoglobulin on their cell surface. They also lose the ability to replicate, making them terminal cells.

Natural killer cells are derived from the same bone marrow stem cell as T and B lymphocytes but lack the same receptor complex (TCR-CD3) and surface antibodies of T and B cells. Natural killer cells are large lymphocytes that are capable of nonspecific killing of tumor- and virus-infected cells. These cells can achieve their immune activity without presensitization. Special surface receptors (killing inhibitory receptors) recognize MHC class I molecules and prevent the attack of these cells. Natural killer cells are stimulated to propagate by IL-12.

Lymphocyte circulation and distribution occur in three major arenas. The first phase involves the migration of stem cells to the various lymphoid organs from their areas of production (fetal liver and bone marrow). The primary lymphoid organs are the areas of differentiation and maturation of the lymphocytes. The lymphocytes are then re-released into the peripheral circulation. Second, lymphocytes migrate back and forth from the lymphatic system to the circulatory system. Third, activated cells migrate to specific organs and body tissues.

Antigen recognition develops from the combination of two sets of genes encoding for the variable regions of immunoglobulins and T-cell receptors. Each genetic region encodes for a variable region (V), a diversity region (D), and a joining region. Variations in the combination of these genes give rise to the ability to recognize an infinite number of antigens. *Maturation* is the term given to the time period when these genetic changes take place.

Each lymphocyte is designed to recognize a single specific antigen. T cells recognize only antigens that have been processed by antigen-presenting cells (i.e., macrophages or dendritic cells). The antigen-presenting cell takes up the antigen and processes it by breaking it down to peptide residues. The peptide fragments are attached to MHC class II molecules and transported to the cell surface. This process is referred to as *MHC restriction*. T-cell proliferation and differentiation follow antigen interaction. T-cell differentiation produces helper T cells and cytotoxic T cells, which have memory cell functions as well. T-regulatory cells (CD4 cells) moderate the immune response by communicating with other immune cells through cytokines and direct contact.

B cells are capable of recognizing antigens that have not been processed by antigen-presenting cells. Specialized receptors on the cell surface enable interactions between the antigen and the B cell. Once this interaction occurs, the B cells proliferate and differentiate into plasma cells, which produce antibodies, and into memory cells. Memory B cells undergo further changes in their genetic makeup to create receptors with a high affinity for a particular antigen. Once memory cells encounter their specific antigen, the immune response that ensues is faster and amplified.

T-cell development occurs through a process of positive and negative selection. Early in the process, large pools of immature thymocytes exist in the cortical region of the thymus gland. These lymphocytes express TCR-$\alpha\beta$ along with CD4, CD8, and CD2 receptors on their surface. Native cells within the thymus gland (macrophages, dendritic cells, interdigitating cells) present self-MHC (class I or II) to the immature lymphocytes. The lymphocytes that have a strong affinity for MHC class II molecules undergo down-regulation of CD8 molecules and up-regulation of the CD4 molecules, becoming CD4 positive. In contrast, the cells that show a strong affinity for MHC class I molecules undergo down-regulation of CD4 and up-regulation of CD8 molecules, making them CD8 positive. T cells that fail to react with self-MHC are destroyed via apoptosis in the process of negative selection. Negative selection eliminates a population of T cells that cannot recognize self-antigens and therefore could mount an immune response to native body tissues (autoimmune disease).

The development of B cells occurs in two arenas, the bone marrow and the lymph nodes. B-cell precursors in the bone marrow have IgM heavy and light chains on their cell surface that serve as receptors. The precursor cells that lack both the receptors are destroyed by apoptosis during positive selection. The precursor cells that survive become immature B cells. These immature B cells migrate to lymph nodes where they undergo negative selection. Cells that interact with self-antigens with high affinity are eliminated by apoptosis. B cells that react weakly with self antigens undergo anergy (fail to develop further).

6
Nitric Oxide

In 1980, it was reported that an acetylcholine-mediated relaxation of vascular rings was affected by a molecule named *endothelium-derived relaxing factor* (EDRF). Later, it was discovered that EDRF is nitric oxide (NO), and its production is dependent on the presence of L-arginine. Nitric oxide is an autocrine and paracrine cellular mediator, which maintains homeostasis. Unlike other bioactive molecules, NO is not stored, and it does not act on a specific extracellular receptor. Instead, it is formed at a basal rate that can be augmented by external stimuli. It then diffuses freely and binds to carrier compounds to act on an intracellular receptor, which is the iron molecule of heme proteins.

Nitric oxide is formed as a byproduct of the stepwise conversion of L-arginine. L-arginine is the sole substrate for NO synthesis. This reaction is catalyzed by a series of enzymes called *nitric oxide synthases* (NOSs). Nitric oxide is a colorless gas with a very short half-life. Although NO acts on many proteins, it is best known for its activation of guanylate cyclase, which produces guanosine 3′,5′-cyclic monophosphate (cGMP). Among several actions, cGMP mediates smooth muscle relaxation and inhibition of platelet aggregation. Nitric oxide synthases exist in several cell-specific isoforms. These forms fall into two distinct categories: constitutive and inducible. Constitutive NOS is present in endothelial cells, platelets, and nerve cells. The inducible form is found in leukocytes, macrophages, Kupffer cells, and hepatocytes. Nitric oxide has a short half-life, a few seconds or less. When the NO free radical interacts with oxygen, the resulting oxidation to nitrite and nitrate inactivates the molecule. It also enables measurement of NO indirectly by the measurement of nitrite or nitrate.

Endothelium-derived NO is involved in the regulation of blood vessel tone. Nitric oxide differentially acts on venous and arterial tissues. Veins are affected to a greater extent than the arteries. Endothelial cells function as mechanoreceptors. The physical forces produced by the blood flow are transduced into biochemical signals to which the vessel wall can respond. Rapid responses are mediated in part by changes in NO production. This may explain the phenomenon of flow-dependent vasodilation that is observed in micro- and macrocirculation. Nitric oxide is also one of several endothelium-derived thromboregulators. It reduces platelet adhesion by activating platelet guanylate cyclase and decreasing intraplatelet Ca^{2+} levels. Nitric oxide is also involved in leukocyte interaction with the vessel wall and can inhibit neutrophil aggregation. The pulmonary vasculature has a similar response to NO. Clinical reports suggest that inhaled NO may prevent the development of adult respiratory distress syndrome. Interestingly, in the absence of hypoxia, inhaled NO has no effect on pulmonary hemodynamics.

Recent studies have observed the importance of endothelium and endothelium-derived NO in therapies to prevent or reverse atherosclerosis. Endothelial cell injury is one of the initiating events in the development of atherosclerosis. Atherosclerosis induces an early impairment of endothelium-derived NO relaxation. Women appear to have a greater resistance to atherosclerosis in the premenopausal years partially because of the estrogen-dependent increase in basal NO synthesis. Endothelial dysfunction is also considered an intrinsic element in the pathogenesis of diabetic angiopathy. There appears to be an impairment of endothelium-dependent relaxation in patients with diabetic angiopathy. Impaired NO-mediated relaxation has also been suggested as the mechanism underlying late vein graft failure. The use of the internal mammary artery in coronary bypass operations produces superior results compared with the use of long saphenous vein. This is likely due to the higher rate of NO formation in the internal mammary artery. Therefore, the internal mammary artery has greater NO and prostacyclin-mediated relaxation and more effective inhibition of platelet activation and leukocyte adhesion.

There is increasing evidence that NO plays a role in acute and chronic inflammation and in the systemic inflammatory response. Nitric oxide enhances vasodilation and edema formation, and inhibition of NO reduces the degree of inflammation. Nitric oxide is likely to come from several sources, including endothelial cells, neutrophils, and macrophages. In the setting of inflammation, the inducible enzyme is activated by cytokines such as tumor necrosis factor. Nitric oxide is a potent inhibitor of leukocyte and platelet adhesion, exerting its effects via activation of soluble guanyl cyclase and generation of cGMP. With regard to platelets, NO has been shown to inhibit the binding of fibrinogen to glycoprotein IIb/IIIa and to limit the expression of P-selectin. Another important anti-inflammatory role of NO free radical is its ability to scavenge superoxide. Inhaled NO moderately reduces the pulmonary hypertension observed with acute respiratory distress syndrome; however, it does not reduce mortality. In endotoxic shock, increased NO production is related to the level of hypotension. Bacterial endotoxins induce NOS and lead to increased production of NO in venous smooth muscles and in cardiomyocytes. This may explain venous pooling and cardiac dysfunction (sepsis-related cardiomyopathy). In the setting of multiple organ dysfunction, NO may be responsible for the associated hepatocellular dysfunction manifested as elevated bilirubin level and decreased serum albumin level.

Part II
Wound Healing

7
Normal Wound Healing

Wound healing can take the form of either repair or regeneration. Repair is the process of restoration of normal function and structure after an injury. Perfect reorganization is sacrificed for the sake of urgent return to function. Regeneration, on the other hand, is the perfect restoration of the original tissue architecture without scar information. Regeneration is found during embryonic development or in certain tissues, such as the liver. The types of wound closures are divided into primary, secondary, and tertiary. Primary, or first-intention, closures are closures for wounds that are immediately sealed with simple suturing, skin graft placement, or flap closure, such as the closure of the clean surgical wound. Closure by secondary or spontaneous intention involves no effort to seal the wound. This type of closure is employed for a highly contaminated wound. The wound eventually seals by re-epithelialization and contraction. Wound closure by tertiary intention is also known as delayed primary closure. In this instance, a contaminated wound is treated with repeated debridement over a certain period of time until infection is well controlled, and then surgical intervention, such as suturing or skin graft placement, is performed. The physiology of wound healing is usually described in phases. These phases blend without distinct boundaries.

Inflammatory Phase

The immediate reaction of the tissue to injury is hemostasis and inflammation. The goal at this phase is to stop the bleeding, seal the surface of the wound, and remove any necrotic tissue, foreign bodies, or bacteria. This is achieved by increased vascular permeability, migration of cells into the wound by chemotaxis, and the secretion of cytokines and growth factors. During tissue injury, blood vessel damage results in exposure of subendothelial collagen to platelets, leading to platelet aggregation and activation of the coagulation pathway. Initial intense local vasoconstriction of arterioles and capillaries is followed by vasodilation and increased vascular permeability. The clotting cascade is initiated through the intrinsic and the extrinsic pathways. Thrombin catalyzes the formation of fibrinogen into fibrin. The fibrin strands trap red blood cells, forming the clot, and seal the wound. The lattice framework that results is the scaffold for endothelial cells, inflammatory cells, and fibroblasts. The increased capillary permeability and the various chemotactic factors facilitate diapedesis of neutrophils into the wound.

Polymorphonuclear cell (PMN) migration requires interactions between integrins and extracellular matrix components. Migration of PMNs stops when wound contamination has been controlled, usually within the first few days after injury. Polymorphonuclear cells do not survive longer than 24 hours. After 24 to 48 hours, the predominance of cells in the wound cleft shifts to mononuclear cells. However, if wound contamination persists, there is a sustained influx of PMNs into the wound. Polymorphonuclear cells are not essential to wound healing, because their role in phagocytosis and antimicrobial defense can be taken over by macrophages. For instance, sterile incisions will heal normally without PMNs.

The macrophage is the one cell that is central to wound healing. Macrophages appear at the time that neutrophils disappear. Wound macrophages release matrix metalloproteinases, which degrade the extracellular matrix and are crucial for removing foreign material, promoting cell movement through tissue spaces, and regulating extracellular matrix turnover. T lymphocytes appear in significant numbers in the wound at around the fifth day, with a peak occurring at around the seventh day; however, B lymphocytes do not seem to play a significant role in wound healing. The macrophage processes foreign debris such as bacteria or degraded host proteins and serves as an antigen-presenting cell to the lymphocytes. This interaction stimulates lymphocyte proliferation and cytokine release. T cells produce interferon (IFN)-γ, which suppresses collagen synthesis and inhibits macrophages from leaving the site of injury. Thus, IFN-γ appears to be an important mediator of the chronic nonhealing wound, and its presence suggests that T lymphocytes are primarily involved in chronic wound healing.

Proliferative Phase

As the acute responses of hemostasis and inflammation begin to resolve, the scaffolding is laid for repair of the wound with angiogenesis, fibroplasia, and epithelialization. Angiogenesis is the process of new blood vessel formation and is necessary to support a healing wound environment. Following injury, activated endothelial cells degrade the basement membrane, allowing migration of cells through this gap. Division of these migrating endothelial cells results in tubule or lumen formation. Eventually, deposition of the basement membrane occurs, resulting in capillary maturation. Angiogenesis appears to be stimulated and manipulated by a variety of cytokines, predominantly produced by macrophages and platelets. Vascular endothelial growth factor, a member of the platelet-derived family of growth factors, has potent angiogenic activity. It is produced in large amounts by keratinocytes, macrophages, and fibroblasts. Both fibroblast growth factor (FGF)-1 and FGF-2, released from disrupted parenchymal cells, are early stimulants of angiogenesis. Fibroblast growth factor-2 provides the initial angiogenic stimulus within the first 3 days of wound repair, followed by a subsequent prolonged stimulus mediated by VEGF from days 4 through 7.

Fibroblasts are specialized cells that differentiate from resting mesenchymal cells in connective tissue; they do not arrive in the wound by diapedesis from circulating cells. After injury, the normally quiescent fibroblasts are chemoattracted to the inflammatory site. After stimulation by macrophage and cytokines and growth factors, the fibroblast, which is normally arrested in the G_0 phase, undergoes proliferation. The primary function of fibroblasts is to synthesize collagen, which is produced during the cellular phase of inflammation. The time required for undifferentiated mesenchymal cells to differentiate into highly specialized fibroblasts accounts for the delay between injury and the appearance of collagen in a healing wound. This period, generally 3 to 5 days, is called the *lag phase* of wound healing. During this phase, the fibroblasts that have migrated into the wound begin to synthesize proteoglycans and collagen, and the wound gains strength. Until this point, fibrin has provided most of the wound's strength. Although a small amount of collagen is synthesized during the first 5 days of the healing process, the rate of collagen synthesis increases greatly after the fifth day. Wound collagen content continually increases for 3 weeks, after which it begins to plateau.

There are at least 18 types of collagen. The ones of primary importance in skin are type I, which makes up 80% to 90% of the collagen in skin, and type III, which makes up the remaining 10% to 20%. A higher percentage of type III collagen is seen in embryologic skin and in early wound healing. A critical aspect of collagen synthesis is the hydroxylation of lysine and proline moieties within the collagen molecule. This process requires specific enzymes as well as oxygen, vitamin C, α-ketoglutarate, and ferrous iron, which function as cofactors. Hydroxyproline, which is found almost exclusively in collagen, serves as a marker of the quantity of collagen in tissue. Hydroxylysine is required for covalent cross-link formation between collagen molecules, which contributes greatly to wound strength. Deficiencies in oxygen or vitamin C or the suppression of enzymatic activity by corticosteroids may lead to underhydroxylated collagen incapable of generating strong cross-links. Underhydroxylated collagen is easily broken down. After collagen molecules are synthesized by fibroblasts, they are released into the extracellular space. There, after enzymatic modification, they align themselves into fibrils and fibers that give the wound strength.

The extracellular matrix exists as a scaffold to stabilize the physical structure of tissues. Cells within it produce the macromolecular constituents, including (1) glycosaminoglycans, polysaccharide chains, usually found covalently linked to protein in the form of proteoglycans; and (2) fibrous proteins, such as collagen, elastin, fibronectin, and laminin. In connective tissue, proteoglycan molecules form a gel-like "ground substance." This highly hydrated gel allows the matrix to withstand compressive forces while permitting the rapid diffusion of nutrients, metabolites, and hormones between the blood and the tissue cells. Collagen fibers within the matrix serve to organize and strengthen it, whereas elastin fibers give it resilience, and matrix proteins have adhesive functions.

Epithelialization of skin involves the migration of cells from the basal layer of the epidermis across the denuded wound area. This migratory process begins approximately 24 hours after wounding. About 48 hours after wounding, the basal epidermal cells at the wound edge enlarge and begin to proliferate, producing more migratory cells. If the normal basement membrane is intact, the cells simply migrate over it; if it is not, they migrate over the provisional fibrin–fibronectin matrix. When epithelial cells migrating from two areas meet, contact inhibition prevents further migration. The cells making up the epithelial monolayer then differentiate into basal cells and divide, eventually yielding a neoepidermis consisting of multiple cell layers. The epithelium never returns to its previous state. The new epidermis at the edge of the wound remains somewhat hyperplastic and thickened, whereas the epidermis over the remainder of the wound is thinner and more fragile than normal. True rete pegs do not form in the healed area.

Maturational Phase

Wound contraction is a powerful mechanical force. Sometimes, the normal biologic process of contraction results in a "contracture," which is a fixed deformity that is an aesthetic and functional disability. Contraction is not limited to the skin. Any type of injury to hollow organs such as the esophagus or common bile duct may trigger the contractile process. The mechanism responsible for wound contraction is entirely clear. Fibroblast-like cells that have smooth muscle components in the cytoplasm as well as fibroblast characteristics are present in contracting skin wounds. These are termed *myofibroblasts*. If colchicine, which inhibits microtubules, or cytochalasin D, which inhibits microfilaments, is added to the tissue culture, the result is minimal contraction of the collagen gels. Myofibroblasts are a constant feature present in diseases of excessive fibrosis, such as hepatic cirrhosis, pulmonary fibrosis, Dupuytren's contracture, and desmoplastic reactions induced by neoplasia.

Certain clinical principles are helpful for the surgical correction of contractures. If there are signs of inflammation remaining, the surgeon must be aware that procedures, such as skin graft or Z-plasty, can result in recurrent contractures because of the cytokines made by these cells and the myofibroblasts still present in the wounds. Before operation, it is important to judge the inflammatory status of the tissue. Mature scar is soft and pliable, whereas immature scar is indurated, hypertrophic, and may be tender. Immature scar still has inflammatory cell components and residual myofibroblasts, which will lead to contracture of the bed under any skin graft that is used to correct the deformity. Therefore, it is preferable to correct the defect with a flap that contains both skin and subcutaneous tissue and, in some cases, muscle. Because a flap is made of composite tissue and supplies the defect with all of the components of soft tissue, contraction is rare. In correcting a mature contracture, a skin graft may be used to fill the defect. The open wound contracts less after the placement of a full-thickness graft than after the placement of a partial-thickness graft. It is not a matter of graft thickness but of whether the graft is full or partial. After skin grafting, it is recommended to splint the wound in a fully open position. Splinting is required until all myofibroblasts and inflammation are gone from the wound, which may take as long as several months.

Approximately 3 weeks after injury, scar remodeling becomes the predominant event. Collagen synthesis is down-regulated, and the wound becomes less cellular. During this phase, there is turnover of collagen molecules as old collagen is broken down and new collagen is synthesized. Collagen breakdown is mediated by several matrix metalloproteins found in connective tissues. The activity of these collagenolytic enzymes is regulated by several tissue inhibitors. During this phase, there is little net change in total wound collagen, but the number of cross-links between collagen strands increases. This highly cross-linked collagen is stronger than the collagen produced earlier during wound healing. The result is a steady, gradual growth in wound tensile strength that continues for 6 to 12 months. However, scar tissue never reaches the tensile strength of unwounded tissue. The rate of gain in tensile strength begins to plateau at 6 weeks after injury. The recommendation that patients avoid heavy lifting or straining for 6 weeks after laparotomy or hernia surgery is based on this fact.

Cytokines in Wound Healing

Cytokines are crucial for wound healing. Interleukin-1 is an endogenous pyrogen that causes lymphocyte activation and stimulation of the hypothalamus, inducing the febrile response. Tumor necrosis factor-α is critical in initiating the response to injury or bacteria. It up-regulates cell surface adhesion molecules that promote the interaction of immune cells and endothelium. Its effects include hemostasis and increased vascular permeability. Interleukin-6 is involved in hepatic acute-phase protein synthesis regulation. Interferon-γ is secreted by T lymphocytes and macrophages. It has been shown to reduce local wound contraction and aid in tissue remodeling. Interferon-γ has been used in the treatment of hypertrophic and keloid scars, possibly by its effect in slowing collagen production and cross-linking, while collagenase (matrix metalloproteinase-1) production increases. Macrophages also release growth factors, which are important in the proliferative phase. Macrophage-secreted platelet-derived growth factor (PDGF) stimulates collagen and proteoglycan synthesis. The PDGF-BB isomer has been studied clinically. The administration of PDGF-BB improved wound closure in diabetic nonhealing ulcers, and it has been approved for use for this purpose. It is being marketed as becaplermin (Regranex®). Platelet-derived growth factor–BB has also accelerated healing when applied topically to pressure sores. Transforming growth factor (TGF)-α and TGF-β are both released by activated monocytes. Transforming growth factor-α stimulates epidermal growth and angiogenesis. Transforming growth factor-β is the most potent stimulant of fibroplasia, and its potent fibroblast mitogenic effects have been implicated in the fibrogenesis seen in disease states such as scleroderma and interstitial pulmonary fibrosis. Enhanced expression of TGF-β1 messenger RNA is found in both keloid and hypertrophic scars. In contrast, fetal wounds have a paucity of TGF-β, suggesting that the scarless repair seen in utero occurs because of absent or small amounts of TGF-β. This important cytokine increases collagen synthesis and inhibits collagenase production and activity. As a result, there is a significant collagen deposition. Therefore, TGF-B is essential for normal healing, and an excessive amount of TGF-β may be important in the pathophysiology of fibrotic states such as keloid. Fibroblast growth factor-2 is a potent angiogenic factor. It induces epithelial cell migration and hastens wound contraction. Epithelial growth factor stimulates epithelial migration and mitosis. It has been shown to hasten re-epithelialization of burn wound graft donor sites.

8
Abnormal Wound Healing

Wound healing is a complex series of events, and many forces can potentially interfere with this process. The most important factor is the balance of collagen formation and degradation. There are certain differences between chronic wounds and incisional wounds. Chronic wounds have greater levels of proinflammatory cytokines. Chronic wounds become colonized by bacteria and may become actively infected. This leads to more inflammation and stimulation of the above cytokines. Bacterial counts more than 10^5 organisms per gram of tissue prohibit wound healing. Wound macrophages are stimulated by endotoxins and release more inflammatory mediators. This seems to provide a vicious cycle that perpetuates nonhealing and leaves the balance favoring collagen breakdown.

Pathologic scars develop from a state of abnormally increased collagen formation. This condition is more common among dark-complexioned people. These scars include hypertrophic scars and keloid scars. Both conditions are the result of collagen deposition exceeding degradation. Keloid scars occur above the clavicles, on the upper extremities, and on the face. Hypertrophic scars can occur anywhere. Unlike keloid scars, hypertrophic scars can be prevented by limiting the amount of tension placed on a wound. Another difference is that hypertrophic scars are limited to the area of the wound, and keloid scars grow beyond the damaged area. Proliferative scar fibroblasts produce increased levels of transforming growth factor-β (TGF-β) and type I collagen. Transforming growth factor-β has been shown to activate fibroblasts. Hypertrophic scars regress over time and seldom need surgical intervention. Keloid scars tend to recur after excision. The intralesional injection of triamcinolone is effective in softening and decreasing the size of keloid scars. Associated symptoms such as itching and burning may also be alleviated.

Several local and systemic factors affect wound healing. Tissue hypoxia limits fibroblast replication and impairs collagen production. Diabetes has a negative effect on wound healing at several levels. Lymphocyte function is altered. Basement membrane thickening leads to decreased tissue perfusion. Collagen is more brittle in diabetic patients than in nondiabetic patients because of glycosylation. Collagen degradation is also accelerated. Radiation adversely affects the vascular endothelium. This results in endarteritis, creating atrophy and fibrosis and delaying tissue repair. Mitotic cells are most sensitive to radiation. Therefore, replicating cells in a healing wound are highly susceptible. Delayed wound healing is more pronounced in the elderly. Wound macrophages are affected mostly at this stage. Malnutrition, which is associated with protein catabolism and hypoalbuminemia, also delays healing. Certain vitamins are integral parts of enzymatic cofactors. Vitamin C is important in collagen synthesis. Vitamin A affects lysosome destabilization.

Certain chemotherapeutic agents can adversely impact wound healing. Doxorubicin (Adriamycin®) is a potent inhibitor of wound healing. Tamoxifen is known to decrease cellular proliferation and appears to have a dose-dependent decrease in wound breaking strength. This is attributed to decreased TGF-β production. Glucocorticosteroid negatively impacts fibroblast proliferation and collagen synthesis. Granulation tissue formation is also decreased. These effects can be reversed by the administration of vitamin A. The affect of exogenous steroids appears to be both time- and dose-related. High doses of nonsteroidal anti-inflammatory drugs have also been shown to decrease wound healing.

A chronic wound fails to heal due to preexisting pathologic conditions. There are many different forms of chronic wounds (ischemic ulcers, venous stasis, diabetic foot ulcers, pressure ulcers), but they all arise from a common pathophysiology. A prolonged inflammatory phase is the main culprit, causing tissue damage and impaired repair. Polymorphonuclear cells invade damaged tissue to rid the wound of bacteria and debris. In doing so, a large number of degradative enzymes and free radicals are released. The prolonged activation of these elements impedes the action of reparative cells.

Venous stasis ulcers are caused by venous obstruction, which creates increased capillary permeability and extravasation of fluid and exudates. Endothelial damage resulting from venous hypertension causes a prolonged inflammatory state. These ulcers are generally positioned superior to the medial malleolus and take on an irregular shape. Pressure ulcers tend to occur over bony prominences. They develop in the deep tissue and spread outward to the skin. Capillary dilatation is seen in this instance as well. Similar to venous stasis, this allows migration of inflammatory cells and exudates into the wound. Damage causing degradative enzymes and free radicals are released into the wound. These wounds progress in stages (stage I, nonblanchable erythema; stage II, partial thickness skin loss; stage III, full thickness skin loss involving subcutaneous tissue; stage IV, full thickness skin loss extending through the fascia involving muscle and/or bone). Diabetic foot ulcers are often caused by neuropathy leading to unrecognized trauma. Diabetic patients are prone to small vessel disease that alters the membrane permeability. Immune response is impaired due to reduced chemotaxis and phagocytosis. The extra-cellular matrix is diminished in diabetic wounds, and collagen fibers are often altered by glycosylation, which alters the function of basement membranes.

A squamous cell carcinoma arising from a nonhealing wound is called a *Marjolin's ulcer*. Dense scar tissue prevents immunologic tissue surveillance from taking place. This leaves the wound vulnerable to the formation of a neoplasm. Conditions associated with this problem include osteomyelitis, pressure sores, venous stasis ulcers, and hidradenitis. The wound takes on an irregular, raised appearance with a white, pearly discoloration. Biopsy samples of the wound may show pseudoepitheliomatous hyperplasia. This is a premalignant state. If discovered on a biopsy specimen, the biopsy should be repeated, because squamous cell carcinoma may be present in other areas.

9
Skin Grafts and Flaps

A skin graft consists of a section of skin including epidermis and dermis of variable thickness that has been completely separated from its blood supply and transplanted to a recipient bed. Skin grafts are organized into two categories, full thickness and partial thickness. A full thickness skin graft contains the dermis and the epidermis. A partial thickness skin graft includes the epidermis and only a small portion of the dermis. The split thickness skin grafts range from 1/1,200 to 1/2,000 of an inch in depth. Thicker grafts are less prone to wound contracture. In general, full thickness grafts are used in places where less wound contraction is desired, such as the face.

Once the skin graft has been harvested, it becomes separated from its blood supply and must revascularize to survive. The vascular bed is recreated in a three-step process: imbibition, inosculation, and revascularization. Imbibition occurs in the first 24 to 48 hours. During this phase, the nutrients diffuse from the underlying wound bed to extracellular fluid and into the capillaries of the graft. The graft begins to fix to the wound bed via fibrin bonds. Inosculation involves the alignment of the donor vascular buds with graft capillaries and establishment of circulation. Revascularization occurs when connecting vessels differentiate into arterioles and venules. Thicker grafts demand more blood supply and require a well vascularized recipient bed to survive. Wounds with exposed bone, tendon, or cartilage or with radiation-damaged tissue offer a poor vascular bed.

There are several reasons for graft failure. The most common cause is loss of contact with the recipient bed because of hematoma, seroma, purulent material, and shearing. Meshing the graft helps to overcome the problem of fluid buildup underneath it. Shearing is caused by movement of the graft against the wound bed. This can be prevented by tie-down compression dressings created by interrupted sutures along the edge of the wound. The ends of the suture are left long in order to tie down a nonadherent dressing on top of the graft. The second most common cause of graft failure is infection. Wounds colonized with more than 1×10^5 bacteria per gram of tissue will be less likely to support a graft.

When choosing the donor site, graft color, thickness, texture, and possible hair growth must be considered. It is best to choose sites that are closest in anatomic match to the area to be grafted. The upper thigh, abdominal wall, and buttocks are often used for split thickness grafts. These harvest sites tend to be concealed by clothing. Full thickness graft harvest sites include the posterior auricular skin, supraclavicular skin, upper eyelid area, hip flexion crease, antecubital crease, and inner arm.

Partial thickness skin grafts are most commonly harvested with the use of a dermatome, which is air driven or electric. Dermatomes can be adjusted for depth of cut as well as width of the skin graft desired. Full thickness grafts are commonly acquired by hand with a scalpel. The incision is made in an elliptical fashion to facilitate wound closure. Securing the skin graft to the recipient bed can be accomplished using staples placed along the circumference of the graft. In addition, interrupted chromic sutures can be placed within the graft to anchor it to the wound bed. Nonadherent dressing as well as sterile absorbent gauze are then placed, and the dressing is left on for 5 days for split thickness grafts and 7 to 10 days for a full thickness grafts. Healing of a split thickness donor site results from epithelialization from epidermal appendages, such as hair follicles, sweat glands, and sebaceous glands that are left behind after the graft is taken. Healing occurs best in an environment that is moist and free from injury and contamination. The process may take up to 21 days. Full thickness donor sites leave no dermis or epidermal appendages behind and, therefore, must be closed primarily or left open to granulate and contract.

The blood supply of the flap is referred to as the *pedicle*. A flap differs from a graft in that it is a section of tissue that comes with its original blood supply. The type of tissue used for flaps are skin, fascia, muscle, bone, nerve, and omentum. Flaps can be characterized according to their blood supply (e.g., random or axial), by their method of transfer (e.g., advancement, rotation, transposition, or free), or by their tissue composition (e.g., musculocutaneous, fasciocutaneous). The blood supply to a random flap is derived from a dermal and subdermal plexus, whereas axial flaps derive their blood supply from cutaneous arteries and veins, which are oriented longitudinally to the flap. Musculocutaneous flaps are composed of skin, fascia, and muscle. The blood supply stems from perforator vessels within the muscle. Fasciocutaneous flaps are composed of skin and fascia. The blood supply is derived from a vascular plexus within the fascia. Free flaps are tissues that are moved from one portion of the body to another where their vessels are re-anastomosed.

Flaps are indicated where there is exposed bone or vessels, implanted devices, or an open joint or in wounds that are too large for primary closure. The advantage to flaps is that they can cover wounds without undue tissue tension. Flaps can also aid in clearing infection from the recipient wound. Muscle flaps have been used in cases such as sternal wound coverage and osteomyelitis.

Part III
Oncology

10
Oncogenes

Oncogenesis is a result of molecular changes occurring in three select stages: initiation, promotion, and progression. The changes that take place involve alteration mechanisms that control normal cellular differentiation and growth (i.e., receptors, growth factors, oncogenes, and signal transduction molecules). Proto-oncogenes are normal genes (nonmutated) that generally have a role in regulating the cell cycle. Oncogenes are genes that were once normal, have been mutated, and now act to form tumors. They can be created by point mutations, translocations, deletions, or amplifications of DNA. Tumor suppressor genes normally function to regulate cell growth. Once they are mutated they lose their regulatory ability, which contributes to tumor development. The accumulation of mutations in proto-oncogenes and tumor suppressor genes leads to malignant transformation. Several families of oncogenes and tumor suppressor genes have been identified (Table 10.1). They are organized according to the function of their protein products.

Ras genes are a family of oncogenes found in solid organ tumors. The gene products of *ras* genes are found in the plasma membrane and are responsible for binding glutamyl triphosphate. This plays an important role in intracellular signal transduction. Their activity arises from point mutations that alter the protein's function. *K-ras* mutations are found in about 30% of lung adenocarcinomas. Tumors that possess the *K-ras* mutation have a less favorable prognosis. The *K-ras* mutation has also been found in colorectal or other cancers but has not proved to be a reliable prognostic marker. Preliminary findings suggest that *K-ras* mutations may be an adjunctive marker in the diagnosis of pancreatic cancer by fine-needle aspiration.

The *bcr/abl* mutation results from translocation of the *c-abl* proto-oncogene from chromosome 9 to the *bcr* locus of chromosome 22. This is also known as the *Philadelphia chromosome* and is associated with chronic myelogenous leukemia. The protein product of this mutated gene has augmented tyrosine kinase activity that results in malignant transformation.

Burkitt's lymphoma results from translocation of *c-myc* from chromosome 8 to chromosome 2, 14, or 22. In addition to lymphoma, the *c-myc* gene is often amplified in small cell cancer of the lung (SCCL) as well as breast and colorectal cancers, although less frequently than SCCL. The *N-myc* and *L-myc* genes encode for proteins that are very similar to that encoded by *c-myc*. About 30% to 40% of SCCL cases have amplification of *c-myc*, *N-myc*, or *L-myc*. The *N-myc* gene amplification can also be found in neuroblastomas and glioblastomas. In neuroblastoma, the presence of *N-myc* gene amplification can often indicate a higher stage (i.e., stage III or IV) tumor. In addition, those patients with lower stage neuroblastomas (i.e., stage II) and *N-myc* amplification have a much less favorable prognosis.

The nonmutated form of the *neu* gene encodes for a membrane-bound growth factor receptor. A single amino acid substitution within the transmembrane region of the protein lends its transforming activity. The gene is most commonly amplified and overexpressed in cancers such as breast, ovary, and stomach. The overexpression of the *neu* gene in node-negative breast cancer imparts a poor prognosis.

TABLE 10.1. Summary of oncogenes identified and their corresponding neoplasm, mutation, and oncogene product.

Oncogene	Neoplasm	Mutation	Oncogene Product
abl	Chronic myelogenous leukemia, acute lymphocytic leukemia, acute myelogenous leukemia	Translocation	Membrane-associated tyrosine kinase
c-myc	Burkitt's lymphoma	Translocation	Nuclear factor
N-myc	Nuclear factor	Nuclear factor	Nuclear factor
K-ras	Colon, pancreas cancer	Point mutation	p21 GTPase
neu (*HER-2*/erb-B2)	Breast, ovarian, gastric cancer	Amplification	Growth factor receptor
Ret	Thyroid cancer (papillary type), thyroid cancer (medullary type)	Chromosome translocation Point mutation	Glial cell-derived neurotrophic receptor tyrosine kinase

11
Tumor Suppressor Genes

The growth of cells has to be controlled by many external signals to maintain homeostasis. Failure of growth inhibition is one of the fundamental alterations in the process of carcinogenesis. The proteins that inhibit cell proliferation are the products of tumor suppressor genes. Mutation of tumor suppressor genes results in loss of their regulatory ability, which contributes to tumor development (Table 11.1).

The *RB* gene was the first tumor suppressor gene discovered. Rb protein is a nuclear phosphoprotein that functions in regulating the cell cycle. It is expressed in every cell type. Mutations of the *RB* gene predispose to retinoblastomas and sometimes osteosarcomas in familial cases. In familial cases of retinoblastoma, the patient is born with one normal and one mutated *RB* gene. A somatic mutation of the normal *RB* in retinoblasts produces the retinoblastoma phenotype. In the sporadic form, both copies of the *RB* gene become mutated and give rise to cancer.

The *p53* gene functions by activating cell arrest and apoptosis and inducing DNA repair genes in the presence of DNA damage. The *p53* protein binds to DNA in the nucleus and controls gene transcription. *p53* mutations are present in a number of human cancers and are the most commonly mutated genes in human cancer. Nearly 50% of human tumors contain mutated versions of this gene. Frequent mutations in *p53* are found in breast, lung, bladder, and brain cancers. The *p53* gene is located on chromosome 17p13.1. Inheritance of one mutant allele predisposes individuals to develop malignant tumors. Individuals affected by the Li-Fraumeni syndrome have a greater chance of developing a malignant tumor by age 50 than the general population. These patients most commonly form tumors such as sarcomas, breast cancer, leukemia, brain tumors, and carcinomas of the adrenal cortex. Compared with sporadic tumors, those that afflict patients with the Li-Fraumeni syndrome occur at a younger age, and a given individual may develop many primary tumors.

APC genes normally function to down-regulate growth-promoting signals. The *APC* gene mutation has been implicated in familial adenomatous polyposis as well as sporadic and nonfamilial forms of colon cancer. Familial adenomatous polyposis is a hereditary condition in which affected people develop more than 100 adenomatous polyps of the colon within the first and second decades of life.

The transforming growth factor (TGF)-β gene encodes for the TGF-β receptor that is absent in up to 70% of hereditary nonpolyposis colon cancers, in sporadic colon cancers, and in gastric cancers. Individuals who posses the mutant genes for the *NF1* allele develop a condition called *neurofibromatosis type 1*. This condition is characterized by the presence of multiple benign fleshy lesions called *neurofibromas*. These benign lesions can later develop into neurosarcoma. These patients also have a greater incidence of gliomas and optic neuromas.

The *NF2* mutations are responsible for neurofibromatosis type 2. This condition is characterized by bilateral schwannomas of the acoustic nerve. The genetic mutation has also been discovered in meningiomas and ependymomas. The gene product is a protein called *merlin*, which functions as a membrane cytoskeletal protein. Cells lacking these proteins are incapable of forming cell-to-cell junctions and do not respond to growth arrest signals from cell contact.

Family history is a well-known risk factor for breast cancer. The greatest risk comes in those who have a history of breast cancer in one or more first-degree relatives. This predisposition has been attributed to *BRCA-1*, which is a highly penetrable autosomal dominant gene. *BRCA-1* is present on chromosome 17q21, and *BRCA-2* is present on chromosome 13q12-13. These mutations increase the risk of breast cancer as well as ovarian cancer. Mutations of *BRCA-1* and *BRCA-2* are associated with nearly 80% of familial breast cancers. *BRCA-2* is also associated with male breast cancer.

TABLE 11.1. Summary of tumor suppressor and corresponding neoplasm, mutation, and gene product/function.

Tumor suppressor	Neoplasm	Mutation	Gene product/function
p53	Lung, colon, and breast cancer; osteosarcoma	Chromosome 17	Nuclear phosphoproteins/apoptosis
RB	Retinoblastoma; breast, lung, and bladder cancer	Chromosome 13q14	Nuclear phosphoproteins/cell cycle regulation
NF1	Neurofibromatosis-1 (neuroblastomas, sarcomas)		
NF2	Neurofibromatosis-2 (schwannomas and meningiomas)		Membrane cytoskeletal protein merlin
TGF-β	Colon cancer	Unknown	Growth inhibition
APC	Colon and pancreas tumors (familial polyposis coli), adenomatous polyposis coli	Chromosome translocation, point mutation	Glial cell-derived neurotrophic factor receptor tyrosine kinase/inhibition of signal transduction
		Chromosome 5	
BRCA-1	Breast cancer	BRCA-1 17q21	
BRCA-2	Ovarian cancer	BRCA-2 13q12-13	

12
Tumor Markers

Clinical Use

Tumor markers are molecules that are manufactured by the tumor or derived from host interactions with the tumor. These molecules are found in serum, body fluids, and the cancer cells themselves. Tumor markers come in many forms, including proteins, carbohydrates, and DNA. Tumor markers result from genetic changes that alter gene expression in the tumor or the surrounding tissues. In some instances, tumor markers are used to diagnose and/or monitor neoplastic disease.

A tumor marker must have several characteristics to be ideal for clinical use.

1. The molecule must be detectable before neoplastic spread begins.
2. The marker must be sensitive (it should be detectable in all patients who have the neoplasm).
3. The marker must be specific (a positive test for the marker should not occur in patients without the neoplasm).
4. The concentration of the tumor marker should reflect the size of the tumor.
5. The testing method should be affordable to facilitate screening of many people.

Tumor markers are measured qualitatively or quantitatively by chemical, immunologic, or molecular biologic methods.

Several confounding factors limit the applicability of certain tumor markers. The sensitivity of a particular tumor marker depends on the assay's ability to detect the marker, the tumor size needed to produce a detectable amount of tumor marker, and the percentage of tumor marker expression for the specific tumor. Specificity depends on the accuracy and reproducibility of the assay used, the number of other neoplasms that produce the same tumor marker, and the number of benign conditions that elevate the marker. Systemic diseases such as liver failure and renal failure disrupt the clearance of tumor

markers. This causes an elevation of tumor marker levels. Manipulation of the tumor mass causes fluctuations in tumor marker levels as well.

Tumor markers are used clinically in a number of ways. They have been used successfully for disease screening (e.g., prostate-specific antigen for prostate cancer), for diagnosing malignancy (e.g., calcitonin for medullary thyroid cancer), for determining prognosis (e.g., cancer antigen-125 for ovarian cancer), and for response to therapy (e.g., carcinoembryonic antigen [CEA] for colorectal cancer). The utility of each tumor marker varies. Some markers, such as CEA, are not particularly useful for screening but are used to evaluate recurrences and to monitor therapeutic response.

The success of the initial treatment and the development of recurrent disease can be evaluated using tumor markers. The tumor marker is measured before intervention and at regular intervals after intervention. In general, progressive disease shows an increasing trend of the tumor marker level (a 25% increase). Disease that is responding to therapy shows a downward trend of the tumor marker (a 50% reduction). A steady state generally reflects stable disease. The success of the intervention can be interpreted from the rate of decrease in the tumor marker level. The half-life of the tumor marker is used to predict the rate of decrease with successful therapy. Unsuccessful treatments are reflected in a slower rate of decrease or in an increase in the level of the tumor marker. Recurrent disease may be indicated by a reduction of the tumor marker level that is still above normal or by an increase in the marker level.

Clinically Relevant Tumor Markers

Alpha-Fetoprotein and β-Human Chorionic Gonadotropin

Alpha-fetoprotein (AFP) is a serum protein that is present in early fetal development. The protein is synthesized from the fetal intestines, liver, and yolk sac. The molecule is useful in classifying the subtypes of germ cell tumors. In general, AFP is absent in seminomas and present in nonseminomas. Yolk sac tumors also cause elevated AFP levels.

β-Human chorionic gonadotropin (β-hCG) is a glycoprotein that is produced by the placenta's syncytiotrophoblasts. Elevated β-hCG levels occur in nonseminomatous germ cell tumors but can be elevated in up to 30% of seminomas. Choriocarcinomas also display elevated β-hCG levels. Embryonal carcinomas can demonstrate elevations of AFP and β-hCG.

BRCA-1/BRCA-2

The *BRCA* mutations are inherited genetic defects in tumor suppressor genes that are associated with an increased risk for developing breast or ovarian cancer. Mutations of *BRCA-1* and *BRCA-2* are associated with nearly 80% of familial breast cancers. Women with a family history of breast cancer (one or more first-degree relatives) should be tested for these genetic mutations. Their identification should prompt prophylactic mastectomy in women with the mutation.

CA 15.3

Cancer antigen (CA) 15.3 is a membrane surface antigen found on breast cancer cells. It is used most often for determining the prognosis of disease.

CA 19.9

CA 19.9 is a glycoprotein that is used to diagnosis and to determine the prognosis of pancreatic carcinoma. Elevations of CA 19.9 can also be caused by cirrhosis, hepatitis, sclerosing cholangitis, and cholestasis.

CA 125

CA 125 is a cell surface antigen that is elevated in patients with ovarian cancer. Its use for the early detection of ovarian cancer is debated. CA 125 is used to differentiate benign from malignant disease. The level of CA 125 is correlated with the extent of disease; therefore, it provides information concerning treatment response.

Calcitonin

Calcitonin is a hormone produced and secreted by the parafollicular C cells in the thyroid gland. Calcitonin plays a role in calcium regulation, and levels are elevated in medullary carcinoma of the thyroid. Serum calcitonin levels are a good marker for determining diagnosis and prognosis and for monitoring the response to treatment.

CEA

Carcinoembryonic antigen is one of the most often used tumor markers in the area of surgery and is an oncofetal protein that in normal cells acts as an adhesion molecule. The molecule is detected on normal mucosal cells of the stomach, intestine, and biliary tract. Tumor cells such as colon and lung cancer express higher levels of CEA. Carcinoembryonic antigen detection is clinically relevant for the prognosis of colon cancer. Poorer long-term survival rates coincide with higher initial CEA levels. In addition, the risk of disease recurrence is greater in patients whose CEA levels fail to decrease postoperatively.

Estrogen and Progesterone Receptors

Breast cancer tumors are evaluated for the presence of estrogen or progesterone receptors. The presence of the receptors lends a more favorable prognosis to the tumor, because this implies that the tumor is somewhat differentiated. The presence of these receptors also offers the possibility of using hormonal therapy against the cancer.

Neuron-Specific Enolase and Squamous Cell Carcinoma Antibody

Neuron-specific enolase (NSE) is a serum marker used to diagnose and monitor treatment response for small cell lung carcinoma. The squamous cell carcinoma (SCC) antibody is detectable in the serum of lung cancer patients. This test is an adjunct to histologic analysis.

Prostate-Specific Antigen and Prostate-Specific Acid Phosphatase

Prostate-specific antigen (PSA) is a proteolytic enzyme that is manufactured by the prostate gland. The enzyme is secreted into the lumen of the gland; however, it can leak into the systemic circulation in cases of prostate cancer, benign prostatic hyperplasia (BPH), prostatitis, and advanced age. Prostate-specific antigen is an effective screening test for prostatic diseases. Therefore, PSA is specific to the prostate organ but is not completely specific for detecting prostate cancer. Benign prostatic hyperplasia can cause elevations above 4 ng/mL. Elevations above 10 ng/mL are generally attributed to cancer. However, some overlap exists between benign and malignant PSA elevation (between 4 and 10 ng/mL). The measurement of free PSA increases the specificity for detecting prostate cancer. Prostate-specific acid phosphatase (PSAP) is a proteolytic enzyme that is a marker of advanced stages of prostatic cancer.

13
Sentinel Lymph Node Biopsy

Sentinel lymph node biopsy is a recently developed procedure in surgical oncology. The technique provides a selective approach that allows patients with lymph node metastases to be treated early in their disease with beneficial adjuvant therapies while sparing patients without nodal metastases an unnecessary lymph node dissection. The concept of the sentinel lymph node is based on the fact that the efferent lymphatic channel draining a primary tumor leads directly to the first, "sentinel" lymph node in the regional basin. Therefore, the sentinel node is the lymph node most likely to harbor metastatic disease if regional nodal metastatic disease is present. If the sentinel lymph node is histologically negative, then the other lymph nodes in the basin are also histologically negative.

Sentinel Lymph Node Biopsy for Melanoma

The presence or absence of lymph node metastases is the single most powerful predictor of recurrence and survival for melanoma patients. Data from the interferon alfa-2β trial indicated that all patients with a melanoma more than 1.0 mm thick should undergo a nodal staging procedure so that adjuvant therapy can be selectively administered. Given the substantial difference in disease-free and overall survival, it is important to offer these patients interferon alfa-2β therapy.

For female patients with melanomas less than 0.76 mm thick, the risk of nodal metastasis is less than 1%; thus, sentinel lymph node biopsy is not indicated. For male patients with a primary site on the trunk, however, the incidence of occult nodal metastases may be as much as 9%, even if the primary lesion is <0.76 mm thick. Therefore, lymphatic mapping may be considered for these patients. For patients with tumors 0.76 to 1.0 mm thick, the risk of nodal metastasis is <6%, and the procedure should be an option. Patients with melanomas of intermediate thickness (1.0 to 4.0 mm) have the most to gain from lymphatic mapping and sentinel lymph node biopsy. For patients with thick (>4.0 mm) melanomas, the rate of occult systemic metastasis is 70%, and the rate of occult nodal metastasis is 60% to 70%. In the past, elective lymph node dissection was not recommended, because there was no survival benefit. However, now that effective adjuvant therapy (interferon alfa-2β) is available, lymphatic mapping and sentinel lymph node biopsy should be offered to these patients as a staging tool.

Patients undergo preoperative lymphoscintigraphy with the injection of 450 μCi in 1 mL of filtered technetium-99–labeled sulfur colloid. Dynamic scans are performed 5 to 10 minutes after injection, and the location of the sentinel lymph node is marked with an intradermal tattoo. In the operating room 2 to 24 hours later, 1 mL of 1% isosulfan blue dye (Lymphazurin) per direction of drainage is injected around the primary site. After 10 minutes is allowed for the vital blue dye to travel to the sentinel lymph node, the radioactive hot spot in the regional basin is identified with the handheld gamma probe, and the in vivo activity ratio is recorded. If shine-through from the radioactivity of the radiocolloid injected at the primary site is a problem, wide local excision of the primary tumor can be performed first.

An incision is made over the hot spot, and small flaps are created in all directions to allow identification of the blue-stained afferent lymphatic vessels. Surgical dissection is aided by visualization of the stained afferent lymphatic vessel leading down to the blue-stained node and by using the handheld gamma probe to direct dissection down to the sentinel lymph node. The entire node is removed by sharp dissection or electrocautery. Afferent and efferent lymphatic vessels entering and exiting the sentinel lymph node, some of which (the afferent vessels) are stained blue, are controlled with hemostatic clips, because electrocautery will not seal these vessels. This decreases the risk of postoperative wound seroma. The radioactivity level in the excised sentinel lymph node is checked with the handheld gamma probe to confirm that the node has been correctly identified as the sentinel lymph node. The residual radioactivity in the basin is then checked to confirm that all sentinel lymph node has been removed. If radioactivity has not fallen to the background level, the probe should be used to direct other dissection to remove additional sentinel lymph node.

Sentinel Lymph Node Biopsy for Breast Cancer

Breast conservation is a viable option for many women. The main physical complaints of patients after surgical operation are related to the side effects of axillary dissection. Preventing node-negative patients from having to experience these side effects is an important therapeutic advantage. Therefore, all women with invasive breast cancer are potential candidates for lymphatic mapping and sentinel lymph node biopsy.

Lymphoscintigraphy is performed in the same way for breast cancer as it is for melanoma except that the radiocolloid is injected into the breast parenchyma around the primary tumor. If the tumor was detected mammographically, localization wires are placed under mammographic or ultrasonographic guidance, and the radiocolloid is injected around the wire and the tumor. The localization wire remains in place to guide subsequent injection of vital blue dye. If the tumor is palpable, injection is done around the circumference of the tumor. If an excisional biopsy was performed, injection is done under ultrasonographic guidance so that the radiocolloid is placed in the breast parenchyma around the biopsy cavity. If the radiocolloid is placed in the tumor or the biopsy cavity, it will not migrate. Alternative injection techniques include injecting the mapping agents either into the subareolar plexus (because the breast lymphatics from all quadrants initially migrate to the subareolar plexus before traveling to the axilla) or into the skin above the tumor. These alternative techniques appear to work as well as intra-parenchymal injection. The timing of radiocolloid injection is not critical as long as enough time (2 to 24 hours) has elapsed between injection and sentinel lymph node biopsy for the mapping agent to migrate into the sentinel node.

Intraoperative lymphatic mapping and sentinel lymph node identification follow the same course for breast cancer patients as for melanoma patients. Patients come to the operating room 2 to 24 hours after the injection of the radiocolloid in the nuclear medicine suite. If the tumor is palpable, 5 mL of 1% isosulfan blue dye is injected around the circumference of the primary tumor 10 to 15 minutes before the surgical procedure. If the tumor is nonpalpable, the dye is injected around the localization wire left in place after preoperative lymphoscintigraphy. After injection of the vital blue dye, the breast is massaged for 5 minutes to facilitate migration of the mapping agents. Before a skin incision is made, a handheld gamma probe is used to identify the most radioactive area in the axilla. A 2 to 4 cm axillary incision is made over the hot spot, dissection is directed with the probe, and the sentinel lymph node is identified. Ideally, the sentinel lymph node should be both hot and blue. A unique feature of breast lymphatic mapping, making it more technically demanding than melanoma mapping, is that breast cancer primary sites are closer to their regional basins than most melanoma primaries are to theirs. As a result, there may be shine-through of radioactivity from the primary site so that imaging of the axilla is impossible. In such cases, vital blue dye mapping becomes more important in identifying the axillary sentinel lymph node. However, radiocolloid mapping takes on a more important role when the axillary sentinel lymph node is full of tumor. In these cases, the node may take up little of the blue dye; however, a radioactive hot spot can usually be identified with the use of the handheld probe in the basin. Once the sentinel lymph node is identified, it is removed. The blue-stained afferent lymphatics are clipped or tied off. The central bed is then re-examined for radioactivity.

14
Systemic Anticancer Therapy

Systemic anticancer therapy is the treatment of a cancer through the systemic delivery of agents that have antitumor effects. These agents are delivered via enteral, subcutaneous, and intravenous routes. Systemic anticancer agents are categorized into three subgroups: chemotherapy, hormonal therapy, and immunotherapy. The purpose of this chapter is to give a simple overview of commonly used agents and how they are classified.

Alkylating Agents

Alkylating agents exert their effects by transfer of alkyl groups to various cellular components, most importantly DNA. Alkylating agents cause cross-linking and strand breaks of DNA, which lead to miscoding during replication.

Nitrosoureas

Carmustine and lomustine are closely related nitrosoureas. They are lipophilic and have excellent central nervous system penetration. Carmustine and lomustine are primarily used to treat brain tumors. Streptozocin is another nitrosourea, which is specifically toxic to the β-cells of the islets of Langerhans. Streptozocin is used in the treatment of insulinomas. The major toxicities of the nitrosoureas are marrow depression and aplastic anemia.

Cyclophosphamide

Cyclophosphamide is used in many chemotherapeutic regimens and is particularly useful in the treatment of breast cancer and Burkitt's lymphoma. A unique toxicity of this agent is hemorrhagic cystitis. Bone marrow depression, nausea, and alopecia are also common adverse reactions.

Chlorambucil

Chlorambucil is used to treat chronic lymphocytic leukemia, Hodgkin's lymphoma, and non-Hodgkin's lymphoma. The major associated toxicities are myelosuppression and bone marrow failure.

Cisplatin

Therapeutic applications include testicular, ovarian, and bladder cancers. The most common adverse reaction is severe nausea and vomiting. However, the major limiting toxicity is dose-related nephrotoxicity.

Procarbazine

Procarbazine is commonly used to treat Hodgkin's lymphoma. Bone marrow depression is the major toxicity, and the drug is highly teratogenic. It is also a monoamine oxidase inhibitor.

Antimetabolites

Antimetabolites are analogs of nucleic acids or nucleic acid precursors. They affect all rapidly proliferating cells and inhibit enzymes important in the production of nucleic acids. As a class, they are most effective against hematologic malignancies but are also used to treat breast and gastrointestinal tumors.

Methotrexate

Methotrexate is structurally related to folate and acts as an antagonist of that vitamin by inhibiting the enzyme dihydrofolate reductase. It is used to treat acute lymphocytic leukemia, choriocarcinoma, breast cancer, and head and neck malignancies. Commonly observed toxicities include myelosuppression, stomatitis, rash, and renal damage. Some of these toxicities can be prevented or reversed with leucovorin. Methotrexate is also highly teratogenic and abortifacient.

Mercaptopurine

Mercaptopurine is used in the maintenance of remission in acute lymphoblastic leukemia. Bone marrow depression is the chief toxicity.

Fluorouracil

Fluorouracil is commonly called 5-FU. Fluorouracil is employed primarily for colorectal, breast, ovarian, pancreatic, and gastric carcinomas. Adjuvant therapy with leucovorin has been shown to improve survival in patients with colorectal cancer. Fluorouracil may also be used topically to treatment superficial basal cell carcinomas. Its major toxicities are bone marrow depression and severe ulceration of the oral and gastrointestinal mucosa. An unusual dermopathy called the *hand–foot syndrome* is seen after extended infusions.

Alkaloids

Alkaloids are plant products that work by binding tubulin and poisoning the assembly of microtubules in the mitotic spindle. They are most useful in the treatment of hematologic, breast, renal, testicular, and head and neck malignancies. Another subgroup of alkaloids works through a slightly different mechanism and is called *topoisomerase inhibitors*. The topoisomerase inhibitors cause DNA strand breaks and structural DNA damage in tumor cells.

Vincristine and Vinblastine

Vincristine and vinblastine are structurally related compounds that bind tubulin through a guanosine triphosphate–dependent pathway. Both are generally administered in combination with other drugs as part of a chemotherapeutic regimen. Interestingly, they have slightly different therapeutic uses and toxicity profiles. Vincristine is used to treat acute lymphoblastic lymphomas, Wilm's tumor, and Ewing's sarcoma. Vinblastine is used to treat metastatic testicular carcinomas. Unique toxicities of vincristine include peripheral neuropathies and gastrointestinal dysfunction. Vinblastine is a more potent myelosuppressant.

Taxol®

Taxol®, a member of the taxane family, is commonly used to treat ovarian cancer and metastatic breast cancer. The major dose-limiting toxicity of the taxanes is neutropenia, which can be treated with granulocyte colony–stimulating factor. Peripheral neuropathy is another commonly observed adverse effect.

Etoposide and Teniposide

Etoposide and teniposide are both classified as topoisomerase inhibitors. Etoposide is predominantly used to treat oat cell carcinoma of the lung and refractory testicular carcinoma. Dose-limiting myelosuppression (leukopenia) is the major toxicity for both drugs.

Antibiotics

As a group, antibiotics are cell cycle nonspecific. They exert their antitumor effects by intercalating in DNA and interfering with nucleic acid synthesis in cancer cells.

Doxorubicin

Doxorubicin (Adriamycin®) is one of the most widely used anticancer drugs. It is used to treat breast and lung cancers, sarcomas, and leukemias and lymphomas. The major toxicity is an irreversible dose-dependent cardiotoxicity. This apparently occurs as a result of the generation of free radicals. Irradiation of the thorax increases its toxicity.

Dactinomycin

Dactinomycin is used in combination with surgery and vincristine to treat Wilm's tumor. The major dose-limiting toxicity is bone marrow depression.

Plicamycin

Plicamycin, also called *mithramycin*, has a specific toxicity for osteoclasts and is used to lower serum calcium levels in hypercalcemic patients with bone tumors or metastases. Other toxicities include hemorrhage, renal toxicity, and bone marrow depression.

Bleomycin

The primary therapeutic application for bleomycin to treat testicular carcinoma in combination with vinblastine. Pulmonary toxicity is the most serious adverse effect. The pulmonary toxicity is progressive, beginning with rales and cough and potentially causing fatal fibrosis.

Hormonal Therapy

The sex hormones and adrenocortical hormones have roles in systemic therapy for various types of cancer. These agents may be used to inhibit the growth of hormonally sensitive cancers. Glucocorticoids have a powerful suppressive effect on lymphoid cells. This makes glucocorticoids useful to treat leukemias, lymphomas, and myeloproliferative disorders. Estrogens suppress androgen production and are a useful adjunct in the treatment of some prostate cancers. Progesterone inhibits the proliferation of endometrial cells and is used to treat endometrial cancer. Progesterone is also used to treat specific progesterone-receptor-positive breast cancers.

In addition to these hormones, tumor growth can be affected by specific androgen and estrogen inhibitors. Two other classes of systemic agents, which alter hormone balance and can affect tumor growth, are gonadotropin-releasing hormone analogs and aromatase inhibitors.

Prednisone

Prednisone is the most commonly used corticosteroid in systemic anticancer therapy. This agent is a potent synthetic corticosteroid with less mineralocorticoid activity than cortisol. It is used primarily to treatment lymphomas. Adverse reactions include bone loss and exacerbation of ulcers.

Estrogens

Ethinyl estradiol and diethylstilbestrol are used to treat certain prostate cancers. These agents inhibit the growth of prostate tissue by blocking the production of luteinizing hormone and thereby decreasing the synthesis of androgens in the testis. Thus, androgen-dependent tumors are affected. Major adverse effects include thromboemboli, myocardial infarction, and gynecomastia and impotence in men.

Tamoxifen

Tamoxifen is classified as a selective estrogen-receptor modulator. The drug binds estrogen receptors, producing estrogenic and nonestrogenic effects. The net result of the drug binding to the estrogen receptor is that the complex fails to induce certain estrogen-responsive genes. This leads to a depletion of estrogen receptors, and the growth-promoting effects of the natural hormone and other growth factors are suppressed. It is most effective for estrogen-receptor-positive and progesterone-receptor-positive breast cancers. Adverse effects include hot flashes, vaginal bleeding, and increased risk for endometrial cancer.

Flutamide

Flutamide is a synthetic nonsteroidal antiandrogen used to treat prostate cancer. Side effects include gynecomastia and gastrointestinal distress.

Leuprolide

Leuprolide is a gonadotropin-releasing hormone analog that acts as a luteinizing hormone-releasing hormone (LHRH) receptor agonist. Leuprolide binds the LHRH receptor in the pituitary, causing desensitization and subsequent inhibition of follicle-stimulating hormone and luteinizing hormone release. Response to leuprolide in prostate cancer is equivalent to orchiectomy with up to 40% regression of the tumor reported. Adverse effects include impotence and hot flashes.

Aromatase Inhibitors

Aromatase inhibitors are a relatively new class of drugs used to treat postmenopausal breast cancers. These drugs reduce the production of estrogens. Adverse reactions include thromboembolism, fractures, endometrial cancer, cataracts, and hypertension.

Immunotherapy

Immunotherapy is a relatively new modality of systemic anticancer therapy that attempts to mobilize the body's natural defense mechanisms against cancer cells. The premise behind immunotherapy is that malignant cells express unique cell surface antigens that can be targeted for destruction by humoral or cell-mediated immune mechanisms.

Interferons

Interferons are used to treat hairy cell leukemia and Kaposi's sarcoma. They are classified as immunomodulators. The exact mechanism of action is unknown and is currently being studied. The most common adverse reactions are related to bone marrow suppression.

Interleukin-2

Interleukin-2 is a cytokine produced by active T cells. Its main function in the immune system is to stimulate the growth of activated lymphocytes. In the clinical setting, interleukin-2 is being used to treat renal cell carcinoma and metastatic melanoma.

Trastuzumab

Trastuzumab (Herceptin®) is a recombinant humanized monoclonal antibody directed against the protein HER-2/neu. It is effective only against breast cancers that over-express HER-2/neu. This drug has its greatest effect when used as part of a chemotherapeutic regimen. Side effects include cardiotoxicity.

Part IV
Imaging

15
Surgical Ultrasound

Background

Ultrasound is a vital diagnostic tool for the surgeon. The basic components of an ultrasound system include a monitor, a transducer, an image recorder, and a keyboard. Ultrasound uses high-frequency sound waves to create images. The ultrasound probe contains piezoelectric crystals. Electrical pulses are applied to the crystals, causing them to distort. The distortion of the crystals creates vibrations (ultrasonic pulsations). The pulsations are reflected by the anatomic structures being examined and are detected by the probe. The reflected pulsations cause distortions in the piezoelectric crystals, and electric signals are produced. The signals are converted to an image. Other components of the transducer aid in image resolution, such as an epoxy resin called *backing material* that absorbs vibrations and, therefore, improves image quality.

The interface between the transducer probe and the skin's surface produces a reflection of the ultrasonic waves. Matching material is applied to the probe and the skin's surface to mediate the transmission of the ultrasound waves across this interface and to limit the reflection of ultrasound waves. The frequency of the transducer is indirectly proportional to the thickness of the piezoelectric crystal. Common frequencies used for diagnostic ultrasound range from 2.5 to 10 MHz. High-frequency ultrasound is unable to penetrate to deeper levels of tissue but has better resolution than low-frequency ultrasound. Low-frequency ultrasound has improved penetration but poor resolution. For example, superficial tissues are best seen with a 7.5 MHz transducer; a deeper structure, such as the abdominal aorta, is best seen with a 3.5 MHz transducer.

Three scanning modes are available for ultrasound: A, B, and M mode. The A mode is amplitude modulation and is the most basic mode of ultrasound. A-mode ultrasound creates one-dimensional images. The strength of the returning signal is plotted along the Y axis, and the time is plotted along the X axis. B mode, also known as brightness modulation, varies the brightness of the image with the strength of the signal. Dense structures appear whiter (i.e., more echogenic), because they reflect ultrasonic waves more efficiently. M-mode ultrasound correlates the amplitude of the wave with structural movement.

Applications

Breast

Ultrasound plays an important part in the diagnosis of breast disease. Ultrasound is easy to use and can be conveniently performed in an office setting. Ultrasound is used in breast disease to evaluate mammographic microcalcifications and nonpalpable masses, to evaluate ductal dilatation and nipple discharge, to distinguish a solid from a cystic mass, to evaluate dense breast tissue to delineate a possible mass, to guide biopsy procedures, and to guide percutaneous aspiration of abscesses or cysts. In addition, ultrasound can be used to guide fine-needle aspiration of axillary lymph nodes and to aid in preoperative needle localization for lumpectomies.

Gastrointestinal Tract

Endoscopic and endorectal ultrasound can augment the preoperative workup for gastrointestinal (GI) malignancies by adding staging information. Endoscopic ultrasound incorporates the use of a high-frequency (12 to 20 MHz) probe attached to an endoscope. This technique provides images of the GI mucosa, submucosa, and surrounding structures to delineate the depth of invasion of lesions. In addition, lymphadenopathy can be detected, and biopsy specimens can be obtained. Endoscopic ultrasound can accurately estimate the stage of a lesion about

90% of the time. Endoscopic ultrasound is used for pre-operative staging for GI neoplasms, localization of pancreatic endocrine tumors (i.e., insulinomas), examination of submucosal GI lesions, and guidance during procedures (i.e., interventions, biopsies).

Rectal diseases can be evaluated with endorectal ultrasound using an axial 7.0 or 10.0 MHz rotating transducer. Endorectal ultrasound creates 360° cross-sectional images of rectal tissues. The transducer is placed in a water-filled latex sheath. As the transducer is gradually removed, the real-time images of the rectal walls are obtained. Ultrasonographic staging is accomplished by correlating the position of the lesion with the layers of the rectum. Benign lesions confined to the middle white line or submucosa may be amenable to submucosal resection. Endorectal ultrasound can accurately estimate the depth of invasion in up to 90% of cases. Tissue inflammation can cause errors in measurements. In addition, microscopic invasion cannot be accounted for. Anal incontinence can be evaluated by endoanal ultrasound. Defects in the internal and external sphincters may be visualized with this modality. The modality is unable to measure sphincter function but can identify disruption of the sphincter. Endoanal ultrasound is used to evaluate distal rectal tumors, perianal abscesses, anal fistulas, and rectal ulcers.

FAST

The FAST (Focused Assessment for the Sonographic examination of the Trauma patient) is a tool used to evaluate patients with potential abdominal injuries. The FAST searches for fluid in the pericardial sac, Morison's pouch, splenorenal recess, and pelvis. Fluid in these spaces may indicate hemorrhage.

Common diagnostic applications include evaluation of soft tissue abscesses, evaluation of biliary disease, identification of fascial defects (i.e., hernias, wound dehiscences), and evaluation of abdominal aorta aneurysms.

Intraoperative

Intraoperative ultrasound has many practical applications. The advantages of intraoperative ultrasound include increased sensitivity and precise visualization of smaller lesions and structure. This modality provides accurate information concerning the resectability of certain lesions (e.g., hepatic and pancreatic neoplasms, common bile duct stones) and can be used in open or laparoscopic procedures. There are two methods for using intraoperative ultrasound. The contact method involves the direct contact between the transducer and the structure of interest. This allows for deep penetration of ultrasound waves and is used primarily to visualize solid organs, such as the liver. The stand-off method involves holding the transducer approximately 1 to 2 cm away from the structure of interest. The ultrasound waves are transmitted through a pool of sterile saline to limit reflection. This method of scanning is used to visualize hollow structures (e.g., blood vessels, biliary ducts, and the spinal cord) without compressing them and distorting the image.

Vascular

The development of color-flow duplex imaging and endoluminal ultrasound allows for diagnosis of vascular diseases such as deep vein thrombosis, arterial disorders (e.g., atherosclerosis, aneurysm, stenosis, and occlusion), arteriovenous fistulas, Raynaud's disease, and thoracic outlet syndrome. Screening or follow-up examinations for abdominal aortic aneurysm can be easily accomplished in the office setting. Vascular ultrasound is often used to assess portal vein and hepatic artery flow after liver transplantation. Venous duplex scans of the lower extremities can be used for surveillance in patients who are at high risk for deep venous thrombosis. Information gained is helpful for deciding when to begin prophylaxis using anticoagulation of inferior vena cava filter placement.

16
Imaging Technology: Magnetic Resonance Imaging and Computed Tomography

Magnetic Resonance Imaging

Magnetic resonance imaging (MRI) is a radiographic modality that relies on the body's magnetic field to create images. In particular, the hydrogen atom of the nucleus is focused on because of the atom's relative abundance in water and adipose tissue. Each hydrogen proton has an axis with North and South Pole orientations. Collectively the hydrogen protons in the body spin about their axes in random north–south orientation. The MRI scanner exposes the body to a strong magnetic field, thus creating uniform alignment of all of the hydrogen protons. Radio wave energy is applied in addition to the magnetic field, causing the hydrogen nuclei to resonate. Manipulations of the magnetic field are produced using a series of gradient electric coils. This causes different cross-sections of the body to resonate when different frequencies are applied.

When the radio wave from the scanner is terminated, the magnetic vector of the body's hydrogen ions return to their resting state (relax). This produces a radio signal that is emitted from the body. Receiver coils that surround the body are used to collect this emitted signal. The intensity of the signal is translated into a gray scale and used to create cross-sectional images.

Multiple radiofrequencies are transmitted in pulse form to emphasize different tissues. Individual tissue forms relax at different rates when the transmitted radiofrequencies are terminated. This creates the distinction between different tissue types. The time required for the proton to return to the resting state is measured in two ways. T_1 measurements determine the amount of time taken for the magnetic vector to return to its resting state. T_2 measurements determine the time taken for resting state resumption of the axial spin. Therefore, an MRI is composed of a series of pulse sequences that each highlights different tissues. The different relaxation times for each tissue allow them to be distinguished from one another. Different tissues can be isolated or excluded from the study. Magnetic resonance imaging is especially sensitive for identifying increased water content, which occurs with most disease states.

Magnetic resonance imaging poses little harm to the body, because it relies on energy forms that people are normally exposed to (i.e., radio waves). Implanted metallic objects, such as artificial valves, pacemakers, and clips, can create a hazard. Prosthetic joints are potentially less of a problem, although they can cause image distortion.

Computed Tomography

Computed tomography (CT) uses an x-ray tube and detectors, which rotate on the long axis of the patient. A thin, fan-shaped column of x-rays is emitted from the detectors, which collect the radiation that transverses the body and organizes it to form images. The images are composed of digital pixels that represent the x-ray attenuation of a specific body tissue. Each pixel is assigned a numerical value, which is based on the difference in the x-ray attenuation of water and a specific material. The numerical value is called a *Hounsfield unit*.

Computed tomography offers many improvements over conventional radiography. Computed tomography produces images with higher resolution and can differentiate overlapping or superimposing structures. Modern CT devices incorporate spiral, helical, or volume technology. Helical CTs obtain image data as the patient is moved throughout the continuously rotating column of x-ray beams. Volumetric CT is described as moving the patient through the scanner the distance of one slice in the time it takes for the x-ray column to make one full rotation. This allows a whole volume of tissue to be analyzed. Slip ring technology allows the continuous rotation of the x-ray tubes and detector systems. Improvements in software have allowed for amazing reconstruction capabilities.

Intravenous contrast is administered to enhance vascular structures and organs. Low osmolar, nonionic intravenous contrast material is commonly used. Contrast material is distributed through the body in three phases that are determined by pharmacokinetics. The bolus phase occurs during contrast injection. This phase is hallmarked by gradual arterial enhancement at a rate proportional to the rate of injection, the iodine concentration, and the cardiac output. Peak enhancement is accomplished at the end of injection. This phase highlights the structures of the arterial system. The redistribution phase occurs approximately 2 to 4 minutes after contrast injection. In this phase, contrast material diffuses from the intravascular to extravascular space. This phase is useful for highlighting organs such as the liver. In the equilibrium phase, intravascular and extravascular contrasts exist in equilibrium.

Computed tomography angiograms are created by accounting for the delivery time of the contrast material. The amount of vascular enhancement is determined by the concentration of contrast, the injection rate, and the patient's cardiac output. Systemic images are obtained after a 30 to 40 second delay, whereas images of pulmonary vasculature are obtained after only an 8 to 10 second delay.

17
Angiography

Contrast angiography is the most accurate method for identifying occlusive lesions. Preoperative arteriograms are used to plan for possible intervention. The arteriogram is generally done by accessing the contralateral vessel, which is distal to the location of the obstruction. The arterial system (femoral or brachial) is accessed percutaneously using a large-bore needle. After the artery is accessed, guidewires and catheters are introduced using the Seldinger technique. Contrast material is injected intravenously, and fluoroscopic images are obtained.

Computed tomography (CT) is also used to evaluate the vascular system. Computed tomography angiography involves the timed injection of intravenous contrast and image acquisition using spiral CT technology. Modern software facilitates three-dimensional reconstructions to view vascular defects (tortuous vessels, stenosis, occlusions, and aneurysms). Computed tomography angiography is used for imaging aortic aneurysms, aortic dissections, and carotid disease. Magnetic resonance angiography (MRA) is a modality that avoids using ionic contrast agents. This provides a good alternative for patients at higher risk for contrast-induced nephropathy. Magnetic resonance angiography is useful for imaging intracranial arteries, major abdominal vessels, and arteriovenous malformations. Lower extremity evaluations are hindered by protracted image acquisition times.

Major complications of arteriography include atheroembolization, bleeding, pseudoaneurysm, and arteriovenous fistula. The passage of the catheter through the arterial system can cause atherosclerotic plaques to dislodge and shower downstream to lodge in distal vessels. This produces ischemia of the distal toes and painful skin lesions. Treatment of these complications varies with the needs of each patient. Stable pseudoaneurysms are treated with ultrasound-guided compression or with ultrasound-guided thrombin injection. Other puncture site complications such as rapidly expanding hematomas, hemorrhage, and large pseudoaneurysms require prompt surgical treatment. Direct exposure of the vessel with primary repair of the injury is required. Prosthetic repairs are seldom needed.

Contrast agent administration can cause adverse effects. Modern contrast agents (nonionic) have a lower osmolarity than older agents. Injections often produce a sensation of heat and a decrease in blood pressure, which are attributable to vasodilation. The effects are grouped into major and minor effects. Reactions occur in approximately 4% of patients, and there is no association with the dose administered. Minor reactions consist of nausea, pruritus, and urticaria. Risk factors include previous history of contrast reaction, shellfish allergies, and asthma.

Renal toxicity is another possible consequence of contrast administration. Theories of how this occurs include direct toxicity to tubular epithelium and renal ischemia from osmotic diuresis. Risk factors include previous renal insufficiency, diabetes, dehydration, age greater than 60 years, and large contrast doses. Proper intravenous hydration and the use of nonionic contrast agents and bicarbonate may lessen renal toxicity.

18
Electrocautery

Electrocautery is a form of electrosurgery that applies high-frequency electrical energy to tissue for cutting or coagulating. The energy can be administered in a unipolar or bipolar mode. The most basic and commonly used method is unipolar electrocautery. In its simplest form, the apparatus consists of a generator and two electrodes. One electrode delivers the current to the tissue. The other returns the current. The patient's body tissue completes the circuit. The amount of heat generated by the device is inversely proportional to the contact surface area. The application electrode has a small surface area to maximize the amount of heat applied to the tissue. In contrast, the returning electrode has a large surface area to lessen the amount of heat and prevent burn injury. There are three main variables that affect the amount of heat generated. These include the current frequency, time of activation, and type of waveform (i.e., continuous or intermittent). The device can be operated in the cut or coagulation mode. In the cut mode, a constant waveform is emitted from the electrode. The heat energy generated is very high, with minimal thermal spread. This causes the device to cut tissue rather than coagulate. The coagulation mode emits energy at a lower frequency, producing a larger area of thermal spread. Tissue dehydration and thrombosis result.

Bipolar electrocautery is perhaps the safest form of electrocautery. With this method, two tissue graspers or forceps are used to conduct energy. The energy travels between the probes and through the tissue. There is no need for a grounding pad in this mode. The amount of thermal spread to the surrounding tissue is minimal. Because compression to the tissue is used with this mode, it is more effective for coagulation. This mode is indicated for areas where the surgeon wants to ensure that no inadvertent tissue injury occurs, such as in the brain.

Potential complications of electrocautery include inadvertent thermal injury, burn, fire, cardiac arrhythmias, and interference with pacemakers. Inadvertent thermal injury is avoided with careful handling of the instruments and by ensuring that the equipment is not damaged (e.g., frayed insulation). Bipolar electrocautery is used when working with delicate areas, such as the brain. Burns to the patient can be avoided by making sure that the operative field stays as dry as possible and using ground pads with full contact to the skin. The electrosurgical units have been designed to operate between 300 kHz and 2 MHz to avoid stimulating ventricular fibrillation. When possible, grounding pads are placed far away from the pacemaker. Bipolar electrocautery is a safer alternative for patients with pacemakers.

Part V
Surgical Research

19
Statistical Tests

The appropriate statistical test depends on the scale of measurement for a particular variable. Variables such as age, blood pressure, and weight are measured on the interval scale. One property of interval scale measurements is that differences are comparable no matter the starting point. For instance, the difference between 5 pounds and 15 pounds is equivalent to the difference between 90 and 100 pounds. If data are not interval but can be ranked from low to high, then the scale is ordinal. The Apgar scale is an example of an ordinal scale measurement. The nominal scale is when there is no ordering of the possible values. The observations are placed into categories. Gender and eye color are measured on the nominal scale.

Nominal data are described by counts and percentages. For interval data, measures of central tendency include the mode, mean, and median. The mode is the value that occurs most often. The mean is the average (sum of the values divided by the sample size). If there are an odd number of values, then the median is the middle value after ranking the data from low to high. If there is an even number of values, then the median is the average of the two most middle points after ranking the data. Of the mode, mean, and median, the mean is the value most affected by an outlier (a value that is much lower or much higher than the other values). There are several measures of data variability. The formal definition of the range is the maximum score minus the minimum score. However, most authors report the minimum and maximum and do not calculate the difference. The formula for the variance is the sum of the squared differences from the mean divided by the sample size minus 1. The standard deviation is the square root of the variance. The standard error of the mean (SEM) is the standard deviation divided by the square root of the sample size.

The normal (bell-shaped) curve has several interesting properties. One is that the mode, median, and mean are all the same value. Another is that the probability a value lies between the mean minus 2 standard deviations and the mean plus 2 standard deviations is approximately 95%. However, this property is not true of most other distributions.

One of the major uses of statistical theory is hypothesis testing. Usually, the null hypothesis states there is no difference in the parameter being tested among the groups. For instance, the null hypothesis for the Student's t-test is that the population means of two groups are identical. The alternative hypothesis is that the means are not identical (if a two-tailed test is chosen). A type I error is said to occur when, at the end of the study, the null hypothesis is rejected when, in fact, it is true. For the t-test, this would occur if the experimenter concludes the means are different when, in fact, they are the same. Alpha (α), the probability of making a type I error, is usually set at 0.05 in the analysis of most medical data. A type II error is made when the null hypothesis is not rejected when, in fact, it is not true. This would occur in the case of a t-test when the experimenter concludes there is no difference in the means of the two groups when, in fact, there is a difference. Beta (β) is the probability of making a type II error. The power of a test is defined as 1 minus β. In planning most medical experiments, the power set should be at least 80%. For a fixed alpha level (e.g., 0.05), the power can be increased by the experimenter by increasing the sample size. For the t-test, the sample size depends on three quantities other than the alpha level. The sample size must be increased as the power is increased. As the standard deviation increases, the sample size must increase. Finally, as the difference in the means of the two groups (sometimes referred to as the *clinically important difference*) decreases, the sample size must increase. When a statistical test is calculated, a *p*-value is usually reported. A *p*-value is the probability of obtaining a result as extreme or more extreme than the actual sample value obtained, given the null hypothesis is true. If the *p*-value is less than or equal to the set alpha level (usually 0.05), the result is said to be statistically significant.

Some statistical tests, known as *parametric tests*, require certain assumptions about the distribution of the data. Examples of such assumptions are that the data are normally distributed and that the variances are equal. The t-test may be the best known of these parametric tests. Multiple two-group comparisons using t-tests should not be performed if there are more than two groups. An extension of the t-test that compares the means of more than two groups is a one-way analysis of variance (ANOVA). The t-tests and analyses of variance require the data from the groups to be independent. In some experimental situations the data are not independent. An example is when the data are measured at more than one time-point on a subject. Similarly, when the subject is measured before and again after being exposed to some intervention, the data are not independent. For this latter type of data, a paired t-test is required. If more than two time-points are measured on the same subject, repeated measures analysis of variance could be used.

For data that are measured on the ordinal scale or data that are not normally distributed, nonparametric statistical techniques are required. For comparing two independent groups, Wilcoxon rank sum test (or an equivalent test called the *Mann-Whitney U test*) is required. When there are more than two groups, the extension of the Wilcoxon rank sum test is called the *Kruskal-Wallis test*. For paired data, the Wilcoxon signed rank test is employed. These nonparametric tests are sometimes known as *distribution free tests*, and their main advantage over parametric tests is that there are fewer requirements on the data to use these tests. Many of these nonparametric tests are performed by ranking the values and then performing a calculation based on the ranks. However, when the assumptions for the parametric tests are met, it is preferable to use them rather than the nonparametric tests. Parametric tests are more "powerful," and, thus, fewer observations are needed to show statistical significance.

For nominal (categorical) data, counts and percentages are used to describe the data. To compare the percents among groups, the chi-squared test is used. If the sample size is small (expected values are less than 5), the Fisher's exact test should be used instead of the chi-squared test.

When describing the relationship between two variables measured on the interval scale, linear regression and correlation can be used when certain requirements about normality and several other assumptions are met. Linear regression is used to determine the best-fitting straight line to the data. This method determines the slope and y-intercept of the best-fitting straight line. Correlation describes how well a straight line fits the data. For interval data, the Pearson's correlation coefficient ranges from a minimum of -1, when the data perfectly fit a straight line with a negative slope, to a maximum of 1, when the data perfectly fit a straight line with a positive slope. A correlation of 0 indicates that the best fitting straight line has a slope of 0. The value of the correlation squared (r-squared) tells the investigator what percentage of the changes in y are explained by linear changes in x. For instance, an $r = -0.8$ would have an r-squared of 64%; however, if the data were on a perfect straight line, the r-squared would equal 100%, since both -1 and 1 squared are 1 (or 100%). For ordinal data, the Spearman's correlation coefficient is used.

If one cannot sample the complete population (or universe), then the "best" estimate of a population mean is the sample mean, assuming the sample is randomly chosen. The best estimate of a proportion in a population is the sample proportion. The sample mean is called the *point estimate* of the population mean. It is a fixed quantity. It is sometimes preferable to calculate a range of values that are consistent with the data and not one fixed number (or point). A confidence interval provides this range. A 95% (99%) confidence interval for the mean is a range such that if random samples were repeatedly chosen and the corresponding confidence intervals were calculated, then 95% (99%) of the intervals would contain the true population mean. Confidence intervals can be calculated for one parameter in the population, such as the population mean, and also for the difference between two parameters, such as the difference of the means of two subgroups. There is a relationship between hypothesis testing at the alpha = 0.05 level and the corresponding confidence interval for the difference. The t-test comparing the means of two groups will be statistically significant ($p \leq 0.05$) if, and only if, the 95% confidence interval for the difference of the two means does not contain the value 0. A similar statement is true about proportions.

In diagnostic testing, a new screening test is compared to a gold standard. The percentage of subjects who have the disease (according to the gold standard) and are correctly judged by the screen to be positive (have the disease) is called the *sensitivity* of the test. The percentage of subjects who do not have the disease (according to the gold standard) and are correctly judged by the screen to be negative (do not have the disease) is called the *specificity* of the test. The percentage of the subjects whom the screen labels as positive who are truly positive (according to the gold standard) is called the *yield* or *positive predictive value*. It is important to remember that the positive predictive value is influenced not only by the sensitivity and specificity but also by the prevalence of the disease. The prevalence is the proportion of people in the population who have the disease at one point in time. If the screen is then applied to a population with a lower prevalence of the disease than the original population tested, the yield will decrease. The percentage of the subjects whom the screen labels as negative who are truly negative (according to the gold standard) is called the *negative predictive value*.

In many prospective observational studies the question of interest is whether the presence of a certain exposure or condition leads to a higher incidence of disease. The incidence is the proportion of the population who develops the disease during some fixed interval of time. One statistic that is reported is the relative risk (RR). It is the ratio of the incidence in the exposed group to the incidence in the unexposed group. For instance, if the mortality rate for smokers is 5% over the time period and only 2% for the nonsmokers, then the relative risk of dying for smokers is 5%/2% = 2.5. That is, the smokers are 2.5 times more likely to die over this time interval. A relative risk of 1 means that the rates are the same for both groups. The null hypothesis for this type of study is that RR = 1. If the 95% confidence interval for the relative risk does not contain the number 1, then the null hypothesis that RR = 1 is rejected. However, if the number 1 is in the 95% confidence interval, then the null hypothesis is not rejected. In a retrospective (case–control) study, the statistic that corresponds to the relative risk is called the *odds ratio*. It is a number that is interpreted in a similar manner to the relative risk. For a retrospective (case–control) study, a group of people with a disease (the cases) are compared with an appropriate group of people without the disease. Data concerning previous exposures are gathered, and the two groups are compared using the odds ratio.

Special types of statistics are required when the analysis will be the time to an event. Examples of such events are death, development of cancer, or the recurrence of cancer. Over time, patients can be lost to follow up, or, for some subjects, the event does not occur during the study time period (censored data). The probability of the event occurring over time can be calculated and graphed using Kaplan-Meier survival curves. The statistical procedure that will yield a *p*-value comparing the curves for two or more groups of subjects is the log-rank test.

The statistical tests discussed previously have one dependent (or outcome) variable and one independent (or explanatory) variable. More complicated procedures can accommodate more than one independent variable. For dependent variables measured on the interval scale, multivariable techniques include two-way analysis of variance (when there are two dependent variables that are nominal), multiple regression (for two or more interval scale–dependent variables), and analysis of covariance (when the dependent variables include both nominal and interval scale measurements.) For a dichotomous dependent variable (yes/no), the logistic regression model can include multiple dependent variables. For time-to-occurrence data, where there may be loss to follow up or censored data, the Cox (proportional hazard) model can be used when there are multiple independent variables.

20
Clinical Trials

A clinical trial is a medical experiment that uses human subjects for the purpose of proving information about the efficacy of drugs, surgery, devices, or other medical therapies. A clinical trial usually has a control group and, for new drugs or new uses of existing drugs, is called a Phase III trial. This contrasts with a Phase I trial, which is used to determine the dosage of the drug, and a Phase II trial, which is used to demonstrate a level of efficacy but usually without a control group.

Most clinical trials have a control group, which consists of subjects not receiving the active treatment. They may receive a placebo treatment, such as an inert drug or saline solution, or they may receive the present standard of care. When the clinical trial has a separate control group, it is called a parallel design. This is in contrast to cross-over studies. In cross-over studies, the patient acts as his own control. At one time-point, the patient receives the active treatment, and, at another time-point, the patient receives the control. The order of treatment and control should be randomized among the subjects. The advantages of the cross-over study design are that the demographics are identical for both treatment and control groups, and, in some instances, a smaller sample size is appropriate. The disadvantages are possible carry-over effects from the treatment to the control period, the need for the patient to return to the baseline condition before starting the second phase, a possible longer time to complete the study, and problems with patient drop-outs.

The gold standard for clinical trials requires that the patients should be randomized to either the treatment group or the control group. If patients or their physicians assign the patients to the treatment or control group, a bias in assignment may occur. The randomization ensures that, on average, the two groups will be similar for the variables that are being studied and for all possible variables that might affect the study. In practice, especially when the sample size is small, the groups may not be balanced on demographic variables or baseline measure-ments. The experimenter should analyze the demographic and baseline variables for both groups. If important differences exist between the groups after randomization, then statistical analysis is needed to account for these differences when comparing outcome variables. A method for guaranteeing equivalence on a particular demographic or baseline measure is achieved using a stratified random sample. In this case, the patients are divided or stratified on a variable, and then a random sample is chosen within each of the strata. For example, if the patients are stratified on gender, then, within the females and males, a separate randomization occurs. This guarantees that the distribution of males and females in the treatment and control groups will be nearly identical. To ensure that the groups remain comparable, many trials are analyzed under an intention-to-treat methodology. This requires that the patients remain in the groups they are randomized to when the data are analyzed, even if they do not complete the treatment and even if they receive the treatment assigned to the other group.

The eligibility and exclusion criteria for the patients need to be rigorously determined before the start of the study. Exclusion, where at all possible, should occur before the randomization process. Sometimes clinicians include only patients at high risk in order to maximize the statistical power of the study. However, this may make the generalizabilty of the study more tenuous in that the results may only apply to a small subset of patients.

Sample size calculations should be made before the ini-tiation of the study to ensure adequate power to make the correct conclusion at the end of the study. Most clin-ical trials attempt to show an improvement compared with a placebo or with the existing treatment. Typically, 80% or 90% power is chosen, and a $p \leq 0.05$ is consid-ered statistically significant. To ensure that a type I error probability is maintained at 0.05, the statistical test ana-lyzing the principle outcome is performed once at the end of the trial, and the null hypothesis is rejected if $p \leq 0.05$.

The experimenter may not repeatedly perform the statistical analysis and stop the study whenever $p \leq 0.05$. The p-values must be adjusted for multiple "peeks" at the data. For instance, the investigator may stop the study at the half-way point and declare a difference in the treatments if $p \leq 0.001$. However, at the second analysis the results are only statistically significant if $p \leq 0.049$, not 0.05.

The goal of some clinical trials is not to prove a new treatment is superior to an existing treatment but merely is the same or not inferior. This might be the case if the new treatment is less expensive or has fewer side effects. Such studies are called *equivalence studies*. It is theoretically impossible to prove that two different treatments are completely identical. However, one can prove that the difference between the two treatments is within a small margin of error. A confidence interval (usually 90%) can be calculated at the end of the study, and if the difference between the two treatments is within the margin of error then equivalence is said to have been proved.

Meta-analysis is the process of systematically combining into one study a number of smaller published clinical trials that compare the same treatments. This is in contrast to a review article where the author comments on past studies and reports his or her opinion. Advantages of a meta-analysis include a method for determining one p-value from the combined data and a possible increase in statistical power by increasing the sample size compared with any of the individual studies. There are a number of potential problems inherent in a meta-analysis. Difficulties may arise if the patient populations, treatment regimens, and outcome measures are not constant across the studies. Also, there may be a bias in that studies with negative or equivocal results for the new treatment may not have been reported or accepted for publication.

Part VI
ICU and Trauma

21
Preoperative Assessment

The preoperative evaluation identifies patients with comorbidities who need further evaluation or treatment. The major components of the evaluation include history, physical examination, and laboratory testing. Of the three components, the history provides the most useful information. The major areas of concern include intravascular volume status, airway abnormalities, cardiovascular disease, pulmonary disease, neurologic disease, renal disease, hepatic disease, nutrition, endocrine, and metabolism. Preoperative assessment involves careful yet economic evaluation of major risk factors. To provide the most valuable information, preoperative testing is stratified against age and gender (Table 21.1).

Examination of the airway is conducted with the goal of identifying factors that may impede assisted mask ventilation and tracheal intubation. A careful history and examination of past anesthesia records made show previous situations of difficult intubation. Physical examination involves frontal and profile evaluations of the airway. The mouth opening, thyromental distance, mobility of the neck, and the size of the tongue in relation to the oral cavity are key areas of evaluation. The Mallampati classification provides a systematic grading system for the upper airway. The patient is evaluated in an upright position, with the head positioned neutrally, mouth open, and the tongue protruded. The grading system predicts the likelihood of being able to successfully mask ventilate and intubate the patient (Table 21.2).

Intravascular volume status can be assessed by clinical signs, such as supine hypotension and oliguria, and by laboratory evaluation. Laboratory tests that may suggest hypovolemia include increased blood urea nitrogen/creatinine level, low urinary sodium level, and metabolic alkalosis.

Cardiovascular disease should be evaluated to judge the risk for perioperative myocardial ischemia or infarction. Major predictors for postoperative myocardial infarction include left ventricular hypertrophy indicated by electrocardiogram, hypertension, diabetes, coronary artery disease, and digoxin use. Comorbidities such as coronary artery disease, congestive heart failure, and arrhythmias pose a significant risk for postoperative cardiac complications. Other factors include stable or unstable angina, valvular disease, history of stroke, and advanced age. Patients who have had a myocardial infarction within 30 days before surgery have the highest risk. Patients who are being medically treated for coronary artery disease pose a higher operative risk than those who have undergone revascularization. The level of exercise tolerance is an accurate indication of cardiac function and reserve. Perioperative β-blockers reduce long-term mortality in high-risk patients. Hypertensive patients should continue to take antihypertensive medications during the perioperative period to avoid intraoperative lability of blood pressure.

Bacterial endocarditis is a risk for patients with preexisting valvular or congenital heart disease. Procedures involving dental work or the respiratory, gastrointestinal, or genitourinary tracts can cause transient bacteremia, which can lead to bacterial endocarditis. Prophylactic antibiotics should be given in these cases.

Pulmonary function is generally evaluated through careful history and physical examination along with laboratory testing. History should elicit information concerning the type of pulmonary disease, the type of treatment, severity of disease, exercise tolerance, and recent exacerbations. Pulmonary function tests and arterial blood gas measurements are not useful for identifying high-risk patient populations. Spirometry may identify patients with obstructive pulmonary disease.

Neurologic conditions (e.g., seizure disorders, neuromuscular diseases) affect the use of anesthetic agents such as neuromuscular blockers. A complete history and neurologic examination are conducted.

Hepatic and renal diseases can alter the metabolism and elimination of many anesthetic agents. Chronic renal insufficiency poses problems because of associated acid–base disturbances, electrolyte abnormalities, and

TABLE 21.1. Recommended preoperative testing for asymptomatic patients scheduled for elective surgery.

Age (years)	Men	Women
<40	None	Hb, Hct, ± pregnancy test
40–50	ECG	Hb, Hct, ± pregnancy test
54–64	ECG, Hb, Hct	ECG, Hb, Hct, ± pregnancy test
65–74	ECG, Hb, Hct	ECG, Hb, Hct
>75	ECG, Hb, Hct, creatinine, BUN, glucose, ± chest x-ray	ECG, Hb, Hct, creatinine, BUN, glucose, ± chest x-ray

BUN (blood, urea, nitrogen); ECG (electrocardiogram); Hb (hemoglobin); Hct (hematocrit).

TABLE 21.3. The ASA classification system.

Classification	Patient condition
ASA I	No organic, physiologic, biochemical, psychiatric disorders
ASA II	Mild systemic disease with no sequelae
ASA III	Severe systemic disease with functional impairment
ASA IV	Severe systemic disease that is life threatening
ASA V	Patient not expected to survive with or without surgery
ASA VI	Declared brain death, undergoing organ procurement
E	Emergent procedure required

ASA (American Society of Anesthesiologists).

coagulopathies (altered platelet function secondary to azotemia). In the case of acute renal failure, surgical procedures should be delayed when possible until the condition is corrected. Patients receiving dialysis should be dialyzed 18 to 24 hours before surgery to avoid the fluid and electrolyte shifts caused by dialysis. Hepatic dysfunction alters the metabolism of many anesthetic agents. In addition, the associated hypoalbuminemia causes elevation of the free form of these agents, making more active drug available. This makes patients more sensitive to the actions of these drugs. Evaluation should include tests to determine synthetic function (albumin, pre-albumin, pro-time, transferrin), metabolic function (liver transaminases, bilirubin), encephalopathy (ammonia), and ascites.

Diabetes poses a significant problem because of associated end-organ effects, altered healing, and lowered immune response. In general, tight control of serum glucose is recommended for the perioperative period. Most patients are allowed nothing by mouth (NPO)

TABLE 21.2. Mallampati classification.

Class I	Soft palate, uvula, fauces, anterior and posterior pillars visualized
Class II	Soft palate, fauces, and uvula visualized
Class III	Soft palate and base of uvula visualized
Class IV	Unable to visualize soft palate

during the perioperative period for variable amounts of time. Therefore, hypoglycemia is avoided by making slight changes to the glucose control management. These changes include substituting long-acting insulin for short-acting insulin, reducing the morning dose of insulin the day of surgery, adding glucose to the intravenous fluids while the patient is NPO, substituting short-acting sulfonylurea drugs for long-acting sulfonylurea drugs, and discontinuing metformin to avoid drug-induced lactic acidosis.

Patients receiving exogenous steroids may be unable to endure the stresses of surgery because of iatrogenic adrenal insufficiency. A stress dose of glucocorticoids is routinely administered to overcome this effect. Typical doses are based on the relative presumed stress of the procedure, the preoperative dosing, and the duration of steroid therapy. In general, patients receive 25 mg of hydrocortisone for minor surgical procedures, 50 to 75 mg equivalent of hydrocortisone for 1 to 2 days for moderate procedures, and 100 to 150 mg of hydrocortisone equivalent for 2 to 3 days for high stress procedures.

Fasting is recommended preoperatively to avoid the rare but very hazardous complication of pulmonary aspiration. The minimum guidelines consist of a 2-hour fasting period for clear liquids and 6-hour fasting period for nonclear liquids and solid food.

The American Society of Anesthesiologists (ASA) classification (Table 21.3) provides risk stratification based on the overall physical condition of the patient. The classification system is independent of the type of procedure and age.

22
General Anesthesia

In the past, anesthesia was associated with high morbidity and mortality rates. Recent improvements in anesthetic agents and equipment have reduced these risks. General anesthesia is a state of unconsciousness that can be reversed. The anesthetized state is composed of the following four components: amnesia, analgesia, noxious reflex inhibition, and muscle relaxation. Routine general anesthesia is produced by using a combination of agents that includes intravenous anesthetics (e.g., sodium thiopental), intravenous analgesics (e.g., fentanyl), and muscle relaxants (e.g., succinylcholine). The selection of the agents is individualized for patients to avoid possible complications.

The preoperative evaluation is of great importance to minimize perioperative and intraoperative complications. The preoperative evaluation is discussed in detail in Chapter 21. In general, the evaluation includes an assessment of the patient's physical status and of potentially confounding disease states (e.g., cardiovascular disease, pulmonary disease, liver failure, and renal failure). The preoperative evaluation also offers the anesthesiologist time to determine the most suitable agents and methods of administration.

The risk of injury or death caused by anesthesia complications depends on many factors. Independent risk factors for anesthesia include gender, age, American Society of Anesthesiologists (ASA) classification, nutritional status, metabolic status, cardiac disease, pulmonary disease, length of procedure, site of procedure, type of anesthetic used, and method of administration. Despite these many risk factors, the complication and death rates, particularly for ambulatory surgical procedures, are low (1:1,366 and 1:11,273, respectively). Major complications associated with general anesthesia include hypotension, respiratory depression, cardiac arrest, and aspiration of gastric contents. Most complications take place during the induction and emergence phases.

Induction

The induction period involves the delivery of anesthetic agents and the securing of the airway. Intravenous induction is a common administration method for surgical procedures for adults. Intravenous agents allow for the induction of anesthesia without exposing the patient to the strong odors associated with some of the inhaled agents.

Preoxygenation using 100% oxygen is done to prevent hypoxia during intubation attempts. At this time, benzodiazepines or opiates may be administered also. Next, an intravenous dose of an anesthetic agent is given. The patient is manually ventilated during this entire period. The next step involves the administration of a neuromuscular blocking agent. After adequate relaxation, the patient is ready for endotracheal intubation. Intravenous agents are used for most patients to induce anesthesia, and maintenance is accomplished using inhaled medications. However, total intravenous anesthesia can be achieved using intravenous agents in conjunction with opiate administration.

The most common intravenous anesthetic agents include sodium thiopental, ketamine, propofol, etomidate, and midazolam. Sodium thiopental is the oldest agent. It provides rapid induction of anesthesia; however, prolonged infusion can cause prolonged somnolence. High doses of thiopental require hepatic elimination (10% per hour) of the drug, thus prohibiting rapid emergence. However, when given in the usual doses, the drug rapidly redistributes to other tissues, allowing for rapid emergence. Other side effects include vasodilation and cardiac depression, which can lead to hypotension in hypovolemic individuals. Bronchospasm is a potential reaction in patients with reactive airway disease. This can be stimulated by endotracheal intubation. Ketamine and propofol are appropriate substitutes for this patient group.

Ketamine produces the effect of dissociative anesthesia. Administration can cause elevated blood pressure, increased heart rate, and decreased bronchial tone. These effects are mediated by an increase in sympathetic tone. Cardiac depression is a possible side effect for patients with an increased sympathetic tone (i.e., compensated hypovolemic shock).

Ketamine is the induction agent of choice for patients with asthma and hypovolemic conditions (given in reduced doses) because it causes less respiratory depression and hypotension. Limitations to ketamine include lack of muscle relaxation, lack of visceral analgesia, and increased intracranial pressures. These limitations prevent its use as the only anesthetic agent for abdominal procedures and for patients with traumatic brain injuries. The tendency for increases in heart rate precludes its use in patients with coronary artery disease. Unpleasant dreams and delirium have often been reported with its use in older children and adults. These side effects generally occur during emergence and can be countered with benzodiazepines or inhaled agents.

Propofol is a short-acting agent that has proved advantageous for use during short-term procedures. This agent also provides the added benefit of bronchodilation, making it excellent for use in asthmatics and smokers. Its side effects include hypotension and pain with administration.

Etomidate offers intravenous induction of anesthesia without producing hypotension. Therefore, it is a good choice for patients with cardiovascular disease. Limitations include pain with injection, myoclonus, and the potential for adrenal suppression in critically ill individuals and with prolonged administration.

Midazolam is a benzodiazepine and is often used for cardiovascular surgery because of its limited effects on the cardiovascular system. Important properties of this agent include rapid onset of action, the production of amnesia, and anxiolytic effects.

Systemic opioids are given in most cases of general anesthesia. The advantages lie in their ability to provide excellent analgesia with little negative impact on the cardiovascular system. Opioids increase the efficacy of other anesthetic agents. When given in conjunction with inhaled agents, such as sevoflurane, opioids reduce the minimal alveolar concentration. They are often combined with local anesthetics to augment their effects in epidural and intrathecal blocks. Opioids diminish autonomic responses (tachycardia and hypertension) to endotracheal intubation and surgical incision. Opioids can provide total anesthesia when given in high doses.

Patients at increased risk for aspiration require rapid sequence intubation. This includes obese and obstetric patients and patients who have a bowel obstruction, have recently eaten, and have gastroesophageal reflux. As the name applies, rapid sequence intubation involves quickly placing a conscious patient into a completely anesthetized and intubated state. The patient is preoxygenated in the conscious state and then given an intravenous anesthetic agent, such as sodium thiopental, followed by a neuromuscular blocker, such as succinylcholine. During the time allowed for the drugs to take effect, pressure is applied to the cricoid cartilage to avoid inadvertent aspiration of gastric fluids. Potential hazards include hypoxia from unsuccessful intubation and inadequate ventilation.

Inhalational Induction

Inhalational induction is a good option for pediatric patients and patients with reactive or difficult airways. The development of new agents has improved the efficacy and safety of inhaled products. Specifically, agents have been created with lower blood/gas solubility coefficients and lower minimum alveolar concentrations. These agents have a faster onset of action and are more potent.

Nitrous oxide has many limitations as a single agent; however, when combined with other agents, it enables smaller doses of anesthetic to be given. A potential hazard of nitrous oxide is its ability to easily diffuse into closed spaces. This makes its use potentially dangerous in small bowel obstructions and pneumothoraces because of its potential to increase the volume in these spaces. Some of the more commonly used agents include isoflurane, sevoflurane, desflurane, and halothane.

The combination of intravenous and inhaled anesthesia provides easy and rapid induction of anesthesia. The airway is maintained with the aid of an oral airway or chin tilt maneuver. The airway can be secured by traditional endotracheal intubation or by laryngeal mask airway. Anesthesia is generally maintained using a combination of opiates, inhaled agents, and nitrous oxide. These agents are titrated according to the level of anesthesia required. Intraoperative monitoring of hemodynamic stability and the respiratory system takes place throughout the surgery. The depth of anesthesia is judged by the monitoring of autonomic signs. Emergence from anesthesia requires the timed withdrawal of inhaled agents, the discontinuation of continuous intravenous agents, and the reversal of neuromuscular blockers (via anticholinesterases). The solubility of the particular inhalational agent and the length of anesthesia are important factors in the time required for emergence. Most patients are extubated when they can follow commands and protect their airway. Deep extubation (extubation while the patient remains deeply anesthetized) is done in patients with a low aspiration risk and high risk for bronchospasm.

23
Local Anesthesia

Local anesthesia provides an effective means of pain control to avoid side effects such as respiratory depression, sedation, and nausea. Neuronal action potentials move across the nerve membrane via an electrical gradient. The movement of sodium and potassium ions establishes the gradient. The application of a stimulus results in the depolarization of the membrane and propagation of the action potential. Local anesthetics work by decreasing the cell membrane permeability to sodium ions and blocking the propagation of neuronal action potentials. The neuronal blockade affects both afferent and efferent limbs of the pain reflex.

Local anesthetics are used in a number of settings, including regional blocks, wound infiltration, intercostal blocks, nerve blocks, spinal anesthesia, and epidural anesthesia. The onset of action is determined by tissue pH, the pK_a of the particular agent used, and the amount of nonionized drug available in the tissue. The duration of action depends on the length of time that the drug binds to the membrane. Side effects include hypotension, cardiac depression, arrhythmias, and cardiac arrest. Clinical symptoms include perioral numbness, restlessness, tinnitus, seizures, and vertigo. These agents are sometimes combined with epinephrine to increase the duration of action and to reduce systemic absorption by causing vasoconstriction.

Local anesthetics are grouped into amides and esters. Esters are local anesthetics with an ester link between the aromatic and amine groups. Examples of esters include procaine, cocaine, and tetracaine. Esters are metabolized in the plasma through hydrolysis by pseudocholinesterases. Amide anesthetics contain an amide link between the aromatic compound and the amine groups. Anesthetics in this class typically have an "i" in their name followed by "caine" (e.g., lidocaine, etidocaine). Amide anesthetics are metabolized in the liver via aromatic hydroxylation, N-dealkylation, and amide hydrolysis.

Commonly used agents include lidocaine, bupivacaine, and ropivacaine. Lidocaine has a quick onset of action and low potential for complications. It can be used as a topical anesthetic and for spinal and epidural pain control. Toxicity occurs when 6.5 mg/kg or more is given. Bupivacaine is often given for epidural pain control in the obstetric setting. Its high protein binding capacity enables the drug to have a long duration of action. Doses greater than 2 mg/kg can cause systemic side effects. Ropivacaine is a newer agent that is less likely to cause cardiac depression.

Regional anesthesia is used when it is not desirable to use general anesthesia. Patients who are poor operative candidates because of overwhelming comorbidities may be able to tolerate a regional anesthetic. Lung complications, thromboembolic events, and blood loss may be reduced. Other potential advantages include a shorter time for resumption of ambulation and decreased hospital stay.

Spinal anesthesia is accomplished through the administration of local anesthetic into the intrathecal space. Blockade of the spinal nerve roots and dorsal root ganglia takes place. Epidural anesthesia is administered into the epidural space. Headache is experienced by some patients after spinal anesthesia. This is due to cerebrospinal fluid leak through the site of injection and loss of pressure in the subarachnoid space. A blood patch is performed by injecting about 5 to 10 mL of the patient's blood into the epidural space at the location of the spinal injection. The coagulation of the blood helps to seal off the cerebrospinal fluid leak. Other complications include hypotension, urinary retention, and risk of hematoma.

Nerve blocks can be used for postoperative pain relief or in cases of trauma. Patients with multiple rib fracture may be able to achieve pain relief through intercostal nerve block. The technique can be labor intensive and is therefore not often used.

24
Neuromuscular Blockade

Neuromuscular blockers are drugs that interfere with the transmission of neuronal signaling at the neuromuscular junction. The result is muscle relaxation and paralysis of skeletal muscles, including the diaphragm. They are used for intubation, mechanical ventilation, and to provide muscle relaxation during surgical procedures. Other uses include treatment of elevated intracranial pressure and status epilepticus. The neuromuscular junction is composed of two interfaces, the presynaptic membrane and the postsynaptic membrane. The presynaptic membrane is located at the end of the nerve ending. When an action potential reaches the nerve ending, an influx of calcium is triggered, causing the release of acetylcholine across the synaptic cleft. Acetylcholine binds to nicotinic cholinergic receptors at the postsynaptic membrane. This triggers the opening of ion channels with ion flow across their gradients. The ionic flow lowers the membrane potential and propagates an action potential through the muscle, resulting in contraction.

The two main types of neuromuscular blockers are depolarizing agents and nondepolarizing agents. Depolarizing agents act as acetylcholine agonists by mimicking the action of acetylcholine at the postsynaptic receptor. Succinylcholine is an example of this type of agent. Pseudocholinesterase enzymes in the plasma are responsible for the metabolism of succinylcholine. The enzyme is not found at the neuromuscular junction. Therefore, succinylcholine is present at the postsynaptic membrane longer than acetylcholine, resulting in a longer depolarization and muscle relaxation. Succinylcholine is generally used for situations that require rapid muscle relaxation for a short time (e.g., intubation). Potential hazards of succinylcholine include hyperkalemia, malignant hyperthermia, increased intracranial and intraocular pressures, and bradycardia. Hyperkalemia results from the up-regulation of receptors outside the neuromuscular junction. This up-regulation occurs in burn patients, immobilized patients, and patients with muscular dystrophy, closed head injury, and spinal cord injury. Activation of the extrajunctional receptors leads to release of intracellular potassium stores, causing hyperkalemia and arrhythmias.

Nondepolarizing agents work by antagonizing acetylcholine at the postsynaptic membrane. These agents are grouped according to their duration of action (Table 24.1).

Side effects of nondepolarizing agents are mediated through histamine release and include tachycardia. Metabolites of these agents (e.g., pancuronium and vecuronium) accumulate in patients with renal failure, producing a prolonged neuromuscular block.

Prolonged muscle weakness is also a potential complication of neuromuscular blockade. It occurs in patients who have been exposed to the agents for days to weeks. Up to 10% of patients demonstrate proximal and distal paresis and respiratory insufficiency. Patients with asthma and patients receiving exogenous steroids or aminoglycosides are more susceptible. Steps to minimize the risk of prolonged muscle weakness include physical therapy, close monitoring of the level of blockade, intermittent holidays of drug administration, and the avoidance of steroid based agents (e.g., pancuronium, vecuronium).

Patients are monitored for the level of neuromuscular blockade to avoid overdose. Peripheral nerve stimulation is the most widely accepted method for monitoring. Electrical impulses are delivered to a peripheral nerve (e.g., facial nerve, ulnar nerve, or posterior tibial nerve) via electrodes. As the level of neuromuscular blockade deepens, the number of twitches from nerve stimulation lessens. The number of twitches is proportional to the percentage of neuromuscular receptor blockade. Generally one to two twitches are the norm corresponding to 85% to 90% receptor blockade. Neuromuscular blockade alone allows the patient to be aware of pain and discomfort; therefore, sedatives and analgesics are given in conjunction with paralytics.

TABLE 24.1. Nondepolarizing agents grouped according to their duration of action.

Short acting (5–60 minutes)	Intermediate acting (60–90 minutes)	Long acting (90–120 minutes)
Mivacurium	Vecuronium	Pancuronium
Rocuronium	Atracurium	Doxacurium

Reversal of blockade can be accomplished by acetylcholinesterase inhibitors such as neostigmine and edrophonium. These agents work by decreasing the breakdown of acetylcholine, thereby increasing their presence at the receptor level.

25
Surgical Microbes

Bacteria are organized into groups according to their physical characteristics (shape), metabolic needs (aerobic or anaerobic), and histologic staining characteristics (Gram's stain). The different species of bacteria have virulent factors that are unique to each organism. The most important groups in relationship to surgery are Gram-positive cocci, Gram-negative rods, and anaerobic bacteria.

Gram-Positive Cocci

The most prevalent species involved with surgical infections in this class are *Staphylococcus* and *Streptococcus*. *Staphylococcus* organisms are anaerobic Gram-positive cocci. These organisms inhabit most body surfaces, especially on moist areas of the body. The most common organism responsible for wound infections is *Staphylococcus aureus*. *Staphylococcus aureus* produces an enzyme called *coagulase* that increases the organism's ability to cause infection. The organism can evade components of the immune system by using a surface capsule (prevent opsonization and phagocytosis) and by producing a slime coat. Extracellular products of the organism are responsible for a number of conditions. The production of enterotoxin has been implicated as a cause of food poisoning. Skin lesions such as exfoliative bullae develop from the production of epidermolytic toxins (e.g., scalded skin syndrome). Toxic shock syndrome (TSS) is the result of inflammatory reaction to the presence of TSS toxin-1.

Staphylococcus epidermidis is a common inhabitant of the skin and mucous membranes. *Staphylococcus epidermidis* is thought to be less virulent than *Staph. aureus*; however, it is still a common cause of infection of prosthetic materials (e.g., intravenous catheters, heart valves, and prosthetic joints).

The streptococci are Gram-positive cocci that occur in chains. The *Streptococcus* genus is characterized according to cell surface markers and hemolytic activity (Lancefield classification). The hemolytic activity is measured by incubating the organism on blood agar plates. There are three grades of hemolysis. Alpha-hemolysis is defined as an area of green discoloration of the agar immediately surrounding the colonies caused by incomplete destruction of red blood cells. The red blood cells in this are found intact. Beta-hemolysis implies complete destruction of surrounding red blood cells and, thus, clearing around the colonies. Gamma-hemolysis is defined as the absence of red cell destruction or change in coloration. The organisms in the genus *Streptococcus* that are most relevant to surgical practice are *pyogenes*, *pneumoniae*, and the viridans group.

Streptococcus pyogenes is a characteristic member of the group A class of streptococci. Virulent factors unique to group A streptococci include M proteins and streptolysins O and S. The M protein is a cell surface protein and is the major virulence factor for group A streptococci. M proteins aid in adherence to epithelial cells and in evasion of phagocytosis. The streptolysin proteins O and S are responsible for hemolytic and cytolytic activities. Streptokinase is also a product of streptococci. Streptokinase activates the fibrinolytic system and allows the bacteria to lyse local clots. Group A streptococci are responsible for infections of the pharynx (pharyngitis), the skin (erysipelas), and heart (endocarditis). Group A streptococci are often the cause of postoperative wound infections, cellulitis, urinary tract infections, and endocarditis.

Gram-Negative Bacilli

Gram-negative bacilli are responsible for a number of diseases. Of the many diseases, intraabdominal peritonitis, abscess, pneumonia, wound infection, and urinary tract infections are the most often encountered in surgical practice. Gram-negative rods contain a substance called *lipopolysaccharide* (LPS) in their cell walls.

Lipopolysaccharide is an endotoxin that triggers the immune system and an extensive inflammatory response. The most prominent Gram-negative rods isolated from surgical infections include *Escherichia coli, Klebsiella, Proteus, Serratia, Enterobacter*, and *Providencia.*

Pseudomonas aeruginosa are obligate aerobic Gram-negative rods. *Pseudomonas* is the causative agent in pneumonia and urinary tract infections. Many infections occur nosocomially, especially in immunocompromised patients. Antibiotic resistance is common, requiring antibiotic therapy with two different agents in most cases.

Anaerobic bacteria thrive in environments with low oxygen tension. These organisms inhabit areas of the gastrointestinal and urogenital tracts. Conditions that lower the local oxygen tension in tissue (e.g., ischemia, malignancy, necrotic tissue, and shock) facilitate the development of an anaerobic infection. Important anaerobic bacteria include *Bacteroides fragilis, Clostridium, Fusobacterium*, and *Peptostreptococcus.*

Clostridia are found in stool and soil. They are the most effective pathogen in the anaerobic class of bacteria and are known for their role in necrotizing soft tissue infections. Local and systemic reactions are produced in response to exotoxin secretion by these organisms. These exotoxins cause cell lysis, hemolysis, and breakdown of matrix components that aid in the spread of the infection. Pseudomembranous colitis is caused by *Clostridium difficile*. This organism arises when broad-spectrum antibiotics have been used, causing the elimination of other competitive bacteria within the colon. *Clostridium tetani* produces a neurotoxin that causes muscle spasms and results in the clinical condition called *tetanus. Clostridium botulinum* is found in contaminated foods. The neurotoxin it produces causes the paralysis that is seen in the condition botulism.

Fungi

Fungi are one of the most basic forms of eukaryotic organisms. They can appear as single-celled organisms (yeast) or as long hyphae. The composition of the fungal cell wall has many more similarities to mammalian cells. Therefore, most antibacterial agents are ineffective against fungi. Fungi can cause opportunistic and primary infections in nonimmunocompromised hosts. Most opportunistic infections are produced by *Aspergillus, Blastomyces, Candida, Coccidioides, Cryptococcus, Histoplasma, Mucor*, and *Rhizopus.*

Candida albicans is the most prominent species responsible for surgical infections. Infections are prone to develop in immunocompromised patients (e.g., malnourished patients, patients taking steroids, and patients receiving immunosuppressant therapy).

Viruses

Viruses are classified according to their size and to the type of genetic material they contain (RNA or DNA). Many viral infections manifest in immunocompromised hosts such as transplant patients. Cytomegalovirus produces the most viral infections in the transplant population. The hallmarks of infection are gastrointestinal ulcers that can cause bleeding or perforation. B-cell lymphomas arise in transplant patients as the result of Epstein-Barr viral infections. The hepatitis viruses (HBV and HCV) and the human immunodeficiency virus (HIV) pose a risk to the surgeon treating patients with these infections. The hepatitis viruses are discussed in Chapter 108.

Human immunodeficiency virus is a retrovirus belonging to the lentivirus family. The virus is composed of a central core containing RNA, core proteins, and RNA reverse transcriptase. The virus is contained in an envelope obtained from the nuclear membrane of the host. Glycoproteins on the envelope surface (gp120) bind to $CD4^+$ receptors of host T lymphocytes. The virus is brought into the T cell when gp120 binds to the $CD4^+$ receptor. Once inside, the virus is uncoated. New DNA is produced using the viral DNA as a template. The new DNA integrates into the host genome where it is transcribed to produce more viral RNA. Once infected, the T cells lose their ability to regulate immune functions. This lowers the patient's immune response, opening the door for opportunistic infections (e.g., fungal, mycobacterial) and the development of malignancies (e.g., Kaposi's sarcoma, lymphoma). $CD4^+$ counts at 200 or less define the illness as acquired immunodeficiency syndrome (AIDS). Human immunodeficiency virus is transmitted from contact with blood or secretions such as semen, vaginal fluid, and breast milk. Populations that comprise the highest risk groups include homosexual/bisexual men, intravenous drug users, hemophiliacs, and children born from HIV-positive women. The risk of transmission from blood transfusion is approximately 1 out of 450,000 to 660,000.

Nonspecific symptoms of malaise, fever, and lymphadenopathy generally accompany initial infection. Antibodies to the virus begin to appear 6 to 12 weeks into the infection (seroconversion). It is during this time that the immune system is still relatively intact, causing a drop in the viral numbers. Acquired immunodeficiency syndrome may not become apparent until 9 to 10 years after infection. At this time, a second rise of viral titers occurs. The number of HIV-infected patients requiring surgery is growing, making them a common occurrence in surgical practice. Pitfalls of surgery in the HIV-infected population include the risk of patient-to-health-care-worker transmission and malnutrition associated with AIDS. Indications for perioperative antibiotics are the same as for patients without HIV.

Exposure risk to health-care employees is reduced by complying with universal precaution guidelines. Post-exposure treatment involves employee counseling and clinical and serologic evaluations. Employees who test negative initially should be retested at 6 week, 12 week, and 6 month intervals. All febrile illnesses during that time period should be investigated. Postexposure administration of zidovudine (AZT) (Retrovir®) has shown to reduce the transmission of the disease. With proven HIV exposure, a regimen of AZT (Retrovir®) and lamivudine (3TC) (Epivir®), with or without indinavir, has been recommended starting 2 hours postexposure. In addition to universal precautions, the practice of double gloving and wearing face shields also minimizes the risk of transmission from skin exposures.

26
Soft Tissue Infections

Soft tissue infections range in severity from minor infections of the epidermis, which are treated medically, to major necrotizing infections, which can cause death if not treated immediately. Cellulitis is a superficial spreading bacterial infection of the skin and subcutaneous tissue. It manifests with erythema, warmth, tenderness, and edema. The organisms most often are responsible for cellulitis are group A *Streptococcus* and *Staphylococcus aureus*. Most cases of cellulitis are treated with antibiotics; however, when the infection is deeply seeded, an abscess forms, which requires surgical incision and drainage.

Folliculitis is the infection or inflammation of a hair follicle, often caused by *Staphylococcus*; however, Gram-negative organisms can cause them also. These infections often resolve without intervention. If folliculitis progresses to the development of a fluctuant nodule, it is termed a *furuncle*. The small abscess usually spontaneously ruptures and resolves. Drainage can be accelerated with warm soaks. If the infection is deep with multiple draining cutaneous sinuses, it is called a *carbuncle*. Treatment of a carbuncle involves either incision and drainage or a wide local excision of the infected tissue and the associated sinus tracts.

Necrotizing soft tissue infections spread rapidly, destroy tissue, and can be associated with septic shock. Classification of these infections is based on the tissue planes affected, extent of invasion, location, and the causative pathogen. The most common type is necrotizing fasciitis, which invades along the fascia deep to the adipose tissue. Necrotizing myositis is less common, involves the muscle, and spreads into the surrounding soft tissues. Necrotizing fasciitis in specific locations has separate names, such as Fournier's gangrene when there is necrotizing fasciitis in the perineum. Despite the different names, the disease process is the same. The most common causative pathogens in necrotizing fasciitis are Gram-positive organisms such as group A *Streptococcus*, *Enterococcus*, *Staphylococcus aureus*, and *Clostridium*. Gram-negative organisms, such as *Escherichia coli*, *Enter-obacter*, *Pseudomonas*, *Serratia*, and *Bacteroides*, can cause necrotizing infections, although they do so much less frequently. Nearly all necrotizing infections are polymicrobial in nature. Risk factors for developing a necrotizing infection are diabetes mellitus, obesity, malnutrition, alcoholism, peripheral vascular disease, chronic lymphocytic leukemia, steroid use, renal failure, cirrhosis, and autoimmune deficiencies.

Treatment for necrotizing infections includes early recognition, broad-spectrum antibiotics, and aggressive surgical debridement. Patients should be admitted to the intensive care unit for aggressive fluid replacement caused by the renal failure that develops due to associated septic shock. Debridement should remove all infected tissue, with additional debridements and reassessments in the operating room as needed. The possible benefit of hyperbaric oxygen treatment is debated; however, there are no definitive data showing benefit.

Hidradenitis suppurativa is another soft tissue infection often encountered by general surgeons. This condition is caused by a defect of the terminal follicular epithelium of the apocrine glands, which leads to blockage of the gland that causes infection. This occurs in areas where apocrine glands are most numerous, including the axillary, inguinal, and perianal regions of the body. There is a genetic component to hidradenitis suppurativa. The expression of the involved gene is under hormonal influence, so it manifests as patients reach puberty. The disease process includes formation of abscesses with repeated draining sinuses. This leads to scarring and pain. The treatment for an acute abscess is application of a warm compress, antibiotics, and drainage. Improved hygiene helps prevent recurrences; however, many patients develop chronic hidradenitis, which requires wide excision of the affected area and skin grafting if the area is extensive.

Pilonidal disease is an infection that begins with obstruction of a hair follicle and the associated pilosebaceous unit in the gluteal cleft. A localized folliculitis occurs, and it spreads and produces an abscess. The abscess often drains spontaneously, producing a sinus tract located just off the midline. The sinus tract is lined with granulation tissue. Over time, the tract epithelializes. Hair and debris enter the tract and cause further foreign body reactions. Infected pilonidal cysts occur primarily in young adults, with males being affected four times as often as females. Treatment for an acute pilonidal abscess is incision and drainage without antibiotics. Because the recurrence rate is high, the chronic sinus tract should be treated by local excision and closure, by wide excision with marsupialization or flap closure, or by tract curettage. Nonsurgical options include shaving the gluteal cleft and careful perianal hygiene; however, these have much greater recurrence rates compared with surgical excision. One rare but possible complication of pilonidal disease is the development of squamous cell carcinoma arising from the sinus tract.

Pyoderma gangrenosum is a rare inflammatory condition of the soft tissue. Although it is not a true infection, it is sometimes confused with one. The lesions caused by pyoderma gangrenosum are rapidly enlarging necrotic skin lesions with an indeterminate border and surrounding erythema. More than half of the patients with these lesions have an underlying systemic disease, such as inflammatory bowel disease, rheumatoid arthritis, a hematologic malignancy, or monoclonal immunoglobulin A gammopathy. Because of the incidence of other serious medical conditions, extensive medical workups are rec-ommended so that diagnosis and comprehensive medical treatment can be started. Treatment consists primarily of systemic steroids and cyclosporine. In cases of slow wound healing, local wound care and skin grafting may be needed.

Staphylococcal scalded skin syndrome manifests clinically with erythema of the skin, bullae formation, and skin loss. It is caused by an exotoxin produced by *Staphylococcus* infections of the nasopharynx or middle ear (in children). The diagnosis is made when a skin biopsy specimen demonstrates a cleavage plane in the granular layer of the epidermis. This lesion can easily be confused clinically with toxic epidermal necrolysis because they have very similar appearances. Toxic epidermal necrolysis is caused by an immunologic reaction to drugs such as sulfonamides, phenytoin, barbiturates, and tetracycline. It is not due to an infectious process. A skin biopsy specimen of toxic epidermal necrolysis shows a cleavage plane at the dermoepidermal junction. Another name for toxic epidermal necrolysis, when less than 10% of the patient's epidermis is detached, is Stevens-Johnson syndrome. Patients with toxic epidermal necrolysis can also have respiratory and gastrointestinal symptoms caused by the sloughing of epithelium along these tracts. Both types of epidermal conditions, toxic epidermal necrolysis and staphylococcal scalded skin syndrome, should be treated like second-degree burns with fluid resuscitation and local wound care with temporary coverage with a biologic dressing for protection while the epidermis regenerates.

27
Acute Respiratory Distress Syndrome

Acute respiratory distress syndrome (ARDS) is the leading cause of acute respiratory failure in the United States. It is not a primary disease but is more a complication that arises when other diseases produce a progressive form of systemic inflammatory response.

The basic pathology of ARDS is a diffuse inflammatory process that involves both lungs. The alveolar spaces contain erythrocytes, leukocytes, and proteinaceous debris. As the condition progresses, this exudative material eventually obliterates the alveolar airspaces. The lung consolidation in ARDS is believed to originate from a systemic activation of circulating neutrophils. The activated neutrophils become sticky and adhere to the vascular endothelium in the pulmonary capillaries. They then release the contents of their cytoplasmic granules (i.e., proteolytic enzymes and toxic oxygen metabolites), and this damages the endothelium and leads to a leaky-capillary type of exudation into the lung parenchyma. Therefore, although ARDS is often referred to as a type of pulmonary edema, it is an inflammatory process and not an accumulation of watery edema fluid. This is an important distinction for the diagnosis and management of ARDS.

Many conditions predispose to ARDS. The common feature in these conditions is the activation of neutrophils in the pulmonary or systemic circulation. The most common predisposing condition is sepsis, which is a systemic inflammatory response (such as fever or leukocytosis) due to an infection. The distinction between inflammation and infection is an important one because inflammation, not infection, produces the lung injury in ARDS.

The earliest clinical signs of ARDS include tachypnea and progressive hypoxemia. The hypoxemia is often refractory to supplemental oxygen. The chest roentgenogram can be unrevealing in the first few hours of the illness. However within 24 hours, the chest roentgenogram begins to reveal bilateral pulmonary infiltrates, which may be more prominent in the peripheral lung fields. Progression to mechanical ventilation often occurs in the first 48 hours of the illness. The diagnostic hallmarks of ARDS are diffuse pulmonary infiltrates, refractory hypoxemia (PAO_2/FIO_2 less than 200), the presence of a predisposing condition, and no evidence of left-heart failure (wedge pressure less than 18 mm Hg).

The other conditions that can mimic the clinical presentation of ARDS include pneumonia, acute pulmonary embolism, and cardiogenic (hydrostatic) pulmonary edema. The severity of the hypoxemia can sometimes help distinguish ARDS from cardiogenic pulmonary edema. In the early stages of ARDS, the hypoxemia is often more pronounced than the chest roentgenogram abnormalities, whereas in the early stages of cardiogenic pulmonary edema, the roentgenogram abnormalities are often more pronounced than the hypoxemia. The presence of high-risk conditions for ARDS may be the best means of distinguishing ARDS from cardiogenic edema. However, many of the conditions that predispose to ARDS also predispose to pneumonia and pulmonary embolism, so the predictive value of these conditions is limited if pneumonia or pulmonary embolism is a consideration.

The management of ARDS is usually designed with the following goals: (a) preventing iatrogenic lung injury, (b) reducing lung water, and (c) maintaining tissue oxygenation. It is important to point out that, although the main management is focused on the lungs, only 15% to 40% of deaths from ARDS are caused by respiratory failure. The majority of deaths are attributed to multiple organ failure. Age is also an important factor, with mortality being as much as five times higher in patients greater than 60 years of age.

There is now considerable evidence indicating that the large tidal volumes used during conventional mechanical ventilation (10 to 15 mL/kg) can damage the lungs. The pathologic changes in ARDS are not distributed uniformly throughout the lungs. Rather, there are regions of lung infiltration interspersed with regions where the lung architecture is normal. These normal lung regions (which may make up only 30% of the lung) receive most of the delivered tidal volume. This results in overdistension of normal lung regions, which leads to alveolar rupture, surfactant depletion, and disruption of the alveolar-capillary interface.

Recognition of the risk of lung injury at high inflation volumes and pressures has led to an alternative strategy where peak inspiratory pressures are kept below 35 cm H_2O by using tidal volumes of 7 to 10 mL/kg. According to this strategy, mechanical ventilation is started at inflation volumes of 10 mL/kg. If the resulting peak inspiratory pressure (PIP) is above 35 cm H_2O, the inflation volume is reduced in increments of 2 mL/kg until PIP falls below 35 cm H_2O. When low inflation volumes are used, external positive end-expiratory pressure (PEEP, 5 to 10 cm H_2O) is added to prevent compression atelectasis and to limit phasic collapse of the distal airways. Inflation volumes of 5 to 8 mL/kg can result in CO_2 retention; however, in the absence of adverse effects, the hypercapnia is allowed to continue (permissive hypercapnia).

The fractional concentration of inspired oxygen (FIO_2) should be kept at 50% or less to minimize the risk of oxygen toxicity. Arterial oxygen saturation (SaO_2) should be monitored instead of arterial PO_2, because SaO_2 determines the oxygen content in arterial blood. An SaO_2 above 90% should be sufficient to maintain oxygen delivery to peripheral tissues. If the FIO_2 cannot be reduced to below 60%, external PEEP is added to help reduce the FIO_2 to nontoxic levels.

The two measures that are advocated for reducing lung water are diuretics and PEEP. Unfortunately, neither measure is likely to be effective in ARDS. Diuretic therapy can reduce lung water by decreasing capillary hydrostatic pressure and increasing colloid osmotic pressure (increased plasma protein concentration). Although this should work in watery hydrostatic edema, the situation is different in ARDS. The lung infiltration in ARDS is an inflammatory process, and diuretics do not reduce inflammation. Considering the pathology of ARDS, the use of diuretics to reduce lung infiltration in ARDS does not seem warranted as a routine measure. The use of diuretics to minimize or reduce fluid overload seems a more reasonable measure but only when renal water excretion is impaired. Whenever diuretics are used, some form of hemodynamic monitoring must be used to make sure that the diuresis is not adversely affecting cardiac output.

The use of PEEP was popularized in ARDS because of the presumption that lung water could be reduced by this maneuver. However, the application of PEEP does not reduce extravascular lung water in ARDS. Furthermore, the prophylactic use of PEEP does not reduce the incidence of ARDS in high-risk patients. In fact, high levels of PEEP can actually *increase* lung water. This latter effect may be the result of alveolar overdistension mentioned earlier or may be the result of PEEP-induced impairment of lymphatic drainage from the lungs. Therefore, PEEP is not considered a therapy for ARDS. Instead, PEEP is a measure that helps to reduce iatrogenic lung injury by allowing ventilation with low inflation volumes and by allowing the FIO_2 to be reduced to less toxic levels.

The ultimate goal of treating respiratory failure is an adequate level of oxygenation in the vital organs. The best measurements available for evaluating tissue oxygenation at the bedside are systemic oxygen uptake (VO_2), venous lactate level, and gastric intramucosal pH (measured indirectly by gastric tonometry). Tissue oxygenation is considered to be inadequate if whole body VO_2 is less than 100 mL/min/m^2, venous lactate is greater than 4 mmol/L, or gastric intramucosal pH is less than 7.32. If there is evidence for impaired tissue oxygenation, certain measures should be taken to improve tissue perfusion.

Central venous pressure (CVP) and wedge pressures tend to overestimate cardiac filling volumes during positive-pressure mechanical ventilation, particularly when PEEP is applied. Thus, a normal CVP or wedge pressure does not necessarily indicate normal cardiac filling volumes during positive-pressure mechanical ventilation. In this setting, CVP and wedge pressure are interpretable only if they are reduced or are less than the level of applied PEEP. If the cardiac output is inadequate (e.g., a cardiac index below 3 L/min/m^2) and the CVP or wedge pressures are not elevated, volume infusion is indicated. If volume infusion is not indicated, dobutamine is used to augment the cardiac output. Transfusion is often recommended to keep the hemoglobin above 10 g/dL, but there is no basis for this recommendation. In fact, given the propensity for blood transfusions to *cause* ARDS, it seems wise to avoid transfusing blood products in ARDS. If there is no evidence of inadequate tissue oxygenation, there is no need to correct anemia.

28
Mechanical Ventilation

The decision to intubate a patient is guided primarily by clinical judgment. That being said, three of the major indications are pulmonary failure, altered mental status, and threatened loss of airway protection. Impending pulmonary failure is indicated by increased respiratory rate, increased work of breathing (excessive use of accessory respiratory muscles), hypercapnia ($PaCO_2 > 45\,mm\,Hg$), and hypoxia ($PaO_2 < 60\,mm\,Hg$).

Intubation is accomplished by orotracheal insertion, nasotracheal insertion, cricothyroidostomy, or tracheostomy. Each method has advantages and pitfalls. Nasotracheal intubation requires the patient to be awake during the procedure, avoiding the need for sedation and paralysis. The nasotracheal route requires the use of smaller tubes than does the orotracheal route. Complications of nasotracheal tubes include sinusitis and pressure necrosis of the nares. Cricothyroidostomy is reserved for emergent situations to gain security of the airway. A midline incision is made over the cricothyroid membrane, which is located inferior to the thyroid cartilage. The ostomy is enlarged with the handle of the knife, and a number 4 or 6 tracheostomy tube is inserted. Cricothyroidostomies are temporary and can only be used for 2 to 3 days before stenosis (glottic or subglottic) takes place. Conversion to a tracheostomy should be undertaken within this time period. Tracheostomies offer the benefit of easier airway clearance, less damage to the vocal cords, and easy connection and disconnection from the ventilator when attempting to wean.

Mechanical ventilators are used for ventilation and oxygenation for a patient who is unable to breathe. Ventilators are classified as either volume or pressure regulated. Volume ventilators are designed to convey a predetermined volume to the patient. Ventilation and oxygenation are adjusted by manipulating four main variables. The ventilatory rate and tidal volume can be changed to adjust the $PaCO_2$. Oxygenation is adjusted by manipulating the concentration of inspired oxygen (FiO_2) as well as the positive end-expiratory pressure (PEEP). The initial rate is generally set around 12 to 15 breaths per minute and then adjusted according to the needs of the patient. Patients capable of taking spontaneous breaths generally breathe at a higher rate than the set rate. Patients incapable of taking spontaneous breaths will breathe at the rate set by the ventilator. The $PaCO_2$ is maintained at or near $40\,mm\,Hg$, with some exceptions (e.g., elevated intracranial pressure). A normal tidal volume in a person at rest is approximately $7\,mL/kg$. Similarly, volume ventilators are initially adjusted to deliver the same amount of volume. Larger tidal volumes result in hyperexpansion of the alveoli and airways, which produces barotrauma. The body is more apt to tolerate hypercapnia before epithelial damage secondary to high lung volumes. Bronchopleural fistulas are exceptions to this rule. In this condition, higher tidal volumes are administered to overcome volume loss from the fistula.

Arterial oxygenation can be adjusted by controlling the fraction of inspired oxygen. Concentrations greater than 60% can lead to toxic side effects (chronic pulmonary fibrosis, loss of respiratory drive in patients with chronic obstructive pulmonary disease). Therefore, FiO_2 levels should be kept at a minimum to sustain oxygen saturations greater than 90%. Positive end-expiratory pressure, another variable that affects arterial oxygenation, is the airway pressure that remains in the ventilatory circuit at the end of the respiratory cycle. It retains patency of the smaller airways and alveoli. It prevents their collapse and the resulting atelectasis. When more airways remain open, more surface area is available for gas exchange. Intubation eliminates the natural or physiologic PEEP that is produced from the closed glottis. Physiologic levels of PEEP are approximately $5\,cm\,H_2O$ and should be provided for the majority of intubated patients; the level can be adjusted as high as $20\,cm\,H_2O$. Positive end-expiratory pressure also helps to minimize the FiO_2 needed. A pitfall to PEEP is decreased ventricular filling resulting in impaired cardiac output.

Peak airway pressures are also increased in proportion to the amount of PEEP applied. In certain patient groups, increased peak airway pressures may lead to airway rupture and tension pneumothorax.

Volume Control Modes

The two basic modes of volume ventilation are assist control and intermittent mandatory ventilation. Assist control is a mode that delivers a predetermined volume whenever the patient initiates a breath. Assist control requires minimal effort by the patient and, thus, greatly limits the amount of work done by the patient. The machine can also give the patient a predetermined number of breaths if the patient fails to initiate them. The drawbacks include poor weaning ability (because the machine does the majority of respiratory work) and hyperventilation if the patient becomes tachypneic. These drawbacks have been addressed through the development of intermittent mandatory ventilation (IMV). The IMV mode delivers machine breaths at a predetermined rate but also allows for spontaneous unassisted breaths by the patient. This mode uses two parallel circuits. One is connected to the ventilator, and the other connects to a reservoir filled with a gas mixture. A one-way valve opens with the patient's spontaneous efforts and allows the patient to breathe from the reservoir unassisted by the machine. Synchronized mandatory ventilation (SIMV) coordinates the predetermined rate of machine breaths with the patient's spontaneous breaths. The set rate of machine breaths can be adjusted to vary the amount of work required by the patient. Weaning can be accomplished by gradually reducing the number of machine breaths.

Pressure Ventilation Modes

Pressure ventilation modes were developed with long-term mechanically ventilated patients in mind to limit excessive tidal volumes and elevated airway pressures. They consist of pressure support and pressure control.

Pressure Support

During pressure support, a predetermined level of pressure is applied to assist with the patient's spontaneous breaths. When the patient initiates a breath by creating a negative pressure in the ventilator circuitry, a one-way valve is opened. The ventilator provides the inspiratory volume at a flow rate just enough to maintain the predetermined pressure. This modality enhances the sponta-

neous breathing of the patient and also decreases the workload by providing enough pressure to overcome the resistance of the ventilator tubing (generally 5 to 10 cm H_2O). Pressure support can be combined with IMV to assist with the patient's spontaneous breaths. General ranges of support vary from 5 to 25 cm H_2O. Pressure support can be a good modality for weaning patients from mechanical ventilation. The patient is asked to do more work of breathing as the pressure support is reduced.

Pressure Control

Pressure control ventilation delivers a continuous pressure during the inspiratory phase of the respiratory cycle. In contrast to volume-controlled ventilation, pressure control ventilation varies the inspiratory flow to maintain a constant pressure. This causes the inspiratory volumes to vary according to the compliance of the patient's lungs. Pressure control allows for adjustment of rate, tidal volume, PEEP, FiO_2, and the ratio of inspiratory time to expiratory time (I:E ratio). The I:E ratio is adjusted from 1:1 to 4:1 to allow for increased time for inspiration compared with expiration. The normal I:E ratio is 1:2 in a person breathing spontaneously. Reversal of the I:E ratio (inverse ratio ventilation [IRV]) is uncomfortable and requires sedation and paralysis. Increasing the inspiratory time is helpful for patients who have deficits in oxygenation and who have decreased lung compliance by preventing alveolar collapse. Drawbacks to this modality include air trapping or the auto PEEP phenomena. This occurs when inspiration is begun for the next cycle before expiration has been completed from the previous cycle. This can cause hyperinflation of the lungs and decreased cardiac output.

Continuous Positive Airway Pressure

Continuous positive airway pressure (CPAP) assists spontaneous breathing efforts by providing a constant positive pressure. In essence, this eliminates the need for generating a negative pressure by the patient to initiate breaths, therefore reducing the work of breathing. Continuous positive airway pressure has proved useful for nonintubated patients and serves as a bridge to elective intubation rather than emergent. Pitfalls include the need for a tight-fitting mask, which prevents the patient from being able to eat and causes poor tolerance of some patients. Continuous positive airway pressure can be administered through specialized nasal masks for patients with sleep apnea. This prevents collapse of the upper airways when negative pressure is generated to breathe.

Weaning

Weaning from mechanical ventilation requires gradually increasing the amount of work contributed by the patient for respiration. As a general rule, weaning is not instituted until the FiO_2 is at or below 40% and the PEEP is 5 cm H_2O. At this point, weaning parameters are obtained to determine the probability of successful discontinuation from the ventilator. Some parameters have greater predictive value than others. The most widely used parameters are listed in Table 28.1. The method of weaning depends on the mode of ventilatory support being provided. Patients supported on IMV mode can be weaned by gradually reducing the set respiratory rate. Once an IMV rate of 4 or less is reached and maintained for period of time, the patient may be given a trial of spontaneous breathing. Spontaneous breathing can be accomplished by placing the patient on T-piece or tracheostomy collar (flow-by oxygen is attached to the endotracheal tube or tracheostomy tube, respectively), or the patient is left connected to the ventilator with only 5 cm H_2O of pressure support and 5 cm H_2O of PEEP (to overcome the circuit resistance). Spontaneous breathing trials are conducted for 30 minutes. During this time, the respiratory rate must be below 25 breaths per minute without labored breathing. Spontaneous breathing trials can be conducted intermittently throughout the day, prolonging each trial until the patient is able to tolerate more than 30 minutes at a time. Patients receiving pressure support can be weaned by gradually reducing the level of pressure support given. Patients may be extubated when they are able to tolerate ventilation with less than 10 cm H_2O of pressure support for more than 24 hours.

TABLE 28.1. Weaning parameters.

Parameter	Normal	Expectable for weaning
PaO_2/FiO_2	>400	200
Tidal volume	5–7 mL/kg	5 mL/kg
Respiratory rate	14–18/min	<40/min
Vital capacity	65–75 mL/kg	10 mL/kg
Minute ventilation	5–7 L/min	<10 L/min
Maximum inspiratory pressure (negative inspiratory force)*	Above –90 cm H_2O	–25 cm H_2O
Rate/tidal volume*	<50/min/L	<100/min/L

*Greatest predictive values.

Extubation

The possibility for extubation is governed mostly by the progress of the patient's underlying disease. Objective parameters for possible extubation include the patient's performance during spontaneous breathing trials and arterial blood gas values. In general, the patient must maintain a respiratory rate of <25/min, a $PaCO_2$ of 42 mm Hg or less, a PaO_2 above 90% on 40% FiO_2 (or less), and a maximum PEEP of 5 cm H_2O. Mental status is another important factor. To effectively protect the airway, a patient must be able to follow simple commands.

29
Coagulation and Anticoagulation

Coagulation involves a complex chain of interactions among platelets, the vascular wall, and circulating coagulation factors in the plasma. The coagulation cascade is initiated by either an intrinsic or extrinsic pathway, both of which eventually result in the formation of a fibrin clot. The intrinsic pathway is so named because all involved components are circulating in the plasma, and no surface is required for activation. The cascade begins with factor XII, which sets off a sequential cascade of activation of factors XI, IX, and then VII.

The extrinsic pathway requires exposure of tissue factor on the surface of an injured blood vessel to initiate the cascade of factor activation, starting with factor VII. Factor VII forms an activated complex with tissue factor, which in turn activates factors X and IX. Both the intrinsic and extrinsic pathways result in the activation of factor X and therefore share the final common pathway of clot formation. Factor X activates factor II (prothrombin), which in turn activates factor I (fibrinogen) into fibrin. Fibrin is the final product needed for clot formation.

The coagulation cascade is self-regulated to allow the proper balance between clot formation and propagation to prevent thrombosis of an entire vascular bed in response to a local insult. There is feedback inhibition of the cascade once the procoagulant factors are activated. Tissue factor pathway inhibitor is normally present in the circulation at low concentrations, and it blocks the formation of the tissue factor/factor VII complex, so factor X is not activated. Antithrombin III is another circulating factor, which neutralizes the procoagulant factors of the intrinsic limb of the coagulation cascade. The third inhibitor to the coagulation cascade is protein C, which is activated by thrombin formation. Activated protein C cleaves factors V and VII, so they are no longer able to participate in the coagulation cascade. Besides the three inhibitors to the coagulation cascade, another major mechanism for preventing excessive clot formation is fibrinolysis. Fibrinolysis is the breakdown of the fibrin clot

by plasmin, which also allows for repair of the injured vessel with connective tissue deposition.

Platelets also play an important role in hemostasis by adhering to the site of injury, aggregating to form a platelet plug, and providing a procoagulant surface on which to deposit fibrin. There are glycoprotein IIb/IIIa receptors on platelets, which are joined to adjacent platelets by fibrinogen. Thromboxane A_2 and ionized calcium are potent platelet aggregators, which are also important to aiding clot formation. Like the coagulation cascade, there is a counterbalance system for platelet aggregation. Endothelial cells produce prostacyclin, which limits the local hemostatic process by increasing adenyl cyclase levels, which in turn increase the platelets cyclic adenosine monophosphate levels, leading to lower available ionized calcium needed for aggregation. Prostacyclin is a potent vasodilator also, which further limits localized coagulation.

Evaluation of bleeding disorders is begun with a thorough history and simple laboratory tests, which evaluate for deficits in the coagulation cascade or platelet function. A platelet count identifies a quantitative deficit in platelets, and a bleeding time evaluates the qualitative function of platelets. Prothrombin time (PT) and activated partial thromboplastin time (aPTT) are the two tests that evaluate the factors of the coagulation cascade. The PT evaluates the factors of the extrinsic pathway (VII, X, V, II, and I), and the aPTT evaluates the intrinsic pathway (factors XII, XI, IX, VIII, X, V, II, and I).

There are many hemostatic defects caused by congenital deficiencies in specific coagulation factors. Hemophilia A is a sex-linked recessive disorder that results in deficient levels of factor VIII, and hemophilia B causes a deficiency of factor IX. The severity of each disease depends on the measurable level of these factors in the plasma. Mild disease manifests with levels between 5% and 30% of normal and typically manifests as prolonged bleeding after minor surgery or major trauma. Moderate hemophilia manifests with a factor VIII or IX plasma level between 1% and 5% of normal. Patients can have spontaneous bleeding, severe postoperative or post-traumatic bleeding, and may develop retroperitoneal hematomas after heavy lifting. Patients with a factor VIII or IX level less than 1% of normal have severe hemophilia, which presents with spontaneous bleeding. Bleeding is usually into joints, intramuscular, retroperitoneal, or from the gastrointestinal or genitourinary tract. Treatment for patients with hemophilia is replacement of the deficient factor. Desmopressin is used for type A, mild to moderate hemophilia with minor bleeds. Desmopressin works by stimulating the release of von Willebrand's factor and associated factor VIII from endothelial cells.

Von Willebrand's disease, an autosomal dominant disease, is the most common bleeding disorder. Patients with this disease have low levels of von Willebrand's factor, which is a glycoprotein produced by endothelial cells that serves as a carrier of factor VIII and is necessary for normal platelet aggregation and adhesion to the subendothelium. These patients typically present with easy bruising and mucosal bleeding. Treatment involves DDAVP (1-deamino-8-D-arginine vasopressin) in mild cases or replacement with infusion of factor VIII concentrates, which also contain von Willebrand's factor. Deficiency in factor XI, also called hemophilia C, is a rare autosomal recessive disease occurring most often in persons of Ashkenazi Jewish descent. This disorder rarely causes spontaneous bleeding, but serious bleeding can occur after surgery or trauma. Treatment is with fresh-frozen plasma. Deficiencies of the other coagulation factors (II, V, VII, and XIII) are rare, and significant bleeding only occurs if the factor deficiency is severe. All can be treated with fresh-frozen plasma.

In addition to the congenital bleeding disorders, there are many acquired bleeding disorders. Patients with a vitamin K deficiency are unable to synthesize prothrombin, factors VII, IX, and X, and proteins C and S. Vitamin K deficiency can be caused by inadequate dietary intake, malabsorption, lack of bile salts, obstructive jaundice, biliary fistula, oral antibiotics (especially cephalosporins, quinolones, doxycycline, and trimethoprim-sulfamethoxazole), or total parenteral nutrition. Treatment is with administration of vitamin K (preferably subcutaneously or intramuscularly) or fresh-frozen plasma for a more rapid correction of coagulopathy.

Hepatic failure, due to trauma, cirrhosis, or biliary obstruction, affects coagulation, because the liver makes all coagulation factors except factor VIII. Patients with hepatic failure also tend to have thrombocytopenia due to decreased platelet production, splenic sequestration, circulating antiplatelet antibodies, and viral hepatitis infection. Prolonged bleeding times are often improved by administration of desmopressin. Renal failure and uremia also cause prolonged bleeding due to platelet dysfunction and can be treated with desmopressin. Hypothermia is a frequent cause of prolonged bleeding and is due to the decreased activity at lower temperatures of the proteolytic enzymes that make up the coagulation cascade.

The other major acquired cause of prolonged bleeding is anticoagulation therapy. Many patients take medications for anticoagulation, including warfarin, heparin, and aspirin. Warfarin works by inhibiting the formation of vitamin K–dependent factors (prothrombin, factors VII, IX, X, and proteins C and S), and therefore prolongs the patient's PT and causes a slight increase in the aPTT. The half-life of warfarin is approximately 40 hours. Reversal is accomplished with vitamin K administration or fresh-frozen plasma infusion for a more rapid reversal. Unfractionated heparin blocks the activation of factor X by binding with antithrombin III. All coagulation tests are affected by heparin, but an increased aPTT is the most sensitive. The half-life of heparin is 6 hours, but this can vary based on hepatic function, body temperature, and shock. Heparin can be reduced with protamine. Heparin causes thrombocytopenia in 5% of patients because of the presence of immunoglobulin G antibodies to heparin platelet factor 4 complexes. When this sudden drop in platelet count occurs, heparin should be stopped and another anticoagulation medication should be used. Low-molecular-weight heparins have more selective anti-Xa activity and are associated with fewer bleeding complications. With these medications, the PT is usually not affected. Aspirin is another medication used for anticoagulation. This medication affects platelets and, therefore, bleeding time. It works by irreversibly inhibiting the enzyme cyclo-oxygenase, which converts arachidonic acid to prostaglandin G_2. In platelets, prostaglandin G_2 is converted to the prothrombotic thromboxane A_2. Reversal usually requires platelet transfusion because of the irreversible nature of aspirin's affect on platelets.

30
Hypercoagulable States

Deep venous thrombosis (DVT) results from thrombosis in a segment of the venous system. Virchow's triad provides the classic description for causes of DVT. The triad consists of endothelial injury, venous stasis, and a hypercoagulable state. The consequences of DVT can be deadly. Propagation is the continued development and proximal spread of a thrombotic segment. Propagation occurs in approximately 30% of hospital patients with DVT. Pulmonary embolism involves the migration of a piece of the thrombus to the pulmonary arteries. This impedes blood flow into a portion of the lungs and causes hypoxia. Pulmonary embolism is potentially deadly. More than 60% of patients who experience venous thromboembolism also develop DVT. Approximately 50,000 to 200,000 deaths per year in the United States are attributed to pulmonary embolism. Another potential complication of DVT is chronic venous insufficiency caused by intraluminal obstruction and damage to the valves.

Patients who have undergone a major surgical procedure are at risk for DVT. The three elements of Virchow's triad are demonstrated in many postoperative patients. Abnormalities in the coagulation and the fibrinolytic systems increase the likelihood of forming clots and thrombi. These inherited forms of hypercoagulability occur in 24% to 37% of patients with DVT. Common conditions that lead to hypercoagulability are listed below. These conditions require lifelong anticoagulation:

- Antithrombin III deficiency
- Antiphospholipid syndrome
- Factor V Leiden
- Homocysteine
- Protein C deficiency
- Protein S deficiency
- Prothrombin genetic mutation

History taking should be directed to information about previous episodes, family history of DVT, and coexisting conditions (e.g., malignancy, pregnancy, trauma, heart failure, or recent surgery). Women should be questioned about oral contraception use, hormone replacement medications, and obstetric history. A medication history is important, because drugs such as heparin are associated with thrombosis. Others, such as phenothiazine, procainamide, and hydralazine, precipitate the production of antiphospholipid antibodies.

Most cases of DVT are asymptomatic; only 40% of patients have symptoms. Symptoms usually do not manifest until the disease is severe (proximal thrombus propagation). The most common manifestations are edema, pain, and warmth. A physical examination provides very few clues to the presence of DVT. A Homan's sign (pain in the calf with foot dorsiflexion) indicates DVT. This observation is used as an indication for further testing; however, the absence of this sign does not rule out DVT. Thrombosis of the iliofemoral veins results in a condition called *phlegmasia alba dolens*. This condition is marked by severe swelling, pitting edema, and pain. The edema can compromise the arterial inflow into the extremity, causing ischemia. At this point, the extremity turns blue and is even more painful (phlegmasia cerulea dolens).

Laboratory tests should include coagulation studies (i.e., prothrombin time [PT], partial prothrombin time [PTT], and international normalized ratio [INR]), complete blood count, liver function tests, and renal panels). The diagnoses of polycythemia and thrombocytopenia are indicated by increased erythrocyte or platelet counts. Blood smears help identify schizocytes and fragmented red blood cells associated with disseminated intravascular coagulation (DIC) or thrombotic microangiopathies.

Testing for all hereditary causes of hypercoagulable states in all patients with DVT is impractical and expensive. Therefore, specific testing is restricted to selected patients. The indications for laboratory testing are listed below.

1. Proteins C and S and antithrombin deficiencies
   - DVT occurring in persons younger than age 50
   - Family history of DVT

- Recurrent DVT
- Women taking oral contraceptives
- Women who are pregnant
2. Factor V Leiden, prothrombin genetic mutation, antiphospholipid antibodies, and hyperhomocysteinemia
   - All Caucasian patients without an obvious reason for DVT (malignancy, trauma, recent surgery)
   - Non-Caucasian patients should undergo limited testing, including investigations into antiphospholipid antibodies and hyperhomocysteinemia

Patients with a clear etiology of DVT (malignancy, lupus, recent major surgery, trauma, inflammatory bowel disease, heparin-induced thrombocytopenia, and myeloproliferative diseases) need not undergo testing for inherited hypercoagulable states.

The timing for specific testing is important, because test results are influenced by other illnesses, anticoagulant therapy, and acute thrombosis. Transient decreases in proteins C and S as well as antithrombin concentrations are observed during acute thrombosis. Heparin causes reductions in plasma antithrombin levels, and Coumadin depresses the levels of proteins C and S. In general, most testing is done at the initial onset of DVT and before anticoagulation begins. Decreased levels of proteins C and S and antithrombin at this time can be erroneous. Therefore, repeated testing is warranted 2 weeks after the conclusion of 3 to 6 months of anticoagulation treatment. If initial testing shows no deficits, then the theory of an inherited coagulopathy is disproved.

Factor V Leiden is evaluated by using clotting assays or by the evaluation of genomic DNA. Activated protein C resistance is diagnosed by coagulation assays and genotyping. Genetic analysis for the prothrombin gene mutation is the only method of evaluation. Coagulation assays are used to test for proteins C and S deficiencies. An antithrombin-heparin cofactor assay is used to test for antithrombin deficiencies. Evaluations into hyperhomocysteinemia require an overnight fasting period. A dose of methionine is given orally, and plasma homocysteine levels are determined 4 to 8 hours afterward. Antiphospholipid antibodies cause an increase in the activated partial thromboplastin time (aPTT). The patient's serum is often tested after mixing it with the serum of a normal patient (1:1). A prolonged aPTT after mixing indicates antibody inhibition of coagulation. Some patients with systemic lupus erythematosus and lupus anticoagulant also have anticardiolipin antibodies. Serologic testing can be done to identify the antibodies.

Duplex ultrasound is the most often used modality to diagnose DVT. The advantages of duplex ultrasound include its noninvasiveness and the avoidance of the complications of angiography. The test evaluates the flow in the venous system and the compressibility of the veins. In a normal venous system (one without thrombi), blood flow increases in response to distal compression. Thrombosed venous systems do not demonstrate augmented flow in response to distal compression. Flow through the system is evaluated with B-mode ultrasound and color imaging. Compressibility of the veins can be demonstrated by applying direct pressure with the ultrasound probe. Veins with thrombi are not compressible. Other modalities used for making the diagnosis include venography, fibrin fibrinogen assays, and magnetic resonance venography.

Prophylaxis against DVT is individualized according to the patient's degree of risk and the presence of contraindications (active bleeding, hemostatic disorders, severe uncontrolled hypertension, and recent surgery). Prophylaxis methods range from mechanical to pharmacologic. Patients who are ambulatory within 24 to 48 hours after surgery are considered at low risk for DVT. Ambulation provides a simple and effective prophylaxis for low-risk patients. The muscular contractions produced from walking improve venous flow and counteract stasis. Sequential compression devices are often used in surgical patients. These devices, usually placed on the lower extremities, compress the calf muscles at time intervals. This causes systemic activation of the fibrinolytic system.

Patients who are determined to be at moderate to high risk for DVT undergo chemical prophylaxis as long as they have no contraindications to their use. Low-dose heparin is often used for prophylaxis. Heparin exerts its anticoagulation effect by potentiating the thrombolytic action of antithrombin III. Low-dose heparin is administered subcutaneously at doses of 5,000 U every 8 hours. It acts by inhibiting the function of factors Xa and IIA and does not require laboratory tests to evaluate its therapeutic efficacy. Studies have also demonstrated that low-molecular-weight heparin can be given safely to patients with head injuries without increasing the incidence of intracranial bleeding. Patients with inherited hypercoagulable states should receive prophylaxis with low-molecular-weight heparin, which should be continued in the postoperative period.

Definitive treatment for DVT is accomplished with chemical anticoagulation. The typical treatment begins with the administration of intravenous heparin followed by Coumadin. Heparin provides initial anticoagulation, because patients actually become hypercoagulable with the initiation of Coumadin. Coumadin interferes with the production of vitamin K–dependent clotting factors produced in the liver (factors II, VII, IX, X, C, and S). Proteins C and S actually exert an anticoagulation effect. Their half-lives are shorter than those of the other vitamin K–dependent factors and therefore render the patient hypercoagulable when their levels decrease. Heparin therapy begins with a bolus of 80 U/kg and continues at an infusion rate of 15 U/kg. Prothromboplastin times of 60 to 80 seconds are the target for heparin therapy. Coumadin therapy should begin the same day as heparin therapy, and dosages are adjusted to achieve a target therapeutic INR of 2 to 3. Coumadin therapy is continued for at least 3 months. Patients with hypercoagulable states require lifelong treatment. Coumadin is a known teratogen, so it should not be taken during pregnancy. Low-molecular-weight heparin is an appropriate alternative. In addition, low-molecular-weight heparin is an effective substitute for traditional heparin for initial anticoagulation. Because low-molecular-weight heparin does not require laboratory monitoring, it can be used in the outpatient setting. Deep venous thrombosis recurrence rates of 6% to 7% have been reported with anticoagulation therapy.

Thrombolytic therapy is rarely instituted for DVT. The only potential benefit is to provide symptom relief for phlegmasia. Thrombolytic therapy avoids the need for surgical thrombectomy for these patients. Thrombolytic therapy has a greater risk of causing bleeding than does routine anticoagulation.

Vena cava filters are mechanical devices placed in the inferior vena cava to prevent embolized thrombus from reaching the pulmonary system. Indications for inferior vena cava filter placement are the following:

- Patients with contraindications to anticoagulation (active bleeding, hemostatic disorders, severe uncontrolled hypertension, and recent surgery)
- Thromboembolism despite anticoagulation therapy
- Propagation of thrombi despite anticoagulation
- Chronic pulmonary embolism producing pulmonary hypertension
- When complications arise from anticoagulation therapy

The device is placed in the inferior vena cava below the level of the renal veins. The procedure is performed percutaneously using a Seldinger technique. Placement is aided by fluoroscopic venogram using CO_2 or iodinated contrast. Patency rates are about 95%, with a 4% rate of embolism recurrence. Complications include hematoma, device migration, and obstruction of the vena cava caused by emboli trapping. Caval occlusion causes hypotension because of reduced venous return. This condition is usually treated with volume resuscitation.

Warfarin-induced skin necrosis is associated with a pre-existing protein C deficiency. Warfarin induces a temporary state of hypercoagulability by reducing the activity of protein C. Patients with known protein C deficiencies and a history of warfarin-induced skin necrosis can be successfully treated with Coumadin. Patients should be fully heparinized, and Coumadin should be started slowly (a 2mg initial dose for 3 days, then increasing by 2 to 3mg a day until therapeutic levels are reached). Other options include protein C replacement with fresh-frozen plasma or concentrate.

Some patients with antithrombin deficiencies are resistant to the effects of heparin because of the suppressive effect that heparin has on antithrombin itself (a 30% reduction in plasma levels). In addition, the stresses of a surgical procedure can lower antithrombin levels for up to 5 days postoperatively. Such patients require greater than normal doses of heparin to achieve anticoagulation. Antithrombin concentrate can be administered to patients with severe thrombosis and to patients who fail anticoagulation therapy. Antithrombin concentrate is generally given in doses of 50U/kg. The goal of therapy is to maintain antithrombin levels greater than 80%.

31
Transfusion Therapy

Blood transfusions have been experimented with since the seventeenth century. During the 1900s, major advances, such as the discovery of blood types and preservative solutions, have made transfusion therapy relatively safe and effective. Blood is composed of many cell types, which serve various vital functions. Although, in the past, whole blood transfusion was common, blood product components such as packed red blood cells, platelets, and fresh-frozen plasma (which contains many of the circulating clotting factors) are now transfused.

Serologic compatibility is necessary for successful transfusion. Therefore, a patient should be typed, which means identifying the A, B, and Rh antigens in his or her red blood cells. To prevent reactions, patients should only be transfused with compatible or cross-matched blood types. Because the Rh factor is somewhat less important and because there is a smaller supply of Rh-negative blood, older men with no prior transfusions can be given Rh-positive blood products. In these cases, Rh antibodies form within 2 weeks. Up to that point, the patient can receive Rh-positive blood. Giving anti-Rh antiserum to Rh-negative patients receiving Rh-positive products will decrease the chance that the patient's immune system will be sensitized and begin producing Rh antibodies. Rh-positive blood should never be given to Rh-negative women of childbearing age because of the future in utero risk to Rh-positive children she may bear. In emergency situations, O-negative blood can be used for transfusion in all patients while waiting for cross-match information. Transfusion of more than four units of O-negative blood into a patient whose blood is not yet typed should be avoided because of the risk of hemolysis.

Many blood products are available for transfusion. Whole blood, for the most part, is no longer available except for autologous previously donated blood, which has a shelf life of up to 40 days. Changes that occur in banked blood include decreased intracellular adenosine diphosphate and decreased 2,3-diphosphoglycerate, both of which cause a shift in the hemoglobin–oxygen dissociation curve and therefore decrease the effectiveness of red blood cell oxygen delivery to tissues. Other changes that occur in banked blood include instability of platelets and clotting factors V and VIII, decreased pH due to increased lactic acid levels, and increased potassium and ammonia concentrations.

Packed red blood cells are generally given to patients who need blood replacement. Leukocyte-reduced and leukocyte-washed packed red blood cells reduce the risk of febrile and nonhemolytic transfusion reactions by filtering out 99.9% of white blood cells and most platelets. There is debate regarding the extra cost of leukoreduction compared with the proposed decreased risk of postoperative infection and multiorgan failure. This product is usually only given to patients with a history of transfusion reactions.

Platelets are given for thrombocytopenia and qualitative platelet disorders. Due to the short lifespan of platelets, they must be transfused within 120 hours of donation. Complications, rates of transmission of infectious diseases, and allergic reactions are similar to those of packed red blood cell transfusions. Leukocyte reduction through filtration can prevent some of the risk of these complications. Fresh-frozen plasma is another blood component transfused. It contains all of the vitamin K–dependent clotting factors and factors II, V, and X.

Indications for transfusion are the need for improvement in oxygen-carrying capacity, volume replacement, and replacement of clotting factors. Acute anemia due to hemorrhage or surgery can be disabling and should be corrected, especially in patients with multiple medical problems or low cardiac reserve. Chronic anemia does not usually require transfusion, because the patients have had time to compensate for the deficiency of red blood cells. For these patients, erythropoietin with iron supplementation is a better treatment option. Volume replacement is the most common indication for blood transfusion for surgical patients. When blood loss is less than 20% of total blood volume, crystalloids alone should be sufficient for treatment. If blood loss is greater than 20% of total blood volume, crystalloid and packed red blood cells should be given. If the blood loss is greater than 50% plasma, albumin and fresh-frozen plasma should be given in addition to the crystalloids and packed red blood cells. This is to overcome the chelating effect of the citrate used to preserve stored blood products on the circulating coagulation factors. Replacement of clotting factors with fresh-frozen plasma or platelets is indicated preoperatively or intraoperatively to correct clotting deficits, such as in patients receiving anticoagulants who need emergency surgery.

Blood transfusions are not without complications, so transfusion should be avoided whenever possible. Hemolytic reactions are the most common of the serious complications associated with transfusion. Nonfatal hemolytic transfusion reactions occur in approximately 1 of every 6,000 units transfused, and fatal reactions occur in 1 of every 100,000 units transfused. These reactions are caused by serologic incompatibility, usually the result of a laboratory or clerical error. Immediate hemolytic reactions are caused by an ABO mismatch. These occur during the infusion and manifest with hemoglobinemia and hemoglobinuria because of the intravascular destruction of red blood cells. Other symptoms in a conscious patient include heat and pain along the vein receiving the transfusion, facial flushing, pain in the lumbar region, constricting chest pain, fever, chills, respiratory distress, hypotension, and tachycardia. In anesthetized patients, sudden hypotension and diffuse bleeding are signs. Free hemoglobin is toxic to the renal system and causes tubular necrosis. Antigen–antibody complexes in circulation can initiate the coagulation cascade and result in disseminated intravascular coagulopathy. The diagnosis is confirmed by a positive Coombs' test, indicating that the transfused cells are coated with the patient's antibodies. Treatment should be immediate discontinuation of the infusion if a transfusion reaction is suspected. A Foley catheter should be placed to monitor urine output, and diuresis and alkalinization of the urine should be initiated to prevent precipitation of hemoglobin in the renal tubules. If anuria develops, fluid intake and potassium should be restricted to avoid renal failure. Dialysis may be needed to treat the intravascular destruction of red blood cells.

Delayed hemolytic transfusion reactions occur between 2 and 10 days after transfusion. The reactions occur because the titers of the patient's antibodies to Rh antigens are low at the time of transfusion and increase after the transfusion. The patient presents with fever, recurrent anemia, jaundice, and low-grade hemoglobinemia and hemoglobinuria. Usually no specific intervention is required other than identification of the antigen to prevent future reactions.

Other complications include febrile or allergic reaction, bacterial sepsis, embolism, superficial thrombophlebitis, volume overload, and disease transmission. Allergic reactions occur in approximately 1% of patients receiving a transfusion and are caused by transfusion of antibodies from a hypersensitive donor or of antigens to which the recipient is hypersensitive. Treatment is usually with antihistamines, although rare anaphylactic reactions occur and require epinephrine. Bacterial sepsis can be caused by contaminated collection bags or poor cleaning of the donor's skin. Gram-negative organisms are the most common cause. Air embolism is a rare complication, because normal adults can typically tolerate a 200 mL embolism of air without a problem. Treatment for air embolism is to place the patient on his or her left side with the head down and feet up. Superficial thrombophlebitis can occur during peripheral vein infusion lasting more than 8 hours. Treatment is discontinuation of the infusion and placement of a warm compress. Volume overload can occur during massive transfusions, particularly in patients with underlying heart disease. This complication manifests with increased central venous pressure, dyspnea, and cough. Treatment is diuresis. A transfusion-related acute lung injury syndrome causes noncardiogenic pulmonary edema. This syndrome often requires intubation and does not respond to diuretics. Transmission of diseases by blood transfusion has been greatly reduced by strict screening of donor blood, but the risk is still present. Cytomegalovirus is the most commonly transmitted virus, followed by hepatitis B and C viruses and human immunodeficiency virus.

32
Shock

Shock is defined as a state of inadequate tissue perfusion. It affects all organ systems, including the kidneys, liver, lungs, brain, and heart. Shock has many causes, but all are associated with a reduction in the effective circulating blood volume. This is the result of loss of intravascular volume (hypovolemic shock), loss of vascular tone (septic or neurogenic shock), or pump failure (cardiogenic shock).

Shock is usually signaled by one or more clinical physiologic markers. Hypotension is a sensitive, but not specific, marker of shock; the absence of hypotension does not rule out shock. Often, the sympathetic response can maintain blood pressure despite being in shock. Tachycardia is often seen as well, but bradycardia may be present, which allows for added time for ventricular filling and coronary perfusion of the myocardium. In most forms of shock, the release of catecholamines and potent vasoconstrictors compensate for what would be profound hypotension. This produces the most sensitive sign of shock, which is pale, cool, and clammy skin. Oliguria, tachypnea, mental status changes, hypoxemia, metabolic acidemia, and myocardial ischemia are also often seen.

Hypovolemic Shock

Hypovolemic shock can be subdivided into hemorrhagic shock, which is due to bleeding, and shock from loss of large volumes of extracellular fluid, which occurs in patients with diarrhea, vomiting, or fistula drainage. There are many compensatory responses to hypovolemic shock. Loss of intravascular volume results in increased vascular tone, elevating peripheral vascular resistance, and redistribution of blood flow among the organ systems. Blood flow to the heart and brain is maintained at the expense of the skin, gut, and kidneys. Cardiac output increases because of increased contractility and venous return, thus maintaining blood pressure. Intersti-

tial fluid leaks back into the capillaries to increase circulating volume, which also decreases blood viscosity. A decrease in the affinity of oxygen for hemoglobin occurs due to increases in 2,3-diphosphoglycerate concentrations and an acidemia that is present from anaerobic metabolism in the tissues. A large release of epinephrine and norepinephrine occurs, which produces vasoconstriction and tachycardia, leading to increased cardiac output and blood pressure. Catecholamines also inhibit insulin release, which then promotes glucose mobilization, protein catabolism, and negative nitrogen balance. Adrenocorticotropic hormone (ACTH) is released that increases cortisol secretion, potentiating the effects of epinephrine and resulting in increased renal sodium and water retention. Antidiuretic hormone is released in response to increased serum osmolarity and hypovolemia, which is the most potent stimulus. It increases water resorption in the kidney and is also a potent splanchnic vasoconstrictor. The rennin–angiotensin system also is stimulated in response to decreased renal perfusion. Renin is released from the juxtaglomerular apparatus and results in increased production of angiotensin I, which is rapidly converted by angiotensin-converting enzyme (ACE) in the lung to angiotensin II, a powerful arterial and arteriolar vasoconstrictor. Also, there is a large release of inflammatory mediators, such as prostaglandins, thromboxane A_2, leukotrienes, and nitric oxide.

The successful resuscitation of patients in hemorrhagic shock depends on two events, restoration of blood volume and therapeutic interventions, to stop hemorrhage. Initially, volume is given in the form of isotonic fluid (either normal saline or lactated Ringer's solution) as a 2 L bolus to adults or a 20 mL/kg bolus to children. Patients who remain hypotensive after this initial bolus will probably require blood transfusion. In an emergency, O-negative blood is given. If the patient is stable, type-specific blood is given. In most cases, solutions containing dextrose or colloids such as albumin should not be given in the acute phase of resuscitation. A metabolic acidosis with an elevated chloride level often ensues after volume resuscitation with crystalloid. After massive blood transfusion, a coagulopathy may develop and should be treated with the appropriate blood products as well as warming the patient and correcting any underlying acidosis.

Septic Shock

Systemic inflammatory response syndrome (SIRS), sepsis, and septic shock are a continuum of human response to infection. Systemic inflammatory response syndrome is defined as a patient with at least two of the following characteristics: temperature >38°C or <36°C, pulse >90, respiratory rate >20, and white blood count >12,000 or <4,000. Systemic inflammatory response syndrome occurs in other conditions that induce systemic inflammation, such as pancreatitis or burns. Sepsis is SIRS plus a clearly established focus of infection. Severe sepsis is sepsis plus signs of organ dysfunction and hypoperfusion, such as hypotension, oliguria, mental status changes, or lactic acidemia. A patient with severe sepsis who is not responsive to resuscitation fluid and requires vasopressor support has septic shock. The most common culprits are Gram-negative bacteria followed by Gram-positive bacteria. The most common sites are the genitourinary system, the respiratory system, gastrointestinal tract, and bloodstream. The early and aggressive use of appropriate antibiotics has a crucial role. Patients with a surgically correctable focus of infection have a more favorable prognosis.

A combination of endogenous and exogenous mediators and host responses to stimuli give rise to the pathophysiology of septic shock. Endotoxin is the bacterial component largely responsible for Gram-negative bacterial sepsis. It induces tumor necrosis factor (TNF)-α production from macrophages. Tumor necrosis factor-α has been implicated in the septic response by increasing the circulating levels of interleukin (IL)-1 and IL-6. Patients with sepsis have also been found to have increased nitric oxide levels and decreased antidiuretic hormone (ADH) levels. The hemodynamic response to sepsis is a hyperdynamic one, with decreased systemic vascular resistance, increased cardiac output, decreased oxygen utilization, tachycardia, and hypotension. Septic patients can also develop a profound capillary leak where a large amount of volume is lost to the interstitial space.

Therapy begins with volume resuscitation followed by the use of vasoactive drugs. Also, broad-spectrum antibiotics should be started until the sepsis-causing organism is known and therapy can be narrowed. If the infectious process requires surgical therapy, an operation should be performed as soon as the patient is stabilized. Invasive hemodynamic monitoring is essential in the management of these patients. Human recombinant activated protein C (Xigris®) has been shown to decrease mortality in patients with sepsis. Steroids and other anti-inflammatory drugs have been shown to be of no benefit in sepsis except for patients who are found to have adrenal insufficiency by the corticotropin stimulation test.

Neurogenic Shock

Neurogenic shock occurs after a disturbance in autonomic innervation of the vasculature by injury to the spinal cord, administration of high spinal anesthesia, or syncope. The loss of arteriolar tone leads to hypotension, and the loss of venular and small venous tone leads to pooling of blood in the venous system followed by hypotension caused by decreased venous return. Patients become hypotensive, relatively bradycardic, and have warm, dry, and sometimes flushed skin. As opposed to patients with other forms of shock, the Trendelenburg position is helpful because it increases venous return to the heart. The next line of therapy is an isotonic fluid bolus followed by vasoconstrictor support, if needed. If the patient is bradycardic, dopamine may be a good choice. If the heart rate is normal or rapid, phenylephrine is probably the drug of choice. If neurogenic shock is caused by an injury, bleeding must be ruled out because the vasopressor can maintain normotension until the patient is extremely hypovolemic.

Cardiogenic Shock

Cardiogenic shock is caused by the heart itself being unable to pump blood to maintain adequate tissue perfusion, with acute myocardial infarction being the most common cause. Other frequent causes are valvular heart disease, cardiomyopathy, and cardiac contusion. Therapy involves minimizing myocardial oxygen demand, optimizing preload, minimizing afterload, correcting arrhythmias, and improving contractility. Often, the first line of treatment is a diuretic, such as furosemide. Morphine, nitroglycerin, nitroprusside, ACE inhibitor, or β-blockers can be used to treat hypertension. Dobutamine or dopamine can be used if the first-line agents fail. If further mechanical support is needed, an intra-aortic balloon pump may be used. It can be inserted at the bedside and will elevate diastolic blood pressure and decrease myocardial work.

33
Abdominal Compartment Syndrome

Abdominal compartment syndrome results from elevated urinary bladder pressures. Normal pressures in the abdomen are between 0 and 10 mm Hg. As the intra-abdominal pressures rise, dysfunction begins in other organ systems, such as the pulmonary, renal, and cardiovascular systems. The syndrome occurs most commonly in patients with severe shock who receive major resuscitation with fluid and blood products. The syndrome often occurs in patients with massive intra-abdominal or pelvic bleeding. Intestinal obstruction resulting in distended bowel, and abdominal distension can cause abdominal compartment syndrome as well. Untreated cases progress to respiratory failure, renal failure, acidosis, and shock. Hallmarks of the syndrome include abdominal distension, oliguria, hypoxia, hypercarbia, and hypotension.

The diagnosis is made through the demonstration of elevated intra-abdominal pressures. This is commonly done by taking readings through a Foley catheter. Clinical signs begin with pressures above 15 mm Hg. Elevated pressures are transmitted to the renal parenchyma, negatively impacting venous return and arterial perfusion. Pulmonary failure results from pressure applied against the diaphragm, limiting its movement and decreasing ventilation. Airway pressures become elevated, which prevents adequate ventilation. Decreased venous return leads to diminished cardiac output and can eventually lead to shock. The need for surgical intervention is based on the degree of pressure elevation and associated symptoms (Table 33.1).

Treatment of abdominal compartment syndrome involves prompt surgical decompression. During the procedure, the abdominal wall is opened by creating a new midline incision or by re-entering the original incision. The abdomen is then closed in a staged fashion, allowing for resolution of bowel edema and secondary organ dysfunction. Temporary closure can be achieved with vacuum dressings, mesh placement, or with use of a Bogota bag (sterilized genitourinary bag). Attempts should be made to have complete fascial closure within 3 to 4 days.

TABLE 33.1. Grades of intervention for abdominal compartment syndrome based on pressure elevation.

Grade	Pressure (mm Hg)	Intervention
I	10–14	Intravenous fluid resuscitation
II	15–24	Decompression if pulmonary, renal, or cardiovascular symptoms occur
III	25–35	Decompression
IV	>35	Surgical exploration

34
Compartment Syndrome

Compartment syndrome is caused by increased pressure within a fascial compartment. The common pathway is tissue edema and ischemia. The most common cause is hemorrhage and edema in the fascial compartment caused by trauma. Venomous toxins from insect and animal bites can also cause extensive soft tissue swelling. Iatrogenic causes include dressings that are too tight, tight fitting casts, and intravenous infiltration. Eschar from burn wounds can become compressive as well. Common sites for compartment syndrome include the forearms and the lower legs because of the well-defined fascial compartments. Swelling from tissue edema causes increased pressure within the compartment. The increased pressure prevents venous capillary flow while arterial blood flow continues, causing a backup of blood flow and higher compartment pressures. Spasmodic reflexes impair arterial flow, and tissue ischemia sets in. Muscle tissue can tolerate only 4 hours of ischemia, after which the muscle dies and contributes to more swelling.

Evaluation for compartment syndrome requires a complete examination, including vascular and neurologic assessments. An early clue to the development of compartment syndrome is pain with passive range of motion of the digits. The diagnosis is made primarily through physical examination. The compartment will often feel tense when palpated. Classic signs include pain, paresthesia, paralysis, poikilothermia, and pulselessness. Muscle is more sensitive to ischemia than nerve tissue; therefore, pain and paralysis manifest sooner than paresthesia. Compartmental pressures can be measured as well. The compartmental pressure is subtracted from the mean arterial pressure. A difference of <40 mm Hg is indicative of compartment syndrome. Pulselessness is a late manifestation. Most patients have intact pulses in the presence of elevated compartment pressures.

Treatment of compartment syndrome involves lessening the external causes of pressure, such as dressings and casts. If the condition fails to improve, fasciotomies must be performed. Fascial decompression of the forearm consists of creating volar and dorsal incisions. The incisions are created longitudinally on the dorsal surface to access the extensor compartment and curvilinear on the volar surface to access the flexor compartment. The volar incision must extend from the proximal portion of the antecubital fossa to the midpalm. The deep intramuscular fascia of the flexor muscle may have to be opened in advanced cases.

Lower leg decompression is achieved by making two incisions as well. The lateral incision is created between the tibial crest and fibula. This decompresses the anterior and lateral compartments. Care should be taken to avoid damage to the superficial peroneal nerve that runs posterior to the lateral compartment. The lateral intramuscular membrane is identified through a transverse incision through the fascia. The medial incision is created 2 cm posterior to the posterior crest of the tibia. This allows decompression of the posterior compartments. Attention must be directed to avoid the saphenous vein and nerve. The septum between the deep and superficial compartments is identified through a small transverse incision. The skin and fascia are then left open. Closure of the wounds can be done at a later date with skin grafting or delayed primary closure.

35
Thermal Injuries

Burns are created by application of cold, hot, or chemical substances to the skin. The depth of tissue injury is directly proportional to the temperature of the substance, the length of application, and the thickness of the tissue. Thermal injuries can result from several etiologies, including scalds, flames, flash burns (e.g., explosions), direct contact, and electricity.

Scalds are the most common type of burn. They result from spills or from immersion into a hot liquid. Scalds caused by immersion generally produce deep burns because of longer contact times with the hot liquid. Substances with higher viscosities (grease, oil, and tar) tend to produce more severe injuries (partial and full thickness burns) because of increased contact times as well. In addition, exposed skin is injured less severely than is skin covered by clothing, because clothing tends to remain hot after exposure and provides longer contact. Flames are the second most common cause of thermal injuries, followed by flash burns from explosions. Most flash burns produce partial thickness injuries unless clothing becomes ignited, causing more severe injuries. Contact burns generally occur from interaction with heated metals, glass, and plastics. They usually involve only a small area of tissue; however, the injuries tend to be deep (fourth degree).

Burn severity is determined by the size and depth of tissue injury. The severity of the burn plays a major role in predicting mortality and complications. Burn size impacts mortality (impacts the physiologic response) most, and burn depth governs the need for surgical resection. A quick estimation of the size of a burn can be made using the rule of nines. The size of a burn is reported as the percentage of total body surface area (TBSA) (Table 35.1).

The depth of the burn is measured in terms of the anatomic layers of the tissue involved and is reported in degrees (first to fourth degrees). Clinical evaluation by an experienced physician is a reliable method for determining the depth of the burn. Accurate assessment of burn depth is important because partial thickness burns heal within 3 weeks when there is no infection. In contrast, full thickness burns require many weeks to heal, leaving them vulnerable to complications such as infection.

First-degree burns are limited to the epidermis. These injuries are typically painful and become erythematous because of vasodilation. The pain and redness resolve over 2 to 3 days followed by sloughing of the injured epithelium (such as peeling of a sunburn). Second-degree burns are divided into superficial partial thickness or deep partial thickness. Unlike first-degree burns, superficial partial thickness burns tend to form blisters. These wounds tend to blanch with direct pressure and have increased sensation. The injury is limited to the upper layers of the dermis. Healing generally takes place within 3 weeks, with minimal incidence of hypertrophic scar formation. Deep partial thickness burns are limited to the reticular layer of the dermis. Characteristics include mottled appearance, blister formation, and decreased sensation. These wounds generally take 3 to 9 weeks to heal, with considerable scar formation.

Third-degree burns extend through all layers of the dermis and are thus known as full thickness burns. Common characteristics include firm, white, red, or black wounds. These wounds lack sensation. The devitalized tissue forms an eschar that eventually separates from the viable tissue below. Fourth-degree burns extend through the skin and into the subcutaneous tissues. These wounds typically have a charred appearance and are often associated with electrocution, immersion, and contact burns.

Immediate care of a burned patient encompasses the use of the basic ABCs. The airway is first evaluated for patency, and patients are given 100% oxygen via a nonrebreather mask. Patients with compromised airways (patients with inhalation injury, edema, and neurologic deficits) should undergo endotracheal intubation. Intravenous access is obtained, and fluid resuscitation is

TABLE 35.1. Demonstration of the size of burns using the rule of nines and TBSA.

Location	% TBSA
Upper extremity	9 each
Lower extremity	18 each
Anterior trunk	18
Posterior trunk	18
Head and neck	9
Perineum	1

started using lactated Ringer's solution (1 L/hr). Clothing and restrictive items are removed before the onset of edema. Small burn wounds can be treated immediately by rinsing in cool (not cold) water to decrease skin temperature and reduce tissue damage.

Major complications of thermal injuries include inhalation injury, carbon monoxide intoxication, infection, compartment syndrome, sepsis, and multisystem organ failure. Inhalation injuries are commonly associated with flame burns and should be suspected in such circumstances. Clues to the presence of inhalation injury include the smell of smoke from the patient's clothing, hoarseness, wheezing on expiration, carbonaceous sputum production, and excessive production of mucus. Serum levels of carboxyhemoglobin should be measured, as well as arterial blood gases. The P:F ratio ($PaO_2 : FiO_2$) can be measured, with a normal ratio being 400 to 500. Ratios of 300 or less are indicative of possible pulmonary compromise. A ratio of 250 or less is an indication for intubation. Bronchoscopy is reserved for cases that are not readily diagnosed by clinical or laboratory evaluation. Fiberoptic bronchoscopy can provide therapeutic value in cases of obstructions or lobar collapse. Supportive therapy is the mainstay of inhalation injury management. Prompt endotracheal intubation is indicated for instances of pharyngeal or laryngeal edema. Patients are left intubated with soft-cuffed endotracheal tubes until the edema subsides. This is evidenced by the ability to breathe around a deflated cuff. Stridor occurs in up to 47% of patients after extubation and may be responsive to nebulized racemic epinephrine and heliox (helium/oxygen mixture). Steroids are avoided.

Compared with oxygen, carbon monoxide (CO) has 200 times the affinity for hemoglobin. Carbon monoxide produced from fires overcomes oxygen and attaches to hemoglobin, forming carboxyhemoglobin (COHb). This disturbs oxygen delivery by preventing oxygen from binding to hemoglobin, shifting the dissociation curve to the left, and binding to cytochrome a_3, impairing intracellular respiration. The severities of symptoms are roughly related to the level of COHb. Patients with less than 10% COHb are usually asymptomatic. Nausea, vomiting, headache, and clumsiness are associated with levels of 20%. Weakness, confusion, and lethargy are caused by COHb levels of 30%. Coma develops at 40%, and death occurs at levels of 60% or greater. The half-life of COHb is inversely proportional to the partial pressure of oxygen. At room air, the half-life of COHb is approximately 4 hours. One hundred percent oxygen decreases the half-life to about 60 minutes. In hyperbaric oxygen at 3 atmospheres, the half-life is reduced to approximately 20 minutes. However, there is no definitive evidence that hyperbaric oxygen therapy offers therapeutic benefit. Carbon monoxide poisoning should be suspected in all persons with a thermal injury that occurred while in an enclosed space. Administration of 100% oxygen through a nonrebreather mask is the standard initial therapy. Carboxyhemoglobin levels should be measured. False elevations cause errors in pulse oximetry readings. Intubation should be avoided when possible. When intubation is needed, patients are given an FiO_2 of 100% along with an increased respiratory rate.

Fluid Resuscitation

Hypovolemia and shock can quickly develop in the setting of thermal injury. Following thermal injury, the total body water volume remains the same, but hypotension occurs as the fluid shifts from one compartment to the next. Extravascular fluid shifts play a major role in the development of hypovolemia. Mechanisms that promote shifts in fluid compartments include increased capillary permeability (secondary to histamine release) and increased intravascular hydrostatic pressure. Changes in cellular transmembrane potentials stem from sodium ion accumulation in the cell. Impaired Na/K-ATPase activity leads to the accumulation of intracellular sodium ions. With no intervention, the alterations in the transmembrane potential eventually lead to cell death. With this in mind, aggressive fluid resuscitation regimens have been designed to decrease mortality following thermal injuries. The timepoint of maximal edema formation is within the first 24 hours following injury. Therefore, aggressive fluid management generally takes place within the first 24 to 48 hours.

Numerous strategies have been developed to approach the initial resuscitative effort, but none has shown a clear benefit over the other. Lactated Ringer's (LR) solution is the most commonly used resuscitative fluid. This is mostly because LR solutions have not been shown to be less efficacious than colloid within the first 24 hours and are less expensive than colloid solutions. It is postulated that widespread increases in vessel permeability render colloid solutions ineffective due to leakage from the vessels. Therefore, the early use of colloid solutions has not been routinely advocated. Similarly, hypertonic saline and dextran solutions have failed to show a benefit in acute resuscitation. A rough estimate of the amount of fluid required for resuscitation can be obtained from the following formula: 4 mL/kg of LR for each 1% TBSA involved in the injury to be given over 24 hours. Half of the total amount of fluid is given within the first 8 hours, followed by the second half over the following 16 hours. Fluid is administered through two large-bore intravenous needles placed in the upper extremities. The lower extremities are avoided because of the risk of septic thrombophlebitis. Urine output provides an excellent measurement of the effectiveness of resuscitation. The urine output is measured closely with a Foley catheter. Adequate urine output for an adult is 30 mL/hr and 1 mL/kg/hr for children. In addition, children require maintenance fluids supplemented with glucose because of lower glycogen and glucose stores.

Wound Care

Initial estimation of the extent of burn injury is completed in order to direct resuscitation. Wounds are dressed loosely in gauze, and the patient is kept warm. The devitalized tissue that results from thermal injury continues to die and form a thickened constrictive area of tissue called an *eschar*. Circumferential eschars can be problematic in the trunk and extremities because of impaired ventilation and blood flow. Circumferential thoracic eschars limit the chest wall movement during respiration, which impairs ventilation. This is shown by increased peak pressures and hypercapnia. Compartment syndrome can manifest within the first 72 hours after injury. Signs and symptoms include decreased arterial pulses, pain with passive range of motion, pallor, and cold extremities. Escharotomy is a procedure in which a relaxing incision is made in the eschar to relieve constriction. Thoracic escharotomies are performed bilaterally by placing incisions along the anterior axillary line. These incisions are extended along the costal margins for circumferential burns such as in the abdomen. Indications for thoracic escharotomy include increased peak pressures and hypercapnia. The manifestation of any of the signs of compartment syndrome is an indication for extremity escharotomy. Incisions are created along the midmedial or lateral aspect of the extremity to avoid transection of any important neurovascular structures. One incision is generally adequate. If a second is needed, it can be placed on the opposing side. Escharotomies can be performed at the bedside without local anesthetic. In addition, incisions can be carried across joints.

Past treatment of burn wounds consisted of multiple washes to debride the wounds, along with dressing them in saline-soaked gauze. Wounds were allowed to heal via secondary intention and granulation tissue formation. Superficial partial thickness burns required an average of 3 weeks to heal, and full thickness injuries required several weeks to heal. Full thickness burns were allowed to spontaneously shed their eschar (2 to 6 weeks) and granulate and then were skin grafted. Infection and poor graft take were common occurrences with these practices. Current techniques employ early excision and grafting of thermal injuries. Eschars are surgically removed within 3 to 7 days (no later than 10 days) immediately followed by wound coverage with skin grafts or flaps. Early excision of eschar has reduced infection rates and overall mortality of the burn patient.

Excisions are performed in one of two basic techniques: fascial or tangential excision. Each technique has advantages and disadvantages. Tangential excisions offer a better cosmetic result but are hindered by increased risk of graft loss and excessive blood loss. Tangential excisions are performed with a scalpel blade or dermatome. Devitalized tissue is removed at an angle tangential to the skin until healthy bleeding tissue is encountered. Fascial incisions provide excellent beds for graft support but can result in poorer cosmesis because of the large amounts of tissue excised. Fascial excisions provide better results for patients with little subcutaneous tissue (e.g., elderly patients). Eschar excisions are indicated in wounds that are projected to require longer than 3 weeks to heal.

Three agents are used for the topical application of burns in order to reduce the risk of infection. These include silver sulfadiazine, mafenide acetate, and silver nitrate (Table 35.2).

TABLE 35.2. Agents used for topical application to burns to reduce risk of infection, their special activities, and their complications.

Agent	Special activities	Complications
Silver nitrate		Hyponatremia Methemoglobinemia
Silver sulfadiazine	Antifungal and antibacterial properties	Neutropenia
Mafenide acetate	Penetrates eschar	Hyperchloremic metabolic acidosis (carbonic anhydrase inhibition) Pain

Hypermetabolism

Thermal injuries create a hypermetabolic state through the increased release of catecholamines. As a consequence, resting energy expenditures are increased as are hyperglycemia, hyperinsulinemia, lipolysis, and proteolysis. Skeletal muscle is broken down at an accelerated rate. In particular, glutamine and alanine are wasted at a greater rate. Thermal injuries require a protein intake of 2 g/kg per day. Enteral nutrition should be started as soon as possible for burn patients with formulas composed of high amounts of carbohydrates and proteins and low fat. The addition of supplemental glutamine, vitamins, and minerals provides added benefits.

36
Cold Injury

Cold injury is classified in a variety of ways, including acute and chronic pernio (chilblains), trench foot (immersion foot), and frostbite. Many of the descriptive terms are derived from military experience.

Pernio, also known as chilblains, occurs in acute and chronic forms and is described as mild injury to the skin and subcutaneous tissues. The classic appearance is red or purple pruritic skin lesions along with edema or blistering. Repeated exposure to cold but not freezing temperatures results in chronic vasculitis. Injuries are generally confined to the anterior tibial surfaces, the face, and the dorsum of the hands and feet. Prolonged exposure causes scarring, ulceration, hemorrhage, fibrosis, and atrophy. Treatment involves removing the patient from the cold environment, elevating the affected body part, and gradually rewarming it to room temperature. Massaging the affected body part should be avoided because it can cause secondary mechanical damage.

Trench foot, also known as immersion foot, is an injury commonly seen in military personnel because of exposure to cold, damp conditions for a prolonged time. Temperatures are typically above freezing, but injury is augmented by the moist environment (i.e., water, mud). The pathophysiology involves alternating vasoconstriction and vasodilation of the extremity. In the beginning, the affected limb is cold and numb. This eventually progresses to hyperemia and intense pain within 24 to 48 hours. The physical characteristics consist of edema, erythema, ecchymosis, and blistering. Injuries can be complicated with infection, lymphangitis, and gangrene. The posthyperemic phase initiates within 2 to 6 weeks and is hallmarked by cyanosis and cold insensitivity. Treatment starts with removal from the hostile environment, elevation of the limb, and exposure to warm, dry air. Again, massage, rapid rewarming, and immersion in warm liquid are not recommended.

Frostbite is the most common type of cold injury affecting the civilian population. It is caused by prolonged exposure to below-freezing temperatures. Exposure to temperatures ranging from −7°C to 7°C for 18 hours or longer is generally sufficient to cause frostbite injury. The pathophysiology of frostbite involves cold injury directly to the tissues and to the vasculature. Patients typically present with pain, pruritus, edema, and limited range of motion. Symptoms progress to numbness and eventually to loss of sensation. The affected area may appear pale, cold, and hard.

Vasoconstriction and arteriovenous shunting with intermittent vasodilation are the initial responses to cold temperatures. This response fades with prolonged exposure to cold temperatures. Cold injury begins at 10°C and becomes irreversible at −5°C. At −2°C extracellular ice crystals begin to form, causing the osmotic movement of fluid into the interstitial spaces and edema. Cells shrivel, become hyperosmolar, and alter enzymatic function. Rapid chilling (>10°C/min) causes intracellular ice crystal formation and cell death.

Vascular damage begins with low-grade vasculitis that proceeds to intimal inflammation, endothelial damage, capillary leak, and extravasation of intravascular fluid into the interstitium, causing edema. Tissue rewarming can induce injury through thrombosis of the microvasculature and release of free radical species. Frostbite injuries are classified according to degree of severity (Table 36.1).

Treatment involves removal from the causative environment, rapid rewarming in warm water (40° to 44°C for 30 to 45 minutes), and elevation to prevent further edema. Analgesics are given because rewarming can cause significant pain. Blisters can be debrided, and antibiotics are given for infection. The injured tissue is dressed in sterile bandages with sterile cotton placed between digits to prevent additional mechanical injury. Adjuncts to therapy include whirlpool baths daily to twice daily, topical aloe vera (inhibits thromboxane), and nonsteroidal anti-inflammatory drugs. Sympathectomy has been used with mixed results to limit vasospasm and to prevent the late complications of chronic pain,

TABLE 36.1. Degrees of frostbite injury classified by severity.

Injury severity	Description
First degree	Hyperemia, edema
Second degree	Hyperemia, edema, blistering
Third degree	Necrosis of skin and subcutaneous tissues
Fourth degree	Full thickness tissue necrosis, gangrene

hyperhidrosis, and cold sensitivity. Tissue damage can initially appear more severe than it actually is. Surgical intervention should be delayed until the devitalized tissue becomes demarcated (this usually requires several days).

37
Electrical Injury

Electrical injury differs substantially from thermal injury in that most electrical injuries are not immediately apparent. Electrical current can enter the body at one point, travel through tissues that offer the least resistance (muscle, nerve, vascular structures), and exit at a grounding point, often the feet. The skin offers a high resistance to electrical current and is usually spared. The internal injury is thermal in nature, resulting from the conductance of current through the affected segment. Low-voltage injuries behave more like thermal injuries, and the effects are local. These are treated with local wound care similar to that for thermal injuries. High-voltage injuries can cause extensive muscle and nerve damage, cardiac arrhythmia, and central and peripheral nervous system injury.

The physical signs of electrical injury include small thermal injury at the entry and exit sites. Cardiac arrhythmia is variably present and should be treated according to Advanced Cardiac Life Support protocols. The heat generated by current conduction can cause extensive myonecrosis with subsequent release of myoglobin. The myoglobin then precipitates in the renal tubules, causing renal failure. Neurologic manifestations include encephalopathy, aphasia, hemiplegia, and peripheral nerve destruction. A unique late complication is the development of cataracts, which can be treated accordingly.

Early, aggressive debridement is needed, with particular attention to deep muscle compartments, which may have sustained substantial damage. Questionably viable tissue can be re-explored in 48 hours. A careful evaluation for compartment syndrome must be undertaken, with early escharotomy or fasciotomy as needed. Alkaline diuresis with mannitol and sodium bicarbonate solution renders the myoglobin pigments more soluble. Urine output should be maintained near 2 mL/kg/hr. Invasive monitoring (central venous pressure [CVP], pulmonary arterial [PA] catheter) may be required to ensure optimal volume status.

The initial evaluation should include electrocardiogram, arrhythmia recognition and treatment, and rhythm monitoring as indicated. Frequent neurologic checks should be made during hospitalization as varying degrees of encephalopathy or peripheral nerve injury manifest. A thorough assessment for associated trauma should be undertaken, because high-voltage injuries (e.g., power-line injuries) are often associated with falls.

38
Sodium

Water exchange between cells is primarily a result of tonicity and osmolarity. Water tends to distribute itself so that tonicity and osmolarity are equal on either side of a cellular membrane. As sodium is the major extracellular cation, the serum sodium is a primary indicator of the relative volumes of the intracellular and extracellular compartments. Sodium fluctuations reflect changes in free water volume as opposed to reflecting true sodium deficit or excess.

Most sodium is reabsorbed in the proximal convoluted tubule of the kidney. Aldosterone causes reabsorption in the distal tubule. Antidiuretic hormone (ADH) affects free water reabsorption in the collecting tubules. Thus, the kidney is primarily responsible for changes in free water and sodium concentration. Changes in sodium are best categorized according to volume status. Euvolemic, hypervolemic, and hypovolemic hypernatremia and hyponatremia have different mechanisms and treatment strategies.

Hypernatremia

Euvolemic

Euvolemic hypernatremia is indicative of free water loss or the loss of hypotonic fluid with isotonic replacement. The most common cause is diabetes insipidus, which is an abnormality in ADH release (low levels in central diabetes insipidus) or activity (decreased renal response in nephrogenic diabetes insipidus). This clinical entity is hallmarked by dilute urine in the presence of plasma hypertonicity. Free water restriction in a normal human results in hypertonic urine production, whereas in diabetes insipidus there is no change, and the urine remains dilute. Central diabetes insipidus requires administration of vasopressin for treatment, whereas nephrogenic diabetes insipidus is resistant to exogenous ADH. The management requires free water replacement over a period

of days to prevent cellular overhydration. Etiologies of central diabetes insipidus include closed head injury, anoxia, and meningitis. Nephrogenic diabetes insipidus can be caused by hypokalemia, aminoglycosides, lithium, and contrast dye.

Hypervolemic

Hypervolemic hypernatremia is uncommon and is usually iatrogenic in nature following aggressive fluid resuscitation with hypertonic fluids (e.g., 3% saline, sodium bicarbonate, excess table salt intake). The treatment is sodium limitation and replacement of urinary losses with hypotonic fluids.

Hypovolemic

Hypovolemic hypernatremia is the most common scenario of hypertonicity encountered in clinical practice. It results from a loss of hypotonic fluid, particularly gastrointestinal. The exception is small bowel and pancreatic secretions, which are isotonic. The most important clinical manifestation is hypovolemic hypoperfusion. Careful attention must be paid to fluid status; fluids should be replaced with isotonic solutions because hypotonic resuscitation can cause cellular overhydration. Hypovolemic hypernatremia can also cause metabolic encephalopathy, which can lead to depressed consciousness, coma, seizures, and death. Volume deficits must be corrected first and quickly to avoid hypoperfusion and shock. A free water deficit is then replaced more slowly (over a period of days) to prevent cerebral edema. A free water deficit can be calculated using kilograms of weight and serum sodium concentration. The formula is as follows:

Free water deficit = $(0.5 \times \text{kg}) \times (1 - 140/\text{serum sodium})$

(0.4 instead of 0.5 for women). Hyperglycemia can cause an aberration in serum sodium levels and is a classic example of hypovolemic hypernatremia. Sodium is corrected by adding 1.5 to 2 mEq/L of sodium to the measured serum sodium for every 100 mg/dL glucose over 100 (normal). Insulin therapy should be withheld until the patient is euvolemic, because insulin aggravates hypovolemia by driving water into cells along with glucose.

Hyponatremia

Hyponatremia is a common occurrence in hospitalized patients, especially in elderly postoperative patients and in patients with AIDS. Hyponatremia is often asymptomatic, but it can manifest with primarily neurologic symptoms (convulsions, coma). Pseudohyponatremia must be ruled out, because plasma protein and triglyceride levels can interfere with measurement of sodium. Sodium concentrations are corrected by the applying the following formulas:

$$\text{Plasma triglyceride} \times 0.002 = \text{mEq/L decrease in Na}$$
$$(\text{Plasma protein} - 8) \times 0.025 = \text{mEq/L decrease in Na}$$

Euvolemic

Euvolemic hyponatremia is caused by a small gain in free water and usually occurs because of inappropriate antidiuretic hormone release or water intoxication. These can be distinguished by measuring urine sodium and osmolarity. Inappropriate antidiuretic hormone release results in increased urine sodium (>20 mEq/L) and high osmolarity (>100 mOsm/kg H_2O), whereas water intoxication has low levels of both (<10 mEq/L and <100 mOsm/kg H_2O).

Hypervolemic

Hypervolemic hyponatremia is common and is a gain of both sodium and water, with the water gain exceeding the sodium gain. The etiology of this disorder can be determined by measuring the urine sodium. Congestive heart failure and hepatic failure cause low urine sodium level (<10 mEq/L), whereas renal failure causes elevated urine sodium level (>20 mEq/L). Diuretics may cloud this picture, because they induce natriuresis.

Hypovolemic

Hypovolemic hyponatremia is a result of loss of sodium and extracellular volume with hypotonic replacement. The distinction to make is between renal and extrarenal losses, which can be made by determination of urine sodium level. Renal loss results in increased urinary sodium level (>20 mEq/L), whereas extrarenal loss results in low urinary sodium level (<10 mEq/L). Renal losses may be caused by diuretic abuse or adrenal insufficiency. Extrarenal losses are usually caused by gastrointestinal losses (diarrhea and vomiting).

Treatment is guided by volume status and by the presence or absence of neurologic symptoms. Symptomatic hyponatremia must be corrected aggressively but cautiously. The goal should be to raise the concentration of serum sodium by no more than 0.5 mEq/L/hr, because higher rates of correction can lead to central pontine myelinolysis. Hypovolemic hyponatremia is corrected with hypertonic saline if symptomatic and with isotonic saline if asymptomatic. Euvolemic and hypervolemic hyponatremia are usually corrected with saline diuresis with or without hypertonic or isotonic saline administration. Calculation of the sodium deficit can be used to guide replacement therapy. The formula is as follows:

Serum sodium deficit =
0.5 × kg weight × (130 − serum sodium concentration)

39
Potassium

Most potassium is intracellular, with only 2% extracellular. Because of this, serum measurement of potassium to determine potassium balance can be quite inaccurate. In addition, the relationship between total body potassium and serum potassium is not directly proportional. It takes large deficits of potassium to be reflected in a change in the serum concentration, whereas potassium excess is reflected with minimal change. This is caused by compensatory mechanisms in individual cells and by the ability of the kidneys to hold on to potassium when necessary.

Hypokalemia

A serum level <3.5 mEq/L indicates hypokalemia. A decrease in serum potassium level can result from a transcellular shift or potassium depletion. The cells have a large store of potassium that can compensate for transient changes in the electrochemical characteristics, the surrounding pH, or immediate metabolic needs of cells. Causes of hypokalemia due to transcellular shifts include β-agonism (albuterol, terbutaline), alkalosis, hypothermia, and insulin response.

Potassium depletion can be either extrarenal or renal. The most common causes of renal potassium losses are diuresis (either spontaneous or medically induced) and hypomagnesemia. Extrarenal depletion is usually caused by gastrointestinal losses from emesis, nasogastric suction, enterocutaneous fistula, biliary drainage, pancreatic fistula, or diarrhea. Diarrhea is the most common cause of colonic secretions, which are high in potassium. The differentiation between renal and extrarenal loss can be determined by a measurement of urinary chloride. Urinary chloride is low (<15 mEq/L) in extrarenal loss (either gastrointestinal or transcellular shift) and high (>25 mEq/L) when caused by diuresis or hypomagnesemia.

Hypokalemia is usually asymptomatic unless it is profound (<2.5 mEq/L) during which mental status changes and asthenia can occur. Hypokalemia alone usually does not cause arrhythmia, but it can cause states that predispose to cardiac rhythm disturbances (digitalis toxicity, hypomagnesemia). Electrocardiographic changes that may be evident include U waves, flattening or inversion of T waves, and QT prolongation; however, these changes are not specific for hypokalemia.

Potassium deficit can be restored by either intravenous or oral potassium administration. The usual infusion is 20 mEq/hr, but higher rates may be used. Potassium administration can be uncomfortable if given peripherally and can cause sclerosis of peripheral veins. The central venous route is preferred, if available, unless high concentrations are used. In this case, split peripheral administration is preferred. It is also important to note that potassium must be administered with care to anuric patients, because impaired renal excretion may lead to life-threatening hyperkalemia.

Hyperkalemia

Although hypokalemia is usually well tolerated, hyperkalemia is not, and it can be a life-threatening emergency. The most important etiologies are transcellular shifts and impaired renal excretions. Two other conditions that also deserve mention are pseudohyperkalemia and hyperkalemia associated with blood component transfusion.

Acidosis leads to a tendency for cells to release potassium and for the kidneys to stop excreting potassium. Not every acidotic condition will lead to hyperkalemia, but it is important to be aware of hyperkalemia compounding the problem of acidosis. Myonecrosis from infection, burns, crush injuries, or vigorous exercise may lead to a transient hyperkalemia that is cleared by normal renal function. Occasionally, these insults result in myoglobin release and damage to renal function, which can impair excretion of potassium and lead to persistent hyperkalemia. β-Blockers and digitalis can also cause hyperkalemia. Digitalis, in particular, can lead to exceedingly high potassium levels (>7 mEq/L), but its use is declining.

Renal insufficiency causes impaired potassium excretion when the glomerular filtration rate is <10 mL/min or urine output is >1,000 mL/day. Exceptions include interstitial nephritis and hyporeninemic hypoaldosteronism (a condition that affects some elderly diabetic patients). Adrenal insufficiency can cause hyperkalemia through direct actions on the kidney effecting an inhibition of excretion, although potassium levels are infrequently life-threatening.

Medications that impair renal excretion are likely the most common causes of hyperkalemia and include nonsteroidal anti-inflammatory drugs, angiotensin-converting enzymes inhibitors, potassium-sparing diuretics, heparin, and pentamadine. These medications (and others) impair the renin–angiotensin–aldosterone system, and, although they infrequently result in life-threatening hyperkalemia, they can promote hyperkalemia, particularly when concomitant potassium replacement is required.

Spurious hyperkalemia is common and can be caused by hemolysis, profound leukocytosis (>50,000 per μL), profound thrombocytosis (>1,000,000 per μL), or muscular release of potassium after tourniquet placement. In a patient with normal renal function, an isolated elevation of potassium may reflect a spurious value and should be confirmed before treatment. Massive blood transfusion may lead to hyperkalemia via several mechanisms. Erythrocytes leak potassium during storage. These transfusions are frequently given to patients with severe hypoperfusion and renal insufficiency (ATN), and the volume of distribution is frequently reduced in patients with severe circulatory compromise. If the renal function is not impaired, the hyperkalemia is frequently transient and cleared by the kidneys.

The most important changes occur in the cardiac conduction system. The earliest cardiac manifestation is peaking of the T waves. As hyperkalemia progresses, there may be P-wave depression, increased PR interval, widening of the QRS complex, sine wave, and eventually asystole.

Treatment of hyperkalemia involves buffering the myocardium, inducing transcellular shifts, and enhancing renal potassium clearance. Treatment is indicated for levels >7 mEq/L or when EKG changes occur. As always, if an underlying etiology is responsible, this must be reversed. Parenteral calcium directly antagonizes the effect of hyperkalemia on the myocardium. Calcium gluconate is indicated as a first-line treatment unless the patient is in shock; in this case, calcium chloride is preferred. Administration of calcium can be repeated once if there is no response. Calcium is contraindicated if hyperkalemia is due to digitalis toxicity. Transcellular shift can be induced by administering glucose and insulin together. The insulin affects cellular potassium channels, allowing for a transient intracellular shift. Sodium bicarbonate is relatively ineffective at treating hyperkalemia and can bind with calcium, negating the effects protective of the myocardium. Excretion of potassium may be enhanced by administering exchange resins (kayexelate) or loop diuretics. These medications can be used for mild hyperkalemia or as an adjunct to the above therapies and require either passage of stool or functional, responsive kidneys to work. Hemodialysis is the treatment of choice for hyperkalemia that is refractory to medical treatment or is associated with renal failure.

40
Magnesium

Magnesium is primarily an intracellular ion with approximately 50% occurring in an active, ionized form. Serum magnesium concentration determination frequently underestimates the presence or magnitude of a total body deficit. The kidney will preserve magnesium in a state of deficiency but normally allows it to be excreted in urine. Deficiency of magnesium is the most common electrolyte abnormality in hospitalized patients. The metabolisms of magnesium and potassium are closely related.

Hypomagnesemia

Hypomagnesemia is a state brought about by predisposing conditions such as diuresis (forced or spontaneous), drug therapy (digitalis, furosemide, adrenergic agents, cisplatin, and cyclophosphamide), malnutrition, chronic alcohol abuse, diarrhea, and myocardial infarction. The mechanisms are similar to potassium deficiency in that increased excretion and transcellular shifts may be responsible.

There are no classically specific manifestations of magnesium deficiency, and the serum concentration may be normal even in the presence of a deficiency. However, associated electrolyte abnormalities are often indicative of magnesium deficiency. Hypokalemia and hypocalcemia, which are refractory to replacement therapy, may be indicative of deficiency and frequently will not correct until the magnesium debt is resolved. Hypophosphatemia is a cause of hypomagnesemia by the enhancement of renal excretion. Hypophosphatemia must be corrected before magnesium replacement is maximally effective.

Magnesium deficiency can lead to cardiac tachyarrhythmias and can potentiate digitalis toxicity. Refractory cardiac arrhythmias occasionally respond to magnesium administration. There are occasional neurologic manifestations of magnesium deficiency. These include seizure, hyperreflexia, and tremors, although these physical findings are too nonspecific to be of any diagnostic value. Reactive central nervous system magnesium deficiency is characterized by ataxia, slurred speech, metabolic acidosis, and progressive obtundation, which can be brought about by loud noises or bodily contact and reversed with magnesium administration.

Urinary magnesium excretion is an accurate indicator of the body's stores of magnesium. In the absence of impaired renal function or renal magnesium wasting, administration of magnesium is followed with urinary magnesium excretion determinations. Recovery of less than 50% of the infused magnesium in urine indicates deficiency. Recovery of more than 80% of the infused magnesium in urine indicates eumagnesemia or excess.

Oral preparations can be used; however, their absorption is erratic, and they can cause diarrhea if taken in large concentrations. Parenteral administration is preferred. Bolus administration (2 to 5 g) of magnesium sulfate is the most common replacement therapy, but continuous infusions can be used (5 g in 500 mL NS over 6 hours). Replacement in patients with impaired renal function should be given at 50% of the usual dosage for patients with normal renal function.

Hypermagnesemia

Hypermagnesemia is most frequently associated with impaired renal function. It can, however, be iatrogenic in patients who are receiving magnesium infusions (e.g., tocolysis). Magnesium is a natural calcium channel blocker, and most of the clinical implications are related to calcium antagonism. Thus, neurologic and/or cardiac manifestations are the most common clinical signs of toxicity. The following levels and side effects are seen: 4 mEq/L, hyporeflexia; >5 mEq/L, prolonged atrioventricular conduction; >10 mEq/L, complete heart block; and >13 mEq/L, cardiac arrest.

Hemodialysis is the treatment of choice for severe hypermagnesemia. Parenteral calcium is used to temporize the cardiac effects. Forced diuresis with fluids and furosemide is helpful if not precluded by renal impairment.

41
Calcium

Calcium is the most abundant electrolyte in the body and is almost entirely extracellular, being found in the bones. In plasma, it is present in three forms: protein bound (usually albumin), ionized (active), and chelated to anions like sulfates and phosphates. The methods of specimen collection can decrease the measurement of calcium. Bubbles of CO_2 can decrease the ionized fraction, whereas anticoagulants such as heparin, citrate, and ethylene diamine tetra-acetic acid bind and chelate calcium.

Hyopcalcemia

The first thing is to verify the hypocalcemia, because serum albumin concentrations can decrease overall calcium but have no effect on the active fraction. This is done by measuring ionized calcium. There are several predisposing conditions that affect calcium metabolism. Magnesium depletion inhibits parathormone release and peripheral activity. Calcium levels typically normalize with magnesium replacement alone. Sepsis causes hypocalcemia by unclear mechanisms and is of unclear clinical relevance. Alkalosis enhances the binding of calcium to albumin. Blood transfusions contain citrate, which acts as a calcium chelating agent. In normal renal function, this agent is metabolized, and the effect is transient. Routine calcium administration with blood transfusions is not indicated unless there is evidence of ionized hypocalcemia. Medications that cause hypocalcemia include aminoglycosides, cimetidine, heparin, and theophylline. Renal failure causes hypocalcemia by phosphate retention (calcium binding) and impaired conversion of vitamin D to its active form. Pancreatitis causes hypocalcemia through several ill-defined mechanisms. Hypocalcemia has been suggested as a prognostic factor in severe pancreatitis.

Symptoms are related to cardiac and neuromuscular changes, as calcium is a factor in the electrochemistry of these tissues. Hyperreflexia, seizures, and tetany can manifest. Chvostek's and Trousseau's signs lack specificity and sensitivity, respectively, as reliable clinical indicators of hypocalcemia. Cardiovascular changes include hypotension, decreased cardiac output, and ventricular ectopy and usually do not manifest unless profound hypocalcemia is present.

Two parenteral forms of calcium are gluconate and chloride. The important difference is that calcium chloride contains three times the calcium of the gluconate compound (272 mg compared with 90 mg in a 10% solution). It takes 200 mg of calcium to raise the serum calcium level 1 mg/dL, but this effect is transient, and continuous infusions should be used. Parenteral calcium has the adverse effect of causing peripheral vasoconstriction and potentiating cell death. It should be reserved for patients with symptomatic hypocalcemia or patients with ionized calcium <0.65 mmol/L. Tums® or Os-Cal® 2 to 4 g/day is used for oral maintenance therapy (tablets contain 500 mg each).

Hypercalcemia

Hypercalcemia is much less common than hypocalcemia. Ninety percent of causes are attributed to hyperparathyroidism or malignancy (paraneoplastic effect, lymphoid malignancy, multiple myeloma, direct invasion from metastasis). Other causes include thyrotoxicosis, medications (lithium, thiazide diuretics), and prolonged immobilization.

The clinical manifestations are usually nonspecific. Gastrointestinal symptoms (nausea, vomiting, constipation, peptic ulcer, ileus, pancreatitis), cardiovascular symptoms (hypovolemia, hypotension, shortened QT interval), renal symptoms (polyuria, nephrocalcinosis), musculoskeletal symptoms (bone demineralization), and neurologic symptoms (confusion, obtundation) have all been described.

Treatment should be instituted when there are associated symptoms or the serum calcium is above 14 mg/dL. The mainstay of treatment is to remove the underlying cause (hyperparathyroidism, drug toxicity) if possible. Other treatments are used to enhance calcium excretion and decrease bone resorption. Hypercalcemia is associated with hypercalciuria, which causes osmotic diuresis and hypovolemia. The goal is to induce a natriuresis and restore and maintain euvolemia. Isotonic saline and furosemide are used to achieve this with the goal of maintaining urine output at 100 to 200 mL/hr. Calcitonin is an osteoclast inhibitor that has rapid onset but is only mildly effective and may lead to tachyphylaxis. Corticosteroids impede growth of lymphoid neoplastic tissue and also enhance vitamin D. Bisphosphonates (pamidronate, zoledronic acid, etidronate) also act as osteoclast inhibitors in a similar fashion to calcitonin; however, they work in a delayed fashion with greater potency. Hemodialysis is effective in removing excess calcium and is usually reserved for patients in renal failure.

42
Phosphorus

The average adult body contains 500 to 800 g of phosphorus, most of which is intracellular, with 85% being in the bony skeleton. Phosphorus participates in numerous vital biochemical reactions, particularly glycolysis.

Hypophosphatemia

The primary cause of hypophosphatemia is transcellular shift, with minor contributions from increased renal excretion and decreased gastrointestinal absorption. Glucose movement into cells is accompanied by phosphorus, which can result in hypophosphatemia, particularly in patients with malnutrition, chronic debilitation, and alcoholism. Respiratory alkalosis stimulates glycolysis, which causes an intracellular shift in both glucose and phosphorus. β-Agonists (albuterol, terbutaline) promote intracellular shifts in phosphorus and potassium. Sepsis causes hypophosphatemia by unclear mechanisms with unclear clinical relevance. Aluminum-containing compounds (Carafate®) cause decreased gastrointestinal absorption of phosphorus by forming insoluble complexes. Diabetic ketoacidosis promotes osmotic diuresis, which promotes urinary loss of phosphorus. The treatment (insulin) promotes intracellular shifts in glucose and phosphorus. Hypophosphatemia is commonly asymptomatic but has adverse effects on aerobic metabolism and oxygen delivery. Cardiac output and contractility are impaired. Erythrocyte structural integrity is impaired, and a hemolytic anemia ensues. The oxyhemoglobin dissociation curve is shifted to the left (higher affinity) as a result of 2,3-diphosphoglycerate depletion. Severe asthenia presents with severe phosphorous depletion. Parenteral phosphorous replacement is recommended for severe depletion or if there is evidence of impaired oxygen delivery, muscle weakness, or respiratory failure. Parenteral phosphorus may be administered with either sodium or potassium as the cation (15 to 30 mmol NaPhos or KPhos). Oral preparations can also be used, but they can be poorly absorbed if sucralfate is being administered, and they can cause diarrhea. The standard daily maintenance dose is 1,200 mg/day.

Hyperphosphatemia

The most common causes of hyperphosphatemia are renal insufficiency and widespread cell death (rhabdomyolysis, tumor lysis). Spurious elevations of phosphorus are seen with diabetes ketoacidosis, but this condition is generally accompanied by phosphate depletion, which becomes evident with insulin therapy. Calciphylaxis is a theoretical concern, but a direct causal relationship has been not been established. Otherwise, hyperphosphatemia is largely asymptomatic. Phosphorous absorption in the gastrointestinal tract can be inhibited with sucralfate. If hypocalcemia is also present, calcium acetate tablets can be used. Hemodialysis is reserved for patients in renal failure and is rarely necessary.

43
Metabolic Acidosis and Metabolic Alkalosis

Metabolic Acidosis

Metabolic acidosis is caused by increased hydrogen ion or bicarbonate loss. Acute compensation occurs via respiratory alkalosis. The greatest increase in minute ventilation occurs because of lactic acidosis, which is one of the most common causes of metabolic acidosis in surgical patients. The initial step in evaluation and treatment of metabolic acidosis is determination of the anion gap (AG), which is performed using the following equation: $AG = [Na] - [Cl - HCO_3]$. The normal anion gap is 8 to 12 mEq/L. Elevation of the AG is caused by methanol, uremia, diabetic ketoacidosis, paraldehyde, isoniazid, lactate accumulation, ethanol, ethylene glycol, and salicylates. Normal gap acidosis is typically caused by gastrointestinal losses, hyperchloremia, and renal tubular acidosis. The base deficit can also be a marker of acid–base status by reflecting the total amount of correction required to restore homeostasis. In the setting of lactic acidosis, it may be used as a marker of the degree of hypoperfusion and in guiding resuscitation measures.

The treatment of acidosis hinges on treating the primary cause. For lactic acidosis caused by hypoperfusion, this involves correcting the source of volume loss and administering crystalloid and/or blood products. For elevated gap acidosis, the treatment is supportive care with or without administration of sodium bicarbonate. The use of bicarbonate in the setting of lactic acidosis caused by hypoperfusion is detrimental in that it blunts the respiratory compensation, leading to cellular acidosis; it increases the affinity of hemoglobin for oxygen (shifting the dissociation curve leftward); and it eliminates the utility of using the base deficit to measure the effectiveness of resuscitation.

Metabolic Alkalosis

Metabolic alkalosis is caused by a loss of hydrogen ions or by the accumulation of bicarbonate. The acute compensation is respiratory acidosis in spontaneously breathing patients. Metabolic alkalosis affects vital biochemical reactions in the body and oxygen delivery by shifting the oxyhemoglobin dissociation curve leftward (increased affinity). Hypokalemia induces an intracellular shift of hydrogen ions, causing intracellular acidosis. This usually reverses with correction of hypokalemia. Volume contraction causes a similar shift at the renal level in an attempt to preserve sodium and water. Gastrointestinal losses (nasogastric suction, vomiting) cause a combination of hydrogen ion loss, volume contraction, and hypokalemia, all of which contribute to metabolic alkalosis. Diuresis, either spontaneous or induced, causes sodium and chloride losses with reabsorption of bicarbonate. Hypochloremic, hypokalemic metabolic alkalosis with paradoxical aciduria is sometimes seen in surgical patients. This is due to loss of gastric secretions with resultant hypovolemia, hypokalemia, and hypochloremia. In an attempt to maintain euvolemia, the kidney preserves sodium and frequently bicarbonate as its anion. Sodium reabsorption occurs at the expense of hydrogen ions, thus acidifying the urine.

The underlying causes must be corrected, particularly hypokalemia and hypovolemia. Patients with metabolic alkalosis are classified as chloride responsive or chloride unresponsive. A determination of urinary chloride predicts which treatment will be the most effective. Low urinary chloride indicates chloride depletion, which should respond to saline, because there is frequently concomitant volume deficit. High urinary chloride typifies chloride-resistant metabolic alkalosis. Treatment options include acetazolamide, ammonium chloride, and hydrochloric acid administration. The latter condition is uncommon, but can be present in hyperadrenalism, either endogenous or exogenous.

44
Acute Renal Failure

Acute renal failure (ARF) is clinically defined as an abrupt decline in glomerular filtration rate within hours to days. Many studies exist that define ARF based purely on changes in serum creatinine level, that is, a doubling of serum creatinine when the baseline creatinine is less than 2 mg/dL or a rise of 1 mg/dL of the serum creatinine when the baseline is greater than 2 mg/dL. Other studies define ARF based on the degree of urine output, degree of metabolic disturbance, or need for renal replacement therapy. Despite the many studies, there is no consensus definition of ARF.

The lack of consensus regarding the definition of ARF makes it difficult to determine the epidemiology of the disease. However, it is estimated that 5% to 25% of all hospitalized patients will develop ARF. The mortality rate for these patients is approximately 45% overall and up to 70% in intensive care unit patients.

The risk factors for developing ARF include underlying chronic kidney disease, age greater than 60 years, diabetes mellitus, coexisting infection, pre-existing chronic diseases, heart failure, coexisting multiorgan failure, and the need for vasoactive medications. Surgical procedures with a high risk of associated renal failure include cardiac surgery, abdominal aortic aneurysm repair, and surgery for obstructive jaundice. Other factors associated with developing ARF include the administration of radiocontrast, use of nonsteroidal anti-inflammatory drugs (NSAIDs), COX-2 inhibitors, acute cyclosporine or FK-506 toxicity, angiotensin-converting enzyme inhibitors, and hypercalcemia.

The treatment of patients with ARF is simplified by classifying ARF as prerenal, intrarenal, or postrenal. Any process that leads to decreased renal perfusion can cause prerenal ARF. The most common prerenal causes are volume depletion, hypotension, heart failure, and liver disease. Intrarenal causes are considered anatomically and include vasculitis, direct vascular injury, stenosis, thrombosis, tubular injury secondary to acute tubular necrosis, drug toxicity, or tubular blockade from uric acid

or myeloma proteins. Postrenal causes are due to obstruction, often caused by a stone or a kinked or occluded Foley catheter. Less often, postrenal obstruction occurs due to injury to the bladder or ureter during the initial operation and may require reoperation.

The high morbidity and mortality rates associated with ARF can be reduced in several ways. Prevention is the best approach. This is most easily accomplished by ensuring adequate hydration. In addition, nephrotoxic drugs such as NSAIDs, aminoglycosides, and amphotericin B should be avoided if possible.

When ARF occurs, simultaneous levels of serum and urine sodium and creatinine should be measured to calculate a fractional excretion of sodium (FENa). This is probably the best method of distinguishing prerenal from renal azotemia. A FENa less than 1% may be normal or indicative of prerenal azotemia. A FENa greater than 1% is indicative of acute tubular necrosis. The urine and plasma levels of sodium and creatinine may also be further compared to determine whether a prerenal state exists. A urine sodium level less than 20 mEq/L or a urine creatinine to plasma creatinine ratio greater than 40:1 indicates prerenal failure. In prerenal failure, a fluid challenge with normal saline may reverse the ARF. Alternatively, 5% dextrose with three ampules of sodium bicarbonate per liter of saline may be used, and it may help avoid the acid load of saline. These solutions are preferable to lactated Ringer's (LR) solution for ARF, because LR contains potassium. If fluid administration does not result in improvement of the oliguria, placement of a central venous pressure or Swan-Ganz catheter is indicated.

When ARF is diagnosed, the treatment must be supportive. The most critical priorities are to reverse hyperkalemia if present and avoid fluid overload. Conservative management of ARF begins with dietary restrictions. Fluid intake is restricted to urine output plus insensible losses, usually 1.5 to 2 L per day. Protein is also restricted to 0.7 to 1.2 g/kg/day to decrease the rise in blood urea nitrogen level. Electrolyte management by restriction of sodium chloride, potassium chloride, phosphorus, magnesium, and aluminum is also critical. Sodium bicarbonate may be used to control acidosis and further prevent protein breakdown when serum bicarbonate levels are less than 20 mg/dL. When the patient fails to respond to fluid and electrolyte management, hemodialysis is warranted. Dialysis can be continued on an intermittent basis until renal function has returned.

Early identification and treatment of ARF is a sound clinical practice and may lessen the associated morbidity and mortality rates for these patients.

45
Head Injury

Initial Evaluation

Both hypoxia and hypotension are detrimental for cerebral oxygenation. Systolic blood pressure <90 mm Hg or hypoxia (arterial oxygen tension <60 mm Hg) is major a predictor of a poor outcome in head injury. Initial care should provide the patient with an adequate airway and ventilation and restore and maintain hemodynamic stability. The ABCs of emergency care (Airway, Breathing, and Circulation) take precedence, regardless of neurologic injuries.

The initial neurologic assessment consists of rating the patient's level of consciousness on the Glasgow Coma Scale (GCS) (Table 45.1) and assessing the width and reactivity of the pupils. Early orotracheal intubation and ventilation are recommended for patients with a GCS score of 8 or lower. Other indications for immediate intubation are loss of protective laryngeal reflexes and ventilatory insufficiency, as manifested by hypoxemia (PaO_2 <60 mm Hg) or hypercarbia (arterial carbon dioxide tension >45 mm Hg). Fluid should be replaced with isotonic solutions such as normal saline, lactated Ringer's solution, or packed red blood cells when appropriate. Glucose-based solutions should be avoided in the acute phase.

Intracranial hypertension should be suspected if there is rapid neurologic deterioration. Clinical evidence of intracranial hypertension, manifested by signs of herniation, includes unilateral or bilateral dilatation of the pupils, asymmetric pupillary reactivity, and motor posturing. Intracranial hypertension should be treated aggressively. Hyperventilation, which does not interfere with volume resuscitation and results in rapid reduction of intracranial pressure (ICP), should be established immediately in cases of pupillary abnormalities. The administration of mannitol is effective, because it not only decreases ICP but also increases cerebral blood flow through modulation of viscosity. Because mannitol is not used to dehydrate the body, all fluid losses through diure-

sis must be replaced immediately or even preventively, especially in patients suffering shock due to blood loss. Arterial hypertension occurring after a severe head injury may reflect intracranial hypertension (Cushing's phenomenon), especially when accompanied by bradycardia. It should not be treated, because it may be the sole mechanism permitting the brain to maintain perfusion despite increasing ICP.

Radiologic evaluation consists of a lateral cervical spine film. After hemodynamic stability is achieved, unenhanced computed tomography of the head should be performed in all patients with persistent impairment of consciousness. In patients with a GCS of 14 or 15 who have experienced transient loss of consciousness or have post-traumatic amnesia, head computed tomography (CT) is probably necessary only when certain specific signs and symptoms are present.

Types of intracranial hemorrhage that are often seen after head injury and that can be detected with CT include contusions and epidural, subdural, subarachnoid, and intraparenchymal hemorrhages. An epidural hematoma characteristically appears as a biconvex hyperdense lesion. Subdural hematomas appear as convex–concave lesions on CT. In many cases, subdural hemorrhage is accompanied by subarachnoid hemorrhage, indicating severe injury. Acute subdural hematomas are hyperdense with respect to the adjacent brain, subacute hematomas are hyperdense to isodense, and chronic hematomas are hypodense. Intraparenchymal lesions appear as an area of increased density on CT scans.

The hematomas are usually associated with extensive lobar contusions. The amount of blood in a lesion determines whether the lesion is classified as a hematoma or a contusion. When blood accounts for at least two-thirds of the lesion, the lesion is classified as an intracerebral hematoma. Contusions, appearing as small hyperdense lesions on CT, usually have a characteristic distribution affecting the frontal poles, the orbital gyri, the cortex

TABLE 45.1. Glasgow Coma Scale.

Test	Response	Score
Eye opening (E)	Spontaneous	4
	To verbal command	3
	To pain	2
	None	1
Best motor response (arm) (M)	Obedience to verbal command	6
	Localization of painful stimulus	5
	Flexion withdrawal response to pain	4
		3
	Abnormal flexion response to pain (decorticate rigidity)	2
	Extension response to pain (decerebrate rigidity)	1
	None	
Best verbal response (V)	Oriented conversation	5
	Disoriented conversation	4
	Inappropriate words	3
	Incomprehensible sounds	2
	None	1
Total (E + M + V)		**3–15**

above and below the sylvian fissures, the temporal poles, and the lateral and inferior aspects of the temporal lobes. Over time, substantial swelling can accompany these lesions, appearing as hypodense areas around the contusion. Diffuse axonal injury appears as punctate hemorrhages and indicates severe head injury. Midline shift and compression of the subarachnoid space are parameters indicating the extent of mass expansion or cerebral swelling.

ICU Management

A GCS score of 8 or less after resuscitation is an indication for admission to a neurosurgical ICU. The focus of ICU management is prevention of secondary injury and maintenance of adequate cerebral oxygenation. To ensure optimal cerebral oxygenation, cerebral perfusion pressure (CPP), hemoglobin concentration, and oxygen saturation should be optimized.

Monitoring of ICP allows calculation of CPP (CPP = mean BP − ICP), an important clinical indicator of cerebral blood flow (CBF). Intracranial pressure monitoring is indicated for patients with a GCS score of 3 to 7 after resuscitation and for selected patients with a GCS score of 8 to 12 and an abnormal CT scan at the time of admission. For patients with a GCS score of 8 to 9 and a normal CT scan, ICP monitoring is indicated if the patient is older than 40 years, has a systolic BP below 90 mm Hg, and exhibits unilateral or bilateral motor posturing.

A CPP of 70 to 80 mm Hg may be the clinical threshold below which mortality and morbidity increase. Cerebral perfusion pressure therapy involves manipulation of both arterial BP and ICP, but its objective is the reduction of ICP. If ICP reduction does not achieve a CPP of 60 mm Hg, arterial hypertension is instituted. Mean arterial BP should be raised first by optimizing volume status. Ample fluids, including albumin (25 to 30 mL/hr), are administered to maintain central venous pressure at 5 to 10 mm Hg. A pulmonary arterial catheter is suggested for patients older than 50 years and for individuals with known cardiac disease, multiple injuries, or a need for vasopressors or high-dose barbiturates. Pulmonary arterial wedge pressure should be maintained between 10 and 14 mm Hg. If necessary, an α-adrenergic drug (e.g., phenylephrine, 80 mg in 250 or 500 mL of normal saline) can be combined with the fluids. As a general rule, ICP values between 20 and 25 mm Hg indicate that therapy should be initiated. The recommended regimen for treatment of ICP starts with drainage of cerebrospinal fluid (CSF) through a ventriculostomy–ICP catheter and continues as necessary in a stepwise fashion with sedation, paralysis, osmotic therapy, hyperventilation, induction of a metabolic coma, and decompressive surgery. Although drainage of CSF has no documented deleterious side effects, it has the potential to aggravate brain shift. Therefore, only a minimal amount should be drained, sufficient to bring the ICP below 20 mm Hg.

Sedation with morphine sulfate, 2 to 5 mg/hr intravenously, is standard treatment. Fentanyl, lorazepam, and midazolam are commonly used alternatives. In some medical centers, propofol is now used for routine sedation. Propofol has a short half-life, which is advantageous for the purposes of neurologic evaluation, but it is expensive and can have deleterious side effects after prolonged use (i.e., >48 to 72 hours). Muscular paralysis is employed by many clinicians as the next step in therapy. Its major downside is that it renders neurologic examination pointless except for assessment of the pupillary response. In addition, the risk of respiratory complications is increased with neuromuscular blockade.

Mannitol is usually administered in IV boluses of 0.25 to 1 g/kg over 10 to 15 minutes until either ICP is controlled or serum osmolarity reaches 320 mOsm/L. It now appears, however, that higher doses (e.g., 1.4 g/kg) may be more effective. Because volume depletion is an important side effect of mannitol therapy, urine losses should be replaced. Hypertonic saline (3% to 10%) may be used in place of mannitol. It appears to be equally or even more effective than mannitol for ICP control, especially in higher concentrations (e.g., 7.5%). In addition, hypertonic saline is not associated with volume depletion and actually increases intravascular volume.

Hyperventilation reduces ICP (by vasoconstriction) and CBF, which may be at ischemic levels in certain parts of the brain. Therefore, hyperventilation (PaCO$_2$ <30 mm Hg) should not be instituted prophylactically but should be reserved for acute decompensation and employed as a short-term temporizing measure until more definitive therapy can be instituted.

The hematocrit and viscosity are directly related, and a balance must be established to optimize oxygenation. If the hematocrit is too high, viscosity increases; if the hematocrit is too low, the oxygen-carrying capacity of blood decreases. Maintaining the hematocrit between 0.30 and 0.35 is recommended. Below 0.30, oxygen-carrying capacity falls without a significant change in viscosity; above 0.35, viscosity increases out of proportion to oxygen-carrying capacity.

Barbiturates appear to protect the brain and to lower ICP through several mechanisms, including alteration of vascular tone, suppression of metabolism, and inhibition of free radical lipid peroxidation. The most important effect may involve coupling of CBF to regional metabolic demands so that the lower the metabolic requirements, the lower the CBF and the related cerebral blood volume (CBV), with subsequent beneficial effects on ICP and global cerebral perfusion. Barbiturate therapy (usually pentobarbital to a blood level of 4 mg/L) is instituted when other measures to control ICP fail.

Propofol is a sedative hypnotic with a rapid onset and a short duration of action. ICP decreases with administration of propofol, but systemic BP usually decreases as well, resulting in a net decrease in CPP. Blood lactate levels do not increase when propofol is administered, indicating that cerebral oxygenation is adequate. If propofol is used, correction of hypovolemia is recommended to prevent hypotension associated with bolus injection. Finally, because of its preservative-free, lipid-base vehicle, there is an increased risk of bacterial or fungal infection, and the high caloric content (1 kcal/mL) may be problematic during a prolonged infusion.

Hypothermia produces a balanced reduction in energy production and use. Protocols for hypothermia include cooling to 32° to 33°C (89.6° to 91.4°F) within 6 hours of injury and maintenance of this temperature for 24 to 48 hours. Hypothermia to 33°C has been shown to be effective for the control of refractory high ICP. The main side effects of hypothermia are cardiac arrhythmias and coagulation disorders, reported after cooling to 32° to 33°C. Other drawbacks of hypothermia include the difficulty of detecting infection because of the lack of warning signs (e.g., spiking and elevated temperature) and the need for specialized equipment (e.g., rotor beds with cooling control) and personnel to induce and maintain the condition. A body temperature between 35° and 35.5°C may be optimal for treating patients with severe traumatic brain injury.

Brain Death

The term *brain death* implies irreversible cessation of activity in the cerebrum and brain stem. Brain death is often a consequence of severe head injury. A qualified physician should determine the occurrence of brain death. The physician should have a clear understanding of the conditions that can mimic brain death, the procedure for the apnea test, indications for confirmatory tests, and the management of physiologic changes associated with brain death. In addition, early identification of potential donor candidates is important.

The clinical diagnosis of brain death requires the following: (1) the presence of a cause that is compatible with brain death, (2) the absence of complicating medical conditions that may confound clinical assessment, (3) the absence of drug intoxication or poisoning, and (4) a core temperature of at least 32°C.

For most patients, a CT scan will document an abnormality that is compatible with brain death. For patients with normal CT scans, the diagnosis should be reconsidered unless there is a relative certainty about the mechanism that has led to brain death (e.g., ischemic-anoxic brain death caused by cardiac arrest or asphyxia). Severe electrolyte, acid–base, and endocrine disturbances should be excluded, and a drug screen test may detect a specific drug or poison.

The core temperature should be at least 32°C, because brainstem reflexes are absent below 27°C. If these conditions are met, clinical testing should follow. The three cardinal features of brain death are (1) coma or unresponsiveness, (2) absence of brainstem reflexes, and (3) apnea.

Coma or unresponsiveness is evaluated by assessing the motor response to painful stimuli, such as either supraorbital pressure or nailbed pressure; this response should be absent. In a brain-dead patient, the pupils are typically in the middle position (4 to 6 mm) and fixed, although pupils can be dilated as well. Many drugs affect pupil size, but the light reflex usually remains intact. Topical ocular instillation of drugs, trauma to the cornea or to the bulbus oculi, pre-existing anatomic abnormalities, and previous surgical procedures should all be considered in the evaluation of the pupils and the pupillary response. The oculocephalic and caloric responses are then tested; these too should be absent. Finally, the corneal, pharyngeal, and tracheal reflexes are tested, all of which should be absent.

If all brainstem reflexes are absent, the apnea test is performed. To minimize confounding factors, such as marked hypotension, severe cardiac dysrhythmias, and desaturations, the following precautions are taken:

1. Core temperature must be 36°C or higher (rewarm the patient if temperature is lower).

2. Systolic BP must be 90 mm Hg or higher (use dopamine if BP is lower).
3. Fluid balance must be positive for 6 hours or more (use vasopressin if this cannot be accomplished).
4. Arterial PCO_2 must be 40 mm Hg or higher (decrease minute ventilation if PCO_2 is lower.
5. Arterial PO_2 must be 200 mm Hg or higher (inspired oxygen fraction = 1.0 for 10 minutes).

Brain death is essentially a clinical diagnosis; testing may be repeated after 6 hours to establish the final diagnosis. In most cases, this clinical diagnosis is sufficient; however, in cases in which the specific components of clinical testing cannot be evaluated reliably (e.g., as a result of drug intoxication, altered metabolic status, shock, or hypothermia), confirmatory tests may be indicated. Accepted tests include electroencephalogram, cerebral angiogram, single-photon emission CT, and, more recently, transcranial Doppler ultrasonogram. Angiography is the most reliable and rapid method to establish brain death. The tests are particularly important when organ and tissue donation are under consideration.

46
Spinal Disc Lesions

The intervertebral disc consists of two parts. The circumferential anulus fibrosus, making up one portion, is composed of dense, fibrous tissue. The central nucleus pulposus consists of fibrocartilage, which has little tensile strength but substantial elasticity. The fibrocartilage can fragment acutely or degenerate gradually. It heals poorly because of limited blood supply. The anulus heals well and is buttressed by heavy anterior and posterior longitudinal ligaments. Intervertebral disc disease occurs at any level from C1 to S1. The lower segments of the cervical and lumbar areas are affected most often. Thoracic disc disease is rare.

Dorsal and ventral nerve roots emerge from the spinal cord separately and pass to their respective intervertebral foramina, where they exit from the spinal canal. The roots join to form a spinal nerve within the neural foramen. In the cervical spine, the roots exit above the corresponding vertebrae; for instance, the C5 root exits above the C5 pedicle. Because there are eight cervical roots, C7 exits above the C7 pedicle, and C8 exits below it. Consequently, all roots below C8 exit below the pedicle of their corresponding vertebra.

Lumbar and sacral roots form the cauda equina below the conus medullaris. The sacral roots are more centrally located adjacent to the filum terminale. Because a lumbar root (e.g., L4) passes laterally toward the neural foramen as it descends in the spinal canal, it crosses the adjacent intervertebral disc (e.g., L4–L5) at its extreme lateral edge, hugging the pedicle of the L4 vertebra laterally. The nerve root that descends to the next lowest foramen (e.g., L5) passes across the disc space (e.g., L4–L5) more medially, making that root more vulnerable to disease involving that disc.

If the nucleus of an intervertebral disc extrudes (herniates) through the anulus, adjacent neural structures can be compressed. In the cervical and thoracic spine, compression of the spinal cord may result in paraparesis or quadriparesis, depending on the spinal segment involved. At all levels, compression of a spinal root can cause weakness and sensory loss in structures innervated by that root. The severity of the clinical syndrome depends on the site and severity of compression by the displaced disc fragment.

Often the nucleus does not extrude, but simply fragments in response to the forces exerted on the spinal column. This is intensified by the concomitant dehydration and loss of elasticity of the disc as it ages. The disc space gradually narrows, the joint becomes loose, and the cartilaginous endplates of the adjacent vertebral bodies abut and wear more quickly. Bony spurs (osteophytes) develop at the joint in reaction to the increased mobility and decreased elasticity. Formation of osteophytes around the joints of vertebrae, termed *spondylosis*, is a common disorder that represents the normal process of aging. If an osteophyte forms in a neural foramen, the nerve root passing through may be chronically irritated and compressed. If the osteophyte develops within the cervical or lumbar canal, the cord or cauda equina may be compromised.

The onset of symptoms and signs of an extruded disc fragment may be acute or chronic. Acute symptoms may or may not be related to trauma. In disc disease of the cervical spine, neck and radicular discomfort occur simultaneously. Spinal cord symptoms are rare. There is usually limitation of neck motion, with loss of normal cervical lordosis. Nerve root compression produces radiculopathy, often characterized by pain and hypoesthesia in the distribution of the involved root. Associated loss of deep tendon reflex with or without weakness can be seen on examination. Cervical cord compression causes myelopathy characterized by progressive spastic quadriparesis or paraparesis, mild to moderate sensory changes in the lower extremities and trunk with cervical dermatomal sensory loss, weak upper extremities, hyperreflexia, and extensor plantar response.

Cervical disc disease must be differentiated from other ailments. These include inflammatory disease of the soft tissues and joints of the arm and shoulder, nerve entrap-

TABLE 46.1. Clinical signs of common lumbar disc herniations

Disc	Nerve root	Pain	Sensory change	Motor deficits	Reflex loss
L3–4	L4	Anterior thigh, anterior leg, and medial ankle	Anterior leg	Quadriceps	Knee jerk
L4–5	L5	Posterior hip and posterolateral thigh and leg	Medial dorsum of foot	Foot and toe extension	None
L5–S1	S1	Hip, buttock, and posterior thigh and leg	Lateral foot and ankle	Plantar flexion	Ankle jerk

ment syndromes, and neoplasms. The pain also must be distinguished from that which accompanies cardiac disease.

Plain radiographs typically demonstrate loss of the lordotic curve of the cervical spine, with narrowing of one or more disc spaces. Osteophyte formation may be seen. In cervical spondylosis, there is usually radiologic evidence of osteophytes and disc space narrowing at multiple levels. In most cases, the anteroposterior diameter of the cervical spinal canal is narrowed. Myelography with computed tomography (CT) is very useful in the diagnostic workup of nerve root compression. The use of intrathecal contrast medium enhances the power of CT to delineate the lesion. Magnetic resonance imaging (MRI) is suitable for investigating myelopathies. In addition to defining the compressive lesion, MRI often shows intrinsic cord abnormalities related to compression. Electromyography may confirm the diagnosis and localize the lesion more specifically, particularly when myelographic defects are multiple.

Painful cervical disc disease can be treated medically as long as there is no evidence of a progressive neurologic deficit (motor loss and bowel and bladder dysfunction being most important). Adequate medical therapy includes immobilization of the neck with a soft or hard cervical collar, analgesics, muscle relaxants, and local heat. These methods, in association with a good physical therapy program, provide relief in most circumstances. Up to 75% of patients with cervical disc disease improve following an adequate trial (10 to 14 days) of medical therapy. Some have recurrence of radicular symptoms on return to full activity. In many cases, these patients can be treated for years with intermittent cervical traction and a cervical collar, but some require surgical therapy. For the 25% who do not respond to conservative means, operation is often helpful.

Herniated lumbar discs often produce some degree of nerve root compression. The severity of the syndrome depends on the degree of root compression. Occasionally, the entire cauda equina is involved, resulting in loss of motor and sensory function, including bowel and bladder sphincter control. Sometimes a disc rupture occurs in the midline, compressing centrally positioned sacral roots preferentially, without involvement of laterally placed lumbar roots.

In the lumbar spine, >90% of clinical problems arise from the L4–L5 and L5–S1 intervertebral discs. Pain is usually chronic, but its onset can be acute when associated with frank herniation. There can be back pain, leg pain, or both. Radiation of low back pain into the buttock, posterior thigh, and calf is usually the same with disease at the L4–L5 and L5–S1 levels. This radiating pain may be exacerbated by coughing, sneezing, or straining. Bending and sitting accentuate the discomfort, while lying down characteristically relieves it. Pain is often described as aching but frequently has a sharp or shooting element and is limited to one lower extremity.

Palpation usually reveals tenderness over the sciatic notch, the popliteal fossa, or both. Paravertebral muscles may undergo spasm. With true nerve root compression, straight-leg raising produces leg pain that is accentuated by dorsiflexion of the foot. Ipsilateral leg pain produced by contralateral straight-leg raising usually indicates lumbar disc herniation. Sensory loss, weakness, and loss of tendon jerks may occur in a variety of combinations and to variable degrees (Table 46.1).

Myelography can be diagnostic in symptomatic lumbar disc disease, but CT alone can delineate the lesion in most cases. Magnetic resonance imaging has replaced myelography and CT at some medical centers in the identification of lumbar radiculopathy. Electromyography may confirm the diagnosis, especially when physical examination is unable to localize the involved nerve root.

Initially medical treatment is indicated for all patients who do not have neurologic deterioration. Bed rest, local heat, analgesics, and skeletal muscle relaxants are usually effective within a few days. Physical therapy and limited exercise often help when the acute episode passes. A back brace partially immobilizes the patient and can minimize muscle spasm. With aggressive conservative treatment, most patients improve sufficiently to return to full activity. Recurrent symptoms may be treated in a similar fashion, often successfully. Surgical treatment is reserved for the patient with an acute or progressive neurologic deficit, chronic disabling pain, or both. The acute onset of weakness or sphincter disturbance constitutes an emergency, demanding prompt diagnosis and early operation. Operation usually entails a unilateral laminotomy with removal of the offending disc fragment.

47
Spinal Cord Injury

Spinal cord injury remains one of the most devastating of all traumatic injuries. Each year, more than 10,000 new spinal cord injuries occur in the United States. Motor vehicle crashes are the most common mechanism for producing spinal cord injuries, followed in descending order by gun shot wounds, falls, and recreational sporting activities. Most of the injured are young males between the ages of 16 and 35 years. The average cost of care for these injuries and their impact on society are staggering.

Injury to the spinal cord most often follows compression or severe angulation of the vertebral spine. These injuries occur due to subluxation of bony elements of the vertebral spine with or without rotation of adjacent vertebral bodies that compress the cord between dislocated bones. In rare instances, severe hypotension will lead to cord infarction, or axial distraction will result in stretch injury to the cord.

Soon after spinal cord injury, there is a temporary loss of function. The initial trauma then initiates a cascade of downstream injury mechanisms, including accumulation of excitatory amino acids, neurotransmitters, vasoactive eicosanoids, oxygen free radicals, byproducts of lipid peroxidation, and activation of programmed cell death pathways. Loss of the blood–cord barrier causes edema and increased pressure that limit the blood supply. Additionally, ongoing hemorrhage can further limit the blood supply to the cord. The resultant ischemia causes more cell damage. The distribution of cord edema, hemorrhage, infarction, and direct injury to the cord dictate the neurologic signs and symptoms present at the time of evaluation.

Evaluation and initial treatment should be started at the scene of injury. The essential priority in the initial care of patients with potential spinal cord injury is to maintain strict immobilization of the entire spine with rigid cervical collars and backboards. Further evaluation of the spine should begin only after the patient is hemodynamically stable and life-threatening injuries have been ruled out. Complaints of neck or back pain make a neurologic injury more likely; however, only 5% of patients with these complaints have a relevant spine injury. Thorough but quick sensory and motor examinations are critical. Sensory examination should evaluate dermatomes, light touch, pinprick, temperature, and perianal sensations. Motor examination should grade the deltoid, triceps, biceps, wrist flexors and extensors, finger abductors and adductors, and grip strength in the upper extremity. In the lower extremity, motor evaluation should test the iliopsoas, quadriceps, hamstrings, hip abductors and adductors, tibialis anterior, extensor hallucis longus, and gastrocnemius–soleus complex. In documentation the terms "moves all extremities" and "feels everything" should be avoided. The physical examination is particularly important because it provides a temporal sequence for potentially evolving neurologic injuries.

Alert, cooperative patients who do not have pain, have normal physical and neurologic examinations, and are not impaired by mind-altering substances are at very low risk for cervical spine injury. A standard trauma radiograph series (anteroposterior, lateral, and oblique) of the cervical spine is sufficient for these patients. Radiographic evaluation of patients with potential neurologic injury includes anteroposterior, lateral, and open-mouth odontoid views of the cervical spine. It is imperative that the C7–T1 junction is adequately visualized on the lateral projection, because injuries at this level are fairly common. A "swimmer's view" may be necessary to adequately visualize this level. A computed tomographic (CT) scan of the C-spine is necessary if the C7–T1 level remains poorly visualized despite a swimmer's view. If radiographic images show no abnormality and the patient still complains of pain or has neurologic symptoms, there may be ligamentous injury. In this case, lateral flexion–extension views may be indicated to evaluate for dynamic instability. In uncooperative or obtunded patients and in patients with persistent symptoms despite normal plain films and CT, a magnetic resonance image (MRI) may be needed. In addition, thoracic and lumbar films may be warranted if the patient suffered a significant mechanism of injury or is symptomatic.

Spinal cord injuries may be classified as complete or partial. In complete injuries, there is permanent quadriplegia or paraplegia, depending on the level of injury. These patients have complete loss of motor function and sensation two or more levels below the bony injury. As a general rule, complete cord lesions are fixed and permanent, with little hope for major recovery of distal function. However, these patients may improve one or, rarely, two motor levels. Recovery of even a single level has an enormous impact on functional outcome. This is especially true in high cervical lesions above C3–C5, where lesions may cause diaphragmatic paralysis and respiratory failure. Additionally, patients with high spinal cord disruption are at greater risk for spinal shock due to physiologic disruption of ascending and descending cerebral impulses. This is manifest by flaccid paralysis with absent deep tendon reflexes. Spinal shock usually lasts 24 to 48 hours and resolves with return of the distal reflex arc (bulbocavernosus reflex). Complete spinal cord injuries can also involve the autonomic system, with disruption of the sympathetic outflow (T1–L2). This entity leads to unopposed vagal tone and hypotension with bradycardia and is called *neurogenic shock*. Other symptoms of neurogenic shock include gastrointestinal dysmotility, bowel and bladder dysfunction, and problems with temperature regulation.

In incomplete spinal cord injuries, the patient exhibits some sensory and motor function below the level of injury. Incomplete injuries have a much better prognosis, and most improve with time. Partial spinal cord injuries include the central cord syndrome, anterior cord syndrome, Brown-Sequard syndrome, cervical cord neurapraxia, and spinal cord injury without radiographic abnormality.

Central cord syndrome is the most common of the incomplete injuries. Patients with this syndrome have motor weakness and sensory loss primarily involving the distal muscles of the upper extremity. Central cord syndrome is thought to be an ischemic lesion, in which hyperflexion or hyperextension of the neck leads to interference with blood flow in the spinal arteries. Typically, this lesion affects older patients with degenerative spine disease and cervical spondylosis. It is usually caused by hyperextension injury during which the ligamentum flavum is thought to buckle, resulting in increased pressure on the central cord as it is compressed anteriorly. The characteristic pattern of injury occurs because the most central portions of the spinal cord contain fibers from the upper extremities.

Anterior cord syndrome is caused by direct or indirect injury to the anterior spinal cord. Direct injury may result due to a crush injury or to compression from a hematoma. Indirect injury may be caused by ischemia

due to compression of the anterior spinal artery. The syndrome is produced by damage to the spinothalamic tracts and corticospinal tracts located in the anterior portion of the cord. The injury is characterized by loss of motor, pain, light touch, and temperature sensations. The posterior columns are preserved, and the patient retains fine touch, vibratory, pressure, and proprioception sensations distal to the injury.

The Brown-Sequard syndrome is a rare spinal cord injury that results in hemisection of the spinal cord. It is usually caused by penetrating trauma. The syndrome is characterized by ipsilateral loss of motor function, vibration, and proprioception below the level of the lesion with contralateral loss of pain and temperature sensation beginning approximately two levels below the lesion. The characteristic pattern of injury is anatomically interesting but uncommon in clinical practice. The prognosis for patients with this syndrome is dismal.

Cervical cord neurapraxia, also called *transient quadriparesis*, is a rare cervical spine injury that is often considered a concussion of the cervical spinal cord. It is thought to be caused by axial loading of the neck in flexion or extension. This injury occurs most commonly in football players. The affected patient experiences sudden, post-traumatic onset of bilateral sensory, motor, or combined neurologic deficits. Sensory findings include burning, numbness, or tingling. Motor findings include weakness or complete paralysis. By definition, these symptoms are transient and resolve within 48 hours.

Spinal cord injury without radiographic abnormality (SCIWORA) was defined in 1982 as an objective sign of myelopathy as a result of trauma in the absence of findings on plain radiographs or CT of the spine. However, with the use of MRI, most cases previously described as SCIWORA actually have demonstrable injury. With the increased use and availability of MRI, SCIWORA may be more appropriately considered spinal cord injury with normal anatomic alignment and no plain-film irregularities. The usual mechanism of injury is acceleration–deceleration or rotation. Transient neurologic symptoms may be the only indication that the cervical spine has been injured. The injury is also more common in children. Current suggestions are to perform MRI for patients suspected of having spinal cord injury despite normal plain films and CT. Several studies have suggested that MRI for this group of patients may be useful in excluding compressive lesions of nerve roots, excluding ligamentous disruption that might warrant surgery, and guiding treatment regarding external immobilization. However, more work is needed to further evaluate the sensitivity and specificity of MRI in identifying this small subset of patients.

Acute therapy for spinal cord injury is dictated by the following principles. First, the injury must be recognized. Second, care must be exercised to prevent further injury. Third, the patient must be maintained in optimal condition to allow the greatest possible nervous system repair and recovery. Fourth, rehabilitation must be actively pursued to maximize the function of the surviving nervous tissue.

Resuscitation of the spinal cord-injured patient parallels that of anyone suffering a major trauma, with the modification that spine alignment must be maintained. In addition, current recommendations by the National Acute Spinal Cord Injury Study 2 and the National Acute Spinal Cord Injury Study 3 are for all adult patients with acute nonpenetrating spinal cord injury to receive steroids. Patients should be given 30 mg/kg of methylprednisolone intravenously within 8 hours and preferably within 3 hours after injury. This should be followed by a continuous infusion of 5.4 mg/kg/hr. Patients treated within the first 3 hours after injury receive the continuous infusion for 24 hours. Patients treated between 3 and 8 hours after injury should receive a 48 hour infusion instead.

Maintenance of adequate blood pressure and ventilation are critical. Patients with cervical cord lesions maintain ventilation only with diaphragmatic activity; if paralytic ileus with abdominal distension occurs or if the patient tires, initial adequate ventilation may deteriorate, requiring the need for mechanical ventilation. Loss of spinal sympathetic pathways can cause hypotension. Low doses of pressors may be used to maintain adequate blood pressure, but these should be used only after the sources of hemorrhage have been ruled out. Surgical intervention is dictated by the degree of deformity and perceived stability of the injury. The goal of surgery in spinal cord injury is to restore spinal canal anatomy, remove foreign bodies, or relieve compression by bone, disc, or hematoma with hopes of limiting further injury. For patients with complete injury, the benefits of early spinal stabilization are related to the prevention of complications of long-term immobilization.

48
Peripheral Nerve Injuries

Each mixed sensory and motor nerve contains 5 to 10 fascicles. Along the course of the nerve, fascicles combine, divide, and rotate within the nerve. Based on this intraneural fascicular anatomy, it is impossible to achieve perfect nerve repair with exact matching between fascicles in the proximal and distal stumps. The axons in peripheral nerves are myelinated to variable degrees. They are maintained by the nerve cell bodies and by the Schwann cells along their course. With nerve injury, the potential for axonal regeneration depends on survival of the neuron. The neuron contains the protein synthesis machinery. Therefore, survival of the neuron is still possible even with the loss of a large amount of cytoplasm that occurs with severance of the axon. With disruption of the axon, there is shifting of the protein synthesis process in the cell body. This results in a decrease in synthesis of proteins required for neurotransmission and in an increase in synthesis of proteins used for axonal growth.

Seddon defined three categories of nerve injuries. Neurapraxia is a physiologic loss of axonal conduction without disruption of anatomic continuity of the nerve. Neurapraxia results from acute nerve compression leading to loss of myelin between nodes of Ranvier (segmental demyelination). As a result, there is blocking of action potential propagation. There is selective deficit of nerve functions with complete motor paralysis, little muscle atrophy, and considerable preservation of sensory and autonomic functions. Recovery of function is rapid and does not depend on nerve regeneration. Surgical repair is not required, and recovery is usually complete. In axonotmesis, the axons are disrupted, but the Schwann cell sheath and the nerve anatomic integrity remain intact. Axonotmesis results in complete motor, sensory, and autonomic deficits. Recovery takes place by axonal regeneration, which proceeds at a rate of 1 mm per day. Surgical repair is not required, and recovery has excellent outcome.

Neurotmesis is an actual disruption of the nerve continuity. Nerve recovery is not possible without surgical repair. Without surgical repair, axonal sprouting begins 10 to 20 days after the injury. Scarring at the site of injury may block axonal entrance into the distal stump. This may lead to coiling of the regenerating axons to form a painful neuroma. On the other hand, if the nerve has been surgically repaired, axonal regeneration proceeds at the rate of 1 mm per day. However, in neurotmesis, functional recovery is always imperfect.

Nerve regeneration depends on several factors. The younger the patient, the faster and more complete the recovery. The type of nerve involved is also important. A pure motor or sensory nerve recovers better than a nerve containing both motor and sensory fibers. Thus, the radial and musculocutaneous nerves, which are primarily motor nerves, recover better than the mixed medial nerves, and the tibial division of the sciatic nerve fares better than the peroneal division. A third factor is the level of nerve injury and the duration of denervation. If regenerating axons take more than 12 months to reach denervated muscle, a significant degree of muscle atrophy will have occurred, and the muscle may remain dysfunctional despite reinnervation. Therefore, the main concern regarding motor dysfunction with peripheral nerve injuries is the risk of muscle atrophy. Muscle atrophy results from disuse and the lack of neurotrophic supply. Muscle cells are completely replaced with connective tissue if reinnervation does not occur in 2 to 3 years.

Nerve injury is the principal factor that accounts for limb loss and permanent disability. Because the upper extremities have more neurologic structures than do the lower extremities, upper extremity injuries are twice as likely to result in nerve damage as are lower extremity injuries. Penetrating injuries from cuts or stab wounds that result in a clean laceration of a nerve are amenable to early intervention and repair. Blunt injuries and penetrating injuries from gunshot wounds are more difficult to assess and treat.

Whenever an extremity is injured, careful assessment of motor and sensory functions is essential. If other life-threatening cranial or truncal injuries are present, evaluation and treatment of nerve injuries may be deferred until these more urgent problems are dealt with. Before any orthopedic manipulation or treatment of vascular injury, an examination must be conducted to assess the integrity of the nerves. A careful neurologic examination is the most important aspect of evaluating peripheral nerve injuries. Clinical examination includes assessment of both sensory and motor functions. It is important to evaluate sensory loss in the autonomous cutaneous zone of the injured nerve. The autonomous zones are defined as areas that are exclusively innervated by a particular nerve without supply from collateral sprouting of adjacent nerves. Therefore, anesthesia in an autonomous zone indicates a complete lesion of that particular nerve. On the other hand, with incomplete nerve lesion, sensation is retained in the autonomous zone.

The autonomous zone for the median nerve is the digital pads of the thumb and index finger and the dorsum of the terminal phalanx of the index finger. The equivalent loss in motor function is the absence of voluntary contraction of the abductor pollicis brevis muscle. This will result in loss of elevation and rotation of the thumb into a grasp position. The radial nerve does not have an autonomous skin zone. However, complete nerve lesion commonly results in loss of sensation on the radiodorsal aspect of the forearm and the dorsum of thumb. There is loss of finger extension at the metacarpophalangeal joints, loss of thumb extension, and wrist drop (loss of wrist extension). The autonomous zone for the ulnar nerve is the distal phalanx of the little finger. There is loss of abduction and adduction of all fingers. Claw hand deformity of the hand results from hyperextension of the metacarpophalangeal joints and flexion of the interphalangeal joints. In the lower extremities, common peroneal nerve injury results in sensory loss over the web space between the great and second toes.

There is loss of eversion and dorsiflexion of the foot (foot drop). The entire sole of the foot is the autonomous skin zone for the tibial nerve.

Pain may also be a consequence of nerve injury. The most important pain syndrome associated with nerve injury is causalgia. Causalgia is a severe burning pain that follows nerve injury and is seen in approximately 2% of incomplete nerve transactions. It is associated with autonomic changes, including smooth glossy skin, tapered digits, and thickened nails. It is postulated that causalgia results from excessive activity in the sympathetic axons that are transmitted to the somatic sensory axons through synapselike connections in the proximal stump neuroma.

For lacerating nerve injuries, surgical exploration is often indicated. Generally, if the wound is clean or minimally contaminated, nerve repair can be considered after the more immediate problems are corrected. If the nerve ends appear to have been sharply divided and there is minimal hemorrhage or contusion, immediate repair is appropriate. If, however, the injury is dirty, or there is significant soft tissue damage, nerve repair should be delayed. In these cases, the wound is cleaned and thoroughly debrided. The divided nerve ends are identified and fixed in proximity to prevent retraction. After the wound has healed, re-exploration is indicated for definitive repair about 3 to 4 weeks after the injury. Closed nerve injuries (i.e., without laceration) are often explored if they do not improve within 6 weeks of injury, whether loss of function is complete or incomplete. Scar tissue at the site of the lesion may prevent axonal regrowth. Neurolysis releases the regenerating nerve fibers from the impinging scar and may improve functional recovery. Prompt institution of physical therapy is also indicated for improvement of muscle function and maintenance of joint motion. It is the best means of minimizing the complications of denervation.

49
Skeletal Injuries

The initial evaluation of skeletal injuries should be directed toward the circulation. Vascular injuries associated with skeletal trauma most commonly present with ischemia rather than bleeding. Certain skeletal injuries are considered high-risk lesions for associated vascular trauma. These include posterior knee dislocation and supracondylar humeral fractures. Popliteal artery injuries occur in up to 40% of cases of posterior knee dislocations. They carry a very high risk of amputation. The popliteal artery is particularly vulnerable because of its restricted mobility in the popliteal fossa. Despite the abundant collateral circulation around the knee joint, popliteal artery injuries have a high risk of distal ischemia due to the fragility of these collateral vessels that make them easily disrupted by the blunt force of trauma.

Distal pulses in the extremities should be carefully examined. If they are present, major vascular injury is unlikely. Injured extremities should be compared with their uninjured counterparts, because pulse assessment may be difficult in the setting of shock caused by systemic injuries. Disparity in peripheral pulses may indicate the presence of vascular injury. If pulses are absent and a joint dislocation or fracture dislocation is present, then gentle reduction of the dislocation should be performed promptly. A pulseless extremity with a dislocation often regains pulses once the fracture or dislocation is reduced. The circulatory examination should be followed by a quick neurologic examination aimed at assessing motor and sensory functions in the hands and feet. Appropriate x-rays should be obtained to include the joints above and below the area of injury. All open wounds in the extremity that are associated with a fracture are by definition open fractures and usually must be explored surgically, ideally within 6 hours of wounding to ensure the removal of contamination. Traumatic penetration of a joint must also be addressed with prompt irrigation of the joint.

Temporary splinting is required when definitive treatment of extensive soft tissue injuries or fractures will be delayed. Stabilization makes the patient more comfortable and facilitates transportation. Immobilization of long bone fractures also helps prevent further soft tissue damage and decreases wound complications.

Open Fractures

Open fractures are classified as type I, II, or III, depending on the associated soft tissue injury. A puncture wound or communication less than 1 cm is a type I open fracture. Type II fractures have a wound larger than 1 cm with moderate associated soft tissue damage. Type III open fractures involve severe soft tissue injury or loss. All open fractures require emergency surgical treatment. Ideally, treatment should begin within 6 hours of injury, because the incidence of infection is directly related to delay in initiating treatment. The most important factors in reducing infection are antibiotic therapy, timely and aggressive surgical debridement, fracture stabilization, and proper treatment of wounds. Tetanus prophylaxis should be given as needed.

For all open fractures, irrigation and debridement in the sterile, controlled environment of the operating room are required. Foreign material should be removed, and all devitalized or contused soft tissue should be aggressively debrided back to clean, bleeding tissue. The fracture ends should be delivered into the wound, inspected, and adequately irrigated. Any devitalized loose bone fragments that are not crucial to reduction or stabilization should be removed. Wound cultures are obtained. The antibiotic regimen is continued for 24 to 48 hours. At this point, if the postdebridement cultures are positive, the drug regimen is modified to cover the infecting organism. If the cultures are negative and the wound appears clean, the antibiotic regimen can be stopped. A patient who has a type III fracture or a type I or II fracture with a positive culture should undergo repeated irrigation and debridement every 48 hours until the wound appears clean.

Femoral Shaft Fracture

Fractures of the femoral shaft are associated with significant blood loss. Because of the shape of the thigh, more than 1 L may be lost into this space with little or no external indication. Therefore, the trauma surgeon must anticipate the blood loss from the fractured femur. The advent of intramedullary nailing has revolutionized the treatment of femoral shaft fractures. With stable femoral shaft fractures that undergo nailing, full weight bearing without crutches is possible within a few days of the operation.

Reapproximation of the fracture fragments with nailing also dramatically reduces bleeding into the thigh. Nailing also lowers the incidence of respiratory distress syndrome, blood loss, and tissue trauma and reduces the patient's need for narcotics. In a multiply injured patient with a fractured femur, nailing should be done immediately to help control hemorrhage to the fracture site and help stabilize the patient hemodynamically. This policy has been shown to result in significant reduction of pulmonary complications and ICU length of stay for those patients.

Compartment Syndrome

One of the most serious complications of extremity trauma or ischemic injury is compartment syndrome. The cardinal signs of pain, pallor, pulselessness, and paresthesias are present to variable degrees. Pain with passive stretch of muscles is one of the more reliable indicators of compartment syndrome, and accurate diagnosis is readily made by measurement of intracompartmental pressures. Pressures in the range of 30 to 40 mm Hg constitute an indication for fasciotomy. For patients with prolonged ischemia due to arterial compromise, prophylactic fasciotomies of all compartments distal to the vascular injury should be done with re-establishment of perfusion. The fasciotomy incisions can be treated with dressing changes and secondary split-thickness skin grafting or with gradual reapproximation of the wound edges using wire sutures or tape strips sequentially tightened daily.

Fat Embolism

Patients with multiple fractures are at high risk for subsequent fat embolism, in which fat droplets from bone marrow enter the systemic circulation and impair pulmonary capillary perfusion. The final common pathway of fat embolism and other injuries that result in pulmonary parenchymal dysfunction after trauma is severe hypoxemia or the acute respiratory distress syndrome (ARDS). Fat embolism generally occurs within 24 to 72 hours of injury and presents with hypoxemia, tachycardia, tachypnea, fever, restlessness, and confusion. The syndrome is fatal in 10% to 15% of patients. Chest radiographic findings are similar to those of other causes of ARDS, with bilateral patchy infiltrates. Petechiae may be present transiently in the axilla, chest, and conjunctiva, and thrombocytopenia may occur. Fat droplets are occasionally seen in blood specimens and in the urine. Fat embolism syndrome is seen most often following femoral fracture.

Treatment of fat embolism syndrome is similar to treatment of ARDS, with administration of oxygen, ventilatory support, and positive end-expiratory pressure. Moderate-dose corticosteroids given prophylactically may reduce the incidence of fat embolism. The other important factor in the management of the multiple-trauma patient that decreases the incidence and severity of fat embolism and ARDS is stabilization of the fractures within the first 24 hours of injury.

50
Pelvic Fractures

Pelvic fractures are a major cause of mortality and morbidity in trauma patients. Hemodynamically unstable patients with pelvic fractures present a real challenge to trauma surgeons. Pelvic fractures can be particularly lethal when they occur in combination with severe injuries to other major organs. The high force required to disrupt the pelvic ring in young patients often results in additional musculoskeletal injuries in up to 80% of patients. Mortality rates for the patient with high-energy pelvic fractures are approximately 15% to 25%. Mortality results from uncontrolled retroperitoneal hemorrhage and other associated injuries. Mortality rate increases nearly 13-fold when the patient also has hypotension. When combined with either a head or an abdominal injury that requires surgical intervention, the mortality rate increases to 50%.

Pelvic ring disruption is classified into two major groups, stable and unstable. A stable pelvis is defined as one that can withstand normal physiologic forces without displacement. This stability depends on the integrity of bony and ligamentous structures. Early recognition of unstable pelvic ring disruptions is essential because they are more likely to be associated with fatal hemorrhage. In addition, these injuries require stabilization to restore the pelvic ring anatomy. Determination of the stability of the injured hemipelvis must be established through a combination of physical examination and review of the anteroposterior radiograph. An anterior defect can occasionally be detected by palpation at the symphysis pubis. Instability can be appreciated by manually compressing and distracting the pelvis through the anterior iliac spines. Vertical instability may also be appreciated when movement of the hemipelvis is detected as manual compression and traction are applied through an extended, uninjured lower extremity. The screening anteroposterior radiograph is then examined. In 90% of cases, this is sufficient to assess stability and guide initial treatment.

Young and Burgess classified pelvic fractures based on the mechanism of injury and correlated this with specific pelvic ring injury patterns. In turn, these patterns are used to predict associated injuries and the propensity of bleeding. Anteroposterior compression (APC) injuries are associated with widening of the symphysis and disruption of the sacroiliac joint (SI) or sacral fractures. They are graded from I to III based on the degree of ring disruption. Anteroposterior compression III injuries are associated with significant bleeding and high blood transfusion requirements. Anteroposterior compression injuries are more likely than other pelvic injury patterns to be associated with thoracic aortic, abdominal, and genitourinary injuries. Lateral compression mechanism involves pubic rami fractures and posterior sacral impaction fractures. These fractures are less likely to bleed, but they may be associated with bladder lacerations. The vertical shear (VS) injury occurs with falling. These injuries involve rami fractures with sacroiliac joint disruption. They are often associated with lumbosacral plexus nerve injury.

The usual cause of hemorrhage in pelvic fractures is from the posterior pelvic venous plexus and bleeding cancellous bone surfaces. Rarely, it can be caused by bleeding from a named artery. Bleeding from a larger artery is even less frequent. Initial treatment should focus on the control of venous bleeding. Reduction and stabilization of the displaced pelvic ring help achieve this. Reduction leads to a decrease in pelvic volume and tamponade of the bleeding vessels through compression of the viscera and pelvic hematoma. Because reduction and stabilization alone usually control venous bleeding, patients who do not respond to these maneuvers are more likely to have arterial bleeding.

Reduction and stabilization of the pelvis can be achieved by a variety of mechanical means. When field personnel detect unstable pelvic ring disruptions on physical examination, they begin treatment by binding the pelvis with a rolled sheet or applying pneumatic anti-shock garments (PASGs). Like the air splints applied to the extremities, the garment functions by compressing the pelvis. However, it blocks access to the patient and restricts excursion of the diaphragm, and there have been reports of gluteal and thigh compartment syndromes developing after its extended use in hypotensive patients. If applied in the field, PASGs should not be deflated until the patient is actively being resuscitated in the trauma room. The standard method for controlling pelvic hemorrhage has been the application of an anterior external fixation frame. Proper application of an anterior pelvic external fixator should provide stability to the pelvis and hematoma while allowing access to the abdomen for surgical procedures. Although this device can be applied in the emergency department, it is frequently deferred until the patient is brought to the operating suite. In these circumstances, the pelvis can remain displaced for many hours with venous bleeding continuing uncontrolled.

If an external fixator cannot be applied expeditiously, another method of provisional stabilization must be employed. Recently, devices called *pelvic C-clamps* have been developed that can be rapidly applied to reduce and provisionally stabilize the pelvis in the emergency department. The design allows for compression of the pelvis through percutaneously inserted pins applied to the outer surface of the ilium. They provide adequate stabilization and easy access to the abdomen or extremities without removal of the device. They can remain in place throughout the resuscitation phase and can be replaced by definitive stabilization methods when the patient is able to undergo these procedures.

The role of angiography in the diagnosis and management of pelvic hemorrhage is controversial. Large series have demonstrated the incidence of arterial hemorrhage amenable to embolization to be approximately 10%. In these cases, arteriography with embolization can be life saving. However, catheterization and embolization of vessels in the pelvis are technically difficult and time consuming. The use of these techniques should be reserved for cases when all other methods of control of hemorrhage have been exhausted. Angiography is therefore indicated for patients with pelvic fractures who continue to have hemodynamic instability after aggressive resuscitation and after other sources of major bleeding, including the chest and the abdominal cavity, have been either excluded or dealt with.

Associated Injuries

Proper management of the hypotensive patient with a pelvic fracture should begin with a search for the cause of the shock. All possible causes of bleeding are explored. Auscultation of the chest and review of the chest radiograph determine the presence of hemothorax and the need for thoracostomy. Once the hemothorax is ruled out as a cause of shock or is controlled by chest tubes, a diagnostic peritoneal lavage or ultrasound of the abdomen is performed. Wounds around the pelvis and in the perineum and bleeding from the rectum, vagina, or urethral meatus are noted. Digital vaginal and rectal examinations to identify tears and fracture fragments are performed.

Proper management of perineal and rectal injuries is crucial to the prevention of infection in pelvic or retroperitoneal hematomas. Evaluation of the rectum in patients with pelvic fractures should include digital rectal examination to determine rectal tone, rectal wall integrity, and position of the prostate. Sigmoidoscopy is indicated if rectal injury is suspected. All perineal tears should be explored and debrided in the operating room. The wound should not be closed primarily because of the need for repeated surgical debridement followed by delayed closure with closed drainage and broad-spectrum antibiotic coverage. Because of the high mortality rate associated with delayed colostomy, immediate complete fecal diversion is mandatory if rectal injury is suspected. Even if no rectal injury is identified, all patients with deep perineal lacerations can be assumed to have rectal injury and should be considered for diverting colostomy.

Diagnostic peritoneal lavage (DPL) has a 12% to 47% false-positive rate in cases of pelvic fractures. However, false-negative DPL is extremely rare. Therefore, negative DPL results are easier to interpret. The high rate of false-positive DPL is attributed to entry of red cells into the peritoneal cavity from the retroperitoneal hematoma via diapedesis or actual rents in the posterior peritoneum. Technical errors involving direct placement of the trocar into the hematoma may also lead to a false-positive DPL. The open supraumbilical technique may eliminate this error. The high false-positive rate of DPL has lead to the recommendation that DPL be considered positive only if gross blood is aspirated on peritoneal tap. Ultrasound examination of the abdomen in the trauma patient is widely used as a tool to determine hemoperitoneum. A computed tomography (CT) scan can determine the nature of intra-abdominal injuries and also evaluate the pelvic ring injury. Therefore, a CT scan should be obtained from all patients with pelvic fractures. This can be performed in the early phase if the patient is hemodynamically stable or later after aggressive resuscitative efforts.

Bladder injuries associated with pelvic fractures should be investigated with cystography. This is performed with 200 cc of contrast to provide adequate bladder distension. Urethral injuries should be suspected if any of the following are present: blood at the urethral meatus, high-riding prostate identified on rectal examination, perineal hematoma, or inability to void. In all pelvic fractures associated with diastasis of the pubic symphysis, urethral injuries must be suspected. In these cases, a retrograde urethrogram must be obtained prior to attempting bladder catheterization.

Overall Management Protocol

Hemodynamically unstable patients with pelvic fractures are endotracheally intubated in the emergency department, and large-bore venous access is secured. Central venous pressure monitoring is initiated along with aggressive crystalloid resuscitation. Ultrasound examination (FAST) of the abdomen is performed to detect hemoperitoneum. Diagnostic peritoneal tap (DPT) is also a valid alternative. An anteroposterior chest radiograph is obtained to exclude intrathoracic injuries. Clinical examination and anteroposterior pelvic radiograph will confirm the presence of unstable pelvic fracture. The pelvic volume is closed by securing sheets tightly around the pelvis and taping the knees and ankles together. Transfusion of packed red cells and fresh-frozen plasma is initiated in a 1:1 ratio, and for every 5 units of packed cells, 5 units of platelets are administered.

In the presence of significant hemoperitoneum (frank blood on DPT or unequivocal positive FAST), the patient should undergo laparotomy. During exploration, associated abdominal injuries are treated, and the pelvis is packed with laparotomy pads. If hemodynamic stability is achieved at this point, the orthopedic surgeon should determine the need for mechanical pelvic fixation. However, if the patient is still unstable, damage control laparotomy is performed. The abdominal packs are left in place, and skin is closed with running nylon suture. The patient is transferred to the angiography suite along with continuing resuscitative efforts. Pelvic angiography is performed with therapeutic embolization if possible. Subsequently, pelvic fixation can be considered, or the patient is directly transferred to the ICU.

If the FAST examination or the DPT is negative for hemoperitoneum, the patient is still hemodynamically unstable, or requires continued blood transfusion, angiography should be performed. After angiography, the patient is either considered for pelvic fixation or transferred to the ICU.

51
The Hand

The hand is supplied by the radial and ulnar arteries. The radial and ulnar arteries divide in the proximal part of the wrist into superficial and deep branches. The corresponding branches then unite to form the superficial and deep palmar arches. The superficial palmar arch is dominated by the ulnar artery. It supplies the digital arteries of the second, third, and fourth web spaces. The ulnar digital artery of the small finger also arises from the superficial palmar arch. The deep palmar arch is dominated by the radial artery. It gives rise to the arteries of the thumb and radial border of the index finger. The radial and ulnar arteries can be assessed for patency by the Allen test, during which they are occluded by the examiner and the patient is asked to open and close the hand a few times. Pressure on one of the arteries is then released, and perfusion is assessed. Capillary refill should occur throughout the entire hand within 5 seconds. The test is then repeated for the other artery.

The median, ulnar, and radial nerves are the principal nerves of the hand. The median and ulnar nerves supply the long flexors of the wrist and fingers in the forearm, and the radial nerve supplies all the extensors. Within the hand proper, the radial nerve is purely sensory and supplies the dorsal aspect of the first web space and the proximal two thirds of the radial three and a half digits. The median nerve supplies motor fibers to the thenar muscles and the first two lumbricals. It also carries sensory fibers from the entire volar aspect and the distal thirds of the dorsal aspects of the radial three and a half digits. The ulnar nerve supplies motor fibers to the hypothenar muscles, all the interossei, the third and fourth lumbricals, the adductor pollicis, and the deep belly of the flexor pollicis brevis. It also carries all the sensory fibers from the ulnar one and a half digits and ulnar border of the hand.

Nerves are assessed for both sensory and motor functions. Sensibility is assessed separately on both the ulnar and radial halves of the pulp by the two-point discrimination test. A bent paper clip can be used to perform this test, and the minimum distance between the two points of the clip that the patient can distinguish as separate is recorded. A two-point sensibility greater than 8 mm suggests nerve injury. Knowledge of the sensory distribution of the various nerves of the hand helps localize the lesion. Regeneration of sensory nerves can be clinically assessed by eliciting Tinel's sign. The injured nerve is percussed along its course from distal to proximal. At the site of regeneration, the patient feels paresthesia along the distal distribution of the nerve. Because nerves regenerate at the rate of 1 mm a day (or about an inch a month), the site at which Tinel's sign is elicited also progresses distally. Such a distal progression of Tinel's sign is taken as clinical evidence of nerve regeneration.

Injury to individual peripheral nerves of the arm results in predictable and defined deficits. A patient with loss of the radial nerve is unable to extend the fingers or wrist, and a wrist drop is noticeable. The sensory loss to the dorsum of the hand is well tolerated. Median nerve dysfunction causes problems with opposition of the thumb and grip of the fingers. Sensory loss is to the radial four digits and can significantly impair use of the hand. An ulnar neuropathy causes dysfunction of the intrinsic muscles of the hand, clawing of the ulnar two digits, and weakness in gripping a key. Sensation is lost along the ulnar side of the hand.

Complete disruption of the nerve is treated by early surgical exploration and repair. An incomplete lesion or questionable disruption of nerve integrity is best treated with close observation, splinting to prevent contractures, and surgical exploration if no recovery occurs. Segmental loss of nerves requires nerve grafts, usually taken from a minor sensory nerve, such as the sural nerve, to bridge the gap. The results of primary repair are better than the results of grafts, and repairs done soon after injury are better than delayed repairs.

Scaphoid Fracture

The scaphoid is the most common carpal fracture and accounts for nearly 60% of all carpal injuries. The patient may present with a diffuse pain over the radial side of the wrist. Examination reveals tenderness over the anatomic snuff box. If a scaphoid fracture is suspected, initial radiographic examination must include posteroanterior, lateral, and a special scaphoid view. Quite often, immediate postinjury radiographs do not reveal a fracture. Computed tomography (CT) may help in such situations, or an empirical splint can be applied and radiographs can be repeated after 2 weeks. Blood vessels enter the scaphoid mainly through its distal half, and fractures through the "waist" can deprive the proximal half of its blood supply, leading to avascular necrosis in as many as 30% of patients. Treatment of nondisplaced fractures is with a long-arm cast, including the base of the thumb. This is called a *thumb spica* and is maintained for 6 weeks, followed by a short-arm cast for an additional 6 weeks. Displaced fractures require open reduction with screw fixation. Nonunion is a notorious problem in the scaphoid and occurs in one third of patients. These can be treated with cancellous bone grafts or pedicled vascularized bone grafts. Electrical stimulation has been shown to be effective in tackling this problem.

Compartment Syndrome

In acute compartment syndrome, increased fluid pressure in the tissues contained in a fascial space increases to a level that reduces capillary blood flow below that necessary for continued tissue viability. When untreated, continued pressure elevation produces irreversible muscle and nerve damage because of ischemia, with secondary necrosis, fibrosis, contractures, and sensibility deficits or chronic pain. Acute compartment syndrome is due to an increase in the volume of fluid within a compartment or limitations on the dimensions of an anatomic compartment. Post-traumatic edema, hemorrhage, hematoma, swelling from infection, and burns increase compartment fluid. Other causes include venous obstruction, strenuous exercise, and constrictive dressings or casts.

Acute compartment syndrome is diagnosed clinically but can be confirmed by measurement of intracompartmental tissue pressure. Clinical observations include a swollen, tense, and tender compartment with pain disproportionate to that expected from the originating injury, peripheral sensibility deficits, and, finally, motor weakness or paralysis. Pain is accentuated by passive stretch of the affected muscle. Peripheral pulses usually remain intact because systolic arterial pressure usually is greater than the dangerously elevated intracompartmental pressure. Although blood flow through the major arteries is not impeded, capillary perfusion is compromised by the elevated pressure (30 to 60 mm Hg) within the compartment. Pressure measurement devices are confirmatory but not infallible, and in treatment decisions clinical concerns should outweigh specific pressure measurements. Threshold pressure measurements of 30 mm Hg or more are consistent with compartment syndrome, and surgical decompression should be prompt. Because tissue perfusion is affected by systemic blood pressure, a lower threshold pressure for fasciotomy should be used in hypotensive patients. Treatment includes removing all occlusive dressings, wraps, layers, and splints and splitting tight casts and cast padding down to the skin. If symptoms are not rapidly relieved, fasciotomy of the affected areas is required. After surgical decompression, the wounds are left open but dressed to prevent desiccation. Skin closure by direct means or with skin grafting is delayed for at least 48 to 96 hours but can be performed after 5 to 10 days as swelling permits.

Volkmann's ischemic contracture develops as a result of myofascial contractures in response to prolonged ischemia. The most common cause for this is an unattended compartment syndrome of the forearm or hand. The involved muscles become necrotic and are replaced by fibrous tissue, which produces contractures that are refractory to passive stretch. The digits are characteristically flexed, and passive extension of the wrist worsens the flexion deformity. This is termed *Volkmann's sign*. If the contracture is mild, passive stretching exercises and serial splinting may solve the problem. If it is severe, the contracture can be released by "Z" lengthening of tendons or by a muscle slide operation.

Carpal Tunnel Syndrome

The carpal tunnel is a tight osseofibrous tunnel at the wrist traversed by the median nerve and all nine long digital flexor tendons. Its floor is formed by the carpal bones and its roof by the flexor retinaculum. Rise in pressure causes progressive conduction blocks in the nerve with subsequent sensory and motor dysfunctions. Pain and paresthesia are the earliest symptoms and characteristically occur more at night or after prolonged activity. Flexor synovitis is the most common cause of carpal tunnel syndrome, but it may also follow traumatic derangement of the carpal alignment. Sensory evaluation may reveal a widened, two-point discrimination and a positive Tinel's sign over the wrist. Holding the wrist in acute flexion may elicit paresthesia along the median nerve distribution. This is called the *Phalen test* and is considered positive if symptoms develop in less than 1 minute. Thenar weakness or wasting is usually a late finding and suggests a severe degree of compression. Nerve conduction studies and electromyography can be useful adjuncts to clinical examination. Initial treatment of carpal tunnel syndrome is nonoperative and includes the use of wrist splints or local corticosteroid injections. Persistence of symptoms is an indication for surgical decompression. This is achieved by longitudinally dividing the flexor retinaculum by open or endoscopic means.

Hand Masses

Ganglia account for 70% of all tumors in the hand. They are formed by an outpouching of the synovial membrane from a joint or tendon sheath and contain a thick jelly-like mucinous substance, similar in composition to synovial fluid. Sixty percent of ganglia occur on the dorsal aspect of the wrist. Volar wrist ganglia are less common. Another frequent site for these tumors is the flexor sheath. They can also occur after osteoarthritis of the distal interphalangeal joints and are erroneously called mucous cysts. Ganglia are more common in women and usually occur around the third decade of life.

By themselves, these tumors are innocuous and can be left alone. Treatment is required only for cosmetic purposes or to relieve pressure effects on adjacent structures. Aspiration of the mucinous substance with a large-bore needle followed by instillation of a corticosteroid into the sac may suffice. If this fails, the ganglion is surgically excised. Particular care is taken to trace and resect the root or pedicle of the tumor down from the joint or sheath from which it arises. The volar wrist ganglion is often very closely related to the radial artery. The Allen test is performed before surgery to determine the adequacy of ulnar arterial flow in order to prevent accidental injury to the radial artery during excision leading to ischemia of the hand. Sometimes it is necessary to leave behind a cuff of ganglion wall attached to the radial artery to avoid injuring it.

Giant cell tumor, also called *pigmented villonodular synovitis* (PVNS), is the second most common hand tumor and arises from the synovial membrane of joints or tendon sheaths. It is yellow-brown on gross appearance and contains multinucleated giant cells on microscopy. The tumor is nearly always benign in the hand and generally asymptomatic, although it can produce notching of adjacent bones by pressure. Giant cell tumors can also envelop digital neurovascular bundles or extend along the tendon sheaths. Treatment is surgical and consists of excision of the tumor along with any involved synovium.

Epidermal inclusion cysts are also called *implantation dermoids* and occur after trauma. Epidermal cells become lodged in the subcutaneous tissue and continue to grow there. They occur more often in men and are usually found fixed to the palmar skin. Symptoms are related to the size and location of the cyst. Treatment is surgical excision, and recurrence is rare.

Pyogenic granuloma is a misnomer for an exuberant outgrowth of granulation tissue at sites of previous trauma. The lesions are highly vascular with a thin epithelial cover and are friable, bleed easily, and can grow rapidly. They occur most commonly on the fingertips and respond to either curettage or simple excision.

Infections

Paronychia refers to infection of the lateral nailfolds and usually results from a penetrating injury. The most common causative organism is *Staphylococcus aureus*. Treatment for early cases is with antibiotics, preferably a penicillin in combination with a β-lactamase inhibitor such as sulbactam or clavulanic acid. Once an abscess develops, surgical drainage is required. Traditionally, this has been achieved by making a longitudinal incision just lateral and parallel to the nailfold; however, recent recommendations are to merely remove the nail and let the pus drain out from under the nailfold.

A *felon* is an abscess of the pulp space and usually accompanies paronychia. Because the pulp space contains rigid fibrous septa fixing the skin to the periosteum of the distal phalanx, collections in this region can lead to a buildup of high pressures that can be very painful. Appropriate treatment is surgical incision and drainage of the abscess followed by appropriate antibiotics. Complications include septic tenosynovitis, skin necrosis, and osteomyelitis of the distal phalanx.

Acute suppurative tenosynovitis most commonly affects the flexor tendon sheaths. They usually arise after penetrating trauma and are caused by *S. aureus*. Kanavel described four cardinal signs in the digit: a fusiform swelling, a flexed attitude, tenderness over the tendon sheath, and pain on passive extension. Early cases may respond to nonoperative treatment, including elevation, warm soaks, and intravenous antibiotics. Unresponsive or advanced cases require surgical drainage. The flexor sheath is opened through two separate incisions proximally at the level of the A1 pulley and distally at the level of the A5 pulley. A small catheter or infant feeding tube is passed down the flexor sheath through these incisions, and the area is continuously irrigated with isotonic saline or lactated Ringer's solution for 36 to 48 hours. Antibiotics are required for at least 1 or 2 weeks. More severe infections or a delay in treatment may lead to necrosis of the tendon sheath, osteomyelitis, and abscesses. These are best treated by debridement through an extensive exposure.

Herpetic infection or "whitlow" of a digit is caused by the herpes simplex virus and frequently occurs in health-care personnel, and the source is usually orotracheal secretions of patients. The organism incubates for 2 to 14 days before forming fluid-filled vesicles on the fingertip. These lesions can sometimes mimic paronychia or felons. The diagnosis is made from a potassium hydroxide prep and Tzanck smear. Viral cultures and immunofluorescence with radioisotope-tagged antibodies can be helpful. Clinically, herpetic infections must be differentiated from bacterial infections. Herpetic infections are self-limiting, and treatment is nonoperative. Surgical incision and drainage can lead to systemic involvement and possible viral encephalitis.

Animal and human bites are quite common on the hand. Of them, human bites carry the worst prognosis. Human bites are contaminated by mixed oral flora and if untreated can lead to severe infection with rapid destruction of local tissue. Common organisms infecting human bites are *Staphylococcus*, *Streptococcus*, *Bacteroides*, and *Eikenella corrodens*. Most human bite injuries on the hand occur when an individual strikes another person in the mouth with a clenched fist. A tooth produces a puncture wound that may even penetrate into the metacarpophalangeal joint. Clinical examination should focus on the possibility of extensor tendon injury and joint penetration. Surgical exploration, debridement, and lavage are mandatory in the treatment of these injuries. Human bite wounds should not be closed primarily and are treated with penicillins or cephalosporins after surgery.

Dupuytren's Disease

Dupuytren's disease is a contracture of the palmar aponeurosis, extending into the digits. It is more common in men and is largely of familial origin, usually affecting those with Scandinavian ancestry. It usually occurs after 50 years of age and is autosomal dominant with variable penetrance. There is some evidence to suggest that it may be more common in patients with a history of epilepsy, alcoholism, diabetes, and myocardial infarction. The disease usually begins in the ring and small fingers, with the index being the least involved of all digits. Slight thickening of the palmar fascia into cords or nodules does not require treatment. Fasciectomy is the surgical operation of choice and is reserved for patients with greater than 30° of metacarpophalangeal joint flexion contracture or any degree of proximal interphalangeal joint flexion contracture. In the palm, this is best accomplished through a transverse incision, whereas in the digits vertical incisions are used. After removal of the offending cords, the transverse palmar incisions can be left open or partly closed, and the longitudinal digital incisions are converted into Z-plasties and closed in a tension-free manner. Frequently, local flaps or skin grafts may be required.

Part VII
Immunology and Transplantation

52
Basic Immunology and Rejection

Immune Response

The primary function of the immune system is to determine self from nonself and to subsequently destroy the foreign nonself material. An elaborate immune system has evolved to ensure host survival. The immune system has two major branches: cell-mediated immunity and humoral-mediated immunity.

Humoral, or antibody-mediated, immunity is characterized by direct interaction of antibody (Ab) produced by plasma cells to the antigen. Antibodies, or immunoglobulins (Igs), are composed of a variable and a constant region. The variable region can bind antigen. There are five different classes of antibodies distinguished by their heavy chains (each antibody has two identical heavy chains and two identical light chains). IgM is the antibody of the primary immune response. IgG is the primary antibody of the secondary response (memory). IgA is found in secretions. IgE mediates type I hypersensitivity reactions. IgD is a membrane-bound receptor.

Cell-mediated immunity is characterized by the interaction of T cells with an antigen. Antigens (Ags) are not recognized directly by the T cells. T cells recognize antigen only when the antigen is bound in a complex with a major histocompatibility (MHC) molecule. The T cell receptor (TCR) then binds this complex along with a costimulation receptor. The purpose of the costimulation receptor is to determine whether to evoke a response that allows for regulation (appropriateness of response).

The MHC (human leukocyte antigen [HLA] in humans) is a cluster of genes encoded by loci on chromosome 6. There are two major classes of MHC, MHC I and MHC II. There are codominate expressions of one haplotype from father and one haplotype from mother for a total of 12 HLA Ags; however, only HLA-A, -B, and -DR are used for tissue typing. The codominate expression allows for genetic polymorphism with different alleles at each locus so that each individual expresses different forms of a single gene.

The MHC I molecules are encoded by HLA-A, -B, and -C and are expressed on all nucleated cells. MHC I molecules are associated with β_2-microglobulin. They function as an activator and target $CD8^+$ (cytotoxic) lymphocytes.

MHC II molecules are encoded by the HLA-DR, -DP, and -DQ loci. They are expressed on B cells, antigen-presenting cells (APC), and the vascular endothelium. They function to activate helper T cells ($CD4^+$), stimulate the mixed lymphocyte reaction, stimulate the antibody response, and act as a possible target for antibody-mediated rejection.

The immune response is the primary determinant of graft viability. Human leukocyte antigen typing, for graft compatibility, is important for renal, lung, cardiac, and pancreatic matching but not for hepatic transplantation (there is no benefit for graft survival). Loci typed are HLA-A, -B, and -DR (6 Ag match). Positive cross-match shows that preformed Abs are present, leading to hyperacute rejection. A complete donor–recipient match is referred to as a *six antigen match* or a *zero antigen mismatch*. The larger the number of HLA-A, -B, and -DR alleles that are matched between donor and recipient, the better the survival rate, particularly in the first year after transplantation. However, current immunosuppressive regimens negate much of the impact of HLA matching.

Most patients on transplant waiting lists submit serum samples that are tested against a panel of typing cells of known HLA specificities. The percentage of cells with which recipient serum reacts is determined, and this number is the panel-reactive antibody (PRA). Most persons have a low PRA value (0% to 5%). Patients who have been pregnant, have received multiple blood transfusions, have had prior transplantation, or have an autoimmune disorder may have a high value (50% to 99%). The higher the PRA, the more likely the chance of having a positive cross-match.

Hyperacute Rejection

Hyperacute rejection occurs within minutes to hours after transplantation. It is the result of preformed antibodies to donor ABO or HLA determinants in the recipient's serum at the time of transplantation. Cytotoxic antibodies bind to the allograft vascular endothelium, resulting in complement-mediated lysis, a procoagulant state, massive hemorrhagic necrosis, graft thrombosis, and, ultimately, graft loss. This type of rejection is irreversible. It does not generally occur in hepatic transplantation (thus, there is no need for preoperative cross-match).

Acute Rejection

Acute rejection occurs as early as 1 week after transplantation but more often occurs in the first to sixth postoperative months (but it can occur at any time). Mediated by T cells, it is also called *cell-mediated rejection*. Histologically, there is an infiltration of the tissue with lymphocytes and macrophages with direct cytolysis and thrombosis. Treatment of acute rejection, unlike hyperacute rejection, most often results in good graft function. Prompt recognition of acute rejection is paramount followed by initiation of high-dose steroids and adjustment of the immunosuppressive regimen to prevent permanent graft damage.

Chronic Rejection

Chronic rejection is poorly understood with insidious onset over time (months to years). It is the result of both antibody- and cellular-mediated attack of the tissues.

There is damage to the vascular endothelium (common to all types of allografts), interstitial fibrosis, thickening of the basement membrane (kidney), and obliteration of the bile ducts (liver). There is a greater incidence of chronic rejection in

1. Grafts that have multiple episodes of acute rejection
2. Grafts that have late episodes of acute rejection
3. Recipients with previous transplantation with development of chronic rejection
4. Recipients with inadequate immunosuppression, including patient noncompliance
5. Graphs with initial delayed function
6. Donor issues such as age and hypertension
7. Organ recovery-related issues, including preservation and reperfusion injury
8. Recipients with diabetes, hypertension, or post-transplant infections

Chronic rejection is the main cause of allograft failure and recipient death following all types of organ transplantation.

Graft-Versus-Host Disease

In graft-versus-host disease (GVHD), donor-derived T and B cells in the vascularized graft are stimulated by host alloantigens. This may result in T cell-mediated lesions such as hepatitis, dermatitis, and gastrointestinal mucosal lesions. The B cells can produce antihost Abs, and, if there is an ABO incompatibility, this can cause hemolytic anemia. This phenomenon is usually self-limited, because these graft donor cells are eliminated by immunosuppression or the host antidonor responses.

53
Immunosuppression

Adrenal Corticoids

Adrenal corticoids bind to cytoplasmic receptors and are then translocated to the nucleus and bind to gene promoters and transcriptional regulators. This results in the inhibition of cytokine gene transcription and cytokine secretion (interleukin [IL]-1, IL-6, and tumor necrosis factor) by macrophages. They also suppress the production and the effect of T-cell cytokines (IL-2 production and binding to its receptor). Adrenal corticoids block the ability of macrophages to respond to lymphocyte-derived signals such as migration inhibition factor and macrophage activation factor. They are used for induction, maintenance, and rejection and are especially effective in treating acute rejection (high doses); however, prolonged use results in severe side effects such as hypertension, weight gain, peptic ulcers and gastrointestinal bleeding, euphoric personality changes, cataract formation, hyperglycemia that can progress to steroid diabetes, pancreatitis, muscle wasting, and osteoporosis with avascular necrosis of the femoral head.

Antimetabolites

Antimetabolites include the following:

1. Azathioprine (Imuran®): Structurally similar to 6-mercaptopurine and inhibits purine synthesis. Azathioprine strongly inhibits the development of both humoral and cellular immunity by interfering with the differentiation and proliferation of the responding lymphocytes. It is helpful in lowering maintenance doses of cyclosporine or glucocorticoids. Its adverse effects include leucopenia, hepatitis, hepatic vein thrombosis, and pancreatitis.

2. Cyclophosphamide (Cytoxan®): Mechanism is alkylation of DNA. It is used in induction and mainte-

nance therapy. Adverse effects include leukopenia, thrombocytopenia, hemorrhagic cystitis, nausea, and emesis.

3. Mycophenolate Mofetil (MMF) (CellCept®): Inhibits purine synthesis and blocks proliferative responses of both T and B cells. Its clinical uses include induction, maintenance, and treatment of rejection. It has almost completely replaced azathioprine, because it reduces the rejection rate. Its adverse effects include thrombocytopenia, leukopenia, neutropenia, and gastrointestinal effects.

Calcineurin Inhibitors

Calcineurin inhibitors include the following:

1. Cyclosporine: A fungal metabolite extracted from *Tolypocladium inflatum* Gams. The mechanism is tyrosine phosphate calcineurin inhibitor, which selectively inhibits T cell-receptor mediated activation events. It is clinically used for induction and maintenance therapy (levels must be monitored). Its adverse effects include nephrotoxicity (most common), hypertension, hyperkalemia, hirsutism, gingival hyperplasia, tremor and other neurotoxicities, diabetogenicity, and hepatotoxicity. The addition of corticosteroids to cyclosporine permits a lowered cyclosporine dosage and decreased nephrotoxicity.

2. FK506 (Tacrolimus, Prograf®): Isolated from the soil fungus *Streptomyces tsukubaensis*. It binds to FK-binding protein (FKBP), resulting in inhibition of calcineurin, which blocks expression of IL-2 receptors. It is clinically used for induction, maintenance, and treatment of rejection (must monitor levels). The side effects of cyclosporine and tacrolimus are similar; however, tacrolimus does not cause hirsutism or gum hypertrophy. FK506 causes alopecia and has an increased incidence of post-transplantation diabetes.

Sirolimus (Rapamycin®)

Sirolimus is a macrolide antibiotic similar to tacrolimus (it binds to FKBP); however, it impairs signal transduction by the IL-2 receptor to the nucleus. Sirolimus has been combined with cyclosporine, tacrolimus, or MMF in attempts to decrease or avoid calcineurin inhibitors with their associated nephrotoxicity. The drug possibly antagonizes B cell lymphomas.

Antibodies

Antibodies include the following:

1. Polyclonal: Antilymphocyte globulin (ALG) and antithymocyte globulin (ATG). Polyclonal antibodies are directed against antigens on lymphocytes. They promote cell clearance through complement-mediated lysis and opsonization. They impair or alter signaling by functionally removing primary effector cells. Polyclonal antibodies are used clinically for short treatment periods; thus, they are used for induction and treatment of rejection. Their adverse effects include allergic reactions to the antiserum (most common), thrombocytopenia, leukopenia, urticaria, and serum sickness, including joint pain, fever, and malaise.

2. Monoclonal:

a. OKT3: Binds with CD3⁺ cells, causing internalization of the T cell receptor and resulting in opsonization of the cell. Blocks cytotoxic effect of activated T cells and naive T cells. OKT3 is used clinically for induction and treatment of rejection. Its adverse effects include massive release of cytokines (high-dose steroids prior to dose), resulting in fever, chills, diarrhea, headache, nausea, vomiting, dyspnea, wheezing, pulmonary edema, aseptic meningitis, seizures, and coma.

b. Rituximab: Anti-CD20 (surface molecule on B cells). Used to decrease antibody production in recipients with high panel-reactive antibody (PRA) or as part of positive cross-match protocols. It is used as treatment for post-transplantation lymphomas.

Interleukin-2 Receptor Inhibitors (Basiliximab and Daclizumab)

Interleukin-2 receptors are directed against CD25 receptors, present only on T cells, leaving the cell with no free receptors for IL-2 to bind. Neither basiliximab nor daclizumab results in the cytokine-release syndrome that occasionally occurs with OKT3 administration or in the serum sickness that occurs with polyclonal antibodies.

Complications of Immunosuppression

Infection

Infection is the most common complication of immunosuppression. Patients often present with subtle signs late in the process due to blunting of the inflammatory response. The increased risk is caused not only by environmental pathogens but also by reactivation of previously controlled internal pathogens. Patients are often given prophylactic medications, including pneumococcal vaccine, hepatitis B vaccine, or lamivudine for hepatitis B–positive serology; trimethoprim–sulfamethoxazole for *Pneumocystis* pneumonia and urinary tract infections; acyclovir, ganciclovir, or valganciclovir for cytomegalovirus (CMV); and nystatin for oral and esophageal fungal infections. Cytomegalovirus is present in approximately 70% of the population and causes substantial morbidity in the post-transplantation patient. This usually appears 6 to 12 weeks after transplantation and again after periods of increased immunosuppression for rejection episodes. Cytomegalovirus reactivation in seropositive patients undergoing transplantation are usually mild and self-limiting and include fevers, myalgias, arthralgias, mild elevation of liver function values, and nonspecific abdominal complaints. Seronegative patients receiving a seropositive organ have a 100% chance of contracting the virus and a 70% chance of a serious infection, including encephalitis, pneumonitis, hepatitis, and necrotizing gastroenteropathy.

Malignancy

Chronic immunosuppression inhibits immune mechanisms that keep transformed cells in check. The incidence of malignancy is related to the amount of suppression over time; however, common neoplasms (lung, breast, prostate, colon, or uterine cancer) have the same incidence rate. Most post-transplantation malignancies are *in situ* carcinomas of the cervix, low-grade skin tumors, or virus-mediated tumors. The incidence of skin cancer, mainly squamous cell carcinoma and Kaposi's sarcoma (human herpesvirus 8), is about 100 times more than in the control group. Human papillomavirus is associated with cancers of the cervix and is 14 times more likely to occur in the post-transplantation population than in the normal population. Lymphomas are 10 to 100 times more common in transplant recipients and are usually related to the Epstein-Barr virus. Treatment relies on reduction or complete cessation of immunosuppression, followed in some cases with chemotherapy (cyclophosphamide, hydroxydoxorubicin, Oncovin, and prednisone [CHOP] and rituximab).

Cardiovascular Disease

Cardiovascular disease is an important cause of morbidity and mortality in transplant recipients. After the first year, the most common causes of death in transplant recipients are (1) allograft loss from chronic rejection and (2) death of the patient with a functioning graft due to cardiovascular death, disease, or infection. Atherosclerotic disease in heart transplant recipients is multifactorial. It can be related to chronic rejection, CMV infection, or classic hyperlipidemia. Cyclosporine and corticosteroids, in particular, are associated with increased coronary artery disease. Adequate pretransplantation assessment of coronary artery disease, including liberal use of coronary angiography, helps identify patients at risk.

54
Kidney Transplantation

The first kidney transplantation was performed by Joseph Murray in the late 1950s and involved identical twins. Insulin-dependent diabetes mellitus, glomerulonephritis, and hypertension are the three diseases most often causing renal failure, which is treated by kidney transplantation (60%). Other diseases that cause renal failure and are treated with transplantation include polycystic kidney disease, Alport's disease, immunoglobulin (Ig) A nephropathy, systemic lupus erythematosus, nephrosclerosis, interstitial nephritis, pyelonephritis, and obstructive uropathy. Ongoing infection and malignancy are contraindications to transplantation, because immunosuppression encourages both microbial and tumor growth. Although having a successfully treated cancer is not a contraindication to transplantation, the general practice is to wait at least 2 years before transplantation.

ABO blood groups and a negative leukocyte cross-match are mandatory. Sensitization to human leukocyte antigen (HLA), indicated by lymphocytotoxic antibodies in the recipient's serum, may occur due to pregnancy, blood transfusions, or previous transplantation. Donor-reactive antibodies, detected by incubation of the recipient's serum with the donor's cells in the presence of complement (a positive "cross-match"), is a contraindication to renal transplantation because of the strong association with hyperacute renal allograft rejection. Serum from patients awaiting cadaveric renal transplantation is periodically screened against a panel of randomly selected HLA-typed lymphocyte donors. Nonreactivity of the patient's serum to the panel cells indicates a likelihood of obtaining a cross-match-compatible donor, whereas uniform reactivity of the patient's serum with panel cells greatly reduces this probability. The importance of matching HLA antigens in the selection of living-related donors for renal transplantation is well established. Excellent graft survival (>95%) occurs when a related donor and a recipient are HLA identical. The graft survival rate is less with one or zero haplotype matches.

During the early days of transplantation, the success of HLA-identical sibling donor grafts was twice that of cadaveric transplants. The short-term results of cadaveric grafts have improved greatly. Currently, 1-year outcomes approach the success of HLA-identical sibling grafts (89% and 96%, respectively). When long-term survival is examined, the importance of histocompatibility is clear. At 5 years, 90% of HLA-identical sibling grafts survive and at 10 years, 65%. Despite advances in immunosuppressive therapy, the survival of cadaveric grafts at 5 years is only 65% and less than 40% at 10 years unless they are matched for the recipient's HLA antigens. This raises the 5-year survival rate to about 73%.

Many other factors influence the results of transplantation, including the age of recipients or donors (<5 or >50 years); interracial grafts; broadly sensitized recipients identified by preformed antibodies against a panel of donor lymphocytes; previous failed transplants, especially if lost from early rejection; delayed transplant function requiring dialysis; poor early function (serum creatinine level >3 mg/dl at the time of hospital discharge); and certain disease states (e.g., hypertensive nephrosclerosis and oxalosis). Despite improvements in cross-matching and immunosuppression, sensitized recipients of first cadaveric kidneys have a 14% greater incidence of delayed graft function and an 8% lower graft survival rate at 5 years. Loss of a previous transplant is also a negative predictor. For recipients of cadaveric grafts, 5-year graft survival rates are 66% for a primary graft and only 62% and 56% for second and third grafts, respectively.

Recipient race is another important factor in graft survival. Late graft loss occurs twice as often in blacks as in nonblack recipients, whether the donor is living or cadaveric. Because of racially associated histocompatibility differences, blacks have also been at a disadvantage for allocation of cadaveric kidneys (the majority of which come from white donors), because the distribution algorithm has been heavily influenced by matching. To address this inequity, the United Network for Organ

Sharing (UNOS) Board of Directors recently voted to discontinue matching at the B locus as a consideration in allocation of cadaveric donor organs. Factors associated with favorable outcome include relatively young donors (aged 6 to 50 years); good histocompatibility (especially complete HLA identity); and living donors (even if not related to the recipient by blood).

The excellent results of transplantation and the donor shortage add to the growing list of patients awaiting transplantation. For older patients, a 3- to 5-year waiting time is a significant portion of their remaining life.

Impatience with long waiting times for cadaveric donor kidneys (during which many dialysis patients die) has led to a substantial increase in living donors. Unfortunately, donation of cadaveric kidneys has increased little, and most of the small increase has been from suboptimal donors, either younger than 5 or older than 50 years. The good success of unrelated-living-donor transplants and the introduction of laparoscopic donor nephrectomy are responsible for much of the increase in living donation. The overall results of transplantation have benefited from this shift to living donors. At 10 years, there is an 18% better survival rate for living-donor compared with cadaveric grafts. For HLA-identical sibling donors, about a 90% 1-year graft survival rate was reported beginning in the mid-1970s; this is now more than 96%. The 1-year graft survival rate for parental or one-haplotype sibling transplants has also steadily improved since about 1980, from about 70% to the current 90% to 93%.

55
Liver Transplantation

Liver transplantation was first described by Starzl and colleagues in 1963 and has evolved dramatically from an experimental procedure with a high mortality rate to an accepted treatment for end-stage liver disease (ESLD). Liver transplantation is now the procedure of choice for a range of diseases that cause acute or chronic ESLD. Indications for liver transplantation include hepatitides B and C, alcohol-induced cirrhosis, cryptogenic cirrhosis, primary biliary cirrhosis, primary sclerosing cholangitis, autoimmune hepatitis, hepatic neoplasm, Budd-Chiari syndrome, Wilson's disease, α_1-antitrypsin deficiency, type I glycogen storage disease, and fulminant hepatic failure (usually drug toxicity).

The Child-Turcotte-Pugh (CTP) score (Table 55.1) was formulated empirically in 1964 as a predictive formula for patients with liver disease undergoing portosystemic surgery. Since its inception, it has also proved to be a useful tool in estimating the risks for both hepatic and nonhepatic surgery for patients with underlying liver dysfunction. The CTP attempts to standardize the severity of chronic liver failure by using criteria that reflect the residual function of the liver. A combination of clinical symptoms and laboratory data are used to provide insight into the severity of the disease and the residual function of the liver. The CTP scoring system was adopted as the standard method for placing patients who have ESLD on the transplant waiting list. The scoring system places patients in class A (4% 3-month mortality), B (14% 3-month mortality), or C (51% 3-month mortality). Waiting time on the list was used to stratify patients in a CTP score group.

In 2002, the United Network for Organ Sharing (UNOS) developed a new system for allocation that is not limited by emphasis on waiting time and subjective clinical parameters (such as degree of ascites or encephalopathy). The overall goal of this major revision to liver allocation was to give priority to the sickest patients using a system based on objective variables. To accomplish this, a statistical model for end-stage liver disease (MELD) was developed and has been shown to have a high predictive capacity for identifying patients with ESLD at greatest risk of dying within 3 months. This tool was developed by physicians at the Mayo Clinic for patients undergoing transjugular intrahepatic portosystemic shunting (TIPS) and is calculated from a validated predictive equation based on the patient's serum bilirubin level, creatinine level, international normalized ratio, and cause of liver disease (alcohol-induced, cholestatic, viral, or other). Studies have shown that outcomes are worse after liver transplantation for patients with low MELD scores. As a result, patients who have a MELD score less than 15 rarely receive a transplant.

The relatively low immunogenicity of liver allografts and the unique ability of the liver to regenerate are probably the main reasons for the excellent long-term outcome. Patients are tested for ABO compatibility; however, preoperative human leukocyte antigen (HLA) matching does not appear to be necessary (there is no benefit for graft survival), and a cross-match is typically only performed for acute dysfunction postoperatively to rule out circulating antibodies as the etiology. The 1-year graft survival rate is 85% to 90%; at 10 years, patient and graft survival rates for adults are 59% and 51%, respectively.

T cell-mediated acute rejection occurs at a rate of 30% to 50% within the first 6 months after transplantation, most often within the first 10 days. Its clinical presentation is variable and may include the development of fever, abdominal pain, liver enzyme levels, and elevated bilirubin. The diagnosis is confirmed by liver biopsy material that demonstrates the presence of a periportal lymphocytic infiltrate that extends into the liver parenchyma as well as the invasion of inflammatory cells into the vascular endothelium. Most rejection episodes are responsive to the administration of high-dose corticosteroids. More potent monoclonal or polyclonal anti–T-cell antibodies are effective against corticosteroid-resistant rejection, leading to the reversal of the acute episode in more

TABLE 55.1. Child-Turcotte-Pugh scoring system.

	Points		
	1	2	3
Encephalopathy	None	1–2	3–4
Ascites	Absent	Slight	Moderate
Bilirubin (mg/dL)	<2	2–3	>3
Albumin (g/dL)	>3.5	2.8–3.5	<2.8
International normalized ratio	<1.7	1.7–2.3	>2.3

Total score: A, 1–6; B, 7–9; C, 10–15.

than 90% of the recipients. Chronic rejection is seen months or years after transplantation. It is manifested by poor synthetic liver function and hyperbilirubinemia. It is usually characterized histologically by loss of bile ducts, atherosclerosis, and fibrosis.

Primary nonfunction occurs in 2% to 10% of liver transplants. Most cases are related to inadequate tissue preservation or to occult organ dysfunction in the donor. The development of primary nonfunction is a surgical emergency and can be successfully treated by early retransplantation. The failure to find a suitable graft within 7 days is associated with high morbidity and mor-tality rates. Hepatic arterial thrombosis occurs in 5% of adults and in up to 25% of children. Postoperative venous thrombosis is much less common, occurring in 2% to 3%. Biliary leakage is a feared complication with a high mortality rate (up to 50%). This may be the result of a concomitant hepatic arterial thrombosis and infection of the leaked bile or the difficulty of biliary ductal repair in the area of inflamed tissue. Infections remain the most significant complications in liver transplantation and are responsible for most of mortalities in the early postoperative period.

Replacement of the liver may not permanently cure recipients of their original disease. Recurrence of viral hepatitis is likely within a short time after transplantation in infected recipients. Human leukocyte antigen compatibility potentiates the inflammation during viral reinfection and increases the chance for clinical recurrence of the original disease. Control of active hepatitis B infection is possible in most patients using lamivudine, which inhibits the virus DNA polymerase, as well as hepatitis B immunoglobulin. In contrast, interferon-α and/or ribavirin are less effective in hepatitis C infection. Reinfection of the liver graft can be mild and in many cases does not cause liver failure. Retransplantation for recurrent hepatitis B or C is debated.

Part VIII
Head and Neck

56
Salivary Glands

The three pairs of major salivary glands include the parotid, the submandibular, and the sublingual glands. Minor salivary glands are scattered throughout the oral and nasal pharynx. Tumors derived from salivary glands are very rare, comprising only 5% of total head and neck neoplasms. Salivary gland tumors are generally slow-growing, well-circumscribed lesions composed of intercalated duct cells or excretory duct cells. Most salivary gland neoplasms are benign. Smaller salivary glands have a higher incidence of malignant tumors than do larger glands.

The key features of malignant tumors include pain, paresthesias, cervical lymphadenopathy, and rapid enlargement. Seventy percent of lesions occur in the parotid gland; 85% of these are benign. In contrast, minor salivary gland lesions comprise only 8% of all salivary gland neoplasms; however, 75% are malignant. Fifty percent of submandibular and sublingual lesions are malignant lesions.

Pleomorphic adenomas are benign tumors of mixed cellular origin. They occur mainly in the parotid gland (70%) and represent one-half of all salivary gland neoplasms. The tumors have a lobulated morphology and are slow growing. They can be large, causing little facial nerve dysfunction. They are more common in women about 50 years of age.

Papillary cystadenoma lymphomatosum (Warthin's tumor) is a benign monomorphic adenoma of the salivary gland. It is the second most common lesion and makes up 5% of all parotid lesions. They typically have a cystic morphology with a papillary-cystic form seen on histology. Men are more commonly affected between 60 and 70 years of age. Other benign lesions include oncocytomas, basal cell adenomas, myoepitheliomas, canalicular adenomas, ductal papillomas, and capillary hemangiomas.

The most common malignant lesion of the salivary gland is the mucoepidermoid carcinoma. The tumors are classified as high-grade or low-grade lesions. High-grade lesions are associated with a poor prognosis because of distant metastasis and a shorter survival time. Other malignant lesions include acinar cell carcinoma, adenoid cystic carcinoma, and squamous cell carcinoma. Malignant mixed tumors can arise from pleomorphic adenomas or de novo. About 1.5% of pleomorphic adenomas give rise to carcinoma within 5 years of discovery. The malignant risk is 9.5% after the lesion has been present 15 years or more. Malignant lymphoma can originate in the salivary gland as well. Non-Hodgkin's lymphomas make up the majority of these lesions. The incidence is increased with pre-existing diseases such as Sjögren's syndrome.

Evaluation in most cases includes physical examination and radiographic imaging. Bimanual examination may reveal fixation of the lesion to surrounding structures, which can be taken as a sign of malignancy. Helpful imaging modalities include computed tomography or magnetic resonance imaging. Irregularly shaped lesions within distinct tissue planes are a clue to malignancy as well. Fine-needle aspiration is of little use when attempting to make a tissue diagnosis. Surgical excision is the method of choice for confirming the diagnosis.

Pleomorphic adenomas are excised completely with a rim of normal tissue. When possible, complete removal of the involved lobe should be performed to offer better cosmetic results. These lesions should not be enucleated due to the higher rate of recurrence. The procedure is conducted through a periauricular incision that extends to the neck. This allows for adequate exposure of the facial nerve. The facial nerve should be left intact when treating any benign lesion. Submandibular lesions are treated with total gland excision.

Surgical excision (superficial lobectomy) with sparing of the facial nerve is the treatment of choice for low-grade parotid tumors. If the nerve cannot be spared, an attempt should be made to reconstruct it with nerve grafting.

High-grade parotid gland tumors are treated with surgical excision, followed by radiation of the primary site and regional lymph nodes. Radical neck dissections are indicated for clinically apparent lymphatic involvement. There is no indication for elective nodal dissection.

Salivary gland carcinomas are staged according to their size:

T1 = <2 cm
T2 = 2–4 cm

T3 = 4–6 cm
T4 = >6 cm

Stage and histologic grade are the most important prognostic factors. The 10-year survival rate for low-grade mucoepidermoid cancers within stage I or II is as high as 80%. In contrast, the 10-year survival rate for high-grade carcinomas of stage III or IV is as low as 30%.

57
Neck Injuries

Neck injuries occur due to penetrating or blunt trauma. The evaluation and treatment may differ slightly based on the mechanism of injury. There are many key structures contained in the neck, making neck injuries potentially life threatening.

Penetrating trauma to the neck is classified by the anatomic level of injury. The neck is divided into three anatomic zones. Zone I is composed of the thoracic outlet. Its boundaries are marked superiorly by the cricoid cartilage and inferiorly by the clavicles. Structures of importance that are contained in this zone include the subclavian arteries and veins, the proximal carotid arteries, and major vasculature of the chest. Zone II is bordered by the angle of the mandible superiorly and the cricoid cartilage inferiorly. Zone III extends from the angle of the mandible to the base of the skull. Zones I and III are the most difficult to gain exposure to. Zone I requires a thoracotomy to access the structures in it; exposure in zone III may require disarticulation of the mandible. Zone II structures are the easiest to access and expose. Blunt trauma to the neck most often results in cervical injuries such as fracture and dislocation, cervical spinal cord injury, vascular injury, and airway injury. Occasionally blunt trauma causes arterial occlusions or airway injuries.

Clinical manifestations of neck trauma depend on the structures involved in the injury. Airway injuries (larynx, trachea) produce hoarseness, stridor, or dyspnea. Subcutaneous emphysema is a pathognomonic sign of airway injury. Injuries to the esophagus manifest as severe chest pain and dysphagia if perforation occurs. Esophageal secretions cause inflammation of the mediastinum (mediastinitis).

Cervical spine injuries are commonly associated with direct trauma or sudden deceleration. Pain and tenderness at the level of the injury are the most common complaints. Arterial injuries can manifest with obvious hemorrhage, hematoma, hypovolemic shock, or a bruit heard on auscultation.

Penetrating trauma to the neck can injure many structures at once. Patients are evaluated by either exploratory surgery or a series of diagnostic tests, depending on the level of neck injury and the stability of the patient.

Exploratory surgery is required for an unstable patient, a patient with a rapidly expanding hematoma, or a patient with uncontrollable hemorrhage. Stable patients with zone I or III injuries usually undergo further diagnostic procedures because of the difficulty of gaining exposure to structures in these zones. Arteriograms are obtained before exploration of these regions to precisely locate the injury and to determine its severity.

Mandatory exploration of zone II injuries was the standard practice because of the ease of exposure of these structures; however, the recent trend favors diagnostic evaluation over mandatory exploration. Patients with penetrating injuries beyond the level of the platysma require the following evaluation: (1) Doppler ultrasound or arteriogram of the carotid artery to rule out injury, (2) endoscopic examination of the upper airways and esophagus, and (3) contrasted study of the upper esophagus to evaluate for esophageal lesions that may have been missed by endoscopy. Cervical computed tomography scans or plain films are used to evaluate for fractures.

Arterial injuries caused by high velocity missiles require debridement along with endtoend anastomosis of the clean ends of the vessel. Interposition vein grafts are used when a primary anastomosis cannot be accomplished. Minor injuries, such as pseudoaneurysms and intimal flaps, may not require intervention if blood flow in the vessel remains intact. The same is true for minor carotid artery injuries. Anticoagulation therapy is indicated to prevent thromboembolic complications. Arterial injuries that result in neurologic deficits should undergo ligation of the arterial vessel. Reperfusion of the ischemic infarction will convert the lesion to a hemorrhagic infarct with deadly consequences. Vertebral artery injuries are difficult to repair because of their bony encasement in the cervical vertebrae. Ligation of the vertebral artery may be the only viable option in situations of massive vertebral artery hemorrhage. Complications of the midbrain and cerebral necrosis sometimes occur in unilateral vertebral ligation (3% left, 2% right). Injuries to the subclavian artery require exposure through cervical and thoracic incisions. Attempt should be made at primary repair, but ligation of the vessels is generally tolerated. Venous injuries are simply ligated. Injuries to the esophagus are closed primarily, and drains are placed. Empiric antibiotics are administered to prevent local infection and inflammation. Minor injuries to the upper airway may need no intervention. Complications such as airway obstruction mandate prompt tracheotomy. Tracheal perforations should be debrided and closed primarily. Tracheal transections should be debrided as well with reanastomosis when possible. Injuries to the thyroid cartilage can be stented with a silastic temporary stent. Cervical fractures are immobilized with hard collars or traction to prevent further injuries.

58
Neck Masses

The possible causes of masses in the neck can be grouped into inflammatory, benign, and malignant. The patient's history can provide valuable information toward making the diagnosis. Key elements to inquire about include duration, rate of growth, location, and recent infections. Benign lesions are generally slow growing in direct contrast to malignancies. Malignant lesions tend to appear more quickly than their benign counterparts. Additional risk factors for malignancy should be assessed, which include previous history of cancer, night sweats, excessive sun exposure, tobacco and alcohol use, and radiation exposure. Signs suggestive of inflammatory causes include tenderness, erythema, and fever. Frequent causes of inflammation include sarcoidosis, fungal infection, trauma, tuberculosis, and dental infections. The location of the lesion is also helpful in making the diagnosis. Whether the cause is congenital, inflammatory, or malignant, these lesions tend to occur in predictable areas. The physical examination may be difficult to accomplish in all areas but provides invaluable information for developing the diagnosis.

Management of Specific Lesions

Infections such as tonsillitis, pharyngitis, and viral upper respiratory infections can frequently result in cervical adenitis. Posterior cervical lymphadenopathy is commonly associated with infection of the oropharynx. Patients should be evaluated for mononucleosis via a monospot test as well as receive therapy for their primary infection. Other inflammatory lesions include abscesses, infected sebaceous cysts, infected inclusion cysts, and carbuncles. In addition, bacterial infections can lead to fascial infections of the neck. These require broad-spectrum antibiotic therapy in addition to surgical drainage. Inflammatory lesions are initially treated with empiric antibiotics.

Chronic cervical lymphadenopathy can result from long-standing illnesses such acquired immunodeficiency syndrome, syphilis, and tuberculosis. Biopsy via fine-needle aspiration is the recommended approach to rule out a neoplastic process.

Benign neck masses can be congenital lesions or nonmalignant neoplasms. Congenital lesions located in the neck are often derived from the thyroglossal duct (thyroglossal duct cyst), the branchial clefts (branchial cleft cysts), the lymphatic system (cystic hygromas), or the vascular system (hemangiomas). Thyroglossal duct cysts arise from remnants of the embryonic thyroglossal duct. During embryonic development, the thyroid gland traverses the thyroglossal duct from the foramen cecum to its final position in the neck. Thyroglossal duct cysts comprise approximately 70% of congenital lesions located in the neck. They are usually discovered within the first 10 years of life and vary in size. They are consistently found in the midline of the neck near or inferior to the hyoid bone but also occur from the tongue base to the suprasternal notch. In addition, the morphology of the lesions ranges from a simple cyst, to a sinus tract, to a concrete cord of thyroid tissue. Thyroglossal duct cysts require surgical excision because of their high rate of recurrence and infection and a small association with papillary cancer (1%).

Branchial cleft cysts occur as masses positioned laterally, anterior to the sternocleidomastoid muscle. They can appear at any age but are generally identified by 2 months of age. These masses are typically painless, exhibit slow growth, and may or may not have an associated sinus tract. Branchial cleft cysts originate from the fetal branchial clefts (most often the second cleft). Patients often give a history of intermittent swelling and tenderness of the mass. Branchial cleft cysts are treated with antibiotic therapy to resolve infection, followed by complete surgical excision of the entire cyst and sinus tract.

Lymphangiomas that develop from lymphatic vessels of the neck are termed *cystic hygromas*. The lesions often manifest by the age of 2 years as painless cysts in the posterior triangle of the neck or in the supraclavicular region. Other locations include the base of the neck, the angle of the mandible, or the midline involving the tongue, mouth, or larynx. The masses are often diffuse and irregular. Cystic hygromas can resemble lipomas; however, unlike lipomas, they are capable of transillumination, release a serous fluid when aspirated, and have less distinct borders. Severe symptoms of tracheal compression and dysphagia can accompany large lesions. Surgical excision is reserved for lesions that fail to spontaneously regress or produce symptoms from mass effect. Recurrences are common because of numerous satellite lesions.

Hemangiomas are congenital vascular malformations that occur early in life (before 1 year of age). The lesions are often warm, blue, compressible, and have an audible bruit and palpable thrill. Angiography is the gold standard modality for making the diagnosis but is seldom necessary. Spontaneous regression often occurs; therefore, observation is recommended, and surgical resection is reserved for lesions that display rapid growth or cause thrombocytopenia.

Benign Tumors

Salivary gland tumors can be typically located anterior and inferior to the ear, at the submandibular triangle, or at the angle of the mandible. The majority of benign salivary neoplasms are asymptomatic. Malignant lesions often manifest with facial nerve impairment and involvement of the overlying skin. Computed tomography or magnetic resonance imaging can demonstrate the degree of salivary gland involvement. Tissue diagnosis is achieved via complete excision of the submandibular gland or superficial parotidectomy. Malignant parotid tumors are treated by complete excision of the superficial and deep lobes.

Thyroid nodules are common neck masses, most of which are benign. However, malignancy should be suspected in certain populations such as children, patients with a family history of thyroid cancer, those with a history of radiation exposure, younger men, and older individuals. Malignant characteristics include solitary, firm, rapid growth and a cold appearance on radioisotope scans (nonfunctional). Symptoms such as dysphagia, hoarseness, and pain are suggestive of malignancy as well. Fine-needle aspiration is the best method for obtaining a tissue diagnosis. Benign masses are managed conservatively with thyroid suppression and observation. Surgical excision of solitary nodules is accomplished through thyroid lobectomy. Enucleations are not advised because of the high risk of leaving residual disease. Subtotal thyroidectomy or total thyroidectomy is an appropriate procedure for either Grave's disease or multinodular goiters.

Lipomas and sebaceous cysts are soft tissue tumors often found in the neck. They are most often diagnosed and definitively treated with complete excision of the mass.

Chemodectomas are neoplasms that arise from chemoreceptive tissue in the head and neck. Carotid body tumors are chemodectomas that arise in the carotid body in the carotid bifurcation. These lesions are characteristically round, firm masses that exhibit slow growth. Auscultation of the mass may reveal a carotid bruit. Palpation of the mass demonstrates lateral to medial, not caudal to cephalad, mobility. Computed tomography scanning is the best modality for confirming the diagnosis. Computed tomography findings consistent with chemodectoma include a vascular mass present at the carotid bifurcation. Carotid body tumors are treated by complete excision without biopsy to remove all possible malignancy and to alleviate pressure symptoms. Radiation therapy is another option for patients who are not good candidates for surgical resection.

Tumors of neurogenic origin such as schwannomas and neurofibromas commonly arise in the head and neck. These lesions often manifest as painless masses in the lateral neck and are known for slow growth and malignant degeneration. Therefore, complete surgical resection is the appropriate form of treatment.

Malignant Tumors

Lymphoma (Hodgkin's and non-Hodgkin's) often manifests as palpable adenopathy involving the cervical lymph nodes. Adenopathy due to lymphoma can be differentiated from adenopathy of metastatic neoplasms due to the soft texture and mobility. Involvement of extranodal sites gives a clue to the diagnosis. Fine-needle aspiration is the easiest way to obtain a tissue diagnosis; however, excisional biopsy of an involved lymph node provides definitive proof.

Thyroid malignancies and skin cancers are two additional types of neck masses. An in-depth description of these primary neoplasms and their treatments appears in Chapters 74 and 149.

Malignant soft tissue sarcomas (rhabdomyosarcoma, chondrosarcoma, fibrosarcoma, liposarcoma, and osteogenic sarcoma) are rare lesions that can arise in the head and neck. Malignant fibrous histiocytoma is the most common type of soft tissue sarcoma in the head and neck. Elderly patients are the most affected by this neoplasm. Malignant fibrous histiocytoma arises from soft tissue or from bone (maxilla and mandible). Malignant fibrous histiocytoma is best treated with wide local excision. Rhabdomyosarcoma occurs most often in children and is the most common form of soft tissue sarcoma. Common locations include the orbit, paranasal sinuses, and nasopharynx. Biopsy of the lesion confirms the diagnosis. Therapy incorporates surgical resection, radiation, and chemotherapy. Radiographic imaging should be used to evaluate for distant disease before therapy is started.

Metastatic Tumors

Metastatic melanomas, adenocarcinomas, squamous cell carcinomas, and unknown primary carcinomas are the most common metastatic lesions in the neck. Selective lymph node dissection of the most susceptible group of nodes along with complete resection of the primary tumor is the standard approach to metastatic squamous cell cancer. Bilateral neck radiation (4 to 6 weeks postoperatively) is instituted when the final pathology reveals lymph nodes positive for metastasis.

Metastatic adenocarcinoma arises from several possible primary sites (thyroid, gastrointestinal tract, salivary glands, genitourinary tract, breast, prostate, and bronchopulmonary tract). Therefore complete evaluation of these areas is warranted before definitive treatment is planned. Neck dissection is reserved for scenarios in which the primary site has been identified and is deemed controllable or when the neck lesion is the only site of disease. Radiation therapy is used postoperatively as an adjunct to surgery.

Metastatic melanomas are treated in the following manner. Lesions that are less than 1 mm thick are treated with wide local excision with 1 cm margins without nodal evaluation (because of the low incidence of nodal metastasis). Lesions between 1 and 4 mm are treated with wide local excision with 2 cm margins as well as nodal evaluation via sentinel lymph node biopsy. Patients with clinical or histologically positive lymph nodes must undergo modified neck dissection. Superficial parotidectomy is completed in addition to neck dissection due to the risk of spread to the parotid gland. Chemotherapy and immunotherapy (IL-2) are useful for patients with lesions greater than 4 mm thick. Melanoma occasionally occurs in a cervical lymph node without evidence of a primary lesion. In this instance, the patient should be re-evaluated with careful examination of the scalp, sinuses, nose, mouth, and eyes. If the evaluation fails to reveal the primary lesion, then a unilateral modified neck dissection should be performed.

Investigation into the source of a metastatic neck tumor includes a complete history and physical examination as well as a thorough review of systems. If the primary tumor is not identified by conventional means, the patient should undergo a complete endoscopic evaluation (nasopharynx, hypopharynx, larynx, esophagus, and bronchial tree) under general anesthesia with biopsy specimens obtained. Metastatic squamous cell carcinoma in cervical lymph nodes originates from a head and neck cancer in 90% of cases. When no primary lesion is identified, the standard management consists of unilateral neck dissection followed by radiation therapy.

Part IX
Thorax

59
Pulmonary Function Tests

Pulmonary function tests provide a means for physiologic assessment of lung disease. These tests can at times be helpful for correlating a patient's lung function with a pulmonary disease category (restrictive vs. obstructive lung disease). Anticipated pulmonary resection is the most common indication for preoperative pulmonary function testing. The most common tests rely on lung spirometric volume measurements, the capacity of pulmonary diffusion, and forced vital capacity maneuvers.

Lung Volumes and Capacities

The lung contains varying volumes of gas depending on the phase of respiration. The total amount of gas in the lung can be broken down into the four nonoverlapping lung volumes. In addition, these volumes can be organized into four different lung capacities. The tidal volume (VT) is the amount of gas that is inspired and expired at rest (normal = 500 mL). The inspiratory reserve volume (IRV) is the amount of gas that can be inhaled in addition to the tidal volume (normal = 3 L). The IRV serves as a functional reserve for times when the tidal volume needs to be increased to meet increased oxygen demands (exercise). The expiratory reserve volume (ERV) is the volume of gas that can be expired after normal expiration (normal = 1.3 L). The residual volume (RV) is the volume of gas that remains after maximal expiration. The RV prevents the collapse of alveoli and is measured via plethysmography or dilutional techniques. The total lung capacity (TLC) is the sum of all four lung volumes. It is the total amount of gas in the lungs after maximal inspiration. The inspiratory capacity (IC) is the combination of the VT and the IRV. It is defined as the maximum amount of gas that can be inspired after a normal expiration. The amount of gas that remains in the lungs after a normal expiration is the functional residual capacity (FRC).

The forced vital capacity (FVC) is a measurement of maximal expiration after maximal inspiration (vital capacity) performed as rapidly as possible. Forced expiratory volume in 1 second (FEV_1) is the volume of the FVC that is expired within 1 second. The FEV_1 is one of the most important measurements to obtain when planning a lung resection. This test can generally predict whether or not a patient will have an adequate amount of remaining functional lung tissue after the procedure. Patients with values more than 2 L should be able to endure a pneumonectomy, and values above 1 L may allow for lobectomy. To improve accuracy and reliability, FEV_1 measurements are adjusted according to the patient's age, sex, and height and then reported as percentage predicted. Patients with values less than 50% of their predicted values are considered to have severe disease. Moderate disease is reported as values ranging from 59% to 75% of the predicted FEV_1, and mild disease is considered above 75%.

The FEV_1% is a ratio of FEV_1/FVC that is used along with the FEV_1 measurement to categorize lung disease as obstructive or restrictive. The principal characteristic of obstructive disease is increased resistance of the airways with reduction of expiratory flow. Patients with obstructive disease will display decreased values for FEV_1 as well as the FEV_1/FVC ratio. Patients with restrictive lung diseases will generally display a decreased FVC along with an increased FEV_1/FVC ratio.

60
Lung Cancer

Twenty-eight percent of cancer deaths are caused by lung cancer. Lung cancer is the number one cause of cancer death in women, surpassing breast cancer in 1987. Mortality from lung cancer for men has decreased, probably because of the effectiveness of smoking cessation programs. The most important risk factor for the development of lung cancer is cigarette smoking. Patients are generally between 50 and 70 years of age. The symptoms include cough, dyspnea, chest pain, and hemoptysis. Systemic symptoms such as fever, weight loss, anorexia, fatigue, and malaise occur in many patients. Local invasion into nearby structures manifests as hoarseness (recurrent laryngeal compression), superior vena cava syndrome (venous distension, facial edema, and plethora), Horner's syndrome (sympathetic nerve compression causing miosis, ptosis, anhidrosis, and enophthalmos), dysphagia, phrenic nerve paralysis, and pleural effusion. Horner's syndrome and invasion of the cervical sympathetic plexus can occur in apical (superior sulcus) lung cancers. These types of tumors are also called *Pancoast's tumors*. Obstruction of the bronchioles can cause obstructive pneumonia due to bacterial overgrowth and impaired airway clearance.

Lung cancers are grouped into large cell or small cell varieties. The subtypes of large cell lung cancer include adenocarcinoma, bronchoalveolar carcinoma, squamous cell carcinoma, and undifferentiated carcinoma. Adenocarcinoma is the most common form of lung cancer (45%). Lung adenocarcinoma develops from mucous cells in the bronchial epithelium. Most adenocarcinomas are located in the periphery of the lung. Early metastasis is characteristic of this cancer. Histologically the cancer cells have a cuboidal or columnar appearance, and some organize into glandular structures. Primary lung cancers may be indistinguishable from metastatic lesions originating outside the lung. The *K-ras* genetic mutation is a common feature of lung adenocarcinoma.

Bronchoalveolar lung cancer is a variant of adenocarcinoma that occurs in the terminal bronchoalveolar area of the lung. Bronchoalveolar lung cancers are highly differentiated and carry a more favorable prognosis. This cancer organizes into nodules (multiple or single) or diffusely infiltrates the lung tissue. Consolidations of tumor nodules can be confused with pneumonia. The key histologic feature of this lesion is its growth among parenchymal tissue without direct invasion. These tumors are often located in the lung periphery.

Squamous cell lung cancer comprises approximately 30% of lung cancers. There is a close association with cigarette smoking. Most are centrally located adjacent to the bronchus. Squamous cell cancers have a tendency to become necrotic and form central cavities. Tumor growth can cause a mass effect and compress nearby bronchi. Microscopic characteristics include intracellular bridging, the presence of keratin, and stratified organization of cells. Squamous cell cancer metastasizes later than adenocarcinoma. There is a strong association with *p53* mutations and squamous cell carcinoma.

Large cell undifferentiated lung cancers do not have the physical characteristics of squamous cancers and adenocarcinomas. These tumors comprise about 10% of lung cancers. Large cell undifferentiated lung cancer tends to localize in the peripheral lung parenchyma and tends to metastasize early.

Small cell lung cancer (also called oat cell carcinoma) is a very aggressive form of lung cancer that is derived from neural crest cells. This form of lung cancer is associated with cigarette smoking, tends to be centrally located, and metastasizes early. Histologically, the tumor cells have small dark nuclei, have a small amount of cytoplasm, and organize into sheets or clusters. The extensive nature of the neoplasm and its tendency for early metastasis make surgical resection impractical in most cases. Therefore, chemotherapy is the treatment of choice. Palliative radiation is given in some cases. Genetic mutations of tumor suppressor genes (*p53* and *RB*) are common.

Carcinoid Tumors

Carcinoid tumors comprise approximately 1% to 5% of total lung cancers. These tumors can be located in the periphery of the lung or centrally. Most lesions remain in the main stem bronchi, while some invade the bronchial wall and peribronchial tissue. They are of low-grade malignant potential and are usually 3 to 4 cm in size. Most display benign behavior and do not metastasize. The lesions are morphologically grouped as typical or atypical carcinoids. Typical carcinoids display minimal mitotic figures (<2 per 10 high-powered fields), little cellular atypia, and little necrosis. In contrast, atypical lesions have higher mitotic figures (2 to 10 per 10 high-powered fields), more cellular atypia, more necrosis, and lymphatic invasion. Common symptoms include cough, hemoptysis, bronchiectasis, and atelectasis caused by bronchial obstruction from intraluminal growth. Symptoms produced from the secretion of vasoactive substances are rare. When they occur, they consist of flushing, diarrhea, and cyanosis.

Metastasis

Lung cancer spreads primarily through the lymphatics, by hematogenous spread, and by direct extension into surrounding structures. Pulmonary and mediastinal lymph nodes are common areas of metastasis. Movement through the lymphatic system progresses from the hilar lymph nodes to the mediastinal nodes. Involvement of contralateral mediastinal nodes occurs in 25% of left lower lobe lung cancers. Metastasis to the adrenal glands, bone, brain, liver, lung, and kidneys occurs through hematogenous spread. Extrathoracic metastatic disease excludes a patient from surgical resection.

Solitary Pulmonary Nodules

The solitary pulmonary nodule is usually a small (<3 cm), well-circumscribed, asymptomatic mass in the lung tissue. Approximately 33% are malignant, with the risk increasing with age (50% risk at age 50 years). Surgical resection for diagnosis is generally recommended but may not be necessary when the mass is unchanged on images over 2 years, the mass is calcified, the mass is associated with an inflammatory disease such as tuberculosis, and when the patient is a poor operative candidate. Fine-needle aspiration (FNA) is seldom used to make the diagnosis and is generally reserved for poor operative candidates. Sputum cytology is also not useful. Failure to make a definitive diagnosis should not prevent surgical resection. Lobectomy is the usual surgical procedure.

Evaluation

History and physical examination are directed toward identifying extrathoracic disease (cervical or supraclavicular lymphadenopathy, paraneoplastic syndrome, and metastasis to the brain, kidney, bone, liver, or adrenals). Many cases are not detected until the disease reaches stages III or IV. The lack of sensation in the lung tissue allows tumors to grow large before becoming symptomatic.

The evaluation includes radiography, endoscopy, sputum cytology, and biopsy. Common imaging modalities include chest radiograph, computed tomography (CT), and magnetic resonance imaging (MRI). Chest radiographs are usually the first imaging modality used. The information gained includes size, location, and shape of the lesion. Pulmonary infiltrates, effusions, pneumonia, and lymphadenopathy can be detected as well. The type of cancer is identified in some instances. Squamous cell carcinomas tend to be large, cavitated, and centrally located; adenocarcinomas appear in the periphery. Small cell cancers are generally centrally located and accompanied by hilar and mediastinal lymphadenopathy.

Computed tomography scans provide superior detail of tumor location, lymphadenopathy, and metastasis. Computed tomography scans for lung cancer should include images of the upper abdominal cavity, including the adrenal glands. Observations on the CT scan dictate whether additional invasive studies are needed. For example, enlarged mediastinal lymph nodes (>1 cm) discovered on CT warrant mediastinoscopy. Magnetic resonance imaging is useful for evaluating the extent of invasion into nearby mediastinal structures or bone. Positron emission tomography scans are used to increase the sensitivity and specificity of CT scans. Additional imaging is recommended based on the patient's symptoms. For example, in patients complaining of bone pain, a bone scan can evaluate this. Brain CT or MRI is suggested for patients with neurologic symptoms.

Invasive testing is used to accurately stage lung neoplasms. The information gained will help select patients for complete surgical resection and patients who require chemotherapy or radiation. The tests include bronchoscopy, mediastinoscopy, FNA, and video-assisted thoracoscopy (VATS).

Bronchoscopy should be performed for patients who are being considered for surgical resection or for patients with positive sputum cytology. The procedure should be conducted by the operative surgeon to gain personal knowledge of the bronchial anatomy in relation to the tumor. Bronchoscopy allows the physician an opportunity to obtain biopsy specimens (primary lesion, mediastinal nodes) and also to search for secondary lesions.

Patients who have enlarged lymph nodes on imaging should undergo mediastinoscopy or VATS, depending on the location of the lymph nodes. These lesions are investigated primarily to rule out causes of lymphadenopathy (pneumonia, inflammation, atelectasis, and bronchitis) other than lung cancer metastasis. More than 70% of enlarged mediastinal nodes contain metastasis, whereas only about 15% of nodes smaller than 1 cm contain metastasis.

Less invasive modalities for obtaining a tissue diagnosis are recommended for poor operative candidates. Sputum cytology is noninvasive and can help make the diagnosis, especially with centrally located tumors (e.g., squamous cell lung cancer). Palpable lymph nodes are investigated with FNA to obtain a diagnosis. Transthoracic FNA of the primary lesion or lymphadenopathy is accurate in up to 95% of cases.

Lung cancers are staged according to the TNM staging system. Three main categories exist based on extent of disease and respectability: (1) Stages I and II diseases are entirely contained in the lung, lending itself to complete resectability. (2) Stage IV is hallmarked by metastatic lesions, which make complete surgical resection impractical. In some cases, partial resection has a palliative benefit. (3) Stages IIIA and IIIB are characterized by locally advanced disease (e.g., ipsilateral mediastinal lymph nodes or structures). In these cases, surgical resection may be possible but cannot address the presence of microscopic disease. Five-year survival rates are as follows: stage I, 65%; stage II, 40%; stage III, 15%; and stage IV, 5%.

Treatment

Large Cell Lung Cancer

Local disease is usually treated with surgical resection, and extensive disease is treated with chemotherapy. Radiation is offered for local control for patients who cannot tolerate surgery. The extent of disease dictates which modalities are used. For example, a favorable response is reported for surgical resection alone of stages I and II large cell lung cancer. Lesions with chest wall involvement should undergo en bloc resection of the lung and involved chest wall and mediastinal nodal dissection. There is increasing evidence to support the addition of perioperative chemotherapy to surgical resection for early-stage lesions. Studies have demonstrated improvements in median and overall survival. Surgery alone is not satisfactory for advanced-stage large cell lung cancer (stages IIIA, IIIB, and IV). Often, the risks of surgery outweigh potential benefits. Investigations are evaluating the potential of neoadjuvant chemoradiation in addition to surgical resection. Unresectable disease encompasses recurrent laryngeal nerve paralysis, superior vena cava syndrome, pulmonary artery involvement, supraclavicular nodal involvement, and tracheoesophageal trachea.

Small Cell Lung Cancer

Chemotherapy is the treatment of choice for small cell lung cancer due to the extensive nature of the disease. Approximately 30% of patients with small cell carcinoma have a complete response. The combination of chemotherapy and radiation therapy is especially beneficial for locally advanced cancers. Radiation is used in certain instances, either preoperatively or postoperatively, for local control. No benefit to survival has been proved.

61
The Pleura

The pleural space is a potential space between the lung and the chest wall. Parietal pleura lines the chest wall, and visceral pleura surrounds the lung. The parietal pleura receives systemic arterial supply and venous drainage as well as somatic innervation. The visceral pleura has systemic and pulmonary arterial supplies, pulmonary venous drainage, and autonomic innervation. Starling forces tend to drive fluid into the pleural space, and approximately 5 to 10 L crosses the pleural space per day. The lymphatics and the parietal pleura are primarily responsible for fluid and protein reabsorption. This balance is affected by gravity, fluid viscosity, membrane thickness, and distribution of lymphatic drainage throughout the parietal pleura. A small change in any of these factors contributes to accumulation of pleural effusion.

Pleural Effusion

The mechanisms include increased hydrostatic pressure, increased negative intrapleural pressure, increased capillary permeability, decreased plasma oncotic pressure, and decreased or interrupted lymphatic drainage. Effusions are classified as either transudates or exudates based on fluid protein and lactate dehydrogenase (LDH) concentrations. Exudates exist when pleural protein/serum protein is >0.5, pleural LDH/serum LDH is >0.6, or pleural LDH is 1.67 times normal serum LDH. The etiologies of transudative effusions include congestive heart failure, cirrhosis, nephrotic syndrome, hypoalbuminemia, fluid retention/overload, pulmonary embolism, lobar collapse, and Meigs' syndrome. The etiologies of exudative effusions include malignancy (through multiple mechanisms), various infections, collagen-vascular disease, esophageal perforation, subphrenic abscess, pancreatitis, chylothorax, uremia, sarcoidosis, radiation, trauma, and asbestosis.

The treatment of pleural effusion is removal of the underlying cause, if applicable, and diagnostic and therapeutic thoracentesis. When the effusion recurs, options include repeated thoracentesis, tube thoracostomy ± pleurodesis, and video-assisted thorascopic surgery (VATS) or thoracotomy ± pleurectomy and/or pleurodesis. Pleurodesis is performed using abrasion (mechanical), talc, or doxycycline and is effective for prevention of recurrent effusion, as it effects an obliteration of the pleural space. If reoperation is necessary, it is made more difficult because of this anatomic change. Occasionally, when pleural effusions become recalcitrant, they cause an inflammatory reaction that entraps the lung in a fibrous rind and inhibits full expansion. This condition is treated by either VATS or thoracotomy with decortication.

Empyema is a suppurative infection of the pleural space and is the most common cause of exudative effusion. The three phases of empyemas are acute (low viscosity, cell count), transitional (increased leukocytes, fibrin deposition), and organizing or chronic (well-defined pleural rind and "trapped" lung). Empyema is usually parapneumonic and is due to a contamination of the pleural space by any of several methods. Parapneumonic effusions are often caused by Gram-negative bacteria and anaerobes. Tuberculous empyema is more common as acquired immunodeficiency evolves. Treatment of empyema is with antibiotics initially. Other treatment options are phase dependent. Transitional-phase empyema is best treated with VATS/thoracostomy, whereas chronic empyema can require decortication. Complications include empyema necessitans (spontaneous decompression through the chest wall), pulmonary entrapment, osteomyelitis or chondritis of the ribs or vertebra, pericarditis, mediastinitis, bronchopleural fistula formation, or central nervous system infection. Chronic empyema can progress to a generalized failure to thrive and anemia. Occasionally, open drainage with rib resection, marsupialization, or chronic tube thoracostomy is required until the empyema cavity obliterates itself, which can take months.

Chylothorax is defined as lymph within the pleural space and can be due to thoracic duct damage, obstruction of lymphatic channels (malignancy, infection), or surgical procedures (lymphadenectomy). The fluid is usually milky white but is clear if the patient's diet is deficient in fats. The treatment is tube thoracostomy and instituting a low-fat diet, which is usually successful. Occasionally, thoracic duct ligation at the diaphragmatic hiatus is required. Treatment of associated malignancies can resolve chylothorax.

Hemothorax arises from accidental or iatrogenic trauma. Blood in the pleural space should be drained with large-diameter tube thoracostomy. Incomplete evacuations can cause a sterile chronic empyema with lung entrapment, requiring VATS or thoracotomy with decortication.

Pneumothorax

Pneumothorax is defined as air in the pleural space and is often caused by trauma or an invasive procedure. If the collection is moderate to large or is symptomatic, tube thoracostomy is indicated. Spontaneous pneumothorax may be primary (unclear etiology) or secondary (underlying pulmonary disease). Both are thought to be caused by spontaneous rupture of pulmonary blebs. Primary spontaneous pneumothorax is characteristically a disorder of tall, thin, young males. The treatment for the first episode is tube thoracostomy for moderate-to-large pneumothoraces, followed by blebectomy or lobectomy by either thoracotomy or VATS.

Pleural Tumors

Localized fibrous tumors of the pleura usually arise from the visceral pleura and are usually benign, although they are occasionally malignant. They are usually identified as an asymptomatic radiographic abnormality. Pleural tumors behave like sarcomas, and the treatment varies according to location. Visceral pleural tumors are amenable to wedge resection or lobectomy. Parietal pleural tumors frequently require chest wall resection. Malignant mesothelioma is associated with asbestos exposure and can be latent for 15 to 50 years before becoming clinically evident. Pleural thickening, effusion, and narrowing of intercostal spaces are seen radiographically. Symptoms include dypsnea on exertion and chest wall discomfort. Diagnosis requires immunohistochemical analysis and, occasionally, electron microscopy. This condition is lethal, and effective treatment has yet to be established. The most widely accepted treatment involves pleurectomy and decortication with postoperative radiation. The median survival is 7 to 16 months, which increases to 25 months with surgery and radiation.

62
Mediastinal Tumors

The mediastinum occupies the space in the thoracic cavity between the lungs. Its borders are delineated laterally by the parietal pleura medial to both lungs, anteriorly by the sternum, posteriorly by the vertebral bodies and rib articulations, superiorly by the thoracic inlet, and inferiorly by the diaphragm. Several designations exist with respect to subdivisions within the mediastinum. However, the frequency with which tumors occur in the anterior compartment extending superiorly prompted a commonly used three-compartment designation, with anterosuperior, middle, and posterior divisions. In this designation, the region posterior to the sternum and anterior to the heart and brachiocephalic vessels defines the anterosuperior compartment. The middle mediastinum is the space containing the heart and pericardium, including the ascending and transverse aorta, brachiocephalic vessels, vena cava, main pulmonary arteries and veins, trachea, mainstem bronchi, and adjacent lymph nodes. The posterior mediastinum is bordered anteriorly by the heart and trachea, extending posteriorly to the thoracic vertebral margin to include the paravertebral sulci containing the descending thoracic aorta, middle and distal esophagus, azygous vein, autonomic ganglia and nerves, thoracic duct, and lymph nodes.

Although differences in the relative incidences of neoplasms and cysts exist in some series, the most common mediastinal masses are neurogenic tumors (20%), thymomas (19%), primary cysts (18%), lymphomas (13%), and germ cell tumors (10%). Mediastinal masses are often located in the anterosuperior mediastinum (56%), with the posterior (25%) and middle (19%) mediastinum being less frequently involved. Malignant neoplasms comprise 25% to 42% of mediastinal masses. Lymphomas, thymomas, germ cell tumors, primary carcinomas, and neurogenic tumors are the most common. The relative frequencies of mediastinal malignancy vary with the anatomic site in the mediastinum. Anterosuperior masses are most likely malignant (59%) relative to middle mediastinal masses (29%) and posterior mediastinal masses (16%). The relative percentages of lesions that are malignant also vary with age. Patients in the second through fourth decades of life have a greater proportion of malignant mediastinal masses. In contrast, in the first decade of life, a mediastinal mass is most likely benign (73%).

Computed tomographic (CT) scanning is the examination of choice for suspected mediastinal tumors and not only precisely defines location but also reliably distinguishes cystic, fatty, vascular, and soft tissue masses. Computed tomographic scans are also important to identify pleural metastases, effusions, and pulmonary lesions. Of note, the most common mediastinal masses consist of metastatic spread to lymph-bearing tissue from the lungs or extrathoracic organs. In general, most primary malignant tumors arising from the mediastinum produce clinical signs and symptoms such as pain, dyspnea, or cough because of relatively rapid growth and local and distant spread. Benign tumors are usually asymptomatic or produce few symptoms.

The anterior compartment contains the thymus gland and contiguous fat anterior to the great vessels superiorly and pericardium inferiorly. The differential diagnosis for masses originating in the anterior compartment is the historically well-known "four-T" acronym, which includes thymoma, teratoma, thyroid lesions, and "terrible" lymphoma. These four conditions comprise >90% of all anterior mediastinal masses. For any young adult male presenting with a mass in the anterior compartment, measuring serum tumor marker (STM) levels, which include β-human chorionic gonadotropin (β-hCG) and α-fetoprotein (AFP) is essential. A significant elevation of either STM is diagnostic of a nonseminomatous germ cell tumor primarily arising in the mediastinum. Symptoms of night sweats and fatigue may indicate a lymphomatous process.

Following initial clinical and CT evaluation, biopsy of the anterior compartment mass may be indicated. The least invasive technique is CT-guided fine-needle aspiration (FNA), although it must be emphasized that cytology is notoriously nondiagnostic and occasionally misleading, particularly with respect to differentiating thymomas and lymphomas. A CT-guided core-needle biopsy can safely be performed if the mass abuts a significant area of the anterior chest wall and therefore can be accessed without traversing lung parenchyma with a large-bore needle. If core-needle biopsy is not possible, anterior mediastinotomy (Chamberlain procedure) is generally the next diagnostic procedure. Video-assisted thoracic surgery (VATS) provides excellent exposure to the anterior compartment for biopsy purposes.

Thymomas are the most common mediastinal tumor and are the most common anterior compartment neoplasm, constituting approximately 40% to 50% of the anterior compartment masses and 15% of all mediastinal masses. It is a rare, slow-growing tumor derived from thymic epithelial cells that is considered malignant because of its potential for local invasion and pleural space dissemination. Obtaining serum antiacetylcholine receptor antibody levels and considering neurologic consultation preoperatively are indicated if myasthenia gravis is suspected, because severe respiratory morbidity can be minimized with appropriate perioperative medical therapy.

Lymphomas constitute the second most common anterior compartment neoplasm in adults and the most common neoplasm in the pediatric population. Lymphomas can manifest as isolated mediastinal disease or more frequently as generalized disease. Hodgkin's lymphoma, and in particular the nodular sclerosing variant, is the most common type of mediastinal lymphoma with predilection for the anterior compartment.

Benign teratomas, seminomas, and nonseminomatous germ cell tumors are a heterogeneous group of benign and malignant neoplasms thought to originate from primordial germ cells that fail to complete migration from the urogenital ridge during embryogenesis. Benign mediastinal teratomas constitute only 5% to 10% of all mediastinal tumors but are the most common mediastinal germ cell neoplasm (60% to 70%).

Although mediastinal goiters comprise only 6% to 10% of all mediastinal masses, nearly all goiters are extensions from their original cervical location and therefore are not true primary tumors of the mediastinum. The most common indication for surgery is to relieve symptoms such as tracheal compression or pain, although resection is occasionally indicated to rule out malignancy if a relatively rapid growth pattern is demonstrated. Parathyroid tumors are usually located on the posterior capsule of the thyroid but can be in ectopic positions. Twenty percent of ectopic parathyroid tumors are located in the mediastinum, with the majority found in the anterior compartment.

The middle mediastinum contains the heart, pericardium, great arteries and veins, trachea, mainstem bronchi, and surrounding lymph-bearing tissue. Lymphadenopathy is the most common visceral mediastinal "tumor," and the differential diagnosis includes a wide variety of benign and malignant conditions. Benign conditions include lymphoid hyperplasia, sarcoidosis, and sequelae from granulomatous infections such as histoplasmosis or coccidioidomycosis, endemic to the Ohio and San Joaquin valley regions, respectively. The most common malignant tumors located in the visceral compartment are actually lymph node metastases from other organs such as non-small cell or small cell cancer of the lung.

Mediastinal cysts usually arise in the middle compartment and are usually congenital abnormalities of foregut origin. The most clinically important are bronchogenic cysts, esophageal duplications, and neuroenteric cysts. Bronchogenic cysts are often located in the subcarinal region and tend to be symptomatic in pediatric patients. Esophageal duplication cysts are usually lined with gastrointestinal epithelium and located in the wall of the distal esophagus. Neuroenteric cysts are rare and are always associated with vertebral anomalies. Therefore, they usually manifest in infancy. Other miscellaneous cysts that also occur in the middle mediastinum include thymic and pericardial cysts.

The paravertebral sulcus contains the proximal intercostal arteries and veins, proximal intercostal nerves, and entire sympathetic chain with associated ganglion and communicating rami to the intercostal nerves. Neurogenic tumors comprise the majority of tumors primarily arising in this compartment. Schwannoma (or neurilemoma), neurofibroma, and malignant nerve sheath tumors arise from the peripheral nerves, whereas ganglioneuroma, ganglioneuroblastoma, and neuroblastoma arise from the sympathetic ganglia. Pheochromocytomas and chemodectomas are the least common and are derived from the paraganglionic cells. Nerve sheath tumors are usually benign and are most common in adults, and sympathetic ganglia tumors are more common in children and are malignant in most patients.

Tumors of the mediastinum comprise a wide variety of benign, primary malignant, and metastatic malignant processes. The surgeon's role in evaluating patients with a mediastinal mass should initially begin with a thorough knowledge of the three mediastinal compartments and the respective differential diagnoses of each compartment. Occasionally, serologic tests, transesophageal ultrasound, and/or magnetic resonance imaging can provide additional critical information.

63
Chest Wall Tumors

Primary chest wall tumors are relatively uncommon, accounting for 1% to 2% of all primary tumors occurring in the body. These chest wall neoplasms are classified as benign or malignant tumors of bone and soft tissue. Approximately 60% of primary chest wall tumors are malignant. Malignant neoplasms arise most often (nearly 50%) from soft tissue rather than from bone or cartilage. Chest wall tumors include tumors originating in the bone, cartilage, or soft tissue of the chest wall. Most bony chest wall tumors arise in the ribs (85%), with the remainder arising from the scapula, sternum, and clavicle. Malignant lesions are further divided into primary or secondary (metastatic) tumors. Although metastatic disease to the ribs is the most common malignant chest wall tumor, primary bone tumors account for 7% to 8% of all chest wall tumors.

Primary chest wall tumors generally manifest as slowly enlarging masses. Initially, most tumors are asymptomatic, although, with increasing growth, invasion of surrounding structures, or the development of pathologic fractures, nearly all malignant tumors and 25% of benign masses are likely to become painful. Tumors of bone and cartilage are usually fixed to the chest wall, whereas soft tissue tumors are more often, but not exclusively, mobile. The correct diagnosis of a chest wall lesion relies on a thorough clinical evaluation (history and physical examination) and radiologic tests. In particular, chest radiography with rib tomograms and chest computed tomography (CT) are helpful in delineating soft tissue or bony involvement. Magnetic resonance imaging (MRI) is used to determine neural and vascular invasion. Bone scanning also may aid in the differential diagnosis to rule out the presence of satellite or metastatic disease. A definitive diagnosis is made only by histologic confirmation. In the past, excisional biopsy was believed to be the best method for diagnosis, because the lesion was entirely removed and included sufficient tissue sampling. Excisional biopsy is appropriate for lesions smaller than 2 cm and for lesions that appear radiographically benign.

Improved cytopathologic techniques have reduced the need for open biopsy. Core biopsies provide significant quantities of tissue that enhance diagnostic accuracy to more than 95% and enable histologic grading. If evaluation of a core biopsy is indeterminate, incisional biopsy is performed to obtain at least $1 \, cm^3$ of tissue.

Benign Tumors

The average age of patients with benign primary tumors of the chest is approximately 26 years. Benign tumors occur more often in men, with the exceptions of chondroma and desmoid tumors. At presentation, most patients have an asymptomatic mass, and only 25% of patients have a painful lesion.

Chondromas account for 15% to 20% of benign chest wall lesions. These lesions occur in the second or third decade of life as asymptomatic, slowly growing tumors at the anterior costochondral junction. Males and females are affected equally. The tumors can arise in the medulla (enchondroma) or the periosteum (periosteal chondroma). On chest radiography, the neoplastic growth appears as a lytic lesion with sclerotic margins that may be difficult to distinguish from chondrosarcomas. As a result, wide excision of the lesion is necessary to rule out a malignant component.

Fibrous dysplasia of bone accounts for more than 30% of benign chest wall tumors. These lesions usually appear in the third or fourth decade of life, with equal frequency in men and women. They are slow growing and asymptomatic and appear as a mass in the lateral or posterior aspect of the rib. Pain may develop as the tumor enlarges and causes pressure symptoms or develops pathologic fractures. The diagnosis is assisted by the appearance of a lytic lesion in the posterior aspect of the rib with a characteristic "soap bubble" or "ground glass" appearance on chest radiography. Excision is indicated for symptom relief (pain) and to confirm the diagnosis.

Osteochondromas originate from the cortex of the rib. Symptoms depend on the direction of tumor growth. Inward-growing tumors are usually asymptomatic, whereas outward-growing tumors appear as a painless mass. Young males are most commonly affected. A characteristic finding on chest radiography is a pedunculated bony mass capped with viable cartilage. Familial osteochondromatosis should be suspected if multiple lesions are noted. Complete excision is the treatment of choice; recurrences are rare.

Eosinophilic granuloma is a benign component of malignant fibrous histiocytosis, which primarily affects men. Patients present with skull and rib involvement that appears as expansile bone lesions on radiographic evaluation. Excisional biopsy is indicated for solitary lesions; radiotherapy is reserved for patients who have multiple lesions.

Aneurysmal bone cysts occur in the ribs and can be due to chest wall trauma. The characteristic pattern of a blowout lytic lesion frequently appears on chest radiography. Complete excision is warranted for relief of pain.

Malignant Tumors

Chondrosarcoma is the most common malignant tumor of the chest wall, accounting for 20% of all bone tumors. These lesions arise in the third and fourth decades of life and may be associated with trauma to the chest or represent malignant degeneration of benign chondromas or osteochondromas. On chest radiography, a poorly defined tumor mass, which is destroying cortical bone, is observed. The anterior costochondral junctions of the sternum are usually involved. Resection with circumferential margins of at least 4 cm is the treatment of choice, with a 70% 5-year survival rate reported for complete excision. Chemotherapy and radiotherapy (RT) have limited roles in the primary treatment of chondrosarcomas; however, they may be warranted for treatment of unresectable or recurrent sarcomas. Postoperative RT is indicated after margin-positive resection.

Ewing's sarcoma is a bone tumor that arises most often in the pelvis, humerus, or femur of young males. It is the third most common malignant chest wall tumor (5% to 10%). A mass that is intermittently painful is a common presentation in this disease. A characteristic onion peel appearance caused by periosteal elevation and bony remodeling is seen on the chest radiograph. Survival is approximately 50% at 5 years with multimodality therapy (chemotherapy, radiotherapy, and surgery).

Osteosarcoma (osteogenic sarcoma) is usually a painful tumor that arises most often in the long bones of adolescents and young adults. It also can occur as a late (more than 10 years) manifestation of prior irradiation. In the chest, osteosarcomas account for 10% to 15% of malignant tumors. Typically, the tumor presents as a rapidly enlarging mass with a characteristic sunburst pattern on chest radiography. Because metastases are common at presentation, a complete radiographic evaluation of the lungs, liver, and bones is indicated. The 5-year survival rate with complete excision and adjuvant chemotherapy approaches 60%.

Solitary plasmacytoma constitutes 6% to 15% of primary chest wall malignant neoplasms. Multiple myeloma is the same tumor arising in more than one location. The tumor commonly manifests as pain without a mass in older men. A diffuse, punched-out appearance of the bone caused by myelogenous deposits appears on chest radiography. Systemic disease can be confirmed using serum electrophoresis, urinalysis (Bence Jones protein), and bone marrow aspiration. Incisional biopsy is used to confirm the diagnosis, although a solitary plasmacytoma should be resected completely. Radiotherapy is the primary method of therapy, with a 5-year survival rate of 30% reported.

Soft tissue sarcomas account for approximately 20% of malignant lesions affecting the chest wall and are more common in men than in women. They can occur from any cell type in the soft tissues and include fibrosarcoma, leiomyosarcoma, liposarcoma, synovial sarcoma, neurofibrosarcoma, malignant fibrous histiocytoma, and angiosarcoma. Soft tissue sarcomas are usually graded as low or high grade based on mitotic rate, cellular pleomorphism, and nuclear-cytoplasmic ratio. Fine-needle or core biopsy is performed to establish the diagnosis, and surgical excision with wide margins is used for definitive therapy. Of note, the pseudocapsule that surrounds the tumor and frequently contains microscopic disease should be avoided during the resection to decrease the chance of local recurrence. Chemotherapy and RT are used as adjuvant therapeutic modalities. Patients with low-grade sarcomas have a 5-year survival rate of 90%, and a 50% survival rate is observed for patients with high-grade tumors. The local recurrence rate is 10% to 30%; therefore, adjuvant RT is usually indicated.

Desmoid tumors are low-grade fibrosarcomas. Unlike other soft tissue sarcomas, they occur more often in women. Although histologically benign, there is a high rate of local recurrence, ranging from 25% to 75% at 5 years. Generally, the risk of local recurrence is greatest during the first year after resection. Postoperative chest wall RT appears to reduce the rate of recurrent disease, primarily with tumors that could not be resected with negative margins. With wide local excision, overall 10-year survival rate is 95%.

64
Thoracic Outlet Syndrome

The space through which the subclavian vessels and the brachial plexus exit the neck to the upper extremity is termed the *thoracic outlet*. Its borders are composed of the chest wall, clavicle, and scalene muscles.

Thoracic outlet syndrome is defined by abnormal compression of vascular and neural structures at the base of the neck. Mechanical compression can result from cervical ribs, ligaments, hypertrophy of strap muscles, and positional changes that affect the first rib. Symptoms rarely appear in childhood but manifest during adulthood. Some patients describe a history of trauma. It is thought that changes in normal structural relationships between the first rib and overlying neurovascular structures develop over time. These abnormal orientations produce intermittent compression of the subclavian or axillary vessels and the trunks of the brachial plexus. Symptoms can be divided into neurologic, arterial, and venous components. Neurologic symptoms such as paresthesia, pain, and numbness are the most overwhelming symptoms. Arterial symptoms include intermittent ischemia. Long-term sequelae of circulatory changes include subclavian artery stenosis, reflex poststenotic dilatation, and emboli. Venous compression causes thrombosis, which leads to edema, cyanosis, and pain. This occurs intermittently, acutely after exertion (effort thrombosis), or as post-thrombotic intermittent obstruction. Common clinical manifestations include numbness, pain, and paresthesias, which are dependent on shoulder position. Symptoms are most aggravated by hyperabduction or downward traction (hyperextension) of the shoulder girdle. A physical examination may demonstrate muscle atrophy of the hand, a bruit over the subclavian artery with abduction, upper extremity edema, or absent pulses. The Adson's test produces a radial pulse deficit with abduction of the arm and rotation of the head to the opposite direction. A positive Tinel's test occurs with reproduction of neurologic symptoms by percussion of the brachial plexus in the supraclavicular fossa.

The evaluation usually includes plain radiographs and angiography. The diagnosis is made by arteriogram with subclavian or axillary artery stenosis with abduction. A poststenotic lesion identified on arteriogram aids in confirming the diagnosis. Venograms of the arms may reveal a beaklike appearance of the vein proximal to the first rib when the arm is in the affected position.

Treatment of thoracic outlet syndrome begins with physical therapy and posture training. Surgical treatment is reserved for patients who fail 3 to 6 months of conservative treatment and for patients with vascular sequelae such as stenosis, aneurysm, and thrombosis. Surgical decompression is composed of transaxillary resection of the first rib with excision of the anterior scalene muscle and fibrous tissue. Surgical reconstruction is warranted in the case of arterial stenosis and aneurysm. Venous thrombosis is treated with thrombectomy plus optional venous reconstruction or stent placement.

Part X
Breast

65
Breast Anatomy

The human breast is located on the anterior chest wall between the subcutaneous fat of the skin and the superficial fascia of the pectoralis muscle. Its superior and inferior boundaries are composed of the second rib and the sixth intercostal cartilage, respectively. Beneath the breasts lie the pectoralis major and minor muscles. The pectoralis minor muscle is enveloped by the clavipectoral fascia that projects into the axilla to combine with the axillary fascia.

The breast tissue itself is composed of stromal supportive elements, glandular epithelium, and adipose tissue. The predominant tissues present in childhood are the stromal elements and epithelium. These are replaced with fat as the female ages. The shape and contour of the breast is produced by dense connective tissue bands called *Cooper's ligaments*. These bands traverse the breast tissue and anchor themselves to the underlying skin and fascia. The breast tissue forms a central disc that lies directly beneath the nipple/areola complex. A tail of breast tissue extends toward the axilla from the central disc called the *tail of Spence*. The nipple is a nodular elevation found in the center of the areola. The areola itself is darkly pigmented in contrast to the surrounding breast tissue. Its surface is lined by tiny nodules called *Montgomery's elevations*. These structures are responsible for sebaceous gland and sweat secretion onto the surface of the areola and nipple. This provides protective immunoglobulin A and lubrication needed for nursing. The dermis of the areola contains smooth muscle and elastic tissue to aid in nipple erection and lactation.

Elaborate systems of ducts are present that extend downward and out in a radial pattern beginning at the nipple/areolar complex. The milk ducts just beneath the areola are enlarged to form lactiferous sinuses. These sinuses connect to a series of 10 to 15 ducts that exit the nipple. The lactiferous sinuses are connected to approximately 40 lactiferous ducts that together form a lobulus. At the lower depths of each lobulus, the elaborate branching network ends in spaces called *acini*.

The acini in combination with the small efferent ductules are called *lobules*. The acini are the functional units for milk production under the influence of prolactin. Myoepithelial cells surround the alveoli and ductal system and contract when stimulated by oxytocin to eject the milk. The basement membrane comprises a continuous layer surrounding epithelial and myoepithelial elements.

Lymphatic flow travels from the nipple and skin to a subareolar complex of lymph vessels called *Sappey's plexus*. The lymphatic drainage then continues through the breast parenchyma via the interlobular lymphatics. Approximately 75% of lymphatic flow from the breast enters the axillary lymph system. The medial lymph node groups drain a small portion of the rest. The axillary lymph nodes are grouped into three levels. Level I encompass the nodes that lie lateral to the pectoralis minor muscle in association with the axillary vein and central axilla. Level II nodes are found beneath the pectoralis minor muscle. Level III nodes are located in the subclavicular and are medial to the pectoralis minor.

The axilla contains many important neural and vascular structures that must be preserved during dissection. The long thoracic nerve travels along the chest wall medial to the axilla. It is responsible for innervation of the serratus anterior. The serratus anterior functions to adduct the scapula. Injury to the long thoracic nerve produces the classic winged scapula deformity (abduction of the scapula). The thoracodorsal nerve arises beneath the axillary vein and courses along the lateral border of the axilla. It is responsible for innervation of the latissimus dorsi. The pectoralis major muscle is innervated by the medial pectoral nerve found at the lateral boundary of the pectoralis minor muscle. The intercostal brachial nerve traverses the center of the axilla and provides sensory innervation to the skin of the upper underarm and chest. Innervation of the breast itself is accomplished through the lateral and anterior cutaneous branches of intercostal nerves 2 through 6. Limited innervation is supplied to the upper breast through the cervical plexus.

The principal blood supply of the breast is derived from perforating branches of the internal mammary artery, the lateral branches of the posterior intercostal arteries, and branches of the axillary artery. The venous drainage follows the same course as its arterial counterparts.

66
Breast Complaints

Gynecomastia

Gynecomastia is defined as the hypertrophy of male breast tissue. Most cases of gynecomastia are idiopathic. The condition tends to occur in males with a bimodal age distribution. Pubertal hypertrophy takes place in males aged 13 to 17 years. Hypertrophy is often bilateral and is seldom painful. Most cases end with regression of hypertrophy; therefore, reassurance is all that is needed. Surgical resection is reserved for cases that fail to regress and are aesthetically unpleasant.

Senescent hypertrophy involves men over 50 years of age and generally involves only one breast. Physical examination reveals a firm, symmetric, disc-shaped mass underlying the areola. The condition can be painful in some cases. These characteristics are in direct contrast to signs of cancer (painless mass, asymmetric, and fixed to surrounding tissue). Development of senescent gynecomastia can be due to systemic disease states (cirrhosis, renal failure, malnutrition) and drug side effects (digoxin, thiazides, phenothiazines, theophylline, and estrogens). No treatment is required due to the self-limited nature of this condition.

Nipple Discharge

Nipple discharge from the breast of a nonlactating female is a common occurrence. Nipple discharge and carcinoma are rarely associated. Important information to elicit from the patient includes unilateral versus bilateral discharge, the number of orifices producing the discharge, and the nature of the discharge (milky or bloody).

Bilateral milky nipple discharge is generally due to galactorrhea. Excess prolactin hormone is responsible for galactorrhea in patients without a recent history of lactation. An elevated serum measurement of the prolactin level confirms the diagnosis.

Unilateral nonmilky nipple discharge from single ductal orifices requires further investigation. Less than 10% these cases are associated with cancer; however, there are several characteristics that increase a patient's risk. These include bloody or hemoglobin-positive discharge, the presence of a palpable mass, and a recent abnormal mammogram. Intraductal papilloma is the most common etiology for unilateral single-duct bloody nipple discharge. Surgical biopsy is warranted to establish the diagnosis.

Unilateral discharge from multiple ductal orifices is caused by a number of benign conditions. The most common condition is subareolar duct ectasia, which is a condition of inflammation and dilation of the subareolar collecting ducts. Fibrocystic change is another benign condition that can be associated with multiple-duct nipple discharge.

Breast Pain

Pain in the breast tissue is a common complaint of women seeking medical treatment. Reassurance of the patient is important, because only about 5% of breast cancer cases are associated with breast pain. Breast pain is often influenced by hormonal fluctuations that accompany abnormal menstrual cycles. Other causes include fibrocystic change, which in the past has been attributed to caffeine, nicotine, and antihistamine use. However, scientific evidence to support these associations is lacking.

Galactocele

A galactocele is defined as a round, well-circumscribed, mobile breast cyst that contains milk. Galactoceles develop 6 to 10 months after lactation ends. The lesions are thought to develop from milk ducts clogged with inspissated milk. The cysts tend to occur in central locations or beneath the nipple. Needle aspiration is generally the only treatment needed. Aspiration frequently produces a thick dark fluid with the consistency of cream. Surgical excision is warranted for lesions that cannot be aspirated or that develop infection.

67
Benign Breast Disease

Fibrocystic disease can manifest as diffuse breast pain that is often bilateral. It affects women mainly in the second and third decades of life and regresses at menopause. Cysts develop from dilated lobules and terminal ductules. They appear as dark unilocular structures that are lined with epithelium. Histologic evaluation of the epithelium may reveal apocrine metaplasia. However, these lesions are rarely associated with malignancy. Multiple palpable tender masses may be present. The pain seems to coincide with menstrual activity. Many patients report cyclic pain that increases during the second half of their cycle and begins to decrease after menses begins. The size of the cyst often fluctuates during the menstrual cycle due to hormonal influence. The cystic component is confirmed by ultrasound. The size of the cysts varies from microscopic disease to several centimeters. Large cysts should be aspirated. Cyst fluid only needs to be sent for cytology if a residual mass is present after aspiration. Cysts that contain bloody fluid should be resected. Frequent aspirations may be necessary. Symptomatic cysts that fail to resolve after several aspirations should be excised. These lesions generally pose no risk of cancer unless they are associated with dysplasia.

Fibroadenomas are benign tumors composed of stromal and epithelial components. They typically occur in young females (teenagers to those in their thirties). Clinically they appear as firm, mobile 2 to 3 cm masses. Giant fibroadenomas are fibroadenomas greater than 5 cm. These tumors have a well-developed capsule separating them from the surrounding breast tissue. They are differentiated from cysts by the absence of fluid on attempted aspiration or by ultrasound. Carcinoma is extremely rare and, when present, occurs in the form of lobular carcinoma *in situ*. Management includes observation or surgical excision. Observation is usually recommend for women in their twenties or younger with an examination consistent with fibroadenomas. Another option is to obtain core-needle biopsy specimens of the lesions. Lesions identified as fibroadenomas without dysplasia can be watched. Surgery to exclude cancer may be indicated for older women (>35 years). Excisions are accomplished through circumareolar incisions to optimize cosmesis.

Sclerosing adenosis has an appearance similar to carcinoma. The lesions are fibrous acinar structures containing microcalcifications, which can be seen on mammography.

Radial scar can resemble breast carcinoma as well. The lesions are composed of deformed lobules with a characteristic radial scar radiating from the center. The lesions can occur in multiple areas of one breast or bilaterally as well. There is no malignant association.

Ductal ectasia is characterized by periductal scar formation caused by inflammation. The ductal system becomes injured by dilation and fibrosis. Clinically, palpable nodules can be detected beneath the nipple/areola complex. Nipple discharge is common. On mammography, calcifications of the ductal structures are seen giving the appearance of malignancy. Women who are approaching menopause or who are in late menopause are affected.

Hamartomas are abnormal collections of normal tissue. Breast hamartomas are composed of tightly grouped lobules with ectatic ducts. They are very similar in appearance to fibroadenomas.

Tubular adenomas are composed of small collections of glands that lack associated stroma. The glands are formed from tubular structures packed closely together. Clinically, they appear as fine nodules. A similar condition occurs during pregnancy, called *lactating adenoma*.

Intraductal papillomas are papillary projections of epithelium that occur within the lumen of large ducts. The masses vary in size and can be multiple or continuous within the duct. The epithelium can exhibit atypical hyperplasia and even ductal carcinoma *in situ*. Unilateral serosanguinous or bloody discharge typically occurs. The malignancy risk is greater when intraductal papillomas are present and even greater when multiple papillomas occur. Management includes ductography to help identify the affected duct. At the time of operation, the breast is palpated to stimulate nipple discharge. A lacrimal duct probe is inserted into the involved duct as a marker. The nipple areola complex is elevated through a circumareolar incision. The ductal complex is excised circumferentially below the nipple.

Nipple adenomas are lesions localized within the nipple. They resemble papillomas and can have hyperplastic characteristics.

68
Invasive Breast Cancer

Ductal carcinoma is the most common malignant neoplasm in the breast. Clinically, most infiltrating ductal carcinomas present as a mass or a density on mammogram. Microcalcifications on mammography are common. Invasive lobular carcinoma originates in the breast lobules and comprises 3% to 15% of invasive breast cancers. Lobular carcinoma presents in an identical fashion to ductal carcinoma and has no distinguishing mammographic features.

The gold standard for evaluation of the breast remains the surgeon's clinical examination and mammography. A bilateral mammogram should be obtained when a patient presents with any breast problem. In addition, ultrasound and magnetic resonance imaging (MRI) have utility in diagnosing breast disease.

For breast biopsy, fine-needle aspiration (FNA) is a simple office procedure and is the least invasive. However, FNA requires an excellent cytologist to interpret the material. Fine-needle aspiration is becoming increasingly popular for sampling clinically or ultrasound-suspicious axillary lymph nodes. Core biopsy provides a histologic diagnosis and has been established as the procedure of choice for breast biopsy. It can be performed in the office on clinically detected lesions, with ultrasound guidance, or with a stereotactic machine for mammographically detected nonpalpable lesions. Based on its minimally invasive nature, core biopsy helps preserve the integrity of the breast. This ensures that lumpectomy and radiation, along with mastectomy and reconstruction, can be performed with maximal treatment and cosmetic effectiveness. Breast integrity is also critical to the accuracy of the sentinel lymph node biopsy. Excisional biopsy should be used only when core biopsy is unsuccessful in obtaining sufficient tissue. Incisional biopsy should rarely be performed.

The pathologic evaluation of breast cancers should specify the tumor size, status of surgical margin, estrogen and progesterone receptor contents, and histologic grade. Modern evaluation also includes measurement of DNA content and an estimation of the proliferation fraction of S phase.

The extensive systemic workup for breast cancer is not appropriate for most early-stage breast cancer patients. A good clinical history and examination, mammogram, chest x-ray, and routine blood studies should suffice as an initial workup for most patients. Should a patient present with evidence of locally advanced disease, have pathologically positive lymph nodes, or raise concerns through clinical symptoms at the initial workup, a metastatic workup is indicated.

Most early-stage invasive breast cancers should be treated with breast conservation, lumpectomy, and radiation therapy. Local recurrence rates are high after lumpectomy if radiation therapy is omitted. Relative contraindications to breast conservation include (1) large breast cancers relative to small breast size, (2) inability to receive radiation therapy, and (3) multicentric disease. Several trials suggest without reservation that lumpectomy with radiation therapy is the appropriate choice for most women with invasive breast cancer. Excising the tumor and obtaining adequate margins around the cancer while preserving cosmetic integrity are the primary goals of the surgeon. A 2 to 3 mm margin is considered minimally adequate. The specimen should be handled carefully so that its integrity and its orientation are maintained. A two-point orientation system in the operating room is recommended, with sutures marking the anterior and lateral aspects of the specimen for the pathologist. The pathologist, using colored ink, then designates six margins, which include anterior, posterior, medial, lateral, superior, and inferior. Positive or close margins can, therefore, be more accurately and efficiently dealt with.

Axillary sampling should be performed in most cases of invasive disease. Sentinel lymph node biopsy has become the standard of care for determining the status of the ipsilateral axilla. All women with stage I and stage II breast cancer without clinically positive lymph nodes should be considered for sentinel lymph node biopsy. An axillary dissection should be performed for a positive sentinel lymph node or for a clinically suspicious axilla.

For patients who meet the requirements for mastectomy, strong consideration is given to immediate reconstruction. Implants and autologous tissue transfers are the mainstay of breast reconstruction. Among autologous tissue transfers, reconstruction of the transverse rectus abdominis muscle (TRAM) flap is widely popular. The type of cancer should have little impact on the decision of the plastic surgeon except in situations of locally advanced cancer in which postmastectomy radiation will be used. Patients with locally advanced breast cancer should delay reconstruction until all treatments for the cancer have been completed.

Systemic Therapy

All women with invasive breast cancer should give consideration to systemic adjuvant therapy for breast cancer. These include chemotherapy and hormone therapy and should be based on the patient's age, menopausal status, general condition, and tumor prognostic factors. The fundamental assumption that underlines the addition of systemic therapy (chemotherapy and hormonal therapy) to local treatment of breast cancer by surgery or radiation is that metastatic disease is the principal cause of death of breast cancer patients. Chemotherapy for operable breast cancer was initially studied in patients with positive lymph nodes. The results showed significant benefit for women undergoing chemotherapy who were younger than 50 years of age. Subsequent studies showed that postmenopausal women also benefit, but to a lesser extent, from chemotherapy.

A significant number of node-negative patients also suffer from recurrence of breast cancer after primary treatment. It is likely that certain characteristics of the primary tumor are associated with greater chance of metastasis and treatment failure. Most studies of adjuvant chemotherapy in node-negative patients are restricted to patients with markers of poor prognosis. These poor prognostic signs include (1) tumor size greater than 2 cm, (2) poor histologic and nuclear grade, (3) absent hormone receptors, (4) high proliferative fraction (S phase), (5) aneuploid DNA content, and (6) content of certain oncogenes such as *erbB-2* (HER2/*neu*).

Neoadjuvant chemotherapy refers to chemotherapy given in addition to surgery or radiation (local therapies), which precedes local treatments. Neoadjuvant therapy can achieve high response rates and may permit conservative surgery in advanced breast cancer. There are reasons to apply this treatment to earlier stages of disease. For lower tumor burden, the probability of drug-resistant cells is theoretically less. Therefore, investigators have treated earlier stage patients with preoperative chemotherapy. However, no survival benefit was demonstrated for patients who received preoperative chemotherapy compared with the same regimen delivered postoperatively. Whereas the preoperative approach may not offer survival advantage, it provides an *in vivo* assessment of tumor response. The magnitude of this response has independent prognostic significance and may guide subsequent systemic therapy. For patients who do not respond adequately, oncologists might consider additional treatment in the form of non–cross-resistant drugs.

For patients with hormone receptor–positive tumors, antiestrogen hormonal therapy is an important component of the treatment plan. Available therapies are aimed at modulating the ability of the estrogen receptor to bind estrogen (tamoxifen) or at decreasing the production of estrogen (ovarian ablation or aromatase inhibitors).

Endocrine organ ablation has been replaced by antiestrogen therapy for most patients. The drug tamoxifen is an estrogen agonist–antagonist and is currently the first-line treatment for estrogen-sensitive breast cancer. Tamoxifen is a weak estrogen agonist. In molar excess, tamoxifen acts like a competitive antagonist of estrogen activity in the breast but not in other estrogen-sensitive tissues. Both the beneficial and unfavorable actions of tamoxifen in tissues other than the breast are caused by its estrogenlike actions. Tamoxifen can replace oophorectomy for premenopausal women with estrogen receptor–positive metastatic cancer, and it is considered the first choice of drug for premenopausal and postmenopausal patients with estrogen receptor–positive or progesterone receptor–positive cancers. Tamoxifen is the only agent that has been recognized as effective for the prevention of contralateral breast cancer and primary cancer in women at high risk, including hormone receptor–positive women who have received local treatment for ductal carcinoma *in situ*. Current recommendations prescribe tamoxifen treatment for women with a 5-year projected breast cancer risk of more than 1.7, as assessed by the Gail model. Tamoxifen has been associated with a number of side effects, including increased vasomotor symptoms and, more rarely, thromboembolic complications and endometrial cancer.

Aminoglutethimide is an aromatase inhibitor that blocks steroidogenesis. It has replaced adrenalectomy in the treatment of advanced breast cancer. Recently, second-generation aromatase inhibitors (anastrozole, letrozole) have been developed. These are more specific aromatase inhibitors that block the conversion of androgens to estrogens without the side effects associated with more global steroid blockade. These drugs have replaced aminoglutethimide and are the second line of agents after tamoxifen for advanced disease.

Guidelines for adjuvant therapy after primary treatment of breast cancer have evolved toward extending treatment recommendations to more patients. Therefore adjuvant chemotherapy is likely to benefit nearly all patients with invasive breast cancers, and hormonal adjuvants probably benefit all breast cancer patients with estrogen receptor–positive or progesterone receptor–positive cancers. A risk/benefit ratio must be estimated for each patient, in which the reduction in risk of recurrence is weighed against the morbidity of treatment. Some form of adjuvant therapy should be considered for nearly all patients with invasive breast cancer. An exception is made for patients with very favorable tumors (<1 cm in size), for whom side effects of cytotoxic treatment may outweigh benefits. For older patients, the benefits of chemotherapy are generally less, and the ability to deliver optimal therapy is made more difficult by other physical impairments. For elderly patients, the decision to administer adjuvant chemotherapy should be made on an individual basis. Adjuvant tamoxifen is recommended for estrogen receptor–positive or progesterone receptor–positive cancers, and treatment is continued for 5 years. Although remarkably free of toxicity, a slightly increased incidence of endometrial cancer and venous thrombosis are the major complications of tamoxifen. Tamoxifen should not be routinely recommended for receptor-negative tumors. Aromatase inhibitors may play a role in the adjuvant treatment of breast cancer, but the current standard remains tamoxifen.

Locally Advanced and Inflammatory Carcinoma

Locally advanced breast cancer generally refers to stages IIIa and IIIb. Central to the concept is the notion that the disease is advanced on the chest wall (T3–T4) and/or in the regional lymph nodes (N1 or N2), but without distant metastasis. The treatment of locally advanced breast cancer is changing. When surgery is used alone, the cancer recurs in 30% to 50% of patients, and the long-term cure rate does not exceed 30%. Similar results are reported with radiation therapy alone. These poor results indicate that locally advanced breast cancer is actually metastatic

in most cases. New approaches use chemotherapy to reduce the size of the primary tumor; this is called *neoadjuvant chemotherapy*. This approach can downstage the primary tumor, improve local control, and treat metastatic disease.

Inflammatory breast cancer presents with erythema and warmth that extends over a large area of the breast. This may or may not be associated with a palpable mass. The pathologic hallmark is dermal lymphatic permeation by the tumor cells and is designated as category T4d in the TNM classification. Axillary nodal metastases are often present. Metastatic disease should be sought with a bone scan and CT. In the past, inflammatory breast carcinoma was universally fatal. New treatment protocols use intensive chemotherapy as the first treatment modality. Objective response rates are in the range of 60% to 80%, and most patients are rendered free of disease after mastectomy and nodal dissection. Therefore, the approach used in many medical centers includes a sequence of chemotherapy, mastectomy, and radiation for inflammatory breast carcinoma.

Metastatic Disease

When breast cancer recurs, it is generally thought to be incurable, with a median life expectancy between 18 and 24 months. Despite aggressive approaches, such as high-dose chemotherapy, distant metastatic disease is probably not curable. Nonetheless, breast cancer is often sensitive to both chemotherapy and hormonal therapy, offering disease control for many patients. Tamoxifen is the first choice among the antiestrogens for patients with metastatic, hormone-sensitive breast cancer. The recent development of new aromatase inhibitors (anastrozole, letrozole, exemestane), with few side effects, has moved these agents to second-line therapy. For most patients with metastatic breast cancer, chemotherapy is indicated. Although more toxic than hormonal therapy, chemotherapy may improve quality of life. In general, cyclophosphamide and doxorubicin are first-line agents. The taxanes (paclitaxel, docetaxel) have essentially replaced other drugs as second-line therapy for most patients because of their considerable single-agent activity and toxicity profiles.

69
Noninvasive Breast Cancer

It is theorized that all cases of invasive breast cancer go through a period in which epithelial cells undergo malignant transformation but do not "invade" the basement cell membrane. The basement membrane is the crucial anatomic structure that defines invasion, and the diagnosis of an *in situ* lesion necessitates multiple sections to exclude invasion. Frozen section is rarely relied on. Noninvasive breast carcinoma includes lobular carcinoma *in situ* (LCIS) and ductal carcinoma *in situ* (DCIS). These entities have distinct clinical, biologic, and therapeutic considerations.

The lobular elements of the breast from which LCIS originates are not present in males, and this form of noninvasive cancer is found only in females. Lobular carcinoma *in situ* is an incidental pathologic finding in breast tissue that has been removed for other reasons. It has no mammographic features and does not manifest as a palpable mass. The average age at diagnosis is 45 years, which is 15 years younger than the average age at which invasive breast cancer is diagnosed. More than 90% of women with LCIS are premenopausal. Lobular carcinoma *in situ* occurs 12 times more often in white women than in black women. The disease process often is observed in breast biopsy specimens that harbor microcalcifications. However, LCIS is not associated with these calcific sites, and it typically occurs in surrounding tissues that are clinically and radiologically normal. This "neighborhood calcification" is a feature unique to LCIS that contributes to its diagnosis. Lobular carcinoma *in situ* is considered a *marker* for increased risk rather than an inevitable *precursor* of invasive disease. It has a known statistically significant rate of bilateralism that has been reported to be as great as 90%. *Multicentricity* refers to occult malignancies located outside the quadrant of the primary (index) tumor. Lobular carcinoma *in situ* has a high rate of true multicentricity that may approach 100%.

The consensus for treatment of LCIS is lifelong surveillance. This entails monthly self-examinations, regular clinical examinations, and annual mammography. The goal of observation is to detect subsequent invasive cancers that develop in a minority of patients. Subsequent malignancy may be lobular or ductal, but most cases are ductal carcinoma, which occurs in both ipsilateral and contralateral breasts. The relative risk of developing an invasive carcinoma depends on the age of the patient at the time of diagnosis. There is a trend toward greater risk in younger patients. This age-related increased risk of developing invasive cancer following the diagnosis of LCIS should be considered when formulating treatment options. There is no demonstrable benefit to widely excising LCIS and obtaining clear margins, because the disease is assumed to diffusely involve all breast tissue as well as the contralateral breast. If operation is chosen, anything less than total mastectomy is inappropriate, because the disease process is diffuse. In LCIS, both breasts are considered a single field at risk for development of invasive carcinoma. Bilateral mastectomy may be considered for women with a family history of breast cancer consistent with *BRCA-1* or *BRCA-2* hereditary patterns.

The clinical implications of DCIS and LCIS are distinctly different. While LCIS is a marker of increased risk for subsequent breast cancer in all breast tissue, DCIS is a malignant lesion requiring surgical treatment. The risk for invasive cancer from DCIS is considered to be in the range of 30% to 50% over 10 years. The future cancers are observed in the ipsilateral breast, usually in the same quadrant as the original biopsy, suggesting that DCIS is a true precursor of its invasive counterpart. Ductal carcinoma *in situ* is the most common histologic variant of noninvasive carcinoma. It is observed predominantly in the female but constitutes approximately 5% of all breast cancers in men. Most patients present with DCIS in early menopausal years. Unlike LCIS, DCIS typically presents as microcalcification on mammographic screening, and it represents up to 5% of palpable breast cancers. In contrast to LCIS, DCIS is associated with only a 10% to 15%

incidence of bilaterality and multicentricity in approximately one-third of patients. The earliest phases of DCIS are characterized by proliferation of the inner cuboidal layer of the epithelial cells in major lactiferous ducts to form papillary ingrowths within the lumen. With growth of the "papillary pattern" of DCIS, ingrowths coalesce to fill the ductal lumen until scattered rounded spaces remain interspersed among solid clumps of cells. This is termed the *cribriform* growth pattern of DCIS. In contrast, a *solid* histologic pattern of DCIS is recognized when cellular growth obliterates these spaces, and the ducts become distended with anaplastic cells. With continued growth, these cells outstrip their blood supply, become necrotic, and lead to the classic *comedo*. In the comedo variant, calcium deposition generally occurs in areas of necrosis, leading to typical DCIS radiographic manifestations.

A two-class system of DCIS classification has been proposed to guide therapy. The system distinguishes comedo from noncomedo subtypes of DCIS. The hallmark of the comedo type of DCIS is the predominant necrosis, large pleomorphic nuclei, and numerous mitotic figures. This pattern of DCIS has a significantly higher degree of nuclear grade, multicentricity, and microinvasion, suggesting that its biologic behavior is more aggressive than the papillary or solid types. Other indicators of aggressive biologic behavior and poor prognosis associated with comedo DCIS are high DNA proliferative activity, *C-erbB-2* oncogene amplification, and overexpression of HER-2/*neu* oncogene activity. Distinction should also be made between grossly palpable and microscopically nonpalpable variants of DCIS to plan appropriate therapy more rationally. Compared with nonpalpable or microscopic presentation, large palpable forms of DCIS have occult invasive rates up to 46%, higher rates of local recurrence, multicentricity, axillary nodal metastases, and poor survival rates. The evaluation of a patient with DCIS should also involve an assessment of the extent of the lesion. Magnification mammography is essential for this evaluation. Conventional mammography underestimates the extent of DCIS by 2 cm in 47% of cases. The use of magnification views reduces this discrepancy. An accurate determination of lesion size allows preoperative selection of those patients who are appropriate candidates for breast preservation and minimizes the number of surgical procedures that are needed to achieve an adequate negative margin. Margin assessment is another facet of determining the extent of DCIS. Postexcision mammography for calcification lesions complements margin assessment to determine the adequacy of the surgical resection.

Treatment options for DCIS include mastectomy, wide local excision with radiation, and wide local excision alone. The recurrence rate after total mastectomy is less than 2%. This is the standard against which breast conservation is compared. Mastectomy for DCIS is simple or total mastectomy without removal of the ipsilateral axillary node. The rationale for total mastectomy is based on the risk of multicentric disease in DCIS. The risk of multicentric disease depends on the size, pathologic extent, and histologic type of the intraductal tumor. All cases of tumors >5 cm are associated with multicentricity. The lowest rate of multicentricity is associated with the solid and cribriform types of tumors. It is prudent to offer mastectomy for lesions that carry a substantial risk of local/regional recurrence and reduced survival (palpable mass > 25 mm, comedo histology, extensive multicentricity, multifocality, high nuclear grade, negative estrogen and progesterone receptor studies, and aneuploid DNA pattern). Two clear indications for mastectomy for DCIS are women with two or more primary tumors or with diffuse malignant-appearing microcalcification and patients with persistent positive margins after reasonable surgical attempts.

Breast-sparing therapy may be offered to women with DCIS when uncertainties and risks are fully discussed. Postoperative radiotherapy is recommended after conservation treatment. However, it is important to remember that postoperative radiation reduces but does not eliminate the recurrence of cancer in cases of positive margins after local excision. No role currently exists for use of cytotoxic chemotherapy in this disease. Comprehensive lifelong surveillance is indicated for the contralateral breast in women previously treated for DCIS. Although there is no uniform management plan for the axilla in cases of DCIS, certain recommendations can be made. The axilla is not treated in patients with DCIS undergoing breast conservation surgery. For patients with lesions large enough to require mastectomy, a sentinel node biopsy can be performed. This is done in case permanent sectioning of the mastectomy specimen shows foci of invasion.

70
Inflammatory Breast Cancer

Inflammatory carcinoma is one of the most aggressive malignancies of the breast. The key features of the condition include rapid onset of erythema, edema, and warmth of the breast. The underlying carcinoma has a diffuse infiltrating pattern without forming a discrete mass. The skin overlying the lesion has the classic "peau d'orange" appearance caused by the invasion of dermal lymphatics. Congestion within the lymphatic system results in edema of the skin. The appearance can be confused with acute mastitis and can delay the diagnosis.

The diagnosis is often made clinically and confirmed with skin punch biopsies. The pathologic hallmark is the presence of tumor cells within the dermal lymphatics. The tumor commonly metastasizes to axillary lymph nodes, causing palpable lymphadenopathy in most patients. Thirty-five percent of patients have obvious metastasis at the time of diagnosis.

The median survival without treatment for this disease is 9 to 12 months. The overall 5-year survival rate with optimal therapy approaches 50%. The best results are obtained with a combination of systemic therapy, radiation, and surgery. The treatment protocol begins with aggressive chemotherapy and proceeds to modified radical mastectomy. The addition of radiation therapy to the regimen decreases the incidence of local and regional recurrences. The response to chemotherapy is an important predictor of survival. Patients without residual tumor following neoadjuvant chemotherapy are predicted to have an 80% chance of being disease-free after 5 years. Breast conservation therapy has been offered as an alternative to radical resection. However, cosmetic outcomes are generally poor, and local recurrence rates are higher than with radical resection.

71
Phyllodes Tumor

Phyllodes tumor of the breast, or cystosarcoma phyllodes, is a soft tissue tumor of the breast. This type comprises only 1% of malignant breast tumors. Phyllodes tumors are characterized by neoplastic growth of stromal and mammary epithelium. The lesions can occur at any age, but they are more prevalent in the sixth decade. Most cases present as a palpable mass. Most of these tumors are benign lobulated masses ranging 2 to 40 cm in size. Similar to fibroadenomas, phyllodes tumors arise from intralobular stroma. Histologically the tumors resemble fibroadenomas, but, unlike fibroadenomas, the stromal component is more cellular, with clefts lined with epithelium resembling leaflike structures.

Biologically, phyllodes tumors can be benign, intermediate, or malignant. Wide local excision is generally adequate therapy for benign and intermediate tumors. Malignant varieties are treated similar to sarcomas with en bloc resection (i.e., total mastectomy). In these cases, axillary lymph node dissection is not required because of the low incidence of nodal metastasis. Features that distinguish malignant from benign tumors include larger tumor size, cellular atypia, and mitotic activity. Eleven percent to 20% of benign tumors recur locally after excision. High-grade malignant tumors have frequent local recurrence as well as distant hematogenous metastasis in one-third of cases.

72
Male Breast Cancer

Breast cancer accounts for less than 1% of all cancers in men. Most breast cancers in men present as patient-detected breast masses. The goals of surgical treatment are local control and disease staging. Late detection of the disease remains a problem and is likely a result of failure to consider the diagnosis, often by both the patient and the physician.

Certain risk factors have been associated with male breast cancer. The incidence of the disease increases with age, with the median age at diagnosis in the midsixties. The disease is more common in persons of Jewish heritage. Hepatic schistosomiasis is said to be associated with an increased risk. Radiation to the chest has also been associated with breast cancer in both men and women. A diagnosis of benign gynecomastia is not associated with increased risk of breast cancer. States of increased estrogen exposure, such as severe liver disease, obesity, and exposure to exogenous estrogens, have been associated with breast cancer in men. Conditions of decreased testosterone have also been implicated. Mumps orchitis after age 20 years, undescended testes, orchitis, and infertility have been associated with a small increase in the risk of breast cancer. Klinefelter's syndrome (47,XXY karyotype) is phenotypically characterized by underdeveloped secondary sexual characteristics, azoospermia, gynecomastia, and low testosterone levels. It is associated with at least a 20-fold increased risk of breast cancer. A family history of breast cancer is elicited from 15% to 20% of men with breast cancer. Both *BRCA-2* and, to a lesser extent, *BRCA-1* gene mutations have been associated with breast cancer in men. Persons with these genetic abnormalities usually have a striking family history of breast cancer, may present at an unusually young age, and may occasionally have bilateral cancers.

Terminal lobules are normally absent in men. As in women, most cancers arise from cells that line the ducts of the breast. The most common histology of breast cancer is invasive ductal carcinoma. This accounts for about 90% of breast cancers in men. *In situ* ductal carcinomas are well described, being often of the papillary type and of low to intermediate grade. In men, about 85% of breast cancers are estrogen-receptor positive, and receptor positivity appears to be more common in older men. As in women, estrogen-receptor positivity is associated with a better prognosis. About 95% of breast cancers in men are androgen-receptor positive. HER-2/*neu* is positive in fewer than 20% of all male breast cancers.

The most common presentation of male breast cancer is a painless breast mass. There is often nipple abnormality, such as nipple retraction, ulceration, discharge, or bleeding. Nipple discharge is uncommon as the sole presenting sign of breast cancer but should always be regarded as pathologic in men. The most common cause of a breast mass in a man is gynecomastia. Gynecomastia is a common benign condition that occurs at any age but is most common in adolescents and the elderly. Gynecomastia often presents as a movable, tender, rubbery mass and can be either unilateral or bilateral. In general, breast cancers tend to have a harder consistency than gynecomastia and, in an advanced stage, can directly invade skin and muscle.

Any breast mass in a man warrants evaluation, with a focus on the history of the mass, family history of cancers, medication history, and possible sources of estrogen exposure. The examination focuses on the characteristics of the mass, including size, consistency, and relationship to the skin and pectoral muscle. The regional nodes are examined. Before biopsy, diagnostic mammography and ultrasound are sometimes useful to further characterize the lesion. Any discrete mass requires a biopsy to establish a definitive diagnosis. A radiologic-guided core-needle biopsy is usually preferred because of its simplicity and accuracy. For a patient with benign disease, it can provide definitive diagnosis without a trip to the operating room. For a patient with cancer, it can make the diagnosis in an office setting so that the cancer can be addressed in a single trip to the operating room. Fine-needle aspiration can be considered when expert cytopathologists are available. If a fine-needle aspiration is indeterminate, core-needle biopsy or excisional biopsy is warranted. A standard chest x-ray and liver enzyme studies are appropriate for systemic evaluation. Bone scans, computed tomography, or other studies are pursued if a patient presents with locally advanced breast cancer, if abnormalities are found in the chest x-ray or liver enzyme studies, or if the patient has concerning symptoms.

The goals of surgical treatment include locoregional control and staging. The primary surgical therapy is usually total mastectomy. Radical mastectomy should be considered only when there is direct extension into the pectoral muscle. The lymph node status is a strong prognostic factor. Because decisions about systemic therapy are often influenced by the node status, investigation of the regional nodes is important. If a patient presents with suspicious palpable adenopathy, preoperative evaluation can be undertaken by ultrasound-guided fine-needle aspiration. For a patient with clinically negative nodes, surgical staging is appropriate. Sentinel node biopsy has been described for male patients and can be undertaken at the same time as the mastectomy. If sentinel node biopsy is unavailable, axillary dissection is reasonable. For patients with positive sentinel nodes, axillary dissection for completion of staging and for regional control is indicated. Locoregional therapy sometimes includes radiotherapy to decrease the risk of local recurrence. Postmastectomy radiotherapy is undertaken when the primary tumor is large, when there are microscopically positive margins, or when there are four or more positive regional nodes.

Postoperative systemic adjuvant therapy is considered for men with a primary tumor of at least 1 cm or with disease metastatic to regional lymph nodes. Because most breast cancers in men are receptor positive, hormonal therapy with tamoxifen or other hormonal agents is often indicated. Side effects of hormonal agents can be problematic. About 20% of patients discontinue tamoxifen because of hot flashes, decreased libido, mood changes, or venous thrombosis. Patients with systemic metastases are generally treated with hormonal therapy if their tumor is receptor positive or with chemotherapy for patients with receptor-negative disease or with receptor-positive disease refractory to hormonal agents.

Part XI
Skin Malignancy

73
Melanoma

Melanoma is a skin and sometimes a mucosal neoplasm generated from neural crest–derived melanocytes. Melanomas comprise only 4% to 5% of all skin cancers but are responsible for most skin cancer deaths. Most lesions are found in the skin (90%). Other sites of origin include the eye (5%); mucosal surfaces such as oropharynx, genitals, and esophagus (1% to 2%); and unknown sites of origin (2%).

The clinical features can be remembered by the "ABCDE" pneumonic:

A = Asymmetric shape
B = Irregular borders
C = Color variation (black, brown, red, blue, or white)
D = Diameter <6 cm
E = elevation

The rapid enlargement of a previously existing mole and itching or pain are other clinical manifestations of melanoma.

The neoplasm occurs more commonly in Caucasians. The lesions often appear within the fourth and fifth decades and increase with age. Men are affected more often than women. Sun exposure increases the risk of developing melanoma. Ultraviolet radiation is the most harmful component of sunlight. Ultraviolet B affects the skin by causing increased melanin production, allowing the skin to burn. Ultraviolet A penetrates to the dermis of the skin, causing changes in the connective tissue leading to loss of elasticity and wrinkling. Early childhood sun exposure and sunburns increase the risk for melanoma. Other conditions that predispose someone to melanoma include dysplastic nevi, giant nevi, congenital nevi, Spitz nevi, xeroderma pigmentosum, family history of melanoma, and history of previous skin cancer types other than melanoma.

Radial and vertical growths are the two major growth patterns. Radial growth involves horizontal spread through the epidermis and superficial areas of the dermis. Vertical growth involves the downward spread of the lesion through the dermis. During this phase of growth the lesion becomes more massive, and metastasis becomes possible.

Melanomas are grouped into four major histologic categories based on their pattern of growth and location. Superficial spreading melanoma comprises 90% of cutaneous melanomas. These lesions appear flat because of their radial growth pattern. Over time, they thicken with vertical growth. Itching, bleeding, and ulceration develop in untreated lesions. Lentigo maligna melanoma occurs most often in older persons with sun-damaged skin. They appear as flat, darkly pigmented lesions that develop slowly over time. The lesions tend to stay superficial and therefore have a better prognosis. Acral lentiginous melanoma appears on the subungual surfaces and the palms and soles as well. Their appearance can be confused with subungual hematomas, which can delay the diagnosis. These lesions occur most often in blacks and have a poor prognosis due to late diagnosis. Nodular melanomas develop with an early vertical growth pattern and become thick lesions. The prognosis is poor for patients with nodular melanomas because of their tendency for vertical growth.

The major prognostic factors for melanoma include thickness, ulceration, number of mitotic figures, degree of tumor-infiltrating lymphocytes, gender, location, and regression. Tumors that are thinner than 1.7 mm, have few mitotic figures, are located on the extremity, possess tumor-infiltrating lymphocytes, have no signs of regression, and occur in women have a better prognosis. Typically melanomas appear on the lower extremities of women and on the trunk, head, or neck of men. The thickness of the lesion (Breslow measurement) correlates directly to local recurrence risk, metastasis, and survival rate.

Clinical evaluation begins with a biopsy of the lesion. Biopsy specimens should be full thickness down to the level of the subcutaneous fat with a 1 to 2 mm margin of normal tissue. The size of the lesion determines the method of biopsy. Biopsy procedures can be done in the office using local anesthesia or as an outpatient surgical procedure. When possible the lesion should be completely excised during the biopsy. Large lesions or lesions located near sensitive areas, such as on the face, can be evaluated using punch biopsies. Punch biopsies must be full thickness with a margin of normal tissue also. If the lesion is large enough, an additional full thickness punch biopsy should be taken through the thickest portion of the lesion. Shaved biopsies should not be used for melanomas, because they do not provide the pathologist with enough tissue to ascertain the depth of the melanoma. Wounds from biopsy procedures on the extremity should be closed longitudinally. Large defects can be closed with rotational flaps or skin grafting.

The thickness of the lesion is one of the most important prognostic factors. Thickness is evaluated using two different scales, the Clark level classification (Table 73.1) and the Breslow classification. The Clark level system classifies tumor invasion with respect to histologic skin layer. The Breslow system classifies tumor invasion according to its vertical depth in millimeters. The Breslow system has been shown to have better correlation with prognosis and is easier to reproduce between pathologists. Melanoma staging is done in accordance with the TNM classification system.

A patient with melanoma should have a thorough evaluation for metastatic disease. This includes a complete history and physical examination along with inspection of regional lymph nodes for lymphadenopathy. Chest x-ray and measurement of lactate dehydrogenase are useful for patients with clinically apparent stage II or III disease. Biopsy of the primary lesion as described above provides useful information for planning the definitive treatment. Lesions that are less than 1 mm thick should be widely excised with 1 cm margins of normal tissue. This treatment is associated with a low risk for local recurrence. Tumors measuring 1 to 4 mm in depth are excised with 2 cm margins of normal tissue. Local recurrence is estimated at 2.1% over 10 years with 2 cm margins compared with a local recurrence rate of 2.6% for 4 cm margins. Therefore, there is no added benefit to resection of margins beyond 2 cm. Similarly, retrospective data have shown that lesions greater than 4 mm deep should be resected with 2 cm margins.

TABLE 73.1. The Clark level system of tumor classification with respect to histologic layer and prognostic factors.

Clark level	Histologic layer	Prognostic factors
1	Limited to epidermis, *in situ*	No metastatic risk
2	Extends to papillary dermis	Low metastatic risk
3	Fills papillary dermis	High risk for metastases
4	Extends to reticular dermis	High mortality
5	Extends to subcutaneous fat	High mortality

In the past, elective lymph node dissection was done routinely in conjunction with wide local excision of the primary lesion. Using recent data, it was determined that tumors less than 1 mm posed little risk for nodal metastasis. Tumors 1 to 4 mm showed a greater risk for nodal metastasis but less risk for distant metastasis. Tumors larger than 4 mm showed a propensity for distant and regional metastasis. The use of sentinel lymph node biopsy has changed the treatment of melanoma and lymphatic disease. Tumors greater than 1 mm in depth routinely undergo sentinel lymph node biopsy for staging and treatment planning purposes. Patients with lymph node metastasis are offered lymph node dissections.

Follow-up treatment for melanoma includes a thorough physical examination at 3 to 6 month intervals over the course of 3 years. Recurrent disease occurs locally, regionally, or systemically. Regional lymph node disease is the most common type of recurrence. Patients develop palpable lymphadenopathy in areas that were previously negative clinically. Fine-needle aspiration (FNA) is the modality of choice for making the diagnosis. When FNA fails to determine the diagnosis, an excisional biopsy should be done. A metastatic evaluation should include a computed tomography (CT) scan of the head, chest, abdomen, and pelvis. Complete lymph node dissection should be performed in patients with lymph node metastases. The 5-year survival rate with regional lymph node recurrence is only about 50%.

Local recurrence is the appearance of an additional lesion within a 5 cm radius of the original lesion. The thickness of the original lesion is the most important prognostic factor for local recurrence. Lesions less than 0.76 mm have a 0.2% rate of local recurrence, lesions measuring 0.76 to 1.49 mm have a 2% risk, lesions measuring from 1.5 to 3.99 mm have a 6% risk, and lesions measuring greater than 4 mm have a 13% risk. The long-term survival rate for patients with local recurrence is dismal, only 20%. Local recurrence is treated with surgical resection with histologically clear margins. Extensive surgical resection has no influence on long-term survival rate because of the high propensity of distant metastasis with these lesions.

Sites for distant metastasis include the brain, lung, and liver. Less common sites of occurrence include the bone, skin, and gastrointestinal tract. The workup should include CT and positron emission tomography (PET) scans. When multiple sites of metastasis are discovered, systemic therapies such as dacabazine (DTIC), interferon-α, and interleukin-2 are appropriate for some patients. Single metastases in areas such as the lung, adrenal gland, and gastrointestinal tract can be resected. Skeletal metastasis can improve with radiation therapy.

Less than 10% of melanomas arise from noncutaneous sites. These include the eye (5%) and mucosal surfaces (1.5%) such as the anogenital region, oropharynx, esophagus, and meninges. Two percent of all melanomas are discovered as metastases with no obvious primary lesion. Ocular melanomas are the most common primary neoplasm of the eye. They are derived from melanocytes within the retina or uvea. Lymph node metastasis is a rare occurrence. Distant metastasis is common in the liver. Local therapy includes photocoagulation and radiation. Surgical excision ranges from partial resection to enucleation.

Mucosal lesions carry a poor prognosis compared with their cutaneous counterparts. This is mainly attributed to delayed diagnosis and advanced disease at the time of discovery. They are generally treated with surgical resection limited to histologically clear margins without lymphatic dissection. Lymph node dissection is reserved for cases of clinically evident lymphadenopathy and for vulvar melanoma. The 5-year survival rate for mucosal lesions is only about 10%.

74
Nonmelanoma Skin Malignancies

Basal cell carcinoma is the most common type of malignant neoplasm in the world. Its incidence, like that of most other skin malignancies, is increasing. There are several patterns or types of basal cell carcinomas, including nodulocystic, pigmented, and superficial. The nodulocystic type accounts for more than 70% of basal cell carcinomas. The lesions are typically well-defined, waxy, cream-colored nodules with rolled pearly edges. Central ulceration and telangiectasias over the surface often occur. Pigmented basal cell carcinomas can range from tan to black, and the appearance can be difficult to distinguish from melanomas.

Basal cell carcinomas are very slow growing and rarely metastasize. Although mortality rates are quite low with basal cell carcinoma, the tumors can grow large and cause extensive local destruction if left untreated. Small lesions frequently are ablated with either curettage or electrodesiccation in an outpatient office setting; however, this practice does not allow for confirmation of the diagnosis or knowledge of appropriate margins. Surgical resection with 2 to 4mm margins is the preferred treatment and often can be done with local anesthesia. Moh's technique can be used for surgical resection. This technique involves serially excising small amounts of tumor with immediate pathologic evaluation with the goal of removing the complete tumor with the least sacrifice of uninvolved tissue. This process, although tedious and time consuming, is beneficial to prevent disfigurement in areas of the face where there is minimal redundant tissue. Another treatment option is injection of the lesion with interferon. Although this treatment is frequently effective in halting the progression of the tumor, rarely does the lesion go away, and it requires several injections. Radiation therapy is another option for people who do not want surgical excision. Studies have demonstrated cure rates similar to surgery; however, there is often damage to the surrounding skin, and the radiated skin is at a higher risk of developing further skin malignancies.

The prognosis for basal cell carcinoma is quite good because it rarely metastasizes. However, when it metastasizes, median survival is less than 1 year. The greatest risk for metastasis is a lesion that has grown large or a lesion that has been repeatedly or incompletely resected.

Squamous cell carcinoma, occurring less often than basal cell carcinoma, has a considerably higher mortality rate due to its tendency to invade surrounding tissues and metastasize. They appear as areas of thickened, red, scaling skin that can be ulcerated. Typically the lesions develop from a proliferation of keratin cells in the epidermis, which clinically appears as small red or pink areas called *actinic keratoses*. These lesions are considered premalignant, although only 1 in 1,000 converts to a malignant lesion. Actinic keratoses can develop into Bowen's disease, which is squamous cell carcinoma *in situ* and appears as a plaquelike thickening. The most common cause of squamous cell carcinoma is excessive ultraviolet radiation from prolonged sun exposure. Other known causes of squamous cell carcinoma are exposure to arsenic, organic hydrocarbon, ionizing radiation, cigarette smoke, and impaired-cell mediated immunity. The *p53* tumor suppressor gene is mutated in over 90% of squamous cell carcinomas.

Treatment for squamous cell carcinoma is basically the same as for basal cell. Surgical excision is the standard treatment, with 1 cm margins being the goal. The thickness of the lesion correlates with the biologic behavior of the tumor. Lesions greater than 4mm deep are more likely to recur locally, and metastasis is more likely if the lesion is greater than 10mm. Squamous cell carcinomas that occur in burn scars (Marjolin's ulcer), areas of chronic osteomyelitis, and areas of previous injury have a tendency to metastasize earlier. Regional lymph nodes are typically the first site of metastasis, and, for that reason, regional lymph node dissections are indicated if there are clinically palpable nodes or if the primary lesion is in a chronic wound. Metastatic disease is a very poor prognostic indicator, with 10-year survival rates of only

13% compared with cure rates of more than 90% with nonmetastatic disease.

Merkel cell carcinoma is a primary neuroendocrine cancer of the skin. It is associated with synchronous or metachronous squamous cell carcinoma in 25% of cases. The lesion appears on the skin as a rapidly growing, red-blue nodule and is most commonly located on the head or neck area. Histologically, the tumor is indistinguishable from small cell carcinoma of the lung, and a chest radiograph is recommended to rule out a primary lung cancer. Merkel cell carcinoma is extremely aggressive, with high rates of local recurrence and metastasis. Treatment involves wide local excision with 3 cm margins with prophylactic regional lymph node dissection and adjuvant radiation therapy, because lymphatic spread has occurred in up to one-third of patients at the time of initial presentation. The prognosis for Merkel cell carcinoma is poorer than for malignant melanoma, with mortality rates reported as 55% to 80%.

Important aspects of all skin lesions are the need for biopsy specimens, excision with appropriate margins, and close clinical follow up for patients with skin malignancies because the 5-year risk of developing additional skin cancers after initial diagnosis is more than 50%. Most skin malignancies have high cure rates if they are treated early.

75
Soft Tissue Sarcomas

Sarcomas are a classification of tumors that usually arise from embryonic mesoderm but can also originate from the ectoderm. Sarcomas are rare, accounting for less than 1% of adult cancers and approximately 7% of cancers in the pediatric population. Soft tissue sarcomas are the most common. The other types are osteosarcoma, chondrosarcoma, Ewing's sarcoma, and peripheral primitive neuroectodermal tumors. More than half of soft tissue sarcomas occur in the extremities, with others occurring (in descending frequency) in the trunk, retroperitoneum, and head and neck. The most common histologic types in adults are (in decreasing frequency) malignant fibrous histiocytoma, leiomyosarcoma, liposarcoma, synovial sarcoma, and peripheral nerve sheath tumors. Rhabdomyosarcoma is the most common type of soft tissue sarcoma in children.

The most important risk factor for developing sarcomas is external radiation therapy, which causes an 8- to 50-fold increase in incidence. Other risk factors include chemical carcinogens, such as home herbicides, Thorotrast, vinyl chloride, and arsenic, as well as genetic mutations. Mutations in the oncogenes *n-myc*, *MDM2*, and *c-erb B2* and in tumor suppressor genes *RB* and *p53* are associated with increased rates of sarcomas.

The clinical presentation is often an asymptomatic mass. The location of the mass usually determines its size and symptoms. Tumors in the distal extremities are discovered while relatively small, whereas masses in the proximal limbs or retroperitoneum can be quite large before they are noticed. Common symptoms of tumors in the limbs include pain and edema caused by compression of the bone and the neurovascular structures. With retroperitoneal masses, obstructive gastrointestinal and neurologic symptoms are caused by the tumor compressing the bowel or pelvic nerves.

The diagnostic workup should include imaging studies, with computed tomography (CT) scan preferable for retroperitoneal masses and magnetic resonance imaging (MRI) for extremity masses. Ultrasonography is used in addition to MRI to delineate the mass from adjacent vascular structures. Once imaged, a tissue biopsy specimen must be obtained by fine-needle aspiration, core biopsy, incisional biopsy, or excisional biopsy. Accuracy rates of fine-needle aspiration are 60% to 96%; however, it requires an experienced cytopathologist. Core needle biopsy usually yields ample tissue and an accurate diagnosis with very small complication rates. Computed tomography guidance is used to increase the positive yield rate and to sample tumors that might be otherwise inaccessible. Incisional biopsy procedures are used when adequate tissue cannot be obtained by fine-needle aspiration or core needle biopsy because the mass is deep or the tumor is greater than 3 cm in diameter. Excisional biopsy can be used for lesions less than 3 cm; however, it provides no benefit over other biopsy techniques.

Staging and prognosis are based on histologic grade, tumor size, and presence of nodal or distant metastasis. In addition, the pathologic classification is important for prognosis, because the metastatic potential is quite different for the different types of sarcomas. The most important prognostic factor is histologic grade, which ranges from well differentiated to poorly or undifferentiated. A tumor size of 5 cm is a prognostic factor. In extremity tumors, the depth of invasion and the relationship to the investing fascial plane are also prognostic factors. Nodal metastasis is quite rare with sarcomas and warrants a stage IV classification. The most common site for metastasis is the lung, which is treated with resection and chemotherapy. Other sites of metastasis include bone, brain, and liver, with the liver being most common when the primary tumor is retroperitoneal. Metastasis usually occurs within 3 years of the initial diagnosis of the primary sarcoma.

Treatment for sarcomas is based on the histologic diagnosis and typically involves a multimodality approach. For tumors less than 5 cm (T1 lesions), wide local excision with a 2 cm negative margin is the primary treatment. If wide margins are not possible due to anatomic constraints, radiation therapy is added for local control. For extremity lesions, limb-sparring procedures with radiation should be attempted. In less than 5% of cases of extremity sarcomas, all of the gross tumor cannot be resected. In these cases, the limb should be amputated. Minimal survival benefit for adjuvant chemotherapy has been reported. Recurrences of the primary tumor should be treated with repeated resection with the same goals of wide margins and removal of all gross tumor.

Retroperitoneal sarcomas are most commonly liposarcomas and tend to be very large. More than half of patients with retroperitoneal sarcomas have masses greater than 20 cm at the time of initial diagnosis. In addition to using the standard imaging studies, lymphoma or germ cell tumors should be ruled out because these also manifest as large retroperitoneal masses. This can be done by looking for symptoms of lymphoma, such as night sweats or palpable lymphadenopathy, by performing a careful testicular examination and by measuring germ cell tumor markers such as lactate dehydrogenase, β-human chorionic gonadotropin, and α-fetoprotein. The 5-year survival rate for retroperitoneal sarcomas is 40% to 50% and is based predominantly on the ability to obtain negative margins at the time of resection. Negative margins are often difficult to obtain due to the size of most tumors and the proximity to vital structures. Chemotherapy and radiation have not been shown to be beneficial for these sarcomas. Retroperitoneal sarcomas are much more likely to have local recurrence than to metastasize.

Gastrointestinal stromal tumors (GIST) comprise the majority of gastrointestinal sarcomas. The interstitial cell of Cajal is believed to be the origin of these tumors. The tumor marker for GIST is *c-kit*. In the past, complete resection with negative margins was the treatment goal. Five-year survival rates ranged from 20% to 75% depending on the tumor stage and the ability to get adequate negative margins. Recently, imatinib mesylate, a selective *c-kit* inhibitor, has been used with great success to treat advanced GIST.

76
Lymphoma

Lymphomas are classified as one of two major types, Hodgkin's or non-Hodgkin's. Both types can occur in any lymphoid tissue or organ, such as the stomach, pancreas, small bowel, or thyroid. Non-Hodgkin's lymphoma has an incidence of 50,000 cases per year. It is a proliferation of any of the lymph cell types, including T cells, B cells, and natural killer cells. Non-Hodgkin's lymphoma is classified by location and course as being nodal or extranodal and indolent, aggressive, or very aggressive. Indolent cases can be asymptomatic, whereas more aggressive lymphomas manifest with pain, fever, night sweats, and swelling caused by vessel obstruction. Diagnosis is made by careful history and physical examination, chest radiograph, abdominal and pelvic computed tomography (CT) scans, biopsy of involved lymph nodes, and a bone marrow biopsy. Surgical staging is not necessary. The only surgical intervention is splenectomy for patients with splenomegaly to relieve mass effect symptoms and improve cytopenias.

Hodgkin's lymphoma is a malignancy of the lymphoid system and is identified by the presence of Reed-Sternberg cells. The incidence is approximately 7,500 cases a year in the United States, with young men accounting for most of the cases. Nearly all patients have supradiaphragmatic lymphadenopathy. Mediastinal nodes can be quite large and cause symptoms of shortness of breath, cough, or obstructive pneumonia. Although occult spread to the spleen is common, massive splenomegaly is rare. Unlike non-Hodgkin's lymphoma, surgical staging is important for Hodgkin's lymphoma, especially for clinical stage I or II disease and no symptoms. The staging procedure involves a wedge liver biopsy procedure, splenectomy, bone marrow biopsy procedure, and sampling of retroperitoneal, mesentery, and hepato-duodenal ligament lymph nodes. The four histologic types of Hodgkin's lymphoma are lymphocyte predominant, lymphocyte depleted, nodular sclerosis, and mixed cellularity. Staging is based primarily on location, with stage I disease being confined to a single anatomic region and

stage II occurring in two or more regions on the same side of the diaphragm. In stage III, there is involvement on both sides of the diaphragm; however, disease is limited to lymph nodes, spleen, or Waldeyer's ring, which is a ring of lymphoid tissue formed by the lingual, palatine, and nasopharyngeal tonsils. Stage IV denotes involvement of the bone marrow, skin, lung, liver, gastrointestinal tract, or any organ or tissue not mentioned in stage III classification. Treatment is based on stage. Early-stage Hodgkin's lymphoma without splenic involvement can be treated with radiation. More advanced disease with splenic involvement requires chemotherapy.

Lymphoma is the most common malignancy in the mediastinum. The mediastinum is the primary site in approximately 50% of patients with lymphoma. The anterior compartment is typically involved, with the middle compartment and hilar nodes occasionally involved. Treatment is nonsurgical with chemoradiation. Cure rates are reported to be 90% for patients with early Hodgkin's and up to 60% for patients with a more advanced disease stage.

Gastric lymphoma is the most common site for lymphoma of the gastrointestinal tract; however, it accounts for less than 2% of lymphomas. Symptoms include vague epigastric pain, early satiety, and fatigue. Anemia is present in half of patients at the time of diagnosis, although overt bleeding is rare. The peak incidence is in the sixth and seventh decades of life, with a 2:1 male to female predominance. Gastric lymphoma can occur in any portion of the stomach but usually arises from the antrum. Risk factors for the development of gastric lymphoma are immunodeficiencies and *Helicobacter pylori* infection. Epstein-Barr virus infection is associated with Burkitt's lymphoma, which is a very aggressive gastric lymphoma affecting younger people and often arising from the cardia. There are many pathologic subtypes of gastric lymphoma, which affect the management and prognosis of the disease. Over half are diffuse, large B cell lymphomas, and 40% are extranodal marginal cell lymphoma. The less common types include Burkitt's, mantle cell, and follicular lymphomas and account for less than 5% of gastric lymphomas.

Gastric lymphomas are often identified on endoscopic examination performed for unresolving gastrointestinal symptoms. Lymphomas present endoscopically as nonspecific areas of gastritis or gastric ulceration, with discrete masses rarely identified. A biopsy specimen should be obtained, although a biopsy can be nondiagnostic because of submucosal growth patterns. Endoscopic ultrasound is also helpful to determine the depth of the gastric wall invasion and to identify patients at higher risk for perforation. *Helicobacter pylori* testing should be performed with histology and, if the result is negative, should be confirmed by serology. A metastatic workup should be started, including an upper airway examination, bone marrow aspirate, and a CT scan of the chest and abdomen. A biopsy should be performed for lymphadenopathy identified clinically or on CT scan.

A variety of treatment options are used. Most treatments rely on a multimodality approach. Currently many patients are treated with chemotherapy plus radiation with little indication for surgical resection. The chemotherapeutic combination used most is CHOP, consisting of cyclophosphamide, hydroxydaunomycin, Oncovin, and prednisone. Radiation is more useful for smaller tumors because of the high rate of late complications such as stricture, enteritis, and secondary tumor formation. In general, there is little role for radiation for younger patients with tumors larger than 6 cm. The only role for surgical resection is for isolated stage IE or IIE disease when the tumor is confined to the gastrointestinal tract or spread is limited to regional lymph nodes and when it is believed that all gross tumor can be resected. Disseminated disease cannot be cured surgically; therefore, surgery is only indicated to obtain a tissue sample for diagnosis, for repairing perforations, or for resecting bulky tumors that cause bleeding or obstruction. Recent studies have shown that early-stage mucosal-associated lymphoid tumors (MALT) and limited diffuse large B cell gastric lymphomas can be treated with *H. pylori* eradication. Careful follow-up studies with repeated endoscopic examination are needed to confirm eradication of the infection and to document regression.

Thyroid lymphomas are usually non-Hodgkin's B cell lymphomas and account for less than 1% of thyroid malignancies. This disease usually develops in patients with chronic lymphocytic thyroiditis, although it can be part of a generalized lymphoma. Patients have a rapidly enlarging, painless neck mass, which can cause dysphonia, dysphagia, dyspnea, or even respiratory distress. The diagnosis is made with a fine-needle aspiration, core needle biopsy, or open biopsy procedure. Thyroid lymphoma should be staged to assess for extrathyroidal spread. Treatment is with CHOP and radiation. Surgical intervention with thyroidectomy and lymph node resection is reserved for symptom relief for patients who do not respond quickly to chemotherapy and radiation. Prognosis is based on the histologic grade of the tumor and on the presence of extrathyroidal spread. The overall 5-year survival rate for thyroid lymphoma is approximately 50%.

Primary lymphomas can occur in the pancreas, although this is rare. Patients with pancreatic lymphoma have symptoms similar to those of pancreatic adenocarcinoma. A percutaneous CT-guided biopsy or endoscopic ultrasound-guided biopsy procedure can be used to make the diagnosis. There is no role for surgical resection. Treatment is with chemotherapy. Endoscopic stenting can relieve jaundice caused by common bile duct obstruction.

Part XII
Gastrointestinal Disorders

77
Esophageal Anatomy and Physiology

The esophagus has three functional components: the upper esophageal sphincter (UES), the esophageal body, and the lower esophageal sphincter (LES). The main function of the esophagus is to transport swallowed material from the pharynx into the stomach. Meanwhile, reflux of gastric contents into the esophagus is prevented by the LES, and the entry of air into the esophagus with each inspiration is prevented by the UES. The UES remains closed by tonic contraction of the cricopharyngeus muscle. The UES is 2.5 to 4.5 cm in length and has a mean basal resting pressure of 42 mm Hg. Its duration of relaxation with swallowing is 0.5 to 1.2 seconds. The striated muscles of the cricopharyngeus and the upper third of the esophagus are activated by efferent motor fibers through the vagus nerve and its recurrent laryngeal branches. Integrity of the nerve supply is essential for the coordinated function of the UES. Intact innervation is required for the cricopharyngeus to relax in coordination with the pharyngeal contraction and to resume its resting tone once a bolus has entered the upper esophagus. Operative damage to the innervation can interfere with cricopharyngeal function and predispose the patient to aspiration. The tonic contraction of the UES is also depressed during deep sleep or anesthesia.

Three types of contractions are seen in the esophagus. Primary peristalsis is progressive and is triggered by voluntary swallowing. Secondary peristalsis is also progressive, but it is generated by distention or irritation, not by voluntary swallowing. Tertiary contractions are nonprogressive, simultaneous contractions that can occur spontaneously between swallows. As the swallowed bolus enters the esophagus from the pharynx, a primary peristaltic wave is activated that transverses the esophageal body and propels the swallowed material from the pharynx into the stomach in a progressive manner. Normally, primary peristaltic contraction follows 97% of all swallows. In contrast to the upper and lower esophageal sphincters, the esophageal body has no motor activity in the resting state. Pressure within the body of

the esophagus is a reflection of negative intrathoracic pressure, being most negative (–5 to –10 mm Hg) during deep inspiration and highest (0 to 5 mm Hg) during expiration. Esophageal peristaltic pressure ranges from 20 to 100 mm Hg.

If the entire swallowed bolus of food does not empty from the esophagus into the stomach, secondary peristaltic waves are initiated. These contractions, like the primary waves, are progressive and sequential. Secondary peristaltic waves begin in the smooth muscle segment of the esophagus and continue until retained intraesophageal contents are emptied into the stomach. Therefore, in contrast to the primary wave, the secondary contraction is not initiated by a voluntary swallow, but is initiated by local distention of the esophagus. Afferent impulses from receptors within the esophageal wall go to the swallowing center. If the esophagus is distended, a wave of contractions begins with closure of the upper esophageal sphincter and sweeps down the esophagus. Continuity of the esophageal muscle is not necessary for sequential activation if the nerves are intact. If the muscles, but not the nerves, are cut across, the pressure wave begins distally below the cut as it stops at the proximal end above the cut. This allows a sleeve resection of the esophagus to be done without destroying its normal function. Anchoring of the esophagus at its inferior end is required for efficient aboral propulsion to take place. Loss of the inferior anchor, as in cases of large hiatal hernia, can lead to inefficient propulsion.

Tertiary contractions are simultaneous, nonprogressive, nonperistaltic waves that can occur throughout the esophagus and represent uncoordinated contractions of the smooth muscle that are responsible for the classic "corkscrew" appearance of esophageal spasm on barium swallow examination. Tertiary waves do not have a physiologic function and are often observed in elderly people and in patients with esophageal motility disorders.

Overall, the antireflux mechanism is composed of three components: a mechanically effective LES, an efficient esophageal clearance, and an adequately functioning gastric reservoir. A deficiency in any of these components can cause reflux, with increased esophageal exposure to gastric juice and mucosal injury. The term *lower esophageal sphincter* may give the impression that there is a defined anatomic sphincter such as the pylorus. Anatomically, no such LES has been defined. However, manometry has defined an elevated distal esophageal resting pressure that is 3 to 5 cm in length. Physiologically, this serves as the barrier against abnormal regurgitation of gastric contents into the esophagus and represents a functional sphincter. Therefore, the LES is more accurately referred to as the *LES mechanism* or the distal esophageal *high-pressure zone* (HPZ).

The factors responsible for maintaining competence of the LES are not entirely clear, but the presence of an intra-abdominal segment of distal esophagus, under the influence of positive intra-abdominal pressure, appears crucial to the success of most antireflux operations. Normal resting pressure within the HPZ ranges from 10 to 20 mm Hg. Mean HPZ pressures less than 6 mm Hg and overall sphincter length less than 2 cm are likely to be associated with incompetence of the LES and gastroesophageal reflux. The sphincter actively remains closed to prevent reflux of gastric contents into the esophagus and opens by a relaxation that coincides with a pharyngeal swallow. The LES pressure returns to its resting level after the peristaltic wave has passed through the esophagus.

The competence of LES depends on several factors. The most significant is its resting pressure. The LES intrinsic myogenic tone is modulated by neural and hormonal mechanisms. α-Adrenergic neurotransmitters and β-blockers stimulate the LES, and α-blockers and β-stimulants decrease its pressure. It is not clear to what extent cholinergic nerve activity controls LES pressure. The vagus nerve carries both excitatory and inhibitory

fibers to the esophagus and sphincter. The hormones gastrin and motilin have been shown to increase LES pressure; and cholecystokinin, estrogen, glucagon, progesterone, somatostatin, and secretin decrease LES pressure. Peppermint, chocolate, coffee, ethanol, and fat are all associated with decreased LES pressure and can be responsible for esophageal symptoms after a sumptuous meal. Of equal importance to its competence is the ability of the LES to respond to variations in intra-abdominal pressure. These elevations normally are transmitted to the sphincter causing it to collapse and remain closed provided sufficient length of the sphincter remains intra-abdominally. Therefore, the overall length of the LES remains an important determinant of its competence.

Not all gastroesophageal reflux is pathologic. During 24-hour esophageal pH monitoring, episodes of gastroesophageal reflux have been detected in healthy individuals. This physiologic reflux is more common when awake and in the upright position than during sleep in the supine position. When reflux occurs, normal subjects rapidly clear the acid gastric juice from the esophagus. There are several explanations for the fact that physiologic reflux in normal subjects is more common in the upright position than during sleep in the supine position. Gastric juice can reflux when a swallow-induced relaxation of the LES is not protected by an oncoming peristaltic wave. The average frequency of these "unguarded moments" or of transient losses of the gastroesophageal barrier is far less while asleep and in the supine position than while awake and in the upright position. In addition, in the upright position, there is a 12 mm Hg pressure gradient between the resting, positive intra-abdominal pressure measured in the stomach and the most negative intrathoracic pressure measured in the esophagus at the mid-thoracic level. This gradient favors the flow of gastric juice up into the thoracic esophagus when upright. The gradient diminishes in the supine position.

78
Esophageal Function Tests

Esophageal function tests are used to evaluate and diagnose esophageal motility disorders. Symptoms warranting esophageal function tests are dysphagia, heartburn, and nonburning chest pain. Esophageal manometry and pH monitoring are the major tests used to diagnose esophageal motility disorders.

Esophageal manometry is used to measure pressures generated in the esophagus and esophageal/gastric junction during swallowing. Indications for its use include diagnosis, clarification of other study results, preoperative evaluation, and postoperative confirmation of successful treatment. The study is performed using a flexible catheter with pressure sensors located at various positions along its length. The catheter is introduced, the lower esophageal sphincter pressure and location are determined, and the other sensors measure the amplitude, duration, and coordination of the esophageal response to swallowing. In the normal esophagus the resting intraesophageal pressure is less than that in the stomach with the exception of the elevated pressure in the lower esophageal sphincter, which is typically located in the last 3 to 5 cm of the esophagus proximal to the junction with the stomach. A normal swallow produces a wave of contraction down the esophagus at a rate of approximately 3 to 4 cm per second. When the peristaltic wave reaches the lower esophageal sphincter, a relaxation occurs in the sphincter allowing for passage of the fluid or solid bolus into the stomach.

Several esophageal motility disorders can be diagnosed with esophageal manometry. Achalasia has a very diminished or even absent peristaltic wave. The lower esophageal sphincter pressure is elevated and relaxes less than 50%. Passing the catheter through the lower esophageal sphincter is often difficult because of the dilated esophagus and the closed gastroesophageal junction. In fact, readings are often misinterpreted because the operator falsely assumes that the catheter is in the lower esophageal sphincter when it is really proximal. Treatment for achalasia is based on lowering the lower esophageal pressure either by surgical intervention or, for less severe cases, with botulinum toxin injections.

Diffuse esophageal spasm is another disorder in which the esophageal contractions are uncoordinated, especially in the distal esophagus. Because the degree of dysmotility can vary from swallow to swallow, definitive diagnosis with manometry can be difficult. Nutcracker esophagus is a dysmotility disorder that presents clinically with episodes of severe chest pain and dysphagia. The manometry studies demonstrate normal peristaltic waves with normal configuration, but the waves have abnormally high amplitudes (greater than 180 mm Hg). Sclerodermatous esophagus is a connective tissue disease affecting the smooth muscle of the esophagus, resulting in uniformly weak or even absent contractions. The manometry characteristics are very similar to those of achalasia except that the lower esophageal sphincter tone is also low or absent. Patients with this disorder are at high risk for developing gastroesophageal reflux disease.

Gastroesophageal reflux disease is not diagnosed based on manometry, but there are findings that can suggest patients are predisposed to developing significant reflux. The lower esophageal sphincter in patients with gastroesophageal reflux disease usually has a lower than normal pressure (approximately 6 mm Hg) and is shorter than normal. In addition, patients with gastroesophageal reflux disease often have nonpropagated contractions in the distal esophagus that can prolong esophageal acid exposure after reflux.

New technologies have been applied to basic esophageal manometry in an attempt to address shortcomings. Provocative studies, such as manometry while swallowing a solid bolus, accurately demonstrate dysmotility. Agents, such as edrophonium, are used during manometry to evoke the chest pain symptoms associated with esophageal dysmotility. Topographic mapping of the esophagus can be done by using numerous and closely spaced sensors to show subtle variations in peristaltic wave progression. Ambulatory esophageal manometry allows for more readings and can record symptomatic episodes that rarely occur during the brief evaluation sessions.

Esophageal pH monitoring studies are used to confirm the diagnosis of gastroesophageal reflux disease when atypical symptoms are present and to measure the response to therapy. Monitoring usually involves placing an acid-sensitive probe in the esophagus 5 cm above the lower esophageal sphincter. The probe usually remains in place for 24 hours for continuous monitoring. A measured pH of less than 4 is considered a reflux event. Normal patients have episodes of reflux, so criteria have been established to determine what constitutes abnormal reflux. The factors considered are the following: the total amount of time the pH is less than 4 during the 24-hour period, the amount of time the pH is less than 4 while the patient is in various positions (supine and upright), the total number of events, the number of events lasting more than 5 minutes, and the longest duration of a reflux episode.

Evaluation of esophageal symptoms often includes both manometry and pH monitoring. The three most common symptoms warranting esophageal function tests are dysphagia, chest pain, and suspected reflux disease. The evaluation for dysphagia should start with a barium swallow to evaluate both structure and function. If this study is abnormal, then manometry, continuous pH monitoring, and endoscopy follow. With chest pain it is first necessary to rule out cardiac disease, lung disease, musculoskeletal pain, and anxiety disorders. If these are ruled out and the patient has symptoms of reflux, a trial of proton pump inhibitors is prescribed. If the symptoms do not resolve, the patient needs manometry and pH monitoring. If these demonstrate severe reflux, the patient should undergo endoscopy and biopsy to evaluate for erosive esophagitis, stricture formation, or Barrett's esophagus. Patients with documented reflux that does not respond to proton pump inhibitors may be candidates for antireflux surgery. Pre- and postoperative pH monitoring are recommended for these patients. If the patient responds to the initial proton pump inhibitor trial, consideration should still be given to endoscopy to confirm that the esophagitis has resolved, especially for patients who require chronic proton pump inhibitor therapy.

79
Esophageal Perforation and Injury

Perforation of the esophagus is a relatively uncommon problem; however, it requires immediate attention and surgical intervention. Historically, mortality from esophageal perforation ranged from 15% to 50%. This number depends on both the site of injury and time from initial presentation to diagnosis and treatment.

Esophageal perforation is an emergency because treatment delay reduces survival. Iatrogenic perforation, spontaneous perforation, and trauma account for most esophageal perforations. Endoscopic procedures are the most common cause of iatrogenic esophageal perforation, with the cricopharyngeal area most often injured. Mid and distal esophageal perforations are usually caused by biopsy procedures to document malignancy or from dilatations. Infrequent causes of iatrogenic esophageal perforation include difficult endotracheal intubation, blind insertion of a minitracheostomy, resection of lung cancer, blind dissection of the abdominal esophagus, operations on the cervical spine, thyroidectomy, and palliative intubation, stenting, or laser treatment of esophageal tumors. Boerhaave's syndrome, esophageal rupture caused by straining, is the most common type of spontaneous perforation. Ruptures usually occur in the left posterior aspect of the lower esophagus and occur five times more often in males. Severe reflux, caustic ingestion, and candidal, herpetic, and immunodeficiency infections also cause pathologic perforations. Destruction of the esophageal wall by carcinoma can cause mediastinal or pleural perforations. Esophageal perforations from penetrating or blunt trauma are often overshadowed by associated injuries and have a poor prognosis if unrecognized. In some studies, up to 60% of patients who sustain esophageal perforation have some underlying esophageal pathology, ranging from benign strictures to malignancy.

Patients with esophageal disruption have a variety of symptoms depending on the mechanism or location of injury and on the time interval from injury to treatment. Symptoms and signs of esophageal perforation (pain, vomiting, hematemesis, dysphagia, tachypnea, tachycardia, fever, subcutaneous emphysema, mediastinal crunch, chest hypersonarity, or dullness) vary with cause, location (cervical, thoracic, or abdominal), and pathway of soilage. Pain is the most common symptom, present in 70% to 90% of patients, usually referring directly to the site of perforation. Severe chest pain after straining and hematemesis occur with postemetic ruptures. Tachycardia and tachypnea are documented in most patients with perforation. Hypotension and shock are present when sepsis or significant inflammatory third spacing has occurred. Subcutaneous emphysema often occurs with cervical perforations but less often with thoracic or abdominal perforations. The Mallory-Weiss syndrome refers to a mucosal laceration (single or multiple) at the esophagogastric junction with hematemesis following retching or vomiting that is not associated with pain. Dysphagia appears late and is usually related to a thoracic perforation.

Chest radiography identifies perforation in 90% of patients but can be normal immediately after perforation. Pneumomediastinum, subcutaneous emphysema, mediastinal widening, or a mediastinal air–fluid level prompt investigation to rule out esophageal perforation. Hydropneumothorax on the left occurs in patients with distal third esophageal perforations. Esophagogram with barium should be used for esophageal perforations that are not expected to communicate with the peritoneal cavity to reveal the primary area of leakage. Water-soluble contrast (such as Gastrografin®) should be used for esophageal perforations expected to communicate with the peritoneal cavity. In summary, barium is inert in the chest, whereas aspirated Gastrografin® causes pneumonitis. However, barium in the peritoneal cavity causes peritonitis, whereas Gastrografin® in the peritoneal cavity is inert. Unfortunately, the rate of false-negative esophagograms is as high as 10%. Chest computed tomography scan often shows mediastinal fluid and air at the site of perforation. If a perforation is suspected during an endoscopic procedure, careful inspection of the esophagus without air insufflation is warranted. Based on our experience, esophagoscopy can miss a perforation hidden in a mucosal fold or aggravate soilage by air insufflation and is not recommended as a primary diagnostic study for esophageal perforations. The estimated mortality rate for patients diagnosed within 24 hours of injury ranges from 10% to 20% in most published series. After 24 hours, the rate jumps to 40% to 66%.

The management of patients with esophageal perforations has evolved over the past three decades. Currently, treatment depends on the site of perforation, etiology, patient condition, and time interval between perforation and diagnosis. Initial resuscitation for a patient with an esophageal perforation should include admission to a monitored care setting. Invasive monitoring devices such as arterial lines, central venous catheters, and urinary catheters should be used to follow hemodynamic and resuscitation status. Broad-spectrum antibiotic therapy should be initiated as soon as possible. A thoracostomy tube should be placed for any moderate effusion, as well as to relieve pneumothorax caused by the perforation. Parenteral nutrition should be instituted for all patients to provide caloric support and intravenous hydration. Finally, some authors suggest placement of a nasogastric tube in addition to placement of a secondary drain at the site of perforation; however, this is difficult to place correctly without enlarging the injury and can cause reflux of gastric contents, thereby exacerbating the inflammatory reaction surrounding the injury.

Approximately 25% of all patients with esophageal perforation can be treated conservatively. These include patients without signs of sepsis at initial presentation, elderly patients, and patients who have multiple comorbid diseases. In general, nonoperative management of esophageal disruption is used in the following instances: instrumental perforation especially in the cervical region; perforation caused by sclerosis of esophageal varices or dilation necessitated by achalasia or peptic or corrosive strictures; and perforations identified several days after injury, with minimal symptoms at presentation. Patients treated nonoperatively should have no enteral intake for a minimum of 7 to 10 days. If they remain stable throughout this course, a Gastrografin® swallow study is used to evaluate esophageal integrity. Extravasation of contrast from the esophagus dictates another interval of rest and parenteral nutrition, followed by repeated swallow studies on a weekly basis; it may take several weeks before resolution occurs. When there is no leak demonstrated by esophagography, the patient can resume enteral intake, starting with clear liquids and advancing as tolerated. If the patient's clinical condition fails to improve or worsens after 24 hours of initial conservative therapy, operative intervention is required.

Appropriate operative therapy for esophageal perforation depends on a number of factors, including etiology, location of injury, presence of underlying esophageal disease, and time interval between injury and diagnosis. Other considerations include the extent of mediastinal and pleural soilage and the patient's age and general medical condition. Options for surgery include simple drainage of the contaminated space, debridement with primary repair of the perforation, esophageal diversion and delayed repair, or esophagectomy. The cornerstone of surgical treatment for esophageal perforation is drainage of the contaminated space. In approximately 15% of cases, drainage alone is sufficient treatment for esophageal perforation and repair is not necessary. For most cases of esophageal perforation, operative debridement with primary repair is undertaken, even in cases identified more than 24 hours after perforation. Although the incidence of complications rises as the time interval between perforation and treatment increases, primary repair of lesions more than 24 hours old has been successfully described by many authors and is standard practice today. However, primary repair should not be performed for carcinoma or megaesophagus from achalasia; esophagectomy should be performed instead.

80
Esophageal Neoplasms

Esophageal neoplasms are nearly always malignant, with less than 1% being benign. Of the benign tumors, leiomyomas account for more than half, followed by cysts and polyps arising from the different cell types in the esophageal wall. Esophageal cancer is the sixth most common malignancy in the world and can be either a squamous cell carcinoma or adenocarcinoma.

Leiomyomas are intramural tumors of mesenchymal cell origin and therefore are considered to be gastrointestinal stromal tumors. These tumors, when benign, enlarge but do not invade surrounding tissues, including the mucosa. Leiomyomas occur in people between the ages of 20 and 50 years, with the average age at presentation being 38 years. Up to 10% of patients have multiple lesions. More than three quarters are located in the middle and lower thirds of the esophagus. Clinically, leiomyomas can produce symptoms of dysphagia, mediastinal pressure, and pain due to the mass effect of the tumor; however, most leiomyomas are asymptomatic. The diagnosis can be made with visualization of a well-localized, noncircumferential esophageal mass or filling defect during a barium swallow test. Others are identified with endoscopy, when narrowing of the lumen without a mucosal lesion is detected. Endoscopic ultrasound is used to confirm the diagnosis by visualizing the lesion arising from the muscularis propria or in the submucosa. Endoscopic biopsy should not be performed, because it complicates surgical resection by violating the uninvolved mucosa overlying the mass. The treatment for leiomyomas is resection if the tumor is greater than 5 cm or is symptomatic. Smaller lesions can be observed, because the risk of malignancy in a small, slow-growing leiomyoma is very low. Resection requires a right thoracotomy if the lesion is in the middle esophagus and a left thoracotomy if the lesion is in the proximal or distal esophagus. With the tumor visualized, a longitudinal incision is made in the overlying muscle layer, the mass is enucleated without interrupting the mucosa, and the myotomy is then reapproximated and closed. If the mucosa is

accidentally violated during the enucleation, it can be repaired primarily. Extremely large or multiple leiomyomas require esophageal resection.

Esophageal cysts can be congenital or acquired. Enteric and bronchogenic are the most common cysts, and both are congenital. Esophageal cysts vary greatly in size and usually occur in the middle to lower thirds of the esophagus. Symptoms if present are similar to those of leiomyomas. Treatment is with enucleation. During enucleation it is important to check for a fistula tract connecting the cyst to the tracheobronchial tree, because failure to close this fistula can result in recurrent bronchopulmonary infections.

Squamous cell carcinoma of the esophagus is the most common type of esophageal carcinoma in the world. Risk factors include smoking and alcohol use, with combined heavy use increasing the risk up to 100-fold. Other causes are long-standing achalasia, lye strictures, tylosis, and human papilloma virus infection. African Americans and males are also at a higher risk. Arising from the mucosa of the esophagus, squamous cell carcinoma is histologically identified by invasive sheets of polygonal or spindle cells with an indistinct stromal–epithelial interface. There are four gross pathologic classifications of squamous cell carcinoma of the esophagus: fungating, ulcerating, infiltrating, and polypoid. Fungating carcinomas grow intraluminally and are extremely friable with a high rate of invasion of mediastinal structures. Ulcerating lesions are characterized by hemorrhagic flat-based ulcers with raised edges and surrounding induration. Infiltrating lesions have a dense longitudinal and circumferential growth pattern. Finally, polypoid lesions, the most rare, have intraluminal growth with a smooth surface and narrow stalk.

The incidence of adenocarcinoma of the esophagus is increasing in North America and has surpassed squamous cell carcinoma as the most common type of esophageal cancer in the United States, especially in younger patients. The gross appearance is similar to that of squamous cell carcinoma; however, microscopically it originates from metaplastic Barrett's mucosa and therefore resembles gastric carcinoma. On rare occasions the carcinoma can arise from submucosal glands and resemble mucoepidermal and adenoid cystic carcinoma of the salivary glands. Gastroesophageal reflux disease is the most important risk factor for the development of adenocarcinoma of the esophagus. Approximately 10% to 15% of patients with gastroesophageal reflux disease develop Barrett's esophagus. The risk of Barrett's developing into adenocarcinoma of the esophagus is 1 in every 100 to 200 patient years, which is 30 to 40 times the risk of a person without Barrett's developing adenocarcinoma of the esophagus.

The clinical presentations of squamous cell and adenocarcinoma of the esophagus are the same. The most common complaint is dysphagia; however, many tumors are asymptomatic and are discovered on surveillance endoscopy or esophagogastroduodenoscopy for upper gastrointestinal symptoms. Dysphagia is actually a late finding, because the esophagus has no serosal layers, allowing the smooth muscle layers to dilate easily. If the tumor is advanced to the stage of invading the tracheobronchial tree, a tracheoesophageal fistula forms, producing symptoms of coughing, choking, and recurrent pneumonias. Other symptoms of advanced disease are vocal cord paralysis caused by invasion of the recurrent nerve by either the primary mass or lymph node involvement.

Staging is based on the TNM system. A T1 lesion is limited to the submucosa, T2 goes into the muscularis propria, T3 goes through the muscularis propria, and T4 invades the adventitia. As for the nodal involvement, N0 refers to no nodal involvement and N1 indicates regional lymph node involvement. This can be assessed preoperatively using computed tomography, endoscopic ultrasound, positron emission tomography, magnetic resonance imaging, video-assisted thoracoscopy, or laparoscopy. The depth of the esophageal wall invasion and the presence of lymph node metastasis influence the prognosis.

Treatment for both types of esophageal cancer is primarily surgical. Unfortunately, because of the late stage when many of these tumors are identified, cure rates are low. When evaluating a patient with esophageal cancer, the main decision is whether to attempt a surgical resection for cure or a palliative operation. This decision is based on the tumor location, the patient's age, his or her cardiopulmonary reserve, the clinical staging, and the intraoperative staging. Low cervical lesions tend to be unresectable because of their early invasion of the trachea and great vessels. Lesions in the middle or upper third of the thoracic esophagus should only be resected if they are not invading mediastinal structures and there is no evidence of lymph node involvement. This is because curative surgery requires en bloc resection, which is difficult because of the proximity to the trachea and aorta. Lower esophageal lesions are amenable to en bloc resection with large negative margins and lymph

node resections. Patients older than 75 years should undergo procedures for palliation only. Acceptable cardiopulmonary reserve is a forced expiratory volume in 1 second >2 L and an ejection fraction >40%. Preoperative clinical criteria that should direct the surgical treatment toward palliation include only recurrent nerve paralysis, Horner's syndrome, spinal pain, paralysis of the diaphragm, fistula formation, malignant pleural effusion, a tumor greater than 8 cm in length, enlarged lymph nodes on computed tomography scan, loss of appetite, and a weight loss of greater than 20%. The intraoperative staging component takes into consideration the degree of penetration through the wall.

Surgical options for palliation depend on the degree of resectability of the tumor. If resection is possible, a simple esophageal resection with cervical esophagogastrostomy can be used to stop the dysphagia and pain and to prevent perforation, hemorrhage, and fistula formation. If resection of an obstructing tumor cannot be performed safely, esophageal intubation or laser ablation can relieve some symptoms.

If surgical resection for cure is the goal, it is very important to optimize the patient's preoperative nutritional status. It may be necessary to place a J-tube for this reason. There is disagreement about the best approach for surgical resection of esophageal cancer. One approach is through a right thoracotomy, left neck, and upper midline abdominal incisions. The right thoracotomy is used for dissection of the distal esophagus and mediastinal lymph nodes and for mobilization of the esophagus proximally to the level of the aortic arch. The abdominal incision is used for dissection of the proximal stomach and associated lymph nodes. Finally, the left neck incision is used for proximal dissection of the esophagus. A second approach is to use a transhiatal esophagogastrectomy to remove the primary tumor only and leave the lymph nodes to be treated by adjuvant chemotherapy and radiation. This option can be used only for adenocarcinoma or squamous cell carcinomas involving the distal esophagus. Once resected, the esophagus can be reconstructed using a gastric pull-up if the tumor does not extend down the lesser curve of the stomach. A colonic interposition can also be used for reconstruction.

The roles of radiation and chemotherapy for esophageal cancers are still unclear. Radiation can be used as palliation of dysphagia, but symptoms usually recur in 2 to 3 months. There is some evidence that preoperative chemotherapy may be effective in shrinking the size of the tumor, thus allowing for better surgical resection. Chemoradiation is used for patients who have had no prior exposure to chemotherapy develop recurrent systemic disease after resection. Despite the various options for treatment, overall survival rate is dismal. The 5-year survival rates for stages I, II, III, and IV are <50%, 30%, 10% to 15%, and 0%, respectively.

81
Esophageal Diverticula

Esophageal diverticula are outpouchings of the esophagus that are classified according to site, etiology, and layers of the esophagus involved. They are termed *pharyngoesophageal, parabronchial,* or *epiphrenic*. They can also be termed *true* when the entire thickness of the esophageal wall is involved or *false* when only the mucosa/submucosa is involved. Finally, they can be caused by pulsion related to increased intraluminal pressure or traction applied by structures external to the esophagus. Traction diverticula were historically caused by mediastinal lymph node involvement in tuberculosis with resultant fibrosis. Today, traction diverticula are rare because of tuberculosis treatment. For pulsion diverticula, the surgical correction must involve treatment of the cause of increased intraesophageal pressure. They are identified by anteroposterior and/or lateral views during a barium swallow test, which can also identify an often present underlying motility disorder.

Zenker's, or pharyngoesophageal, diverticula are the most common type. They are false, pulsion diverticula and occur in people older than 60 years as their pharyngeal muscle tone and elasticity decreases. They form in Killian's triangle between the pharyngeal constrictors and the cricopharyngeus muscle on the posterior side of the pharyngoesophageal junction. This is sometimes termed *cricopharyngeal achalasia*, because the cricopharyngeus muscle fails to relax. These are usually asymptomatic and are found incidentally. However, a progression of symptoms may occur from cough, increased salivation, and solid dysphagia to regurgitation, halitosis, cervical dysphagia, gurgling, chest pain, and respiratory difficulty. These patients may apply pressure to the neck to facilitate swallowing. Symptoms progress as the diverticulum enlarges and can lead to significant aspiration. Lateral x-rays on barium swallow are essential, because these are posterior outpouchings. Manometry shows no abnormality. Endoscopy is indicated when signs of malignancy (such as masses or ulcers) are detected during barium swallow or when the patient has dysphagia or weight loss.

Cricopharyngeal bars are the result of long-term cricopharyngeal constriction and are associated with gastroesophageal reflux disease (GERD).

The treatment for Zenker's diverticula is surgery. Many techniques are described; however, all involve a 7 to 10 cm extramucosal esophagomyotomy to ensure all cricopharyngeal fibers are transected. If the diverticulum is resected without esophagomyotomy, a fistula is likely to form. Because these diverticula are in the upper esophagus, a left cervical incision is used. Some surgeons opt for a transverse cervical incision. The diverticulum is typically resected; however, if smaller than a few centimeters are resected, it may be left in place. Alternatively, it can be suspended from surrounding tissue with the mouth in a dependent position to facilitate draining of contents. If GERD is present, it should be evaluated after surgery for the diverticulum.

Parabronchial, or midesophageal, diverticula were historically traction diverticula but are now more often due to pulsion and an underlying motility disorder. They are often relatively wide mouthed, on the right side, singular, and less than 5 cm in size. They are typically asymptomatic but can cause symptoms similar to those of Zenker's diverticula. A distinct difference is the possible formation of an esophagobronchial fistula. Again, cancer must be ruled out, and motility disorders should be investigated with manometry. Because these are midesophageal, they are approached from the right side.

Epiphrenic, or supradiaphragmatic, diverticula occur within 10 cm of the gastroesophageal junction on the right side and are due to pulsion forces. They are typically asymptomatic but can produce symptoms similar to the previous types. A distinguishing feature is the presence of epigastric pain. During barium swallow, transient outpouchings can be seen in areas lacking peristalsis proximal to the diverticulum. These require that motility disorders, stricture, or tumor be investigated. They can also be associated with trauma or congenital disorders such as Ehlers-Danlos. Treatment is based on symptoms and size. If there are minimal or no symptoms and the size is less than 3 cm, no treatment is necessary. Otherwise, a diverticulectomy with extramucosal esophagomyotomy from the aortic arch to the gastroesophageal junction is performed. Although these are typically on the right side, the distal esophagus is approached through a left thoracotomy or video-assisted thoracoscopy. The operative mortality rate is approximately 10%. If reflux is a significant symptom, a partial fundoplication should be performed.

82
Gastric Anatomy

The stomach is a hollow, distensible organ with a mean volume of 1,500 cc that resides in the upper abdomen. The stomach is divided into three major segments. The fundus is the most superior portion of the stomach, which sits to the left of the gastroesophageal junction and rests just below the left hemidiaphragm. It has a high concentration of parietal cells and is the acid-producing section of the stomach. The body of the stomach is bordered superiorly by the fundus and distally by the antrum. A line projecting from the incisura angularis (a subtle indentation on the distal lesser curve) to an indentation on the distal greater curve is the transition between the body and antrum. The antrum is populated by gastrin-secreting G cells.

Although the stomach is a very compliant organ, it sits in a relatively fixed position. It is attached superiorly to the esophagus at the gastroesophageal junction. The serosa and fat circumferentially surrounding the gastroesophageal junction are attached to the crura and diaphragm and anchor the superior stomach to the hiatus. These attachments also are a barrier between the peritoneal cavity and the mediastinum and are liberated during foregut procedures such as antireflux surgery, paraesophageal hernia repair, and Heller myotomy. The pancreas and retroperitoneum form the posterior border of the stomach. The lesser sac is the space between the posterior wall of the stomach and the anterior surface of the pancreas. The lesser sac is usually void of adhesions, although posterior gastric arteries originating from the splenic artery and inflammatory adhesions from pancreatitis can obliterate this space. The anterior wall of the stomach is bordered by the left lobe of the liver and the anterior abdominal wall. Laterally the stomach is connected to the spleen by the gastrosplenic ligament, which runs from the greater curve of the stomach to the spleen and contains the short gastric vessels. The lesser curve of the stomach is attached to the liver by the gastrohepatic ligament, or pars flaccida, which contains the hepatic branches of the vagus nerve.

Ten percent of patients have an aberrant left hepatic artery, which originates from the left gastric artery and courses transversely with the hepatic vagal fibers. The pylorus is the distal aspect of the stomach, which connects to the duodenum.

Although rare, the stomach can rotate and form an acute volvulus. This usually occurs in the setting of chronic gastric dilation or a large hiatal hernia, both of which stretch the normal attachments. Organoaxial rotation, the most common type of volvulus, has a vertical axis of rotation with the greater curve moving in a superior/medial direction. Ultimately, the greater curve rests anterior and medial to the lesser curve. Mesenteroaxial rotation occurs around a horizontal axis with the distal stomach and pylorus moving in an anterior, superior, and lateral direction.

The stomach is perfused by five major vascular arcades, all of which trace their origins to the celiac axis. The left gastric artery is a direct branch of the celiac artery and is located in the superior aspect of the lesser curve. The right gastric artery is located more distal on the lesser curve, near the pylorus as it branches from the hepatic artery. The greater curve is supplied by the gastroepiploic arteries. The right gastroepliploic artery originates from the gastroduodenal artery and feeds the distal greater curve. The left gastroepiploic artery is a branch of the splenic artery and supplies the upper, proximal greater curve. The proximal greater curve is also perfused by the short gastric arteries, which arise from the splenic artery and/or the left gastroepiploic artery. The short gastric arteries are divided during antireflux procedure, gastrectomy, and splenectomy.

The vagus nerves, which provide parasympathetic innervation to the stomach, parallel the esophagus and enter the abdominal cavity at the esophageal hiatus. The anterior, left vagus courses along the anterior aspect of the lesser curvature where it divides into hepatic, gastric, and pyloric branches. The terminal branches of the left vagus that innervate the antrum are called the *crow's feet.*

The right branch of the vagus courses posterior to the gastroesophageal junction. The first branch of the right vagus is the criminal nerve of Grassi, which innervates the posterior fundus. During a truncal vagotomy, this branch must be identified and ligated. The main branch of the right vagus parallels the left vagus as it runs on the posterior aspect of the lesser curve, sending branching fibers to the stomach and celiac region. A highly selective vagotomy preserves the main left and right vagus nerves on the lesser curve while dividing the smaller branches that arc toward the stomach, thus preserving pyloric innervation and function.

83
Gastric Physiology

The stomach stores food and facilitates digestion through a variety of secretory and motor functions. Important secretory functions include the production of acid, pepsin, intrinsic factor, mucus, and gastrointestinal hormones. Important motor functions include food storage (receptive relaxation and accommodation), grinding and mixing, controlled emptying of ingested food, and periodic interprandial "housekeeping."

Hydrochloric acid (HCl) stimulates both mechanical and biochemical breakdown of ingested food. In an acidic environment, pepsin and HCl facilitate proteolysis. Gastric acid also inhibits the proliferation of ingested bacteria and stimulates secretin release when it enters the duodenum. Parietal cells secrete HCl when one of three membrane receptor types is stimulated by acetylcholine (from vagal nerve fibers), gastrin (from G cells), or histamine (from enterochromaffinlike [ECL] cells). Somatostatin from mucosal D cells inhibits gastric acid secretion. The enzyme H^+/K^+-ATPase is the proton pump that is stored within the intracellular tubulovesicles and is the final common pathway for gastric acid secretion. Although electroneutral, this is an energy-requiring process, because the hydrogen is secreted against a gradient of at least 1 millionfold, which explains why the parietal cell is the most mitochondria-dense mammalian cell (about one third by volume). During acid production, K^+ and Cl^- are also secreted into the secretory canaliculus through separate channels.

Food ingestion is the physiologic stimulus for acid secretion. The acid secretory response occurs in three phases: cephalic, gastric, and intestinal. The cephalic or vagal phase begins with the thought, sight, smell, and/or taste of food. These stimuli activate several cortical and hypothalamic sites, and signals are transmitted to the stomach by the vagal nerves. Acetylcholine is released, leading to stimulation of ECL cells and parietal cells. The cephalic phase accounts for 30% of total acid secretion in response to a meal.

The gastric phase begins when food reaches the stomach and lasts until the stomach is empty. It accounts for 60% of the total acid secretion. The gastric phase of acid secretion has several components. Amino acids and small peptides directly stimulate antral G cells to secrete gastrin, which is carried in the bloodstream to the parietal cells and stimulates acid secretion in an endocrine fashion. In addition, proximal gastric distention stimulates acid secretion via a vagovagal reflex arc, which is abolished by truncal or highly selective vagotomy. Antral distention also stimulates antral gastrin secretion. Acetylcholine stimulates gastrin release, and gastrin stimulates histamine release from ECL cells. Enterochromaffin-like cells play a key role in the regulation of gastric acid secretion. A large part of the acid-stimulatory effects of both acetylcholine and gastrin are mediated by histamine released from mucosal ECL cells. This explains why H_2-blockers are effective inhibitors of acid secretion, even though histamine is only one of three parietal cell stimulants. The mucosal D cells release somatostatin, which inhibits histamine release from ECL cells and gastrin release from D cells. The function of D cells is inhibited by *Helicobacter pylori* infection and leads to an exaggerated acid secretory response.

The intestinal phase of gastric secretion is poorly understood and is thought to be mediated by an unknown hormone from the proximal small bowel mucosa in response to luminal chyme. This phase starts when gastric emptying begins and continues as long as nutrients remain in the proximal small intestine. It accounts for about 10% of meal-induced acid secretion.

Interprandial basal acid secretion is 2 to 5 mEq of HCl per hour, about 10% of maximal acid output, and it is greater at night. Basal acid secretion probably contributes to the relatively low bacterial counts found in the stomach. Basal acid secretion is reduced 75% to 90% by vagotomy or H_2-receptor blockade.

Pepsinogen secretion from chief cells is primarily stimulated by food ingestion; acetylcholine is the most important mediator. Somatostatin inhibits pepsinogen secretion. Pepsinogen I is produced by chief cells in acid-producing glands; pepsinogen II is produced by chief cells in both acid-producing and gastrin-producing antral glands. Pepsinogen is cleaved to the active pepsin enzyme in an acidic environment and is maximally active at a pH of 2.5. The enzyme catalyzes the hydrolysis of proteins and is denatured at alkaline pH. Activated parietal cells secrete intrinsic factor in addition to HCl. Intrinsic factor binds to luminal vitamin B_{12}, and the complex is absorbed in the terminal ileum via mucosal receptors.

Gastric Mucosal Barrier

The stomach's durable resistance to autodigestion by caustic HCl and active pepsin is multifaceted. When these defenses break down, ulceration occurs. The mucus and bicarbonate secreted by surface epithelial cells form an unstirred mucous gel with a favorable pH gradient. Cell membranes and tight junctions prevent hydrogen ions from gaining access to the interstitial space. Hydrogen ions that occasionally break through are buffered by the alkaline tide created by basolateral bicarbonate secretion from stimulated parietal cells. Any sloughed or denuded surface epithelial cells are rapidly replaced by migration of adjacent cells via a process called *restitution*. Mucosal blood flow is crucial in maintaining a healthy mucosa by providing nutrients and oxygen for the cellular functions involved in cytoprotection. "Back-diffused" hydrogen is buffered and rapidly removed by the rich blood supply. When barrier breakers such as bile or aspirin lead to increased back-diffusion of hydrogen ions from the lumen into the lamina propria and submucosa, there is a protective increase in mucosal blood flow. If this protective response is blocked, gross ulceration can occur. Important mediators of these protective mechanisms include prostaglandins, nitric oxide, intrinsic nerves, and peptides such as calcitonin gene–related peptide and gastrin. Misoprostol is a commercially available prostaglandin E analogue that prevents gastric mucosal damage in chronic nonsteroidal anti-inflammatory drug users. In addition to these local defenses, there are important protective factors in swallowed saliva, duodenal secretions, and pancreatic and biliary secretions.

Gastric Hormones

Gastrin is produced by antral G cells and is the major hormonal stimulant of acid secretion during the gastric phase. A variety of molecular forms exist: the large majority of gastrin released by the human antrum is G_{17}. Luminal peptides and amino acids are the most potent stimulants of gastrin release, and luminal acid is the most potent inhibitor of gastrin secretion. The inhibitor effect is mediated in a paracrine fashion by somatostatin released from antral D cells. Gastrin also is trophic to gastric parietal cells and to other gastrointestinal mucosal cells. Important causes of hypergastrinemia include pernicious anemia, acid-suppressive medication, gastrinoma, retained antrum following distal gastrectomy and Billroth II surgery, and vagotomy.

Somatostatin is produced by D cells located throughout the gastric mucosa. The major stimulus for somatostatin release is antral acidification; acetylcholine from vagal nerve fibers inhibits its release. Somatostatin inhibits acid secretion from parietal cells, gastrin release from G cells, and histamine release from ECL cells. The primary effect of somatostatin is mediated in a paracrine fashion, but an endocrine (bloodstream) effect is possible also.

Gastrin-releasing peptide (GRP) in the antrum stimulates both gastrin and somatostatin release by binding to receptors on the G and D cells. Nerve terminals end near the mucosa in the gastric body and antrum, which are rich in GRP immunoreactivity. When GRP is given peripherally it stimulates acid secretion, but when it is given centrally into the cerebral ventricles of animals, it inhibits acid secretion, apparently via a pathway involving the sympathetic nervous system.

Ghrelin is a small peptide that is produced primarily in the stomach. Ghrelin is a potent secretagogue of pituitary growth hormone but not adrenocorticotropic hormone, follicle-stimulating hormone, luteinizing hormone, prolactin, or thyroid-stimulating hormone. Ghrelin appears to be an orexigenic regulator of appetite. When ghrelin is elevated, appetite is stimulated, and when it is suppressed, appetite is suppressed. The gastric bypass operation is associated with suppression of plasma ghrelin levels and appetite.

Gastric Motility and Emptying

Gastric motor function has several purposes. Interprandial motor activity clears undigested debris, sloughed cells, and mucus. When feeding begins, the stomach relaxes to accommodate the meal. Regulated motor activity breaks down food into small particles and controls the output into the duodenum. The stomach accomplishes this via coordinated smooth muscle relaxation and contraction of the proximal, distal, and pyloric gastric segments. Smooth muscle myoelectric potentials are translated into muscular activity, which is modulated by extrinsic and intrinsic innervation and hormones.

The intrinsic innervation consists of ganglia and nerves constituting the enteric nervous system with a variety of neurotransmitters. Important excitatory neurotransmitters include acetylcholine, the tachykinins, substance P, and neurokinin A. Important inhibitory neurotransmitters include nitric oxide and vasoactive intestinal peptide. Serotonin has been shown to modulate both contraction and relaxation. A variety of other molecules affect motility, including GRP, histamine, neuropeptide Y, norepinephrine, and endogenous opioids.

Specialized cells in the muscularis propria, interstitial cells of Cajal, also are important modulators of gastrointestinal motility. They amplify both cholinergic excitatory and nitrergic inhibitory input to the smooth muscle of the stomach and intestine.

84
Peptic Ulcer Disease

Peptic ulceration is the consequence of tissue erosion through the mucosa into the submucosa. Peptic ulcers can appear in any portion of the gastrointestinal (GI) tract that is exposed to pepsin or acid. Common sites include the stomach, duodenal bulb, esophagus, small intestine, and Meckel's diverticulum. Peptic ulcers generally develop with cyclic patterns of healing and relapse. Areas of scar and previously healed ulcers are often seen in affected patients. Approximately 2% of the U.S. population is affected by peptic ulcer disease. Young to middle-aged individuals exhibit predominantly duodenal ulcerations, and individuals 40 to 60 years of age are more likely to have gastric ulcerations. Men are affected more often than women.

The two most common etiologies of peptic ulcer disease are *Helicobacter pylori* infection and the use of nonsteroidal anti-inflammatory drugs (NSAIDs). The central theme of both etiologies is altered epithelial protection, leaving the mucosa vulnerable to acid exposure and ulcer formation. It was previously believed that acid hypersecretion was the central cause of peptic ulcer disease, but further understanding of *H. pylori* infection and NSAID use has altered this thinking.

Helicobacter pylori colonization results in chronic inflammation of the gastric mucosa. The organism has a tendency to occupy the nonacid-secreting region of the gastric antrum. The infection of this region alters the function of local somatostatin-producing D cells. The decrease in gastrin inhibition by somatostatin causes increased acid production. Antral colonization with *H. pylori* predisposes the patient to duodenal ulcer formation. When the duodenum becomes exposed to increasing amounts of acid, a metaplastic change occurs in the duodenal mucosa that resembles gastric mucosa. The areas of metaplasia are also susceptible to *H. pylori* colonization. When this occurs, the production of protective bicarbonate secretions is altered. This leaves the duodenal mucosa vulnerable to ulceration.

Nonsteroidal anti-inflammatory drugs lead to peptic ulcer formation by diminishing the production of protective prostaglandins by the mucosa. These drugs inhibit cyclo-oxygenase, the enzyme found in the prostaglandin synthesis pathway.

Peptic ulcers present in a variety of ways from no symptoms, to dyspepsia, to acute peritonitis, to hemorrhage. The most common presentation is that of recurrent epigastric pain. Patients often describe the pain as a burning sensation in the epigastrium. The pain radiates to the patient's back and sometimes is relieved by eating. More specifically, pain that occurs several hours after eating a meal is generally associated with ulceration. Other symptoms include retrosternal burning, acid regurgitation, nausea, vomiting, and diarrhea. Diarrhea with duodenal ulcers may indicate Zollinger-Ellison syndrome. Complications of peptic ulcer disease include bleeding, perforation, and obstruction.

The diagnostic evaluation is performed in one of two ways, depending on the severity of symptoms and the patient's age. The first method involves empiric treatment only for patients who are less than 45 years of age with apparently uncomplicated peptic ulcer disease. A 4- to 6-week course of proton pump inhibitor or H_2-blocker is prescribed. In addition, noninvasive testing for *H. pylori* can be done. The presence of ulceration is less likely in patients who are *H. pylori* negative.

The second method involves the use of contrasted radiologic studies or endoscopy to make the diagnosis. This method is reserved for patients who fail empiric acid-lowering therapy, are *H. pylori* positive, or present with complicated peptic ulcer disease (i.e., bleeding and obstruction). Contrasted radiographs such as upper GI studies have been replaced by endoscopy because of its reliability in detecting ulcers and the ability to perform biopsy procedures during endoscopy; therefore, endoscopy is the modality of choice for making the diagnosis.

Once peptic ulceration has been identified, the cause of the ulceration can be determined. *Helicobacter pylori* testing can be conducted in several invasive and noninvasive ways. Serologic testing evaluates blood serum for antibodies against *H. pylori*. The antibodies tend to remain detectable up to 8 months after eradication of the organism. Urea breath testing is based on the detection of *H. pylori* urease activity. The test is negative within 1 month after *H. pylori* eradication. Urease testing along with Giemsa staining and culture are commonly done with endoscopic mucosal biopsy procedures.

Hypersecretory etiologies such as gastrinoma (Zollinger-Ellison syndrome) and antral G cell hyperplasia are best evaluated with serum gastrin measurement and provocative testing. This method of testing is indicated when ulcers fail conservative therapy, when symptoms of diarrhea are associated with ulceration, and when ulcers have characteristics such as enlarged gastric folds and extension beyond the duodenal bulb. Gastric analysis involves the quantification of gastric acid output via intubation of the stomach. Samples of gastric secretions are obtained to ascertain the basal level of secretion as well as the level after stimulation (pentagastrin given subcutaneously).

Initial management of peptic ulcer disease involves medical therapy aimed at decreasing acid production. The mainstays of treatment include H_2-blockers and proton pump inhibitors. *Helicobacter pylori* therapy is initiated simultaneously with triple drug therapy for 14 days (e.g., lansoprazole, amoxicillin, and clarithromycin).

Surgical therapy is used infrequently because of the success of medical therapy. Indications for surgery include ulcers refractory to medical therapy, patients not capable of adhering to medical treatment, and treatment of complications (i.e., bleeding, perforation, and obstruction). The goal of surgical treatment is to reduce acid production. Surgical treatments include vagotomy, antrectomy plus vagotomy, and subtotal gastrectomy.

Truncal vagotomy is performed by interruption of each vagal trunk on the distal esophagus. From 1 to 2 cm of each trunk is resected. Removing the vagal influence of the stomach decreases acid production but also alters the emptying mechanism of the stomach. Therefore, a drainage procedure is required to aid in gastric emptying. This is most often accomplished by performing a pyloroplasty. Selective vagotomies can be performed to avoid side effects of altered gastric emptying, dumping, and diarrhea. During a parietal cell vagotomy, all the vagal nerves that innervate the proximal two thirds of the stomach are divided. This spares the main vagal nerves (nerves of Latarjet) and innervation to the gastric antrum. Although drainage procedures are often unnecessary after a parietal cell vagotomy, the addition of pyloroplasty produces fewer recurrent ulcers. Ulcers recur in about 10% of patients.

Antrectomy and vagotomy involve resection of 50% of the distal stomach high on the lesser curvature of the stomach. The remaining stomach is either anastomosed to the duodenum in a Billroth I procedure or to the proximal jejunum in a Billroth II procedure. Truncal vagotomy is accomplished as described earlier. Marginal ulcers occur in 2% of cases. Subtotal gastrectomy is rarely preformed. It involves the removal of up to 75% of the distal stomach. A Billroth II procedure is done to restore continuity.

Complications of peptic ulcer surgery are divided into early and late. Early complications include duodenal stump leakage, gastric obstruction, and bleeding. Late complications include recurrent ulceration, fistula, dumping syndrome, alkaline gastritis, anemia, diarrhea, and gastroparesis. Vagotomy and pyloroplasty carry an associated ulcer risk of 10%. The risk of recurrence with antrectomy and vagotomy is 2% to 3%, which is similar to subtotal gastrectomy. Recurrent ulcerations are treated similar to the initial ulcer. Fistulas can form between the stomach and colon after the erosion of an ulcer into the colon. This occurs more often in recurrent ulceration after procedures that involve creating a gastrojejunal anastomosis. The predominant clinical manifestations include diarrhea and weight loss. Stools are loose and watery and often contain undigested food. Malnutrition is another common complication. Barium enema is the most reliable test for making the diagnosis. Treatment goals are resuscitation with correction of electrolyte abnormalities and surgical excision of the affected colon and ulcerated gastrojejunal segment with partial gastrectomy. In addition, a vagotomy is performed to prevent future ulcer development. The excised tissue should be evaluated to rule out possible malignancy.

Dumping syndrome is a result of the stomach's inability to regulate emptying. The syndrome is manifested in cardiovascular and gastrointestinal symptoms. Symptoms occur early (10 to 30 minutes) or late (2 to 4 hours after eating). Patients complain of palpitations, tachycardia, abdominal cramping, diaphoresis, dyspnea, flushing, nausea, vomiting, and diarrhea within a short time after eating a meal. Fluid shifts due to a sudden release of high osmotic load into the intestine with subsequent release of vasoactive substances (5-hydroxytryptamine and vasoactive intestinal peptide) are thought to be the principle causes of early symptoms. Late symptoms are caused by increased glucagon secretion with subsequent insulin response.

Operative procedures that alter the pyloric function can cause reflux of duodenal secretions into the stomach, causing alkaline gastritis. Symptoms are hallmarked by postprandial abdominal pain. Diagnosis is based on endoscopic evidence of gastritis along with biopsy. Conversion to Roux-en-Y is indicated for patients with intractable pain.

Anemia can occur in up to 30% of patients within the first 5 years after partial gastrectomy. Patients presenting with anemia should be evaluated for occult bleeding from sources such as a marginal ulcer or neoplasm. B_{12} deficiencies with megaloblastic anemia are other possible causes. Anemia can be treated pharmaceutically with supplemental iron (i.e., ferrous sulfate or ferrous gluconate). Diarrhea is associated with truncal vagotomy in up to 10% of cases. Symptoms tend to occur episodically and can be controlled with antidiarrheal agents.

Chronic gastroparesis occurs in some patients postoperatively. Some cases are treated successfully with prokinetic agents; other cases refractory to medical treatment require total gastrectomy with Roux-en-Y esophagojejunostomy.

The success of medical therapy has limited the surgeon's involvement in peptic ulcer disease to mostly management of complications. Hemorrhage occurs in 5% to 10% of patients with active ulcer disease. Initial treatment is aimed at fluid resuscitation and correction of underlying coagulopathy. Endoscopy is initiated as soon as the patient is hemodynamically stable. Endoscopy is useful for identifying the source of bleeding and for providing therapeutic intervention (sclerotherapy, argon beam, and heater probe or injection of vasoconstrictive agents). Ulcers that appear to be oozing, have a visible vessel, or have fresh clot have a higher chance of rebleeding within the first 24 to 72 hours after intervention. Surgical intervention is required for patients who continue to bleed or re-bleed.

Perforation occurs acutely and involves spillage of gastric contents into the abdomen. The classic presentation includes peritonitis, fever, leukocytosis, and free air seen on upright abdominal plain films. This condition requires prompt surgical intervention with excision of the ulcer rim and closure (e.g., modified Graham patch). Definitive ulcer procedures are generally not conducted unless it is thought that the patient cannot comply with medical therapy postoperatively. The resected tissue is evaluated for possible neoplasm and *H. pylori* infection.

Chronically scarred ulcers involving the pylorus and duodenal bulb can cause gastric outlet obstruction. The common manifestations are nausea and vomiting. Initial treatment consists of endoscopy with possible balloon dilation, antiacid secretion therapy, and formal peptic ulcer surgery for severe cases.

85
Gastric Polyps

Gastric polyps are grouped according to histologic characteristics, such as hyperplastic or inflammatory. Polyps occur as solitary or multifocal lesions. Hyperplastic polyps are the most predominant, comprising 80% of cases. They are made up of epithelial overgrowth and therefore are not true neoplasms. Epithelial overgrowth may be a response to local inflammation or regeneration from ulceration. These types of polyps often occur with chronic gastritis.

Hyperplastic polyps tend to be small, sessile lesions located in the antrum of the stomach. Their sizes vary, with some as large as several centimeters in diameter. Multiple lesions exist in 25% of cases. Adenomatous polyps comprise 5% to 10% of polypoid stomach lesions. The lesions are thought to arise from chronic gastritis with intestinal metaplasia and autoimmune gastritis. Adenomas have an element of proliferative dysplastic epithelium and therefore have some malignant potential. Adenocarcinoma is present in up to 30% of adenomatous polyps. Similarly, adenocarcinoma in other regions of the stomach can coincide with an adenomatous polyp (20%).

Gastric adenomas can appear sessile or pedunculated. They most commonly appear in the antrum as single lesions. Gastric adenomas can be as large as 3 to 4 cm before detection. The risk of cancer developing in the polyp is directly proportional to its size. Characteristics of favorable lesions include pedunculation and size less than 2 cm in diameter. Ten percent of benign adenomatous lesions develop into malignant lesions. Gastric adenomas occur most often in the elderly population (during the seventh decade).

Inflammatory fibroid polyps (eosinophilic granuloma) are submucosal growths composed of inflamed vascularized fibromuscular tissue with a prominent eosinophilic infiltrate. They arise anywhere in the alimentary tract but typically arise in the distal stomach. Occlusion of the pyloric channel can occur as they protrude into the lumen, causing acute gastric outlet obstruction.

Gastric polyps can manifest clinically as anemia because of chronic blood loss or decreased iron absorption. Achlorhydria is present in as many as 90% of patients. Endoscopy is the most useful tool for making the diagnosis. Non-neoplastic lesions cannot be distinguished from adenomatous polyps by endoscopic means. Therefore, histologic examination of gastric polyps through the collection of endoscopic brushings is essential. Snare excision through the endoscope can be accomplished for most polyps. Laparotomy or laparoscopic resection is indicated for lesions larger than 1 cm in diameter or when cancer is suspected. Single polyps can be excised through a gastrotomy and a frozen section performed. Gastrectomy is indicated when carcinoma is discovered in a biopsy specimen. Partial gastrectomy should be performed in cases of multiple polyps of the distal stomach. An antrectomy should be performed if 10 to 20 polyps are discovered spread throughout the stomach. Symptomatic diffuse multiple polyposis may require total gastrectomy.

86
Gastric Cancer

Tumors of the stomach include gastric adenocarcinomas, lymphomas, carcinoids, and mesenchymal tumors. Worldwide, gastric carcinoma is the second most common neoplasm. The prevalence of disease is higher in certain areas of the world, including Japan, South America, Russia, and Bulgaria.

Helicobacter pylori infection produces a chronic gastritis that is associated with a sixfold increase in the formation of gastric carcinoma. Chronic gastritis, bacterial proteins, and the local immune responses incite mucosal changes such as intestinal metaplasia, dysplasia, and ultimately the development of carcinoma. Hypochlorhydria secondary to chronic gastritis provides an environment conducive to bacterial growth. Diets that are low in fresh fruits and vegetables yet high in preserved foods (i.e., smoked, cured, salted) have been implicated as contributors to gastric carcinoma development. Host factors such as autoimmune gastritis, race (African Americans, Native Americans, and Hawaiians), and blood group A are associated with an increased incidence of disease.

There are two major classification systems for gastric carcinoma. The Lauren classification divides the disease into intestinal and diffuse subtypes. The intestinal form is characterized by tumors composed of glandular structures that resemble colonic adenocarcinoma. Intestinal forms occur most often in high-risk areas. Precursor lesions are often seen before the intestinal type developments. Overall, prognosis is better for intestinal than for diffuse subtypes. The diffuse subtype is characterized by infiltration of poorly differentiated, gastriclike mucous cells. The malignant cells are distributed throughout the mucosa and wall of the stomach as single cells or small clusters. Malignant cells take on a classic "signet ring" appearance because of mucin production and displacement of the nucleus toward the periphery.

The WHO classification organizes gastric cancer into five categories based on morphology. Ulcerating carcinoma accounts for 25% of lesions. These are composed of deep lesions that traverse all layers of the stomach. Surrounding organs can be involved through direct extension of the tumor through the wall of the stomach. Polypoid carcinomas make up 25% of gastric carcinomas as well. These large tumors grow in the stomach lumen. Metastasis is a late occurrence with these tumors. Superficial spreading tumors (15%) are considered early gastric cancer. The lesion is limited to the mucosa and submucosa. There is a 30% risk of metastasis associated with this lesion, and it has a more favorable prognosis. Linitis plastica (10%) is a diffuse lesion of the stomach penetrating all of its layers. The diffuse involvement of the stomach causes it to stiffen and lose flexibility through desmoplastic reaction and fibrosis. Advanced carcinoma is seen in 35% of cases. This lesion is characterized by large tumors that occupy the inside and outside of the stomach. The typical distribution of lesions within the stomach includes the antrum and lesser curvature (40%), the cardia (25%), the body or fundus (30%), and the entire stomach (5%).

The natural history of gastric carcinoma involves penetration of the lesion through the gastric wall beyond the serosa. Spread to regional and distant lymph nodes occurs. In particular, metastasis to supraclavicular lymph nodes (Virchow's node) may be the first sign of carcinoma. Sister Mary Joseph nodules are the result of tumor metastasis to the periumbilical region. Krukenberg tumors form after metastasis to the ovaries. Other areas of metastasis include the pancreas, duodenum, retroperitoneum, liver, and lungs.

The depth of invasion is the single most important factor for determining prognosis. Early gastric cancers are limited to the mucosa and submucosa. Such lesions occur with or without lymphatic invasion. Early gastric cancers are only discovered when aggressive surveillance is practiced. Mass screening programs instituted in high-risk areas such as Japan have a 30% to 35% detection rate of early gastric carcinoma. In contrast, only 10% of patients in the United States are diagnosed at the early stage. Early gastric cancers have a more favorable prognosis. Five-year survival rates approach 90% after definitive treatment for this lesion.

Clinical manifestations may not become apparent until late in the course of the disease. Typical symptoms begin with early satiety and a sensation of abdominal heaviness after a meal. The most common complaint is weight loss. Anorexia, vomiting, hemorrhage, and dysphagia can occur as well. A physical examination may reveal a palpable epigastric mass in one quarter of patients. Other signs include hepatomegaly (10%) and hemoccult-positive stools. Laboratory testing shows anemia in 40% of cases. Carcinoembryonic antigen level is elevated in 65% of patients and is a marker of extensive tumor spread. An upper GI series may facilitate the diagnosis in many cases. The drawback is its inability to distinguish between malignant ulcerating tumors and peptic ulcers. Endoscopy with biopsy of the gastric lesion confirms the diagnosis.

Surgical resection offers the only chance for cure of gastric carcinoma. The goal is to remove all possible tumor along with a 6 cm normal margin of stomach, duodenum, and regional lymphadenectomy. Frozen sections are obtained of potential proximal margins to ensure adequate resection. Antral tumors require a distal gastrectomy along with omentectomy and excision of the lymph nodes below the pylorus. A Billroth I (gastroduodenostomy) or II (gastrojejunostomy) procedure can be preformed to restore continuity. Total gastrectomy with splenectomy is the procedure of choice for proximal tumors and linitis plastica. Reconstruction is accomplished via creation of a Roux-en-Y esophagojejunostomy. Tumors within the cardia require esophagogastrectomy with splenectomy and intrathoracic esophagogastrostomy. Palliative resections are conducted to avoid gastric outlet obstruction in patients who are expected to live longer than 1 to 2 months. Adjuvant chemotherapy has not shown usefulness.

87
Gastrointestinal Lymphoma

The most common location for gastrointestinal lymphomas is the stomach. Gastric lymphomas account for less than 15% of gastric malignancies. Clinical manifestations generally include epigastric pain, early satiety, and fatigue. Anemia from occult bleeding is present in half of patients. Gastric lymphomas occur most often in men during the sixth and seventh decades. The most common location is in the antrum of the stomach, which is similar to gastric carcinoma.

Gastric lymphoma typically invades the mucosa or superficial submucosa. In the mucosa-associated lymphoid tissue (MALT) lymphoma, lymphocytes invade the lamina propria surrounding and destroying gastric glands. Diffuse large B-cell lymphoma (55%) is the most common form of gastric lymphoma. Other forms occurring less frequently include extranodal marginal cell lymphoma, Burkitt's lymphoma, and mantle cell and follicular lymphomas. Diffuse large B cell lymphomas are usually primary lesions derived from MALT lymphomas. Immunodeficiency and *Helicobacter pylori* infection are two important risk factors for its development. *Helicobacter pylori*–induced chronic gastritis occurs in 80% of patients with gastric lymphoma. Successful remission can be achieved in 50% to 75% of gastric lymphomas with eradication therapy for *H. pylori*. Patients undergo endoscopy 2 months after eradication of the organism and then twice a year for 3 years.

Burkitt's lymphomas of the stomach are very aggressive lesions that are associated with Epstein-Barr virus. These lesions tend to occur in younger patients and are usually located in the cardia or body of the stomach.

Endoscopic evaluation is the standard method for making the diagnosis. Prominent findings include nonspecific gastritis and gastric ulcerations without obvious masses. Endoscopic biopsy specimens can be nondiagnostic in some cases because of the submucosal growth of the lesion. Endoscopic ultrasound is a useful adjunct for determining the depth of invasion. Metastatic disease is evaluated by bone marrow biopsy, computed tomography (chest and abdomen), and examination of the upper airway. Suspicious lymphatic enlargement should be biopsied. *H. pylori* infection is diagnosed through endoscopic biopsies and serologic testing.

Multimodality treatment programs consisting of chemotherapy and radiation are the standard therapy. CHOP (cyclophosphamide, hydroxydaunomycin, Oncovin®, prednisone) is the standard chemotherapy regiment. The benefit of surgical resection is debated. Previous studies have demonstrated that surgery combined with chemoradiation provides disease-free 5-year survival rates equal to chemoradiation alone for early-stage (stage IE, IIE) disease (82% and 84%, respectively). Chemotherapy is the only viable treatment option for late-stage disease.

Gastric lymphoma may be discovered incidentally at the time of operation. Intraoperative frozen sections are used to confirm the diagnosis. Early disease encountered during surgery (i.e., stage IE or IIE; see Table 87.1 for staging system) should be resected. For widespread disease, surgical intervention is limited to obtaining tissue for diagnosis and repair of perforations.

TABLE 87.1. Staging systems for primary gastrointestinal non-Hodgkin's lymphoma.

IE	Lesion limited to gastrointestinal tract
IIE	Lesion spread to regional lymph nodes
IIIE	Lesion associated with distal nodal involvement (para-aortic, iliac)
IV	Lesion spread to other intra-abdominal organs (liver, spleen) or beyond abdomen (chest, bone marrow)

88
Digestion and Absorption

The body's fuel comes from carbohydrates, fats, and proteins and small amounts of vitamins and minerals. The basic step in the digestion of these fuels is hydrolysis. For carbohydrates, hydrolysis turns disaccharides and polysaccharides into monosaccharides. For fats, it turns triglycerides into glycerol plus free fatty acids. Proteins are hydrolyzed into their constituent amino acids. All the digestive enzymes are proteins. Absorption occurs by two main mechanisms, active transport and diffusion. Active transport requires energy to transport against a gradient, whereas diffusion requires no energy to transport along a gradient. The small bowel has the capacity to absorb several kilograms of carbohydrates per day, 500 g of fat, 700 g of protein, and 20 L or more of water. The colon can then absorb even more water and ions, but no nutrients.

Carbohydrates

Carbohydrates in the diet come from three main sources: sucrose, lactose, and starches. Carbohydrate digestion begins in the mouth with the enzyme ptyalin (an amylase), secreted by the parotid gland, which hydrolyzes starch into maltose and other smaller glucose polymers. Because food spends only a short time in the mouth, very little hydrolysis occurs. In the stomach, digestion continues in the body and fundus before the food is mixed with gastric secretions that inactivate the salivary amylase because of the low pH. By this point, about one-third of the starches will have been hydrolyzed to maltose. Most of the digestion of starches occurs when the chyme reaches the pancreatic secretions in the duodenum because of the high content of amylase in the pancreatic juice. Essentially all of the starches are converted to maltose and other very small glucose polymers by amylase. The microvilli brush borders of the enterocytes of the small bowel contain four important enzymes: lactase, sucrase, maltase, and α-dextrinase. These enzymes can split the disaccharides into their constituent monosaccharides.

Monosaccharides, and rarely disaccharides, are the breakdown products of carbohydrates that get absorbed. The most abundant monosaccharide is glucose, because it is the breakdown product of starches. Galactose from milk and fructose from cane sugar are the other two common monosaccharides. Glucose is absorbed in a cotransport mode with the active transport of sodium. Once inside the enterocyte, the glucose is transported to the interstitial space by facilitated diffusion. Galactose is absorbed by almost the same mechanism. In contrast to glucose and galactose, fructose is transported by facilitated diffusion all the way into and out of the enterocyte. Because it is not an active process, the transport of fructose is about half that of glucose or galactose.

Proteins

Proteins are large strings of amino acids held together by peptide bonds. Pepsin, secreted by chief cells in the stomach, begins protein digestion. Pepsin is most active in an acidic environment like the stomach. Pepsin digests collagen, a major player in the connective tissue of meats. Pepsin activity accounts for about 20% of protein digestion. Most protein digestion occurs in the proximal small bowel secondary to the proteolytic enzymes from pancreatic secretions. Trypsin, chymotrypsin, proelastase, and carboxypolypeptidase are the major proteolytic enzymes from the pancreas. They mainly break the proteins down into dipeptides, tripeptides, and some larger molecules. Several peptidases are found in the brush border of the microvilli of the duodenum and jejunum. They split the remaining larger polypeptides into tripeptides, dipeptides, and some amino acids, which are all transported into the enterocyte by a sodium cotransport mechanism. Some amino acids do not require this sodium cotransport and enter the enterocyte by facilitated diffusion. Once inside the enterocyte, the remaining dipeptides and tripeptides are broken down into amino acids and then passed into the bloodstream.

Fats

Triglycerides are the most abundant fat in the diet. Lingual lipase, an enzyme secreted by the lingual glands in the mouth, performs a small amount of digestion in the stomach. This is really inconsequential because essentially all fat digestion occurs in the small intestine. Initially, emulsification, or breaking of the fat globules into small sizes so that the water-soluble digestive enzymes can act on globule surfaces, occurs by the contractions of the stomach. The main contributor to emulsification is bile. It contains bile salts and lecithin, which are very important substances. They help to break the fat globules into smaller fragments, thus increasing their surface areas. Pancreatic lipase is the main enzyme of triglyceride digestion. It splits triglycerides into free fatty acids and 2-monoglycerides.

Bile salts, which aid in emulsification, also form micelles, polarized spheres that act as transporters of the monoglycerides and free fatty acids. These micelles go to the brush borders of enterocytes where the monoglycerides and free fatty acids diffuse immediately through the cell membrane to the interior of the cell. They are then recombined to form new triglycerides in the endoplasmic reticulum. The triglycerides are transferred to the Golgi apparatus where, combined with cholesterol and phospholipids, they form a polarized globule called a *chylomicron*, which is released from the Golgi and excreted by exocytosis out of the cell into the lymph. Chylomicrons travel in the lymph, emptying into the neck veins via the thoracic duct.

Other Substances

Water enters the enterocytes by diffusion, which means that it can be transported either way based on the concentration of the chyme. If the chyme is dilute, water will flow into the cells; if it is concentrated, it will flow out of the cells into the chyme until it is isosmotic with the plasma. Sodium diffuses into the cell and is actively transported out the basolateral membrane into the interstitium. The osmotic movement of water follows the sodium ions through the cells into the paracellular spaces. The absorption of sodium is greatly enhanced by aldosterone, which is secreted when dehydration is sensed. Aldosterone increases the absorption of sodium and chloride ions and water. It allows virtually no loss of sodium and little water loss in the feces. The large secretion of bicarbonate by the pancreas and bile is reabsorbed as CO_2 into the blood. Calcium ions are actively absorbed in the duodenum under the control of parathyroid hormone and vitamin D. Iron is also actively absorbed in the small bowel. Vitamins A, D, E, and K are the fat-soluble vitamins and are absorbed in the terminal ileum.

The colon also has a role in absorption. It can absorb up to 7L of fluid per day. Most of the remaining sodium and chloride that enter the colon are absorbed in the proximal colon. The colon secretes bicarbonate in exchange for chloride ions. This absorption of sodium and chloride creates an osmotic gradient for water to follow.

89
Gastrointestinal Hormones

The gastrointestinal (GI) hormones behave in a variety of fashions (endocrine, paracrine, and autocrine and as neurotransmitters). These hormones play important roles in the coordination of digestion efforts and provide a trophic effect on the GI system itself. Many GI hormones exert their effects through interactions with transmembrane receptors on the target cell surface. These transmembrane proteins are coupled to G-proteins that transduce the signal through the cell. Details concerning the specific actions, locations, and stimulators of each hormone are outlined.

Cholecystokinin is produced from the I cells of the duodenum and jejunum. It is responsible for eliciting gallbladder contraction, relaxing the sphincter of Oddi, and stimulating the pancreatic acinar cells to secrete enzymes. It also has a trophic influence on the small intestinal and pancreatic mucosa, stimulates the release of insulin, and encourages small bowel motility. Cholecystokinin is released by the interaction of amino acids and fatty acids with the small intestinal mucosa.

Enteroglucagon is produced from the L cells of the small intestine. It responds to the presence of glucose and fat by stimulating insulin release and limiting the release of pancreatic glucagon.

Gastric inhibitory polypeptide is derived from the K cells of the duodenum and jejunum. Fat and carbohydrates are the primary stimulants for its release. Gastric inhibitory polypeptide inhibits gastric acid and pepsin secretion and stimulates insulin release during hyperglycemia.

Gastrin is manufactured and secreted by the G cells of the gastric antrum and duodenum. Gastrin stimulates the secretion of gastric acid and promotes growth of the gastric mucosa. Peptides and amino acids present in the stomach stimulate the secretion of gastrin. Other major stimulators include antral distension, vagal stimulation, and gastrin-releasing peptide. Gastrin inhibitors include somatostatin, decreased pH (<3), and prostaglandins.

Gastrin-releasing peptide stimulates most GI hormones (except secretin). In addition, it has a trophic influence on the pancreatic, small, and large intestinal mucosa and stimulates motility in the GI tract.

Motilin is a peptide that is produced in the jejunum and duodenum that inhibits gastric emptying, stimulates the migrating motor complex of the GI tract, and induces changes in the lower esophageal sphincter. In effect, it coordinates the motor efforts of the lower esophageal sphincter, stomach, and small bowel during periods of fasting. Major stimulators include gastric distension and the presence of fat.

Neurotensin is widely dispersed throughout the intestinal tract with a primary focus in the distal portion of the ileum. Neurotensin promotes the secretion of water and bicarbonate from the pancreas in the presence of fat. Other functions include the inhibition of gastric secretion and the promotion of intestinal (small and large) mucosal growth.

Peptide YY is found in the distal small bowel and proximal portion of the large intestine. It is released in response to the presence of fat in the colon. Its principle action is to inhibit pancreatic secretion, inhibit gastric secretion, and promote mucosal growth within the small intestine.

Secretin is produced by S cells present in the mucosa of the duodenum. It acts upon the pancreatic ductal cells to secrete water and bicarbonate. In short, secretin helps to create an environment that favors the digestion of fat. Additional influences of secretin include inhibition of gastrin, gastric acid secretion, and gastric motility and stimulation of bile flow. In disease states such as gastrinoma, secretin has the opposite effect of stimulating gastrin releases. Therefore, it has been used for provocative testing of gastrinomas. Stimulators of secretin include the presence of fatty acids, decreased luminal pH, and bile salts.

Somatostatin is a peptide that is primarily responsible for inhibiting the release of most GI hormones. The D cells of the pancreas, the antrum, and duodenum produce somatostatin. Its universal inhibitory function is used in the management of intestinal fistulas and esophageal varices. Major stimulators include fat, protein, carbohydrates, increased acidity, and cholecystokinin.

Vasoactive intestinal polypeptide (VIP) functions as a neuropeptide. This peptide has several actions, which include vasodilation, the promotion of intestinal and pancreatic fluids, and the inhibition of gastric acid. Vagal stimulation is a major stimulator of VIP secretion. In disease states such as VIPomas, excess VIP produces watery diarrhea.

90
Crohn's Disease

Crohn's disease is an inflammatory condition involving the gastrointestinal tract. The disease can affect any part of the alimentary tract from the mouth to the anus. The most common areas affected are the small intestine and colon. Abdominal pain, diarrhea, fever, malaise, and weight loss are the most common symptoms. Typically, patients experience symptoms intermittently, with the periods of remission becoming shorter over time. Crohn's disease has a bimodal distribution, affecting people in the second to third decades of life and the fifth decade as well. The risk of developing Crohn's disease is equal across genders. Smokers have twice the incidence of disease compared with nonsmokers. The incidence of disease is highest in Jews and lower in African blacks. The greatest is familial association.

The cause of the disease is unknown. The most likely causes include infections, genetic influences, and immunologic dysfunction. Two infectious agents implicated are mycobacteria and measles. Immunologic dysfunction has been demonstrated in patients with Crohn's disease as well. Studies have revealed humoral and cell-mediated reactivity to intestinal cells. Inflammatory cytokines (interleukins [IL]-1, IL-2, IL-8, and tumor necrosis factor-α) have been implicated as mediators of the immune response. A genetic cause seems to be very probable. Studies have identified a gene on chromosome 16 that may have some involvement in Crohn's disease. The gene has been named *NOD2* and encodes for an apoptosis regulatory protein.

Crohn's disease has many key pathologic features. The most common sites affected are the small and large intestines. More than 50% of patients with the disease show involvement of both. One-third of patients have perianal and perirectal disease. Crohn's disease should be suspected when a patient presents with a history of multiple perianal fistulas and abscesses. Unlike ulcerative colitis, the rectum is usually spared from disease. The disease pattern is segmental, with some areas of bowel affected between normal segments called "skip areas." Again, this is in contrast to ulcerative colitis, which affects the bowel in a continuous fashion with no skip areas. The affected segments are often thickened and take on a dull appearance. Most notable is the presence of "creeping" mesenteric fat, fat that surrounds the entire circumference of the bowel. Loops of diseased bowel may juxtapose one another or other viscous organs and tend to form fistulas. Multiple areas of aphthous ulceration can be seen within the bowel mucosa. These areas enlarge in a linear fashion and coalesce together with normal areas of mucosa interspersed between. This gives the mucosa a cobblestone appearance. The ulcerations of Crohn's disease are transmural, in contrast to ulcerative colitis, which is restricted to the mucosa.

The diagnosis should be suspected for any patient with a history of intermittent crampy abdominal pain, diarrhea, weight loss, fever, and malaise. The abdominal pain is present commonly in the lower abdomen and, at times, may mimic acute disorders such as appendicitis. The diarrhea associated with Crohn's disease occurs with less frequent stools than ulcerative colitis. The stools also rarely contain mucus, blood, and pus when compared with ulcerative colitis. Radiographic studies often suggest the diagnosis, but it must be confirmed by endoscopy and biopsy. Contrasted barium studies may reveal a cobblestoned appearance of the mucosa, narrowing in the terminal ileum, or fistulas. Computed tomography usually reveals transmural thickening of the bowel. Endoscopy findings include aphthous ulcerations, cobblestoning, and skip areas. Colonoscopy should include inspection of the terminal ileum and biopsy. Certain serologic markers may aid in making the diagnosis. Perinuclear antineutrophil cytoplasmic antibody (pANCA) and anti-*Saccharomyces cerevisiae* (ASCA) are autoantibodies that have been linked to inflammatory bowel disease.

The complications of Crohn's disease are mainly obstruction and perforation. Chronic fibrosis and narrowing of the bowel lumen eventually lead to obstruction. Perforation can occur freely into the peritoneum, resulting in peritonitis, or can fistulize into adjacent structures. Fistulization is far more common than free perforation because of the inherent fibrotic nature of Crohn's disease. Abscesses also occur at areas of perforation. Patients with Crohn's colitis may present with toxic megacolon, which is marked by colonic distension, abdominal tenderness, fever, and leukocytosis. The incidence of cancer of the colon and the small intestine is also increased in patients with long-term Crohn's disease. Cancer of the small bowel is often detected late in its course. The risk of developing colon cancer is greater for patients with ulcerative colitis than for patients with Crohn's disease. Nevertheless, patients with Crohn's should undergo aggressive surveillance with colonoscopy.

Extraintestinal manifestations of the disease may develop as well. The most common site affected is the skin, resulting in erythema nodosum and pyoderma gangrenosum. Arthritis, arthralgias, ankylosing spondylitis, uveitis, iritis, hepatitis, pericholangitis, and aphthous stomatitis are other possible manifestations.

Management of Crohn's disease is based on the disease severity and the presence of complications. The aim of therapy is to treat acute episodes and to maintain remission. Medical treatment is the first line of therapy, with surgical methods reserved for complications. For mild to moderate disease forms, medical therapy includes the use of salicylates (i.e., mesalamine and sulfasalazine) and antibiotics (i.e., metronidazole and ciprofloxacin). Corticosteroids and immunosuppressants (i.e., azathioprine, methotrexate, cyclosporine, and mercaptopurine) are reserved for moderate to severe cases. Infliximab is an antibody to human tumor necrosis factor-α, which has been shown to be effective in maintaining remission. Most patients with long-standing Crohn's disease will require some form of surgical intervention. However, surgery is only palliative and offers no chance of curing the disease. Indications for surgery include failure of medical therapy, intestinal obstruction, abscess, fistula, perforation, hemorrhage, cancer, and perianal disease.

91
Ulcerative Colitis

Ulcerative colitis (UC) is an inflammatory disease of the rectum and colon. The disease is characterized by mucosal ulcerations beginning in the rectum and extending proximally to the colon. A continuous pattern of inflammation is present in contrast to the skip lesions found in Crohn's disease. The etiology has been attributed to dietary factors, immune dysfunction, and genetics, and patients with UC have elevated levels of inflammatory cytokines. The disease occurs equally in both sexes and can appear in any age group. However, there are peak onsets occurring during the second and fourth decades.

The disease pattern of UC is quite characteristic. Rectal involvement is nearly always present, with variable extension into the colon. The inflammation is limited to the mucosal and submucosal layers, which is in contrast to the transmural nature of Crohn's disease. The mucosa takes on a granular and swollen appearance or can appear denuded in the case of long-standing disease. At times pseudopolyps may be seen, which represent areas of regenerated inflamed mucosa. Microscopic features include polymorphonuclear infiltration into the crypts of Lieberkühn, multiple crypt abscesses, and mucosal ulcerations.

Diarrhea and rectal bleeding are the most common presenting symptoms. Stools occur frequently and tend to be bloody and mucoid in nature. Nocturnal diarrhea is associated with extensive disease. Other symptoms include left lower quadrant abdominal pain (caused by involvement of the left colon), fever, weight loss, fecal urgency, and tenesmus.

Complications of the disease include strictures, toxic megacolon, colon cancer, and extraintestinal manifestations. Strictures can have two etiologies, benign and malignant. Benign strictures are the result of muscularis mucosa hypertrophy. Features suggestive of malignant strictures include occurrence late in the disease, proximal location to the splenic flexure, and associated large bowel obstruction. Because of the increased risk of cancer with

UC, it must be assumed that the cause is malignant until proven otherwise. The risk of developing colon cancer increases with the extent of disease, disease duration, presence of dysplasia, and presence of primary sclerosing cholangitis. The risk for colon cancer increases by 1% to 2% each 10 years with pancolitis. The degree of dysplasia also has a directly proportional increased risk of cancer (i.e., low grade ~10%, high grade ~40%). Fibrosis of the extrahepatic and intrahepatic biliary ducts results in primary sclerosing cholangitis. It is associated more so with UC than Crohn's disease; furthermore, 70% of patients with primary sclerosing cholangitis also have UC. The presence of primary sclerosing cholangitis indicates a fivefold greater risk of cancer than UC alone. Toxic megacolon is a potentially life-threatening complication of UC. Patients generally present with a septic picture, including abdominal distension, tenderness, fever, tachycardia, and leukocytosis. Extraintestinal manifestations consist of peripheral arthritis affecting the knees and ankles and ankylosing spondylitis. These conditions tend to dissipate after colectomy.

Complete blood cell count, erythrocyte sedimentation rate, and stool studies are ordered to rule out other causes. Upper gastrointestinal imaging with small bowel follow-through should be completed to help differentiate between Crohn's disease and UC. Perinuclear antineutrophil cytoplasmic antibodies are serologic markers that have shown to be specific for UC. The diagnosis of UC is confirmed by colonoscopy. Endoscopic findings include friable-appearing mucosa to complete ulceration with edema and bleeding. Multiple sequential biopsy specimens are taken every 10 cm to inspect for dysplasia.

Surgical management has offered the only cure for UC. This is in contrast to Crohn's disease, which cannot be cured surgically. Medical therapies generally consist of mesalamine, corticosteroids, antibiotics, and immunosuppressants. Routine surveillance colonoscopy is recommended every 1 to 2 years for pancolitis with duration greater than 8 years. For patients with disease not extending beyond the left colon, surveillance may be delayed until 15 to 20 years after presentation. Indications for surgery include disease refractory to medical therapy, toxic megacolon, massive hemorrhage, the presence of dysplasia, and cancer.

The choice of surgical procedure is determined by the extent of disease and by the presence of complications. The most common indication for surgery is intractable disease. In this case, a total proctocolectomy with ileal pouch anal anastomosis is the gold standard and offers the advantage of avoiding a permanent stoma. In the case of toxic megacolon, surgery is undertaken only after failure of medical therapy (intravenous hydration, broad-spectrum antibiotics, steroids, and immunosuppressants).

The basic approach is a staged procedure beginning with abdominocolectomy, ileostomy, and, if possible, rectal mucous fistula. The mucous fistula decompresses the rectum and makes identification of the rectum easier at a later time. After recovery, the proctocolectomy can be completed with removal of the rectum along with ileostomy take down and ileal pouch anal anastomosis. The delayed procedure reduces the risk of pelvic sepsis that may occur if proctectomy is completed in the presence of toxic megacolon. The confirmed discovery of high-grade dysplasia in biopsy material is an absolute indication for total proctocolectomy. It remains controversial whether to recommend surgery in the presence of low-grade dysplasia.

92
Small Bowel Neoplasms

Small intestinal primary neoplasms are a rare occurrence. The propensity for tumor growth is much more likely in the large intestine than in the small bowel. Theories about why this occurs emphasize decreased exposure to carcinogens in the small bowel.

Small bowel tumors are classified as either benign or malignant. The list of benign tumors is long (adenomas, hemangiomas, fibromas, leiomyomas, and hamartomas). Benign tumors can arise from epithelial or connective tissue. Adenomas are the most common benign tumor of the small bowel and are generally discovered incidentally during autopsy. They occur in three varieties: villous, Brunner's gland, and true adenomas. Most are solitary and asymptomatic. When symptoms occur, they are usually obstruction or bleeding. Brunner's gland adenomas occur in the submucosa of the duodenum and develop from exocrine glands. The tumors can produce symptoms similar to peptic ulcer disease. Villous adenomas appear most often in the duodenum. They take on a characteristic soap bubble appearance on contrast imaging and can be associated with pain, bleeding, or obstruction. The malignancy risk of the lesions is about 55%. Leiomyomas occur less often than adenomas but are more likely to produce symptoms. These are tumors that arise from smooth muscle and are present most often in the jejunum. Obstruction can be caused by tumor growth into the lumen. Bleeding can result from the tumor outgrowing its blood supply and necrosis. Lipomas occur as small solitary lesions in the submucosa of the ileum and are a common cause of adult intussusception. Hamartomas of the small bowel are always associated with Peutz-Jeghers syndrome. This is an autosomal dominant disease characterized by multiple pigmented lesions of the skin and buccal mucosa, as well as polyposis of the gastrointestinal tract. Intermittent intussusception causes colicky abdominal pain. Hemangiomas are abnormal proliferations of blood vessels most often found in the submucosa of the jejunum. Hemorrhage is the most common manifestation of intestinal hemangiomas.

Malignant tumors include lymphomas, adenocarcinomas, carcinoid, and leiomyosarcomas. Lymphomas are typically found in the ileum where there is a large aggregation of lymphoid tissue. True primary intestinal lymphomas lack associated peripheral lymphadenopathy, mediastinal lymphadenopathy, and disease within the liver or spleen. In addition, these patients have normal white blood cell counts. There are three varieties of small bowel lymphomas: the western type (focal lesions), immunoproliferative small intestinal disease (diffuse intestinal spread of malignant lymphoid cells), and childhood abdominal lymphoma. Adenocarcinomas are typically found in the duodenum and proximal jejunum. Fifty percent of duodenal adenocarcinomas involve the ampulla of Vater. Symptoms range from jaundice to obstruction. Leiomyosarcomas can be found throughout the small bowel. These tumors form central ulcers and have a propensity to bleed.

Carcinoid tumors develop from Kulchitsky cells (enterochromaffin cells) and occur in the foregut, midgut, and hindgut. Most originate from the midgut and secrete serotonin, substance P, neurotensin, gastrin, somatostatin, motilin, secretin, and pancreatic substances. The most common site is the appendix, with the small intestine being second. Less than 2% of tumors smaller than 1 cm metastasize. Tumors of 2 cm have an 80% chance of metastasis. Carcinoid syndrome can manifest in up to 10% of patients with carcinoid tumors. Hallmarks of the syndrome include cutaneous flushing, diarrhea, bronchoconstriction, and right-side valvular disease. Symptoms are generally present until hepatic metastasis has occurred. Normally the liver metabolizes bioactive secretions from the carcinoid tumor. When the liver becomes involved with disease, these substances are secreted directly into the bloodstream.

Patients with small bowel tumors often seek medical help for nonspecific symptoms, including nausea, vomiting, abdominal pain, diarrhea, and occult bleeding. Malignant tumors are more likely to be symptomatic.

Obstruction is a possible complication of tumor growth. Malignant tumors tend to grow in a circumferential pattern, causing obstruction. Benign tumors can serve as a lead point and are the most common cause of adult intussusception.

Diagnosis is often made with radiographic imaging or endoscopy. Endoscopic examination is usually limited past the ligament of Treitz. Therefore, the most reliable test is an upper gastrointestinal series with small bowel follow-through. Enteroclysis is a technique in which a catheter is advanced to the small bowel and contrast is administered. This technique aids in visualizing small mucosal defects, which may help make the diagnosis. The diagnosis of carcinoid tumors can be confirmed with measurement of urinary 5-hydroxyindolacetic acid levels.

Bleeding and obstruction are the most common indications for surgery. Benign tumors of the small bowel are treated with segmental resection and primary anastomosis. Smaller lesions may be amenable to simple resection through an enterotomy. The remainder of the small bowel must be explored at the time of surgery to search for contiguous lesions. Malignant tumors are resected with 10-cm margins of both sides. The associated mesentery is removed as well. An end-to-end anastomosis is performed along with closure of the mesenteric defect. Duodenal periampullary carcinomas may require a pancreatoduodenectomy. When complete resection is not obtainable, a palliative resection should be attempted to prevent future complications of bleeding and obstruction. Carcinoid tumor requires a small bowel resection along with lymphadenectomy. Hepatic metastases should be resected whenever possible. When resection is not possible, hepatic metastases may be targeted with hepatic artery embolization or chemotherapy infused through the hepatic artery.

93
Intestinal Physiology

The small intestine is composed of the duodenum, jejunum, and ileum. Total length is approximately 600 cm. The duodenum is the most proximal portion, extending from the pylorus to the ligament of Treitz. Forty percent of the remaining intestine is jejunum, and 60% is ileum. Distal small bowel differs from more proximal small bowel in that it is smaller in circumference and has fewer plicae circulares (mucosal folds), more fat in the mesentery, and shorter vasa rectae. This reflects the difference in functional absorption.

Small bowel has four layers: mucosa, submucosa, muscularis propria, and serosa. The mucosa is the absorptive layer, and it is made up of villi and the crypts of Lieberkühn. In addition, lymphoid follicles (Peyer's patches) are present and increase in number distally. Epithelial cells differentiate into enterocytes, goblet cells, enteroendocrine cells, and Paneth cells. They are recycled every 2 to 5 days. Immunologic cells are also present. The submucosa carries the blood supply, lymphatics, and nerve fibers of the small intestine, as well as the ganglion cells of the submucosal (Meissner's) plexus. The muscularis propria consists of an outer longitudinal and inner circular layer, with the ganglion cells of the myenteric (Auerbach's) plexus interposed. The serosa is a single layer of cells and is a component of the visceral peritoneum.

The major function of the small intestine is nutrient digestion and absorption. Na^+ is absorbed via active transport, and water follows via its osmotic gradient. Carbohydrates are initially broken down by salivary and pancreatic amylase. They are then further digested into monosaccharides by brush border enzymes found in the duodenum and proximal jejunum. Of these monosaccharides, glucose and galactose are absorbed via Na^+-coupled active transport, whereas fructose is absorbed via facilitated diffusion.

Protein digestion begins in the stomach with the action of pepsin. Once in the duodenum, the presence of bile acid causes enterokinase to be released from the intestinal brush border. Enterokinase then causes the activation of tripsinogen to trypsin. Trypsin, in turn, activates itself and other pancreatic proteases. These pancreatic proteases, as well as enterocyte brush border enzymes, break down proteins into amino acids and oligopeptides. Of these amino acids, glutamine provides the primary fuel source for enterocytes.

Fat digestion begins with gastric and pancreatic lipase. The products of lipolysis then form mixed micelles with bile acids. The lipids then dissociate from the micelles in the brush border of the proximal jejunum. Fatty acid-binding protein facilitates diffusion of long chain fatty acids, and cholesterol is actively absorbed. Once in the enterocyte, short and medium chain fatty acids are directly absorbed, while long chain fatty acids are packaged into chylomicrons and then secreted into lymphatics.

Vitamin B_{12} is initially bound by R protein from the saliva. This complex is then hydrolyzed in the duodenum where gastric intrinsic factor then binds vitamin B_{12}. This complex is then absorbed in the terminal ileum. Water-soluble vitamins are absorbed via specific carrier-mediated transport. The fat-soluble vitamins (A, D, E, and K) are absorbed via passive diffusion, although vitamin K is also absorbed via a carrier-mediated uptake. Calcium transport is mediated by the calcium-binding protein calbindin, which is found within the enterocytes. Its synthesis is regulated by vitamin D. Other peptides produced by the intestine include the following:

Somatostatin → inhibits secretion and motility
Secretin → stimulates pancreatic and intestinal secretion
Cholecystokinin → stimulates pancreatic secretion and gallbladder emptying and inhibits sphincter of Oddi contraction
Motilin → stimulates intestinal motility

With more than 70% of the body's immune cells in the small intestine, the small bowel plays an important immunologic role. First, it serves as a barrier to invading organisms. Second, M cells overlying Peyer's patches transfer microbes to antigen-presenting cells.

Peristalsis is the propulsion of intestinal contents. It occurs via coordinated contraction of the outer longitudinal muscle layer, which results in small bowel shortening, and contraction of the inner circular layer, which results in intestinal narrowing. This process is regulated via both intrinsic pacemaker cells and external hormonal signals. Acetylcholine and substance P are stimulatory signals, whereas nitric oxide, vasoactive intestinal peptide, and adenosine triphosphate are inhibitory.

94
Colorectal Anatomy

The colon originates in the right lower quadrant as a blind pouch, the cecum, into which the ileum dumps its effluent via the ileocecal valve. The cecum is also identified by the appendix, present at the junction of the three taenia. The colon continues its clockwise course through the abdomen as the ascending colon, hepatic flexure, transverse colon, splenic flexure, descending colon, and sigmoid colon, which transitions into the rectum. The total length of the colon is 150 cm. Although continuous, the proximal colon to the splenic flexure is embryologically derived from the midgut, and the splenic flexure and distal colon are hindgut derivatives. This corresponds to its vascular supply, with the midgut portion supplied by the superior mesenteric artery and the hindgut portion by the inferior mesenteric artery.

The cecum is an intraperitoneal organ. The ascending colon, however, is fixed to the abdominal wall and has peritoneum on its anterior surface only. The transverse colon is the longest segment of colon and is again intraperitoneal. Because of its mobility, the positioning of the transverse colon within the abdomen is variable. The transverse colon is positioned between the layers of transverse mesocolon, which contains the middle colic artery. The transverse mesocolon also attaches to the lower border of the pancreas. The greater omentum fuses to the anterosuperior portion of the transverse colon. The splenic flexure is markedly superior to the hepatic flexure and is tethered to the diaphragm via the phrenocolic ligament. The descending colon is again fixed in position and does not have peritoneum on its posterior surface. The descending colon then becomes the sigmoid colon, which is again intraperitoneal. Classically described as S shaped, the course and length of the sigmoid colon is highly variable. Its length can range from 15 to 50 cm, and its mobility allows it to occupy any location in the pelvis or lower abdomen. It runs from the pelvic brim to the sacral promontory, at which point it becomes the rectum.

Like other areas of the gastrointestinal tract, the layers of the colon wall can be divided into the mucosa, sub-mucosa, muscularis, and serosa. The mucosa contains the glands of Lieberkühn, lamina propria, and muscularis mucosa. The submucosa contains lymphatics, blood vessels, and Meissner's plexus. The muscular layer is divided into the inner circular layer, where Auerbach's plexus lies, and the outer longitudinal layer. In the colon the outer longitudinal muscle layer is condensed into three bundles, the taenia coli. These bundles spread out to become continuous in the rectum. The outer layer, the serosa, is absent in the rectum. The colon is also identified by the presence of haustra and epiploic appendages. The cecum is the widest part of the colon, and the remaining colon tapers throughout its length until becoming the rectum, where it again widens.

The blood supply of the colon is highly variable. The first colonic branch of the superior mesenteric artery is the middle colic artery, which enters the transverse mesocolon and divides into right and left branches. The last branch of the superior mesenteric artery (SMA) is the ileocolic artery, which divides into an ascending and a descending (ileal) branch. More variable is the right colic artery, which may or may not be present. It classically arises from the SMA, but it may be a branch of the middle colic or ileocolic arteries. The left colon is supplied by the inferior mesenteric artery (IMA), which gives rise to the left colic artery and multiple sigmoidal arteries. All of the major colic arteries are connected via an anastomosing network; the colic arteries all feed the marginal artery of Drummond, which runs along the mesenteric border of the entire colon. The arc of Riolan, or meandering mesenteric artery, is present in 7% of individuals and is an arterial loop connecting the superior mesenteric system to the inferior mesenteric system. It may be an important collateral in instances of arterial disease. The superior mesenteric vein follows the course of the SMA. The inferior mesenteric vein receives tributaries from the left colon, sigmoid, and superior rectal vein. It joins the splenic vein, which then joins the superior mesenteric vein to become the portal vein.

Lymphatic drainage follows the arterial supply of the colon. Colonic lymph nodes are classified as follows:

Epicolic: on the colon or within the epiploices
Paracolic: between the colon and the marginal artery
Intermediate: along the major colic arteries
Main/principal: along the SMA and IMA

The rectum begins at the sacral promontory and is characterized by the merging of the taenia. It is 12 to 15 cm in length and has no mesentery, epiploic appendages, or haustra. It contains the valves of Houston at the points where the rectum curves. The valves of Houston are projections of the bowel wall including the circular but not longitudinal muscle layers. Because the projections are not full thickness, biopsy specimens taken from these areas have a lower risk of perforation. The rectum becomes the anal canal at the level of the levator ani musculature. Waldeyer's fascia is the rectosacral fascia and contains branches of the sacral splanchnic nerves and may have branches of the sacral vessels. Denonvillier's fascia lies anteriorly and separates the rectum from either the prostate or vagina. The lateral ligaments of the rectum run from the peritoneal reflection to the levator ani and may contain the middle rectal artery and pelvic splanchnic nerves. Blood supply is via the superior rectal artery, which is the terminal branch of the IMA, and the middle and inferior rectal arteries, which arise from the pudendal artery.

The anal canal runs from the anorectal junction (at the level of the levator ani) to the anal verge, approximately 4 cm. The musculature of the anal canal can be thought of as two cylinders. The innermost cylinder is made up of the smooth muscle of the intestinal wall and contains the internal sphincter, while the outermost cylinder is skeletal muscle under voluntary control and contains the external sphincter. The dentate line is located at 2 cm and is characterized by the columns of Morgagni and columnar epithelium proximal and squamous epithelium distal. This demarcation is also significant, because sensation is present distal to the dentate line.

95
Colonic Polyps

Colonic polyps are elevations in the colonic mucosa. They are clinically significant because of their potential to transform into a malignancy and to cause bleeding, obstruction, and alterations in bowel habits.

Colonic polyps are identified during a diagnostic or screening colonoscopic examination. The overall prevalence is 20%, and this increases to 33% by age 50. All areas of the colon and rectum can be affected. All polyps identified during a colonoscopy should be biopsied or resected when size permits. Patients with adenomas identified on colonoscopy should undergo another colonoscopy in 3 years. When this examination is normal, an every-5-year screening schedule can be resumed. When more than three adenomas are found or when pathology reveals a high-risk adenoma (dysplasia or carcinoma in the polyp or villus or size larger than 1 cm), screening colonoscopy should be continued every 3 to 5 years for life.

Polyps are histologically classified as hyperplastic or adenomatous. Hyperplastic polyps are small, sessile, and flat. They do not have an increased cancer risk, so they do not alter the routine screening regimen. However, because they cannot be distinguished from adenomas during endoscopy, they should always undergo biopsy. Adenomatous polyps are classified as tubular (87%), villous (5%), or tubulovillous (8%). Adenomas with a greater than 25% villous component have more risk of malignant transformation. The risk of malignancy increases with polyp size. A 1-cm polyp has a 2% cancer risk; a 2-cm polyp, 20%; a 3-cm polyp, 43%; and polyps larger than 3.5 cm have a 76% risk of malignancy.

Cancerous polyps are classified according to Haggitt level:

Level 0 = carcinoma *in situ*
Level 1 = submucosa in the head of the polyp
Level 2 = submucosa in the neck of the polyp
Level 3 = submucosa in the stalk of the polyp
Level 4 = submucosa beyond the stalk

Polyps classified as Haggitt level 3 or lower have a less than 1% likelihood of lymph node metastasis and can be treated with polypectomy alone when they meet the following pathologic criteria: (1) The specimen margins are greater than 2 mm; (2) there is no evidence of lymphovascular invasion; and (3) the tumor is well differentiated. Haggitt level 4 polyps have a 12% to 25% risk of lymph node metastasis and should be treated with segmental colectomy.

Juvenile polyps are 1 to 3 cm, are pedunculated, and occur in individuals less than 20 years of age. When they are solitary, they do not increase the cancer risk. Bleeding followed by intussusception is the most common manifestation. Patients with diffuse juvenile polyposis have a 10% risk of cancer, and colectomy is recommended.

Peutz-Jeghers syndrome is an autosomal dominant syndrome associated with colonic polyps and gastrointestinal hamartomas. Large polyps and hamartomas are resected to reduce the risk of intussusception. There is no increased cancer risk associated with these polyps, so prophylactic colectomy is not indicated.

96
Colon Cancer

Colorectal cancer is the second leading cause of cancer death, lung cancer being the first. It is the third most common malignancy and comprises 10% of all cancer diagnoses and 11% of all cancer deaths. An average person has a 6% lifetime risk of developing colorectal cancer. Colorectal cancer can manifest with occult or gross rectal bleeding, a change in bowel habits, or unintentional weight loss. Advanced disease can manifest with obstruction or perforation as the first sign.

Colorectal cancer screening for average-risk individuals should begin at age 50. Average-risk individuals include those who are asymptomatic (no change in bowel pattern, unexplained anemia, or rectal bleeding) with no personal history of colon cancer or inflammatory bowel disease and no family history of colorectal cancer. Screening colonoscopy is the gold standard and should be undertaken every 10 years following negative examinations. Because of the invasive nature and limited availability of colonoscopy, alternative screening protocols include annual fecal occult blood tests paired with either barium enema or flexible sigmoidoscopy every 5 years.

Colon cancers develop from the predictable sequence of adenomatous polyp → dysplasia → cancer. This is true for both the sporadic and hereditary forms of the disease. The two major forms of hereditary colon cancer are familial adenomatous polyposis (FAP) and hereditary nonpolyposis colon cancer (HNPCC).

Familial adenomatous polyposis is an autosomal dominant mutation in the tumor suppressor gene adenomatous polyposis coli (APC). Affected persons develop carpeting of their colon with polyps and have a 100% lifetime cancer risk if untreated; 50% develop adenomatous polyps by age 15 years and 95% by age 35 years. Surveillance requires annual colonoscopy beginning at age 10 years. When colonoscopy is not begun until a patient develops symptoms, two-thirds already have colon cancer. Prophylactic proctocolectomy with either ileoanal anastomosis or permanent ileostomy is needed by age 20 years. Patients require routine upper endoscopy as screening for duodenal polyps. Variations of FAP include Gardner's syndrome, which is associated with soft tissue and bony abnormalities, and Turcot's syndrome, which has a rare association with central nervous system tumors. In an attenuated form of FAP, polyps develop late in life and are not as numerous (<100). Annual surveillance is required, with colectomy indicated when the polyp burden surpasses 20, dysplasia is identified, or annual colonoscopy is difficult or not feasible.

Hereditary nonpolyposis colon cancer, formerly called *Lynch syndrome*, is also an autosomal dominant disorder characterized by a mutation in DNA mismatch repair genes. Hereditary nonpolyposis colon cancer demonstrates 80% penetrance, and tumors tend to be proximal in the colon and are characterized by microsatellite instability. Type I HNPCC is associated only with colorectal malignancies; type II is associated with other malignancies, especially uterine. The Amsterdam criteria are used for diagnosing HNPCC. They require three relatives (at least one first-degree) spanning two generations to be affected, with at least one relative having colorectal cancer before age 50. The Bethesda criteria are less stringent guidelines to identify individuals who should be evaluated for HNPCC. The Bethesda criteria include colorectal cancer before age 50, the presence of synchronous or metachronous HNPCC-associated tumors, two or more first- or second-degree relatives with HNPCC-associated tumors, or any first-degree relative with colorectal cancer before age 50. Screening should begin for affected individuals with colonoscopy at age 25 or 5 years before the age of onset of the earliest affected relative. Colectomy with ileorectal anastomosis is indicated when multiple adenomas are present or any lesion with microsatellite instability is identified. Segmental colectomy should be avoided, because 50% of affected individuals will have a second colon cancer within 10 years. There is a 12% risk of rectal recurrence, and proctocolectomy should be considered for patients with rectal adenomas. Patients with a rectum require continued endoscopic surveillance. Prophylactic hysterectomy and bilateral salpingo-oophorectomy should also be considered for women when childbearing has ended.

Nonhereditary colon cancer is treated with segmental colectomy with at least 5 cm margins. When possible, colonoscopy should precede resection, because 5% of patients have synchronous colon cancers, and 30% have polyps that warrant evaluation. If this is not possible (i.e., resection was emergent for perforation or obstruction), colonoscopy should be performed within 3 months. Preoperative testing includes a carcinoembryonic antigen (CEA) level test and a full metastatic work-up, because, at initial treatment, 17% of patients already have metastatic disease. Liver function should be measured, and abdominal computed tomography (CT) should be considered. The chest is evaluated with either plain film or chest CT. When metastatic disease is identified and the primary tumor is left *in situ*, 30% of patients require resection due to bleeding, obstruction, or perforation. Following resection, patients should have a colonoscopy every 3 to 5 years for life and CEA measured every 3 months for the first 2 years.

Colorectal cancer is staged using the TNM system, with nodal metastasis indicating stage III colon cancer and distal metastasis stage IV. Chemotherapy for colon cancer is indicated for all with stage III disease and is considered on a case by case basis for stage IV disease or stage II disease with unfavorable pathology. Chemotherapy consists of treatment with 5-fluorouracil and leucovorin with or without oxaliplatin. For stage III disease, chemotherapy has been shown to decrease recurrence and increase survival rate by approximately one-third. Radiation therapy is rarely used for treatment of colon cancer; however, it can be considered for T4 tumors.

97
Rectal Cancer

Rectal cancer comprises 30% of all colorectal cancers, with 42,000 new cases a year. Although rectal cancer shares the behavior and the adenoma–carcinoma progression sequence of colon cancer, it warrants special consideration because of the unique challenges rectal anatomy presents. In colon cancer, margins are discussed in terms of proximal and distal. Rectal cancer is unique in that the most difficult margin to manage is the lateral margin, because the rectum is surrounded by other vital structures. Obtaining an adequate distal margin may require choosing between a sphincter-sparing procedure or the creation of a permanent ostomy.

The most common presentation of rectal cancer is rectal bleeding. Rectal bleeding is often incorrectly attributed to hemorrhoidal disease. Even in the presence of hemorrhoids, if bleeding persists, a colorectal malignancy must be ruled out. Rectal cancers can also present with pain, tenesmus, urgency, or fistula-in-ano, all of which portend a poor prognosis.

The preoperative workup should include a metastatic workup (computed tomography of the abdomen and pelvis and chest x-ray) and a carcinoembryonic antigen (CEA) level test. A colonoscopy should be performed to rule out synchronous lesions, which are identified in 2% to 8% of patients. The lesion can be assessed by endorectal ultrasound (ERUS) or magnetic resonance imaging; ERUS can detect nodes larger than 5 mm and provides information on the depth of a lesion.

Rectal cancers are treated with surgery and often chemoradiation. Neoadjuvant therapy has been shown to decrease the rate of local recurrence and to increase the number of tumors amenable to sphincter-preserving therapy. Neoadjuvant chemoradiation is generally recommended for stage II and III diseases and may be appropriate for T2 lesions. Postoperative chemoradiation is recommended for all stage II and III lesions.

Transanal local excision is considered for tumors that meet the following criteria:

<8 cm from the anal verge
<4 cm in size
less than one-third of the rectal circumference
mobile
T1 or T2
no lymphovascular or perineural invasion
no mucinous characteristics
moderately or well-differentiated

Excision should be full thickness down to the perirectal fat with 1 cm margins. Lesions that do not meet these criteria are removed via a low anterior resection (lesions in the proximal two-thirds of the rectum) or an abdominoperineal resection. This should include total mesorectal excision with 2 cm tumor margins.

Postoperative surveillance consists of measuring the CEA level every 3 to 6 months for 2 years and colonoscopy annually (if polyps are present) or every 3 years (if polyps are not present).

98
Anal Cancer

Anal cancers are divided into anal margin and anal canal neoplasms, because this anatomic difference often indicates the type of cancer that develops and dictates the treatment. The anal canal is approximately 4 cm in length, from the anorectal ring (the level of the levator ani musculature) to the intersphincteric groove. The anal margin is the area from the anal verge extending out 5 cm. As a general rule, anal canal lesions are more aggressive. Location dictates lymphatic spread. Lymphatic drainage above the dentate line is to the superior and inferior mesenteric lymphatics. The area around the dentate line drains to the internal pudendal, obturator, and hypogastric lymphatics and distal to the dentate line drains to the inguinal and femoral regions. Risk factors for anal carcinomas generally include smoking, chronic inflammatory conditions, human papilloma virus and other sexually transmitted diseases, immunosuppression, and human immunodeficiency virus.

Anal canal lesions are given a variety of names (squamous, cloacogenic, etc.), behave in a similar manner, and are thus treated the same. Preoperative studies should include a metastatic workup (computed tomography of the abdomen and pelvis and chest x-ray) and imaging (endoscopic ultrasound or magnetic resonance imaging) to assess the extent of local invasion. Stage I lesions do not extend beyond the sphincters; stage II lesions extend to the perirectal fat; stage III lesions have lymph node involvement; and stage IV lesions have distant metastasis. Twenty-five percent of patients present with stage III disease and 6% with stage IV disease.

Anal canal lesions amenable to local resection are well differentiated, are less than 2 cm, are freely movable on examination, and have no evidence of sphincter involvement on imaging studies. One centimeter margins are recommended. With the exception of these lesions, treatment is chemoradiation with the Nigro protocol (radiation plus 5-fluorouracil and mitomycin). Follow up is recommended every 3 months after treatment is completed. Local recurrences are treated with either additional chemoradiation or abdominoperineal resection (APR). Survival rates are 80% for patients with tumors less than 2 cm and less than 50% for patients with tumors greater than 5 cm.

Anorectal melanomas have a particularly poor prognosis, with a 5-year survival rate of only 10%. Abdominoperineal resection has not been shown to increase survival rate; however, it is occasionally considered for patients who are thought to have a relatively favorable prognosis. Therapy consists of wide local excision for local control and chemotherapy. Lymphadenectomy is performed only in the presence of clinically positive nodes.

Anal canal adenocarcinomas are rare tumors with a very poor prognosis. They arise from the anal glands. They are treated with excision (local or APR) and the Nigro protocol.

Anal margin tumors encompass a broad spectrum of skin cancers. Bowen's disease is an intraepidermal, *in situ* squamous cell carcinoma. Contrary to previous beliefs, it is not associated with other gastrointestinal tract neoplasms. It is generally indolent, with only 5% of tumors progressing to invasion and metastasis. Patients with Bowen's disease can present with pruritus and/or burning but can be asymptomatic. The classic appearance is that of a scaly, erythematous rash, but this is highly variable and is diagnosed via punch biopsy. Treatment is with excision and intraoperative frozen sections to confirm negative margins. The degree of disease extension may require flap reconstruction. Abdominoperineal resection is reserved for tumors that invade the sphincters.

Paget's disease is an intraepithelial adenocarcinoma. Unlike Bowen's disease, Paget's disease is associated with other neoplasms 50% to 80% of the time. Therefore, colonoscopy is required. If a synchronous lesion is not identified, the treatment is a wide local excision. If rectal adenocarcinoma is found, the treatment is an APR.

Basal cell carcinoma of the anal margin is treated with local excision, similar to basal cell cancers in other locations. Verrucous carcinoma, also called giant *condyloma acuminata* or *Buschke-Löwenstein tumor*, is considered an intermediate neoplasm between condyloma acuminata and invasive squamous cell carcinoma. It is treated with wide local excision with 1 cm margins. If foci of invasive squamous cell carcinoma are identified in the specimen, chemoradiation should follow. Squamous cell carcinoma of the anal margin is treated with wide local excision, similar to squamous cells in other locations. Kaposi's sarcoma is treated with local radiation therapy. Leukoplakia is followed clinically with biopsy specimens taken from the affected region to rule out malignant progression.

99
Intestinal Obstruction

Small Bowel Obstruction

Obstructions of the small intestine can be produced by three different mechanisms. Adhesions, malignancy, or abscesses cause extraluminal obstructions. Lesions within the bowel wall cause intrinsic obstructions. Finally, gallstones, fecaliths, undigested particles, and foreign bodies cause obstructions of the luminal orifices. Sixty percent of small bowel obstructions are caused by adhesions. Adhesions are primarily the result of previous surgery (especially pelvic procedures). The remainder of small intestinal obstructions are caused by malignancy (20%), hernias (10%), Crohn's disease (5%), and other causes (2% to 3%; intussusception, gallstones, foreign bodies, and bezoars). Intra-abdominal malignant lesions metastasize to the peritoneum, creating implants. Peritoneal implants cause intestinal obstruction through local adhesion formation of direct compression of the adjacent bowel. Ventral and inguinal hernias can cause obstructions due to bowel incarceration and strangulation. Internal hernias predominantly result from previous surgery. Small bowel obstructions are classified as simple or strangulated. A simple small bowel obstruction is a mechanical obstruction without ischemic intestinal tissue. A strangulated obstruction encompasses impaired vascular flow leading to tissue ischemia.

In the early phases of obstruction, the bowel becomes hyperactive with increased peristalsis on either side of the obstruction. The bowel proximal to the obstruction eventually tires and becomes dilated. Intraluminal fluid and electrolytes collect within the bowel lumen, leading to dehydration and electrolyte abnormalities (i.e., hypochloremia, hypokalemia, and metabolic alkalosis). The third spacing of fluid eventually leads to hypovolemia, oliguria, azotemia, and, in severe cases, shock. Increased intra-abdominal pressure develops, which can impair venous return and compromise ventilation. Increased intraluminal pressure is another consequence of obstruction that can reduce mucosal blood flow, a

prelude to ischemia. This is especially true with closed loop obstructions (twisting of the bowel on itself) where there is no outlet for decompression. Closed loop obstructions are particularly hazardous because of occlusion of arterial blood flow, ischemia, and perforation. Stagnant intraluminal fluid allows for increased bacterial concentrations (i.e., *Escherichia coli*, *Streptococcus*, and *Klebsiella*) in intestinal loops that are normally sterile.

Clinical manifestations depend on the level and severity of the obstruction. The most common symptoms include abdominal pain, distention, nausea, vomiting, and obstipation. Proximal obstructions cause more frequent nausea and vomiting than those located distally. Feculent emesis is the result of bacterial overgrowth from a long-standing intestinal obstruction. Obstipation occurs late in the course of disease; the early phases of disease may be accompanied by diarrhea caused by increased peristalsis. Most cases are diagnosed through history, physical examination, and plain radiographs. Physical examination should include investigation for possible hernias (i.e., incisional, inguinal, femoral, and obturator). Common clinical findings include tachycardia, hypotension, hyperactive bowel sounds with audible rushes (borborygmi), and abdominal distension. Laboratory tests may show hypochloremia, hypokalemia, increased blood urine nitrogen/creatinine levels, hemoconcentration, and leukocytosis. It is important to note that no single clinical sign, symptom, or laboratory test has been shown to predict the severity of obstruction. That being said, there are some clinical parameters that indicate strangulation; however, these are not predictable in every patient. These include fever, peritonitis, leukocytosis, and tachycardia.

Sixty percent of intestinal obstructions are identified with abdominal plain films. Common findings include dilated small bowel loops and air–fluid levels seen in a stair-step pattern. Computed tomography is a helpful adjunct to plain films for ascertaining the diagnosis. Computed tomography can help determine the location of the obstruction, the cause of the obstruction (i.e., malignancy, abscess, and inflammatory disease), and the severity of the obstruction (i.e., complete, strangulation, or intestinal ischemia). It is also useful for diagnosing postoperative bowel obstructions; however, plain films are not generally helpful. Enteroclysis is an imaging method that employs intubation of the small intestine to administer air or barium contrast to the small intestine. This modality is helpful in the setting of low-grade intermittent obstructions, which are clinically puzzling. Ultrasound is useful for pregnant patients to avoid excess radiation, and magnetic resonance imaging is of little use.

The treatment of small bowel obstructions is either surgical or conservative. Treatment begins with the institution of supportive measures along with intestinal decompression. Resuscitation with isotonic intravenous fluids is necessary to correct dehydration. Serum electrolytes should be measured routinely and corrected as needed. Complete blood counts are used to evaluate for leukocytosis and hemoconcentration. Foley catheters are placed to closely monitor urine output as a gauge of resuscitation. Central venous catheters are used in severe cases to provide better access for resuscitation and to monitor central venous pressure.

Intestinal decompression is accomplished by the placement of either a nasogastric tube or a long intestinal tube. Both methods provide adequate decompression; however, long intestinal tubes are associated with a higher rate of ileus and longer hospital stay. From 60% to 85% of partial small bowel obstructions are alleviated with conservative treatment. Therefore, an initial attempt at nonoperative treatment should be made for patients having a probable partial obstruction. Nonoperative management is also appropriate for patients with widely disseminated malignancies causing obstruction. The acute inflammation and edema caused by Crohn's disease may respond favorably to conservative therapy.

Surgical management is indicated for patients who have failed conservative management (i.e., who experience clinical deterioration or increased intestinal distension), for patients with complete obstructions, and for patients with suspected intestinal compromise (i.e., strangulation, infarction, or perforation). Surgical treatment can be safely delayed for up to 24 hours to allow for resuscitation and hemodynamic optimization of the patient. The surgical procedure is tailored to the etiology of the obstruction. Lysis of adhesions should be performed for obstructions caused by adhesive disease. Hernias should be manually reduced and the hernia defect repaired. The viability of the involved intestine is best determined by clinical judgment. The suspected segment should be revived with warm saline sponges for 20 minutes after being freed. A second look operation may be indicated in 24 hours to inspect the segment of bowel. Fluorescein fluorescence or Doppler ultrasound

can be helpful in borderline cases. In the case of chronic Crohn's disease, stricturoplasty or resection of the diseased segment may be needed. Abscesses stemming from diverticular disease can be drained percutaneously. The laparoscopic approach is useful for patients with mild abdominal distension, proximal obstructions, single-band adhesions, and partial obstructions.

Complications include recurrent obstruction, small bowel enterotomies, fistulas, and death. Many methods have been used to reduce adhesion formation. Among the most effective is the practice of good surgical technique, which includes gentle handling of bowel, limited dissections, removal of foreign bodies (glove starch, using absorbable materials, limit sponge and gauze use), proper irrigation, and placement of omentum over the operative site. The recent advent of bioabsorbable membranes composed of hyaluronate (Seprafilm®) has been shown to reduce the severity of postoperative adhesion formation.

Large Bowel Obstruction

Obstructions of the large bowel can be grouped into mechanical and adynamic causes. Mechanical obstructions are the most common. Typical causes of mechanical obstructions include colon cancer, volvulus, and diverticular disease. Left-side colon cancers occur with obstruction more often than right-side cancers. A volvulus occurs when the colon twists upon its mesentery, producing a proximal and distal obstruction. This usually occurs at the sigmoid colon (80%) and cecum (15%). Volvulus of the transverse colon happens in only about 5% of cases. In the situation of a sigmoid volvulus, the colon twists in a counterclockwise fashion, whereas a cecal volvulus generally occurs with a clockwise twist. Colonic volvulus can be associated with chronic laxative use, high-fiber diets, pregnancy, and previous abdominal surgery. Pericolic abscesses or adherent small bowel loops can produce colonic obstruction in diverticular disease.

Ogilvie's syndrome (colonic pseudo-obstruction) is an example of an adynamic obstruction. The condition develops when impaired autonomic function leads to massive dilation and distension. Predisposing factors include trauma, recent pelvic or spinal procedures, metabolic changes, chronic debilitation, and certain drugs (i.e., calcium channel blockers, narcotics).

Intraluminal pressures increase proximal to the obstruction as air, gas, and colonic secretions build up. As the intraluminal pressure approaches the systolic pressure, the venous outflow from the bowel wall becomes impaired. This accentuates the third spacing of fluid and electrolytes into the bowel lumen, producing dehydration, azotemia, and electrolyte abnormalities. Further increases in intraluminal pressure compromise the intestinal flow, producing mucosal ischemia, infarction, and possible perforation. Septicemia can be caused by bacterial migration through lymphatic channels into the systemic circulation. According to Laplace's law, the cecum is the area of the colon with the greatest risk of perforation due to its large diameter and high wall tension.

Common manifestations include abdominal pain, distension, and obstipation. Fever and peritonitis occur with perforation. Bloody stools may suggest ongoing mucosal ischemia or malignancy. Symptoms can be sudden when caused by colonic volvulus, whereas malignancy will cause a slow onset of symptoms over months. As with most conditions, the evaluation begins with a history and physical examination. Serum electrolyte levels and complete blood counts are obtained as well. An obstruction series (i.e., chest, upright, and supine abdominal films) may show dilated segments of colon without rectal air. Cecal dilation to 10 to 14 cm (high risk of perforation) and free intra-abdominal air (perforation) are serious findings. Contrasted enemas can be used to identify the cause, severity, and level of obstruction. Suspicious findings include apple core lesion (rectal cancer) and the bird's beak sign (volvulus). Computed tomography can be helpful when malignancy or diverticular disease is the suspected cause.

Management begins with intravenous resuscitation to correct dehydration and address electrolyte abnormalities. The gastrointestinal tract is decompressed with the placement of a nasogastric tube. Urine output is measured with a Foley catheter to gauge resuscitation. In the case of colonic volvulus or pseudo-obstruction, endoscopic interventions (i.e., sigmoidoscopy, colonoscopy, or proctoscopy) can decompress the colon, allowing time for proper bowel preparation and a semielective surgical procedure later in the hospitalization. Endoscopic decompression has a 79% success rate with colonic volvulus; however, up to 90% recur. A rectal tube is left in place to facilitate continued decompression.

A successful endoscopic decompression of a sigmoid volvulus should be followed by bowel preparation and a definitive resection of the redundant colon. A sigmoidectomy with primary anastomosis is usually performed, but some surgeons recommend a subtotal colectomy in the case of widespread colonic dilation. Failure of preoperative decompression mandates an urgent laparotomy. Intraoperative colonic lavage can be performed in a viable unprepared colon, followed by resection and a primary anastomosis. Mesosigmoidoplasty involves creating an incision in the sigmoid mesentery spanning from the base to the top. The mesenteric incision is then closed in a transverse fashion. This method eliminates the need for resection and anastomoses in an unprepared colon and is associated with only a 1.6% risk of recurrence. Hartmann's procedure is performed for free perforations

and gangrenous tissue. The procedure of choice for cecal volvulus is a right hemicolectomy with ileocolic anastomosis. In cases of perforation or when gangrene has set in, an ileostomy and colonic mucous fistula should be created. Other alternatives are less attractive because of their poor success rates and morbid complications. Cecopexy is associated with a 30% rate of repeated volvulus. Cecostomy has many morbid complications, including fistula, abscess, wound infection, and abdominal wall sepsis.

Prompt surgical treatment is warranted for any patient with peritonitis, suspected perforation, or a failed attempt at endoscopic decompression. The goals of emergent laparotomy are to release a volvulus, inspect the tissue for ischemia, and decompress the colon. A 12-gauge needle is inserted obliquely into the tenia of the transverse colon and connected to suction to decompress the colon.

Right-side colon cancers that are discovered at the time of surgery should be treated with a right hemicolectomy and primary anastomosis between the ileum and transverse colon. Nonperforated cancers of the left colon are managed with colonic mobilization and intraoperative colonic lavage (a Foley catheter placed through the appendix to administer saline, a distal catheter through the level of obstruction to collect saline). After complete lavage of the colon, a subtotal colectomy with or without a primary anastamosis can be done. Patients in a malnourished state, with a free perforation, or taking immunosuppressant drugs should undergo a Hartmann's procedure.

Nonoperative management is the first line of therapy for colonic pseudo-obstruction (i.e., nasogastric decompression, intravenous fluid resuscitation, electrolyte correction). Decompression can be accomplished with the use of intravenous neostigmine or with endoscopic decompression. Recurrent pseudo-obstruction occurs in up to 15% of patients decompressed endoscopically. Neostigmine stimulates the parasympathetic system, causing contraction in the dilated colon. Patients must be placed on cardiac monitors while the drug is being administered because of possible bradycardia. Prolonged episodes of bradycardia can be counteracted with atropine. The typical dose is 2.5 mg given over a 3-minute continuous infusion. Decompression occurs within minutes of receiving the medication. Surgical intervention is reserved for cases refractory to conservative measures and cases complicated by perforation. Primary anastomoses are avoided because of the ischemic nature of the tissue. The creation of an ileostomy as well as a loop colostomy within the same stoma (end loop stoma) is preferred. Other alternatives include the formation of an ileostomy with a separate colonic mucous fistula and cecostomy.

100
Meckel's Diverticulum

Meckel's diverticulum is a congenital anomaly that is created when the vitelline duct fails to involute. The vitelline duct is an embryonic structure that connects the developing intestinal lumen to the yolk sac. This results in an outpouching of the intestinal wall called a *diverticulum*. The shape of a Meckel's diverticulum varies from a small outpouching to a long blind pouch and less commonly to a fistula. The anomaly is present in 2% of the population and is generally located within 2 feet of the ileocecal valve on the antimesenteric border of the bowel. The pluripotent cells line the inside of the vitelline duct, giving it the ability to form heterotrophic tissues. Fifty percent of Meckel's diverticula contain gastric mucosa, fewer contain pancreatic mucosa, and a very few contain colonic mucosa.

Meckel's diverticulum commonly manifests as bleeding or obstruction. Gastrointestinal bleeding is the most common manifestation for children. The bleeding can vary from occult bleeding causing anemia to acute hemorrhage. Gastric mucosa contained within the diverticulum is responsible for acid production that erodes the surrounding ileal mucosa, forming an ulcer. Intestinal obstruction may occur by way of volvulus, intussusception, or incarceration of the diverticulum within an inguinal hernia (Littre's hernia). Diverticulitis is a less common manifestation that mimics the symptoms of acute appendicitis. This presentation occurs more often in adults. Without intervention, perforation and peritonitis may follow. Neoplasms are very rarely associated with Meckel's diverticulum. Most associated tumors are benign.

Meckel's diverticula are often discovered incidentally at the time of laparotomy or at autopsy. The diagnosis is generally elusive. Routine imaging studies provide little aid in making the diagnosis. Sodium ^{99m}Tc-pertechnetate scintigraphy is the most reliable test for making the diagnosis. This test relies on uptake by the mucous-producing cells of gastric tissue. Gastric mucosa can often be found within the diverticulum and should demonstrate the accumulation of substrate at its location. The test is more reliable in the pediatric population because of the higher prevalence of ectopic gastric tissue. Administration of pentagastrin, glucagon, or H_2-blockers increases the accuracy of the test.

Surgical intervention is indicated for any symptomatic diverticulum. Segmental small bowel resection, including the diverticulum, is necessary for cases with gastrointestinal bleeding. Simple resection of the diverticulum is sufficient for cases not complicated by bleeding. The distal ileum should be inspected during a negative laparotomy for suspected appendicitis. An incidentally found diverticulum should be resected in children and in adults less than 80 years of age when it can be safely done.

101
Liver Anatomy

The average adult liver weighs approximately 1,200 to 1,600 grams. The liver is located in the right upper quadrant beneath the rib cage. The inferior border of the liver is the costal margin, and the superior portion lies just beneath the diaphragm. The liver is located at the level of the fifth rib on the right and the sixth rib on the left. Most of the liver is encapsulated except for the gallbladder bed, the porta hepatis, and the posterior surface adjacent to the inferior vena cava (IVC). Ligaments are formed from peritoneal reflections. The major ligaments supporting the liver are the coronary ligaments (attach liver to diaphragm), the triangular ligaments (attach liver to diaphragm), the falciform ligament (connects liver to diaphragm and anterior abdominal wall), the ligamentum teres (contains the left umbilical vein), the gastrohepatic ligament, the hepatoduodenal ligament (contains the portal vein, common bile duct, and hepatic artery), the hepatocolic ligament, and the hepatorenal ligament.

The functional unit of the liver is the hepatic lobule. Lobules are composed of a central vein surrounded by four to six terminal portal triads (portal vein, hepatic artery, and bile duct) to form a polygon-shaped unit. Hepatocytes are placed single file, radiating outward from the central vein. Endothelial-lined sinusoids run between each row of hepatocytes. The lateral walls of the hepatocytes form bile canaliculi, which flow toward the portal triads. The hepatocytes are divided into three zones traveling from the perimeter of the lobule to the center. Zone 1 (periportal zone) is located at the perimeter closest to the portal triads. This zone is rich in oxygen and nutrients and is the least susceptible to hypoxic injury. Zone 2 (intermediate zone) is located in the middle. Zone 3 (perivenular zone) is the most distant from the portal triads and, thus, has the least amount of oxygen and nutrients. It is this zone that is primarily affected during hypoxic insults (i.e., centrilobular necrosis).

Blood is delivered to the liver from the portal venous system and from the systemic system via the hepatic artery. Blood is drained from the hepatic sinusoids to the hepatic veins and then back to the systemic system through the IVC.

The portal vein forms from the connection of the superior mesenteric vein and the splenic vein. The portal vein runs in a superior direction behind the duodenum to enter the posterior portion of the hepatoduodenal ligament. The portal vein branches into a right lobar and left lobar branch at the porta hepatis. The right lobar branch runs through the liver tissue and then makes anterior and posterior divisions. These vessels divide further into anterosuperior, anteroinferior, posterosuperior, and posteroinferior segments. The left lobar branches run through the liver tissue for some distance before dividing into superior and anteroinferior branches. The anteroinferior branch is the larger of the two. It continues to divide into a lateral inferior branch and makes medial superior and medial inferior divisions.

In most cases, the common hepatic artery originates from the celiac axis off of the abdominal aorta. At the superior edge of the duodenum, the common hepatic artery gives off the right gastric artery as well as the gastroduodenal artery. From here, the common hepatic artery continues on as the proper hepatic artery within the anterior medial portion of the hepatoduodenal ligament. The proper hepatic artery divides into the left and right hepatic arteries at the porta hepatis. The right hepatic artery gives rise to the cystic artery before entering the hepatic parenchyma. The hepatic arteries tend to follow the same course as the portal tributaries within the liver itself. The medial hepatic artery arises from the left hepatic artery where it enters the quadrate lobe. Common variations in the arterial anatomy include the origin of the right hepatic artery from the superior mesenteric artery (17%) and the origination of the left hepatic artery from the left gastric artery (23%).

The central hepatic veins of the hepatic lobule interconnect to form sublobular veins. The sublobular veins coalesce to form collecting veins. The collecting veins unite to form three major hepatic vein conduits (i.e., the left, right, and middle veins). The right hepatic vein drains the right posterolateral segments and superior portion of the anteromedial segments. The right hepatic vein empties separately into the IVC. The left hepatic vein drains the left superolateral and inferolateral segments of the liver and then empties directly into the IVC. The middle hepatic vein drains the inferior portion of the right anteromedial segments as well as the left inferomedial portions of the liver. The middle vein unites with the left hepatic vein in 60% of cases.

The division of the intrahepatic biliary system follows the course of the portal vein divisions. On the right side, the right anterosuperior and anteroinferior ducts unite to form the right anterior bile duct. Likewise their posterior counterparts combine to form the right posterior bile duct. The right hepatic duct is formed when the two anterior and posterior segments unite before the porta hepatis. The left hepatic duct is formed from the union of the lateral duct and the medial duct. The lateral duct is composed of the superior lateral and inferior lateral ducts. The medial duct arises from the union of the medial superior and inferior ducts. The right and left hepatic ducts join outside of the liver at the porta hepatis to form the common hepatic duct. The common hepatic duct travels within the hepatoduodenal ligament and then joins with the cystic duct to form the common bile duct.

Original descriptions of liver anatomy were based on lobar divisions. The lobes were defined by ligamentous attachments as well as fissures and grooves. Modern descriptions organize the liver anatomy according to the arrangement of hepatic vasculature and bile ducts (Couinaud's system). Couinaud's system provides a better anatomic road map for hepatic surgery. In this system, the liver is divided into eight segments, each with its own pedicle (portal vein, hepatic artery, and bile duct). The segments are organized further into four sectors determined by the hepatic veins. The sectors are separated by three scissurae that run in the course of the hepatic veins. The four sectors can be grouped into components of the right and left liver. The middle scissura (also called *Cantlie's line*) runs anterior to posterior between the gallbladder fossa to the left of the IVC. It divides the liver into the left and right hemiliver. The middle scissura contains the middle hepatic vein. The right scissura contains the right hepatic vein and divides the right liver into anterior and posterior segments. The anterior portion contains liver segments V and VIII. The posterior portion contains segments VI and VII. Likewise the left liver is divided into anterior and posterior segments by the left scissura. The left scissura contains the left hepatic vein and is located posterior to the ligamentum teres. The anterior portion is composed of segments III and IV, and the posterior segment is made up of only segment II. Segment I (the caudate lobe) is located on the under surface of the liver anterior to the IVC. The caudate lobe receives vascular inflow and biliary drainage from both the left and right systems. The caudate lobe drains venous blood directly into the IVC via multiple small venules.

102
Hepatic Anatomy and Physiology

Hepatic Anatomy

The liver is the largest solid organ in the body, weighing about 1.5 kg in an adult. It lies in the right upper quadrant of the abdomen completely protected by the thoracic rib cage. It extends from the nipple line at the 4th intercostal space down to the costal margin in the midclavicular line. It is completely surrounded by a peritoneal membrane (Glisson's capsule) enveloping the portal triad structures as it enters the liver. The cephalad aspect is in contact with both hemidiaphragms, and the caudal surface is in contact with the stomach, duodenum, and colon. The posterior aspect is in contact with the right kidney and adrenal gland. The gross anatomic landmarks include the falciform ligament and the ligamentum teres hepaticus (round ligament of the liver) separating the left lateral segment of the liver (segments II and III) from the remaining liver. The round ligament, a remnant of the umbilical vein, is an external marker for the intrahepatic portion of the left portal vein. The ligamentum venosum, remnant of the ductus venosus, runs from the intrahepatic portal vein to the vena cava. It marks the border between the caudate lobe (segment I) and the left lateral sector. The gallbladder lies on the caudal surface of the liver. The left and right triangular ligaments secure the liver to the retroperitoneum. The gastrohepatic omentum connects the caudal surface with the lesser curvature of the stomach.

The functional anatomy is composed of eight segments, each supplied by a single portal triad (pedicle) composed of a portal vein, hepatic artery, and a bile duct. The liver is divided into sectors by longitudinal planes by scissurae drawn through each hepatic vein to the vena cava and further divided into segments by a transverse plane at the level of the main portal vein bifurcation. Segments are numbered clockwise on frontal view. The main scissura contains the middle hepatic vein that runs in an antero-posterior direction from the gallbladder fossa to the left side of the vena cava (Cantlie's line) and divides the liver into right and left sides. The right liver is divided into an anterior (segments V and VIII) and a posterior (segments VI and VII) sector by the right scissura containing the right hepatic vein. The left liver is split into an anterior (segments III and IV) and posterior (segment II—the only sector composed of a single segment) sector by the left scissura, which runs posterior to the ligamentum teres and contains the left hepatic vein. Segment I, the caudate lobe, is located on the posterior aspect of the liver not visible on frontal view and receives its blood supply from both the left and right portal pedicles; bile ducts from segment I also drain into the right and left hepatic ducts.

The portal vein is a valveless structure formed by the confluence of the superior mesenteric vein and the splenic vein. The portal vein provides approximately 75% of the total liver blood supply by volume. In the hepatoduodenal ligament, the portal vein is found most commonly posterior to the bile duct and hepatic artery. The normal pressure in the portal vein is between 3 and 5 mm Hg. Because the portal vein and its tributaries are without valves, increases in venous pressure are distributed throughout the splanchnic circulation. In the setting of portal venous hypertension, portosystemic collaterals develop secondary to the increased pressure. The most clinically important portosystemic connections include those fed through the coronary (left gastric) and short gastric veins through the fundus of the stomach and distal esophagus to the azygos vein, resulting in gastroesophageal varices. Recanalization of the round ligament/umbilical vein leads to a caput medusa around the umbilicus. Portal hypertension through the inferior mesenteric veins and hemorrhoidal plexuses can lead to engorged external hemorrhoids.

Most of the venous drainage occurs through three hepatic veins. The right hepatic vein drains segments V, VI, VII, and VIII and enters directly into the vena cava. The middle hepatic vein drains segments IVA, IVB, V, and VIII and enters into a common orifice with the left hepatic vein that drains segments II and III. A scissural branch of the left hepatic vein may run underneath the falciform ligament. A number of small, short hepatic veins enter directly into the vena cava from the undersurface of the liver in segment I.

The hepatic arterial anatomy is part of the portal triad and follows the segmental anatomy. The extrahepatic arterial anatomy can be highly variable. In 50% of the population, the common hepatic artery arises from the celiac trunk, giving off the gastroduodenal artery followed by a right gastric artery. The proper hepatic artery gives rise to the right and left hepatic arteries. There is great variation in hepatic artery anatomy that is important to understand and recognize during cholecystectomies, portal dissections, and liver resections. Replaced hepatic arteries are lobar vessels that arise from either the superior mesenteric artery (replaced right hepatic artery) or left gastric artery (replaced left hepatic artery). The left hepatic artery, regardless of its origin, enters the liver at the base of the round ligament. A replaced or accessory left hepatic artery will run in the lesser omentum anterior to the caudate lobe and is typically very easily identified. Accessory right hepatic arteries often supply the posterior sector of the right lobe (segment VI and VII). An accessory left hepatic artery typically supplies the left lateral segment. The cystic artery most commonly arises from the right hepatic artery but has a variety of common anomalies as well.

The spaces of Disse and clefts of Mall produce lymph fluid at the cellular level that is collected through sub-Glissonian and periportal lymphatics draining into larger lymphatics and emptying through the porta hepatis into the cisterna chyli. The anatomy and physiology of lymphatic drainage is important in the development of ascites and in the process of tumor metastasis. Evaluation of portal lymph nodes must be included during surgical operations for hepatic malignancies to exclude the presence of extrahepatic nodal disease.

Parasympathetic fibers from the hepatic branches of the vagus nerve and both parasympathetic and sympathetic fibers derived from the celiac plexus innervate the liver and gallbladder, the latter traveling along the hepatic arteries. Irritation or stretching of the Glisson's capsule or the gallbladder causes referred pain to the right shoulder through the third and forth cervical nerves.

The microscopic anatomy of the liver is characterized by the acinar unit involving an afferent portal venule, hepatic arteriole, and a bile ductule flowing antegrade along plates of hepatocytes. Portal venous blood flows along sinusoids and contacting hepatocytes through a perisinusoidal space of Disse; blood in these sinusoids flows toward a hepatic venule. Concentration gradients of oxygen and solutes occur along the sinusoidal spaces; three zones have been described, with zone one being closest to the portal triad and zone three being closest to the terminal hepatic vein. Hepatic arterioles are closely adherent to biliary ductule structures and play an important role in bile homeostasis. Hepatic arterioles ultimately feed into the sinusoids and contribute to the oxygen gradient across zones one, two, and three. The liver is also the largest repository of the reticuloendothelial system. Kupffer cells (tissue-based macrophages) line the sinusoidal spaces and are exposed to portal venous blood.

Hepatocytes are highly metabolically active, polarized cells found in platelike orientations in the acinus. They are covered with microvilli and are in close proximity with each other, allowing their common membranes to generate vital canaliculi. They also are in close proximity through the perisinusoidal space to sinusoidal endothelial cells and blood. Sinusoidal endothelial cells are highly permeable, allowing free flow of both large- and small-molecular-weight substances into the hepatocyte.

Hepatic Physiology

The liver is the center of metabolic homeostasis. It serves as the regulatory site for energy metabolism by coordinating the uptake, processing, and distribution of nutrients and their subsequent energy products. The liver is crucial to the production and release of a variety of circulating factors critical to the coagulation cascade. The most sensitive tests of liver function are measures of coagulation function: international normalized ratio, factor VII level, and factor V level. The liver also synthesizes a wide variety of plasma proteins; most important, albumin constitutes one seventh of total protein synthesis. The liver also makes a variety of acute-phase proteins and cytokines that have important interactions with a variety of inflammatory, infectious, and regulatory processes. The liver also synthesizes a large number of proteins, enzymes, and vitamins that participate in a tremendously broad range of bodily functions.

The liver is the critical intermediary between dietary sources of energy and the extrahepatic tissues. The liver accounts for about 4% of total body weight, yet it consumes approximately 28% of the total body blood flow and 20% of the total oxygen intake. The liver also expends about 20% of the total kilocalories used by the whole body. The liver receives dietary byproducts through the portal circulation, sorts them, metabolizes them, and distributes them to the systemic circulation. It also has a major role in regulating systemic sources of energy, such as fatty acids and glycerol from adipose tissues and lactate, pyruvate, and amino acids from skeletal muscle. The liver releases two major sources of energy into the extrahepatic circulation: glucose and acetoacetate. Glucose is derived from glycogenolysis of stored glycogen and from gluconeogenesis from lactate, pyruvate, glycerol, propionate, and alanine. Acetoacetate is derived from the oxidation of fatty acids. Storage lipids, such as triacylglycerols and phospholipids, are synthesized and stored as lipoproteins by the liver. These can be transported in the systemic circulation to the peripheral tissues. These complex and essential functions are regulated by hormones, by the overall nutritional state of the organism, and by the needs of obligate glucose-requiring tissues. The liver also is a critical storage site of glycogen and is essential to the maintenance of systemic glucose homeostasis through a complex process involving broad interactions with lipid metabolism. The liver also metabolizes lactate, and the Cori cycle is important in maintaining peripheral glucose availability in the setting of anaerobic metabolism. It also is an important modulator of lipid metabolism, performing a critical role in the synthesis of lipoproteins, triglycerides, gluconeogenesis from fatty acids, and cholesterol metabolism. In humans, cholesterol is synthesized in the liver and is used most importantly for bile salt synthesis.

The excretion of bilirubin, a product of heme metabolism from erythrocytes, occurs in bile. Bilirubin circulates bound to albumin in the blood. It is actively taken up by hepatocytes, where it is glucuronidated and actively secreted into bile. Benign disorders of bilirubin metabolism include Dubin-Johnson and Rotor's syndromes, which produce conjugated (direct) hyperbilirubinemia. Unconjugated hyperbilirubinemia is seen in Crigler-Najjar type II and Gilbert's syndromes. Crigler-Najjar type I syndrome causes neonatal kernicterus and invariably is fatal. The liver has an immense capacity to metabolize bilirubin, such that correction of jaundice in hilar biliary obstruction requires drainage of only one liver sector. Even with complete lobar biliary obstruction, the serum bilirubin level may be normal.

103
Hepatobiliary Imaging

Abdominal Plain Films

Abdominal plain films are usually used in the initial evaluation of disease. Specific information concerning hepatobiliary disease cannot generally be gained from plain films. This being said, important information can be gained from plain films. This information includes calcifications and gas shadowing. Calcifications can be associated with hemangiomas, granulomatous disease, and metastatic neoplasms. Chronic cholecystitis can be associated with gallbladder wall calcification, called *porcelain gallbladder*. The risk of gallbladder cancer is greater with a porcelain gallbladder.

Overlying gas shadowing can indicate a number of hepatic conditions. Portal venous gas can indicate an ischemic process such as bowel infarction, necrotizing enterocolitis, hemorrhagic pancreatitis, or ulcerative colitis. The portal venous system is generally demonstrated in the periphery of the liver as branching linear gas shadows. Abscesses can appear as large collections of overlying gas. Pneumobilia can be the result of an incompetent sphincter of Oddi or a gastroduodenal ulcer or can occur after enteric anastomosis.

Oral Cholecystography

Oral cholecystography is an older imaging technique that requires the patient to drink oral contrast. Once ingested, the contrast material is absorbed through the intestines and excreted into bile. The gallbladder concentrates the contrast material contained in the bile. This method allows for visualization of stones or wall abnormalities that appear as filling defects. Gallbladder dysfunction is evident through the failure to opacify the gallbladder and failure to contract. The accuracy of oral cholecystography for diagnosing gallbladder disease approaches 100%. The technique has largely been abandoned as other modalities such as ultrasound, computed tomography (CT), and magnetic resonance imaging (MRI) have improved.

Radionuclide Imaging

Liver scintigraphy is used to evaluate a variety of hepatic diseases, ranging from malignancy to cholecystitis. The technique is limited by its lack of resolution and its higher cost. Other modalities, such as CT, MRI, and ultrasound, are less time consuming and less expensive. ^{99m}Technetium-labeled sulfur colloid can be used to evaluate for hepatic metastases. Hemangiomas may be visualized with tagged red cell scans (^{99m}Tc-labeled red blood cell). Hepatobiliary iminodiacetic acid (HIDA) scans can provide some important information concerning gallbladder function when evaluating patients for suspected biliary colic or cholecystitis. These scans involve the administration of iminodiacetic acid labeled with ^{99m}Tc (such as diisopropyl IDA or DISIDA). This radionucleotide is taken up in the liver and excreted within the biliary system. The test is commonly used to evaluate the contractibility of the gallbladder, the gallbladder ejection fraction (normal is 55% to 75%), and the patency of the biliary system. Failure to opacify the gallbladder signifies biliary obstruction, and decreased ejection fractions (<55%) suggest biliary dyskinesia. There are many factors that can cause false-positive results, including hepatitis, cirrhosis, pancreatitis, prolonged fasting, and hyperalimentation. The study is also helpful for evaluating for postoperative bile leaks and congenital disorders such as biliary atresia. Radionucleotide imaging is also helpful in the workup of malignant diseases. Neuroendocrine tumors can be located using radioactive somatostatin analogues (^{111}-indium octreotide). This is especially useful for localizing gastrinomas preoperatively.

Ultrasound

Ultrasound is the most common noninvasive test of the liver. Ultrasound is close to 100% accurate for evaluating gallbladder and biliary disease. Gallstones are intraluminal in ultrasound images. Characteristics commonly associated with acute cholecystitis include a thickened gallbladder wall, pericholecystic fluid representing edema, distention, gallstones, sludge, and sonographic Murphy's sign. In addition, the biliary tree (intra- and extrahepatic) can be evaluated for signs of obstruction and dilation. Common bile duct dilatation (<6 mm) can be seen with ultrasound, although the cause may not always be identified (i.e., common duct stones or malignancy). Ultrasound is quite good for evaluating gallbladder and biliary disease but begins to lose accuracy when examining hepatic masses, especially with cirrhosis. Hepatic metastasis can be overlooked in 50% of cases. Therefore, ultrasound of the liver is a poor tool for excluding liver metastasis. When a focal mass is seen in a cirrhotic liver, the chance of malignancy is about 98%.

Doppler ultrasound is a useful tool for evaluating the hepatic vascular system. Its use is indicated for conditions such as portal vein thrombosis, evaluation after liver transplant, and follow up after transjugular intrahepatic portal-systemic shunt (TIPS) placement. Portal vein thrombosis is diagnosed by the absence of flow through the portal vein seen on Doppler ultrasound. Other associated findings include dilation of the vein or the presence of echogenic material within the lumen. In some instances the portal vein is replaced by venous collaterals when thrombosis is long standing. Pulsatile blood flow from within the venous thrombosis can be a sign of neoplastic invasion.

Doppler ultrasound helps exclude extrahepatic portal vein obstruction and determine baseline flow velocities before TIPS placement is attempted. The function of the TIPS is evaluated at regular intervals (every 3 months for 1 year) with Doppler ultrasound to monitor for hepatic vein stenosis. Velocities less than 60 cm/sec suggest stenosis. Many institutions implement routine Doppler ultrasound evaluation of hepatic vasculature after liver transplantation. In particular, the hepatic artery is examined for signs of stenosis caused by the associated morbidity and mortality. The most common indication of stenosis is an intrahepatic tardus parvus waveform (i.e., prolonged systolic acceleration time [>0.1 second] and low resistive index [>0.5 second]). Thrombosis of the hepatic artery is indicated by the absence of arterial waveforms in the hepatic artery and liver. Postoperative edema can produce false-positive results. Thrombosis may be predicted when a series of Doppler ultrasound examinations show normal hepatic artery flow initially that progresses to loss of diastolic flow, then to decreased systolic velocity, and finally to the entire loss of arterial waveforms.

Computed Tomography

Parenchymal imaging of the liver is better with CT than with ultrasound. The specifics and background of CT are discussed in Chapter 16. Computed tomography scans of the liver can be done as noncontrasted or as single-, dual-, or triple-phase intravenous contrast studies. The type of study needed is determined by the specific disease process being evaluated. Diffuse hepatic diseases may be better detected with noncontrast imaging. Intravenous contrast can obscure diseases such as hemochromatosis and choledocholithiasis.

Single-phase studies are done to visualize focal hepatic lesions (e.g., trauma, malignancy). Single-phase studies acquire images approximately 1 minute after contrast is administered (peak enhancement of the liver). Intrahepatic masses enhance at a lower intensity than does the normal surrounding liver tissue. Single-phase studies are used for demonstrating biliary dilatation.

In dual-phase studies, images are acquired before and after intravenous contrast enhancement. This allows for imaging of the liver during hepatic artery enhancement and portal venous enhancement. This technique is helpful for staging malignancies and determining the resectability of hepatic lesions. The evaluation of hepatocellular carcinoma is easier than more laborious methods such as iodized oil CT (poppy seed oil uptake by hepatocellular carcinoma) and CT arterial portography. Triple-phase studies involve capturing images before and during arterial and portal venous phases of enhancement.

Computed tomography can also be useful for detecting abnormalities of the biliary system. Dilated bile ducts can be clearly seen with single-phase contrast imaging. Primary sclerosing cholangitis is associated with beaded dilations of the intrahepatic ducts. Cholangiocarcinoma often appears with central duct obstruction along with intrahepatic ductal dilation.

Magnetic Resonance Imaging

Magnetic resonance imaging is used primarily as an adjunct to other imaging modalities. The basic concepts behind MRI are discussed in greater detail in Chapter 16. Magnetic resonance imaging relies on the variations in water content among tissue types to differentiate them. Hepatic malignancies tend to have higher water content than the surrounding liver parenchyma, which produces a relatively low signal on T1-weighted images. Unfortunately, the liver parenchyma also tends to produce a low signal on T1 images, making the distinction between normal and neoplastic tissue difficult to resolve. T2-weighted scans are generally done following T1 to provide better contrast between the two tissues (i.e., bright signal in tumor, low signal in normal liver) and in conditions such as fatty infiltration of the liver, which can be confused with a neoplasm. Alterations in the signal frequency suppress certain tissues, such as fat, and lower the intensity of fat in the image.

As with CT, MRI also has the capability of providing intravenous contrast enhancement of images. Gadolinium is a paramagnetic intravenous contrast agent used to accentuate MRI images. Gadolinium is commonly used in magnetic resonance angiography (MRA) in which images are obtained with contrast in the vascular system. This modality is often used to image the portal venous system. The second most common use for gadolinium is with dynamic multiphase imaging of hepatic parenchyma. Obtaining images with administration of contrast is similar to that of CT (i.e., single, double, or triple phase). Contrast agents that have a specific affinity for liver tissue have been developed but are rarely used because of their potential for causing lumbar back pain and hypotension.

Magnetic Resonance Cholangiopancreatography

Magnetic resonance cholangiopancreatography (MRCP) is an excellent alternative to endoscopic retrograde cholangiopancreatography (ERCP) for imaging the biliary system. The complications associated with ERCP (i.e., pancreatitis, cholangitis, bleeding, and perforation) can be avoided with MRCP because it is noninvasive. It is an attractive alternative for patients with previous biliary/enteric surgery (i.e., choledochoenterostomy). Magnetic resonance cholangiopancreatography employs T2-weighted images gathered in volume or in slices to view the ductal structures. Extrahepatic ducts can be seen with 100% accuracy; however, visualization of the intrahepatic ducts is limited to the outer one-third of the liver with approximately 90% accuracy. Pancreatic ducts, with exception of the ampulla, can be imaged in most patients. Conditions such as pancreatic divisum and abnormal common channels can be visualized with MRCP. It is also used for detecting choledocholithiasis in preoperative patients. Stones as small as 2 mm are detected in most cases. Obstructing gallstones causing acute pancreatitis are detected in 50% of cases. Strictures, ductal dilatations, and other signs of acute and chronic pancreatitis can be seen on MRCP. Biliary obstructions due to cholangiocarcinoma can be evaluated with MRCP. The entire biliary tree proximal and distal to the level of obstruction can be examined in detail. Additional information concerning the spread of the tumor can be obtained, which is useful for staging the malignancy.

Invasive Imaging Procedures

Cholangiograms are indicated for the evaluation of stones, tumors, strictures, and leakage. Cholangiography can be performed during surgery, through a T-tube, or via percutaneous technique. An adequate cholangiogram consists of a scout image of the right upper quadrant before administration of contrast, images of contrast filling the biliary system (i.e., right and left hepatic radicals and common bile duct), and delayed images showing contrast emptying into the duodenum. Intraductal stones commonly appear as filling defects within the lumen. Pitfalls of stone detection include air bubbles, which can be introduced into the biliary tree and mimic filling defects and blood clots. A diluted iodinated contrast agent is generally used at a 1:1 ratio of contrast to saline. The use of densely concentrated contrast or dilute contrast can obscure the stones in the ducts.

Operative cholangiography can be conducted during open or laparoscopic cholecystectomies. It involves the administration of iodinated contrast to the biliary system through a surgically created opening of the cystic duct or gallbladder. The study can be done with 93% success and 100% accuracy in most cases. When intraoperative cholangiogram is used selectively (e.g., for patients suspected of having choledocholithiasis or who have elevated liver function tests, dilated common bile duct, or jaundice), the risk of leaving retained stones after surgery is about 1%. Intraoperative cholangiograms are also helpful for evaluating aberrant ductal anatomy before committing to ductal transection.

A T-tube cholangiogram uses a surgically placed biliary drainage catheter to deliver contrast media to the biliary system. The study is used to evaluate for stones, malignancy, stenosis, to follow up on interventions, and to inspect biliary anastomoses. Contrast is allowed to enter through the tube by gravity or by hand injection. T-tubes generally remain in place for 4 to 6 weeks to allow for maturation of a transperitoneal tract. This prevents free spillage of bile into the peritoneum, which occurs with premature tube removal. The development of a mature tract is essential before an interventional procedure is undertaken. Confirmation of proper tract maturation can be made using a contrast tract-o-gram. In this study, the T-tube is removed over a guidewire, and contrast is administered through the exit site at the skin. Images are obtained as the contrast material travels through the tract. Extravasation of contrast material indicates an immature tract and requires replacement of the T-tube.

Percutaneous Transhepatic Cholangiography

During percutaneous transhepatic cholangiography (PTC) the biliary tree is accessed with a small-gauge needle (21 or 22) that is passed percutaneously through the liver parenchyma. Radiographic contrast is administered through the needle to visualize the bile ducts. Noninvasive studies have largely replaced the use of PTC. The technique is now generally reserved for percutaneous bile duct dilatations, for biliary decompression proximal to obstructing lesions, or when noninvasive techniques are not feasible. Percutaneous transhepatic cholangiography is contraindicated when conditions prevent safe access to the liver, such as overlying loops of bowel. Relative contraindications include ascites, coagulopathy, contrast allergy, and the presence of vascular tumors. The procedure must be conducted using analgesia, sedation, and hemodynamic monitoring. Prophylactic antibiotics are given to avoid biliary sepsis. Potential complications include biliary sepsis, bleeding, bile leak, and pneumothorax. The technique can be performed successfully in nearly 100% of patients with dilated bile ducts and about 90% in nondilated patients. The overall risk of major complications is approximately 3%.

Allergic reactions to contrast agents manifest with rashes, facial or glottic edema, laryngospasm, bronchospasm, arrhythmias, and hypotension. Patients with a history of an allergic reaction receive low-osmolar contrast and steroid prophylaxis (Table 103.1).

TABLE 103.1. Regimen for patients with allergic reactions to contrast agents.

Intravenous (IV)	By mouth (po)
Methylprednisolone 32 mg IV × 2 doses (12 and 2 hours before contrast)	Prednisone 50 mg po × 3 doses (13, 7, and 1 hour before contrast is given) Benadryl 50 mg po 1 hour before contrast

104
Jaundice

Jaundice is a condition that involves yellowing of the mucous membranes, skin, and sclerae by bilirubin accumulation in these tissues. Jaundice usually develops when bilirubin levels exceed 2 mg/dL. Bilirubin is the natural product of the breakdown of hemoglobin from aged red blood cells. Unconjugated bilirubin is insoluble and is bound to serum albumin. Unconjugated bilirubin is transported to the liver where it is conjugated in the hepatocytes by uridine diphosphate-glucuronyl transferase. The bile canaliculi collect the conjugated bilirubin and empty it into the intestine by way of the biliary tree. Bilirubin enters the terminal ileum and colon and is converted to urobilinogen. It is urobilinogen in the feces that imparts its dark color. Approximately 10% to 20% of urobilinogen is reabsorbed by the portal system. Urobilinogen is eliminated either by the kidneys or by excretion into the bile.

Causes of jaundice can be grouped into unconjugated (indirect) or conjugated (direct) hyperbilirubinemia. On rare occasions, elevations in both fractions occur. Indirect hyperbilirubinemia is the consequence of increased bilirubin production or decreased hepatocyte uptake. Examples include hemolytic anemia, transfusion reactions, and sepsis. Direct hyperbilirubinemias can be subdivided into hepatic and posthepatic causes. Hepatic causes of jaundice involve decreased hepatocyte transport or conjugation. Causes include certain drugs (rifampin, quinacrine), hepatitis, sepsis, cirrhosis, and cholestasis. Biliary obstruction is an example of posthepatic jaundice. Posthepatic jaundice is characterized by an elevation in the direct (conjugated) fraction of bilirubin. Direct hyperbilirubinemia due to biliary obstruction is a primary concern of the surgeon.

Clinical manifestations of jaundice include yellow discoloration of the sclerae, oral mucous membranes, the palms of the hands, and the soles of the feet. The differentiation between direct and indirect hyperbilirubinemia can be made using history and physical examination. A history of jaundice with normal colored urine and stools suggests a mostly indirect hyperbilirubinemia. Symptoms of dark urine along with pale stools are suggestive of a direct hyperbilirubinemia. The latter can be attributed to the absence of urobilinogen in the feces due to hepatocellular dysfunction or biliary obstruction. Of note, painless jaundice with a slow onset weight loss may indicate a malignant cause.

Cholestatic syndrome is a constellation of symptoms that are brought about by a long-term decrease in bilirubin excretion to the intestine. This change may be the result of hepatocellular dysfunction (no conjugation or excretion by hepatocytes) or by obstruction of the biliary system. Symptoms include steatorrhea, pruritus, dark urine, and light-colored stools.

In addition to physical examination, there are several laboratory tests and imaging modalities that are helpful for making the diagnosis. A history of hepatitis viral infection, alcoholism, or portal hypertension suggests a hepatic etiology of the jaundice. Abdominal pain, pruritus, rigors, and hepatomegaly may be indicative of a posthepatic etiology. More specifically, cholelithiasis produces right upper quadrant pain, and choledocholithiasis produces signs of cholangitis (fever, transient jaundice). Routine laboratory tests include complete blood count, fractionated bilirubin (indirect and direct), liver transaminases (aspartate transaminase [AST] and alanine transaminase [ALT]), alkaline phosphatase, γ-glutamyltranspeptidase, and amylase. Imaging is used in this evaluation to identify biliary obstruction. Some of the most commonly used modalities include cholangiography (endoscopic retrograde cholangiopancreatography [ERCP] or percutaneous transhepatic cholangiography [PTC]), ultrasound, hepatobiliary iminodiacetic acid (HIDA) scan, magnetic resonance cholangiopancreatography (MRCP), and endoscopic or conventional ultrasound. Conventional ultrasound is approximately 95% accurate for detecting extra- and intrahepatic ductal dilatation. Ultrasound is quick, noninvasive, and inexpensive and is generally the first test employed. Cholangiography is the gold standard modality for diagnosis and possible intervention of biliary obstruction.

A hemolytic workup is warranted for patients who have an indirect hyperbilirubinemia. Direct hyperbilirubinemias require a thorough workup to differentiate between hepatic and obstructive causes. When intrahepatic disease is the suspected etiology, a hepatitis viral panel and a possible liver biopsy procedure are needed to search for definitive evidence of cirrhosis.

Extrahepatic biliary obstruction can be the result of a benign or malignant process. Ultrasound is the first test used to confirm ductal obstruction. Patients with gallstones and suspected choledocholithiasis with dilated ducts on ultrasound should undergo ERCP for possible stone extraction and then laparoscopic cholecystectomy. Preoperative ERCP is 95% successful at clearing common duct stones causing jaundice. Alternatively, patients can undergo intraoperative common duct exploration in conjunction with laparoscopic cholecystectomy. Patients with gallstones and normal ductal diameters of the biliary tree on ultrasound can be further evaluated with MRCP. When choledocholithiasis is discovered with MRCP, the physician may use preoperative ERCP before laparoscopic cholecystectomy.

Malignant lesions are suspected in patients with ongoing weight loss, abdominal or back pain, fatigue, and jaundice in the absence of cholelithiasis. Computed tomography scanning is required in addition to ultrasound to determine the etiology and the level of obstruction. Endoscopic retrograde cholangiopancreatography is the modality used to evaluate proximal obstructions and for decompression when indicated. Biliary strictures discovered at the time of cholangiography should be biopsied, or cytologic brushings should be taken. Pancreatic lesions can be biopsied by endoscopic ultrasound and fine-needle aspiration when possible. Lesions distal to the hepatic bifurcation are best approached through PTC. The specific treatments for biliary strictures and pancreatic neoplasms are discussed in Chapters 116 and 124.

Postoperative Jaundice

Jaundice manifests in approximately 1% of all postoperative patients. The condition is the result of many ongoing processes related to intraoperative or postoperative events. Jaundice that develops after hepatobiliary procedures can be due to retained common duct stones, biliary leak, common duct injury, or postoperative stricture. The timing of the onset of jaundice is also important to determining the diagnosis. The development of jaundice by postoperative day 2 can be caused by hemolysis and red blood cell turnover. This is especially true in the case of massive blood transfusions, hematoma reabsorption, or transfusion reactions. Underlying hemolytic anemias can be caused by the administration of certain drugs (glucose-6-phosphate dehydrogenase deficiency and sulfa drugs). Congenital disorders such as Gilbert's syndrome or Dubin-Johnson's syndrome may manifest in the early postoperative period. End-organ damage caused by decreased perfusion can result in conjugated hyperbilirubinemia 5 to 10 days postoperatively. Renal failure decreases the elimination of conjugated bilirubin, thus increasing its serum levels. Complications due to anesthetic or antibiotic agents manifest 7 to 10 days after a surgical operation. Cholestasis can be a consequence of intra-abdominal sepsis, total parenteral nutrition (TPN), biliary sludge, and acalculous cholecystitis. Cholestasis associated with TPN is more prevalent with TPN formulas containing high carbohydrate content and with prolonged use. Viral hepatitis infections from blood transfusions are also a source of late-onset jaundice.

105
Liver Abscesses

Liver abscesses are generally bacterial, amebic, or echinococcal. Liver abscesses are the second most common cause of fever and right upper quadrant abdominal mass; the first is cholecystitis.

Bacterial Abscess

Bacterial (pyogenic) abscesses of the liver are caused by ascending biliary tract infections, hematogenous spread from the portal system, and hematogenous spread via the hepatic artery to the liver secondary to septicemia, trauma, and direct extension from intraperitoneal infection. The most common cause is biliary tract infections stemming from biliary obstruction (by gallstones or malignancy). Hematogenous spread from the portal venous system is the second most common cause. The portal system can become seeded with bacteria from diverticulitis, inflammatory bowel disease, or a perforated appendicitis. Most pyogenic abscesses occur in the right lobe. Abscess sizes range from 1.5 to 8 cm, and only about 20% exceed 8 cm. Abscesses can be solitary or multifocal.

The diagnosis can be made through abdominal ultrasound in most cases. When biliary obstruction is implicated, biliary duct dilatation can occur along with the abscess cavities. Ultrasound can delineate abscess cavities as small as 2 cm in diameter. Computed tomography scanning can evaluate lesions as small as ~0.5 cm in diameter. In addition, it can detect abscesses that may be present near the hemidiaphragms. Endoscopic retrograde cholangiopancreatography (ERCP) and percutaneous transhepatic cholangiography (PTC) are used only when malignancy or biliary stones is the suspected etiology. Blood cultures are positive in up to 50% of cases. There is a strong association between visceral abscesses and *Streptococcus milleri*–positive blood cultures.

Percutaneous drainage accomplished through ultrasound or CT guidance is the treatment of choice. Drainage catheters can be left in place, or serial needle aspirations can be performed. Serial imaging is used to ensure that the cavity is collapsing. Catheters typically remain in place for 2 to 3 weeks. This method is associated with a failure rate of 15% and a complication rate of 4%. Surgical drainage procedures are reserved for cases that are not amenable to or fail percutaneous drainage. The procedure can be accomplished openly or laparoscopically with good success. Multiple abscesses may require a partial hepatic resection. Antibiotic treatment should cover anaerobic and aerobic species. Common microbial isolates include *Escherichia coli*, *Klebsiella*, *Pseudomonas*, and *Streptococcus*. Antibiotic treatment is usually instituted for 3 to 4 weeks once an abscess cavity has been resected, for 4 to 8 weeks after drainage of a solitary abscess, and for 8 weeks when multiple abscesses have been drained. Liver abscess formation with malignancy is a bad prognostic sign, with 28% mortality.

Amebic Abscess

Amebic abscesses are generally caused by infestation with *Endameba histolytica*. The organisms gain entry into the gastrointestinal tract and enter the portal system through intestinal ulcerations. From there they reach the liver to form abscesses. Liver abscesses are generally solitary, predominantly occurring in the right lobe. They contain a characteristic red-brown anchovy paste fluid. They are generally organized by a surrounding wall of granulation tissue, an intermediate zone with destroyed hepatic parenchymal cells, and an inner necrotic core. Fever and right upper quadrant pain are the usual presenting symptoms. Left lobe abscesses can cause epigastric tenderness. Diarrhea occurs in adults and children who often have bloody mucous stool. A history of recent travel to an endemic area (Mexico, Central America, and Southeast Asia) is helpful when determining the diagnosis. Complications develop from abscess rupture or bacterial infection (72%). Abscess fluid can travel to the pleural, pericardial, or peritoneal cavity.

The diagnostic workup begins with laboratory testing. Leukocytosis is evident in most cases. Liver function tests are not useful when making the diagnosis. Amebas are present in stool samples in only 15% of patients. Indirect hemagglutination tests are helpful, as is polymerase chain reaction (PCR). Aspiration fluid from the abscess cavity may allow visualization of the organism.

The initial approach to treatment involves medical therapy. Metronidazole is the drug of choice, administered at 750 mg three times a day for 10 days. Improvement in the size of the abscess cavity may be seen as soon as 1 week after treatment is initiated. Metronidazole has proved effective in treating the intestinal and hepatic phases of infection. A residual cavity of no consequence may persist for up to 2 years. Percutaneous or surgical drainage is reserved for failed medical therapy. Secondary bacterial infections are treated similar to pyogenic abscesses.

Echinococcal Abscess

Echinococcal abscesses are derived from infections by *Echinococcus granulosus* or *Echinococcus multilocularis*. The diagnosis is made by the combination of serologic testing (indirect hemagglutination tests and enzyme-linked immunosorbent assay [ELISA]) and ultrasound evaluation of the cyst. If the diagnosis is suspected, aspiration of the cavity should be avoided to prevent anaphylaxis associated with cyst spillage. Abdominal plain films may show calcification of the cyst. Surgical excision is recommended for secondarily infected or symptomatic echinococcal cysts. Antiparasitic therapy alone is of little help. However, mebendazole or albendazole is instituted 1 month before surgical drainage and is continued postoperatively to reduce the risk of recurrence or intraoperative spread. Marsupialization and complete excision are the procedures of choice.

106
Hepatic Malignancies

Hepatocellular Carcinoma

The most common hepatic malignancy is hepatocellular carcinoma (HCC). The incidence is higher in geographic areas (Southeast Asia and Africa) with endemic hepatitis B infection (HBV). The disease occurs more often in males than in females (8:1). Other contributing factors include alcohol use, cirrhosis, and smoking. Hepatitis C viral infection (HCV) can also cause HCC, but there is a stronger association with HBV infection. Certain carcinogens such as aflatoxin (*Aspergillus*-produced hepatotoxin) and chemicals such as vinyl chloride, pesticides, hydrocarbons, and nitrites have also been implicated.

The condition most commonly manifests in men between the ages of 50 and 60 years. Patients often complain of right upper quadrant abdominal pain and weight loss. A palpable mass is identified in some instances. Most patients tend to present late within the course of the disease. Rupture with acute-onset abdominal pain and shock due to hemorrhage is a rare but possible presentation. Obstructive jaundice, Budd-Chiari syndrome (obstruction of the hepatic veins), hemobilia, and fever of unknown origin are other rare possibilities. Approximately 1% of cases demonstrate paraneoplastic syndromes manifested by hypercalcemia, hypoglycemia, and erythrocytosis.

Computed tomography or magnetic resonance imaging is the first step in using radiographic imaging to make the diagnosis. A key radiographic feature is demonstration of tumor hypervascularity. In addition, these imaging modalities are helpful for searching for peritoneal metastasis, nodal involvement, and invasion of vascular or biliary structures.

α-Fetoprotein (AFP) levels are measured to help confirm the diagnosis as well as to monitor patients during treatment. Preoperative biopsies are not required to plan for definitive treatment. Percutaneous biopsies expose the patient to the risk of tumor spillage, rupture,

and bleeding. The diagnosis of HCC can be secured through imaging and AFP measurement.

Patients with HCC often have associated cirrhosis. Long-term survival depends on the characteristics of the tumor and on the condition of the patient's liver. In fact, both factors are included in the staging of the disease. The preoperative workup evaluates the extent of liver disease and the presence of metastases. Hepatocellular carcinoma commonly spreads to the lung, bone, and peritoneum. Computed tomography scanning evaluates the primary lesion (i.e., macrovascular invasion, multifocal disease) and looks for spread elsewhere in the abdomen. Chest x-rays are obtained routinely to search for pulmonary metastases. A bone scan is done only when a patient has symptoms (i.e., bone pain or pathologic fractures).

Liver resection is the treatment of choice for patients who can tolerate it. Patients with cirrhosis are categorized according to the Child-Pugh classification system to determine the extent of disease and associated mortality with surgery. It is generally accepted that Child-Pugh C patients are not candidates for liver resection. Child-Pugh B patients are considered borderline candidates; Child-Pugh A patients may be able to tolerate a liver resection. In addition, other factors such as coagulopathy, thrombocytopenia, and hyperbilirubinemia must be considered. Laparoscopic staging adds more information concerning the extent of disease. In addition, it may prevent nontherapeutic laparotomies in one of five patients selected for resection.

The Okuda staging system is the most widely accepted system for classifying HCC. This system accounts for tumor size, total bilirubin and albumin levels, and the presence of ascites. Histologic grades of HCC include well differentiated, moderately differentiated, and poorly differentiated. However, histologic grading has shown no influence on clinical outcome. The histologic growth pattern of the individual tumors may be more important than differentiation. The three different growth patterns include the hanging type, the pushing type, and the infiltrative type. The growth patterns are important, because they relate to the ease of resectability of the tumors. The hanging-type lesion contains a small vascular stalk that connects it to the liver and makes the lesion easier to resect. The pushing type is confined to a fibrous capsule. Surrounding vascular structures become displaced rather than invaded as the lesion grows. The infiltrative type has a tendency to invade surrounding vascular structures. Clear margins are difficult to obtain when resecting this type of tumor. Multifocal lesions can develop through the periportal spread of satellite lesions. Multifocal tumors are usually encountered in end-stage disease.

There are many different treatment options available for HCC. Complete tumor excision via partial liver resection or liver transplantation is the only chance for cure. Only 10% to 20% of patients present with resectable disease. Liver resections are recommended mostly to patients with Child-Pugh A liver disease. Child-Pugh B and C cases are recommended for transplantation. Short-term and long-term survival rates for liver resections are 58% to 100% for 1 year, 28% to 88% for 3 years, 11% to 75% for 5 years, and 19% to 26% for 10 years. Factors that negatively impact survival include tumor size, infiltrative growth pattern, vascular invasion, metastasis (lymph node or intrahepatic), <1 cm margins, multicentric disease, and absence of a capsule. The outcomes of liver transplantation for HCC have improved through better patient selection. In general, patients with single tumors 5 cm or smaller or patients with no more than three tumors that are 3 cm do well with transplantation.

Nonsurgical therapies for HCC include percutaneous ethanol injection for small tumors (2 to 5 cm). The technique involves single or multiple injections of ethanol into the tumor, depending on the size of the lesion. Ethanol injection causes tumor cell dehydration, thrombosis, and coagulative necrosis. Long-term survival is estimated at 24% to 40%. Percutaneous acetic acid injection works in a manner similar to ethanol injection. It is a more powerful necrotizing agent, making it useful for septated tumors.

Thermal ablation involves the use of cold or heated probes to destroy tumor tissue. Cryotherapy employs a probe introduced into the tumor to generate a freeze–thaw cycle that results in tissue destruction. The procedure can be conducted through open laparotomy, laparoscopically, or percutaneously. The 2-year survival rate is reported at 30% to 60% for this technique. In radiofrequency ablation, alternating high-frequency currents heat the tissue surrounding the probe. Temperatures reach 60°C, allowing the treatment of lesions up to 7 cm in diameter. Both techniques are limited by the heat-sink effect of adjacent blood vessels.

Transarterial chemotherapy and transarterial embolization are therapies that use blood flow from the hepatic artery to direct the therapy. Transarterial chemotherapy involves the infusion of 5-fluorouracil–based drugs through the hepatic artery and to the tumor. An infusion pump is placed via laparotomy to access the hepatic artery. Up to 60% of cases respond to this technique. A limitation of this method is hepatic toxicity. Arterial embolization has success rates of 50%. Radiation therapy and systemic chemotherapy are not effective in the treatment of HCC.

Cholangiocarcinoma

Cholangiocarcinoma is a malignancy that arises from the biliary tree. Lesion can occur anywhere within the biliary system, including the intrahepatic ducts. The confluence of the right and left hepatic ducts is the most common location for disease (40% to 60%) and is the location for Klatskin tumors. Only 10% originate from the intrahepatic ductal system. Intrahepatic lesions are the second most common primary hepatic lesion. Common risk factors include primary sclerosing cholangitis, choledochal cysts, and recurring cholangitis. Patients present with right upper quadrant pain and weight loss, with jaundice seen in 25% of patients. Serum levels of AFP are normal; however, carcinoembryonic antigen (CEA) level may be elevated. Computed tomography or magnetic resonance imaging reveals a hepatic mass associated with biliary dilatation. Spread along the biliary tree to regional lymph nodes and within the liver is common. The best treatment option is complete surgical resection, which is accomplished in 60% to 90% of cases. The 5-year survival rate for completed resections approaches 44%. Chemotherapy and radiation play little roles in the treatment of intrahepatic cholangiocarcinoma.

Hepatoblastoma

Hepatoblastoma rarely occurs in adults; however, it is the number one primary hepatic tumor in the pediatric population. The median age of onset is 18 months, with a few cases presenting after 3 years of age. Tumors arise from fetal or embryonic hepatocytes. The condition manifests most often as a nontender abdominal mass. Thrombocytopenia and anemia may be present. Elevations of serum AFP are present in 80% to 90% of patients. Neoadjuvant chemotherapy has been used to down-stage tumors before resection. However, complete excision of the tumor offers the best chance at cure. About one-half of patients with lung metastases are cured with a combination of hepatic tumor resection and chemotherapy with or without resection of lung metastases.

Sarcomas and Lymphomas

Angiosarcoma is the most dominant primary sarcoma of the liver. This lesion has a strong association with vinyl chloride and thorotrast exposure. Lesions are commonly multifocal and have an overall poor prognosis. Lymphomas may appear in the liver as primary neoplasms in the form of non-Hodgkin's lymphoma.

Metastatic Tumors

Metastatic lesions are the most common form of hepatic malignancy. A plethora of primary tumors metastasize to the liver, including lung, breast, colon, prostate, kidney, pancreas, stomach, cervical, and ovarian cancers. The most significant is colon cancer because of the possibility of curative resection. Contraindications to resection of hepatic metastases include extrahepatic disease and the inability to perform a complete hepatic resection of liver lesions. In addition, lymphadenopathy associated with a primary colon tumor, synchronous lesions, tumor in both lobes, multicentric disease, and CEA level >200 ng/mL are all poor prognosticators. Recurrent disease is common, with 50% occurring in the liver. Only 5% of patients have recurrent lesions amenable to resection. The 5-year survival rate for these patients is between 30% and 40%. Adjuvant chemotherapy may be used postoperatively, but there has been no proven role for its use. Hepatic artery infusion with chemotherapy has shown the most promising results.

Neuroendocrine tumors often metastasize to the liver, where they secrete their biologically active substances into the systemic circulation. The tumors are generally slow growing and have little effect on overall mortality; however, they may become debilitating once they are active. For this reason, surgical resection is considered when the tumor is solitary and isolated. Common tumors include glucagonomas, gastrinomas, insulinomas, and carcinoid tumors. Medical therapy with long-acting somatostatin analogues and embolization procedures may be of benefit.

107
Benign Hepatic Neoplasms

Benign hepatic neoplasms are present in approximately 10% of the population of developed countries. They tend to occur in younger to middle-aged females. The tumors are detected with increasing frequency because of improved radiologic technology. Most are found incidentally and are diagnosed with radiology alone. A triple-phase computed tomography (CT) scan can usually make the diagnosis; however, some may require resection for histologic diagnosis. Hemangioma, focal nodular hyperplasia, and hepatic adenoma are the most common lesions; however, many other benign lesions occur rarely.

Hemangiomas are the most common benign liver tumor. They often are found in females in the fifth decade. They are congenital vascular malformations composed of endothelial-lined, blood-filled spaces with thin fibrous septa, and they grow by ectasia. Hemangiomas may involute and form scar. There is no risk of malignant degeneration. They can be classified as small capillary hemangiomas, cavernous hemangiomas (often associated with focal nodular hyperplasia, which is another vascular malformation), or giant hemangiomas (greater than 5 cm in size). Hemangiomas are often found incidentally; however, patients may have vague upper abdominal complaints. The hemangioma is usually not the etiology of these abdominal symptoms; therefore, they should not be attributed to the hemangioma without investigation of other causes. Liver function tests and tumor markers are usually normal. The diagnosis is made via CT or magnetic resonance imaging (MRI) with slow filling of intravenous contrast from the edges inward. Percutaneous biopsy is not recommended. A special circumstance is Kasabach-Merritt syndrome in which hemangiomas are associated with thrombocytopenia and consumptive coagulopathy. Hemangiomas are stable with generally a low risk of rupture, but they can grow rapidly, rupture, or thrombose. If the patient has no symptoms, observation is appropriate. If the patient has symptoms with rupture, enlargement, or Kasabach-Merritt syndrome, resection is performed via control of vascular inflow and enucleation

of the lesion. Hemangiomas are common in children, and mortality rate is 70% if symptomatic and untreated. They are often multifocal and involve other organs. Small, asymptomatic lesions usually resolve; however, larger lesions may become symptomatic, even causing congestive heart failure. Such issues are treated medically, and the hemangiomas are treated with embolization and/or chemoradiation. They may ultimately require resection.

Focal nodular hyperplasia (FNH) is the second most common benign liver tumor, often occurring in young females. These lesions are typically less than 5 cm in size and are surrounded by normal hepatic parenchyma. Lesions look like a spoke-wheel with central fibrous scar with radiating septa. They have cords of benign hepatocytes with scattered atypical bile duct epithelium and without normal vasculature. The α-fetoprotein (AFP) level is normal, and liver function tests may be mildly elevated. The etiology is not known but may be a congenital vascular malformation. Focal nodular hyperplasia is a benign and indolent process with no risk of malignant degeneration. Like hemangiomas, they are often an incidental finding. If symptomatic, vague abdominal pain is the usual complaint. Focal nodular hyperplasia is diagnosed with a contrasted CT or MRI showing lesions with central scar, and they rarely require resection for diagnosis. If no central scar is seen, they can be differentiated from hepatic adenoma by technetium nuclear scan. If the patient is asymptomatic and the radiologic diagnosis can be made, no treatment is required. With symptoms, other etiologies should be investigated. If FNH is the cause, serial imaging is appropriate, because the symptoms usually resolve. If symptoms are persistent or the lesions are increasing in size, resection is appropriate.

Hepatic adenoma is a rare lesion occurring in females in the third to fifth decades in which cords of hepatocytes with increased glycogen and fat proliferate within an otherwise normal liver. They are associated with chronic oral contraceptive use. Tumor markers are usually normal. As with other benign hepatic tumors, these are normally found incidentally but may cause upper abdominal pain. Hepatic adenomas are diagnosed with CT or MRI as a well-demarcated heterogenous mass, with MRI showing fat or hemorrhage in the lesion. On nuclear scan, they do not take up tracer. These lesions can rupture with possible intraperitoneal hemorrhage, cause mass effect, or undergo malignant transformation. Patients with hepatic adenoma must stop oral contraceptives and can never resume use. If the patient has no symptoms, serial AFP values and imaging may be used to surveil the lesions. With symptoms, resection is appropriate. Emergent resection or embolization may be necessary if the adenoma ruptures. The decision to resect is made when the risk of surgery is outweighed by the risk of leaving the lesion. Margins are unimportant. Hepatic adenomas are typically singular; however, multiple lesions can be present. The occurrence of 10 or more lesions is termed *adenomatosis*. This is not associated with oral contraceptives and has a decreased association with the female gender. In adenomatosis, large lesions are resected, and a liver transplant may be required.

108
Viral Hepatitis

Viral hepatitis is the most common cause of liver disease. Five major viruses are responsible for the majority of cases of viral hepatitis. These include hepatitis viruses A (HAV), B (HBV), C (HCV), D (HDV), and E (HEV). Hepatitis B virus is the only one composed of a DNA genome that has the ability to integrate into the host genome. The others are composed of RNA. Hepatitis D virus does not have the mechanism for replication and requires the presence of HBV to replicate.

Hepatitis A virus and HEV are spread through fecal–oral transmission, most often after contact with contaminated drinking water and food supplies. Hepatitis A virus usually causes acute, self-limited infections. Fulminant disease develops in 1% to 5% of infected patients. Infected patients under the age of 2 years old are asymptomatic. Most symptomatic patients are over the age of 5 years. Hepatitis E virus infection generally has an acute, self-limited course, with jaundice present in 90% of affected patients. Pregnant women tend to have a more severe disease course.

Hepatitis B virus and HDV are transmitted primarily through sexual contact and intravenous drug use. Perinatal transmission of HBV has been demonstrated in endemic areas. The risk of HBV transmission through blood transfusion is approximately 1 in 63,000. Chronic HBV infections most often occur in the young patient groups (30% in children and 90% in infants).

In the United States, the most common cause of chronic liver disease is HCV infection. Hepatitis C virus is transmitted via parenteral routes and through sexual contact. The risk of acquiring the virus through blood product transfusion is approximately 0.001% to 0.0001%. Most patients with HCV remain asymptomatic for years. Chronic infections can slowly lead to the development of cirrhosis and hepatocellular carcinoma over several decades (mean, 28 years). Concomitant abuse of alcohol has been shown to increase the progression rate of cirrhosis.

Viral hepatitis has a varied range of clinical manifestations. When symptoms occur, they often include malaise, anorexia, abdominal pain, fatigue, and jaundice. A physical examination may show jaundice, hepatomegaly, splenomegaly, and tenderness to palpation over the liver. Elevations in serum bilirubin and liver aminotransferase levels (10 times above normal) are commonly seen. Infections can be self-limiting or occasionally can progress to fulminant hepatic failure (1% to 2%). Fulminant disease is hallmarked clinically by encephalopathy, persistent or worsening jaundice, and ascites. Prolongation of prothrombin time signifies decreased synthetic function seen with hepatic failure. Hepatitis A virus, HBV, and HDV infections are most often associated with fulminant disease. Complications include chronic infection, cholestatic hepatitis, and extrahepatic manifestations. Extrahepatic symptoms are rare but can include headaches, seizures, meningitis, nephritic syndrome, and arthritis.

The clinical course of acute infections generally takes place in three phases: an incubation period, a preicteric period, and an icteric period. The length of the incubation period ranges from 2 weeks to 20 weeks. The virus can be detected via serologic testing during this phase. Antibodies directed against the virus are not present and neither are abnormalities in liver function tests.

Symptoms begin to appear during the preicteric phase. The most common manifestations include fatigue, nausea, anorexia, and abdominal pain. From 10% to 20% of patients develop a syndrome similar to serum sickness that is characterized by rash, hives, fever, and arthralgias. During this phase, antibodies specific for viral particles become detectable, and abnormalities in liver function tests begin to develop. The icteric phase is characterized by darkening of the urine and the development of jaundice. Severe forms of infection are accompanied by pruritus, acholic stools, anorexia, and weight loss.

Histologic characteristics consist of scattered areas of necrosis among diffuse parenchymal inflammation. Inflammatory cells such as macrophages, lymphocytes, and histiocytes infiltrate the hepatic tissues. The host immune reaction is implicated in most of the damage done during infection. Cytotoxic T cells interact with viral antigens that are expressed on infected hepatocytes. Other factors that are responsible include inflammatory cytokines, natural killer cell response, and antibody-mediated damage to cells.

Serologic testing plays an important role in diagnosing the cause of acute hepatitis as well as in monitoring response to treatment and determining recovery from infection. Acute infections of HAV are diagnosed with the detection of anti-HAV immunoglobulin M antibodies. Hepatitis B virus infection can be initially diagnosed by detecting the hepatitis B surface antigen. Surface antigen levels tend to remain for 4 to 6 months after infection and then begin to disappear, which signifies the recovery from infection. Chronic infections display persistent elevations of HBV surface antigens. Antibodies that develop against the hepatitis B core antigens can be detected during early infection and continue to be present during chronic infections. The hepatitis E antigen is produced during viral reflection and indicates active infection. The infection begins to resolve once antibodies are produced against the hepatitis E antigen. The diagnosis of HCV depends on the detection of antibodies to numerous viral antigens as well as on the detection of viral RNA. Hepatitis D virus is diagnosed through the detection of RNA. Hepatitis E virus can be detected by antibody determinations and by finding traces of it in the patient's stool.

Hepatitis prevention depends on improvements in sanitation, immunoglobulin administration, and vaccination. Effective vaccinations have been developed for HAV and HBV. Hepatitis B virus vaccinations are routinely given to high-risk people, such as health care workers. Serum immunoglobulin provides passive immunity for HBV and HAV postexposure prophylaxis.

Hepatitis A virus and HEV infections are often self-limited and thus need only supportive care. Interferon-α and nucleoside analogues such as lamivudine have been used with some success for HBV patients. Corticosteroids may be given in addition to interferon-α. Contacts of patients infected with HAV should receive prophylactic immunoglobulin. Vaccines should be given to any household contacts of HBV-infected patients. Sexual partners should receive immunoglobulin prophylaxis. Prompt referral for liver transplantation is recommended for patients displaying signs of fulminant hepatic failure. The CDC requires that all cases of acute hepatitis be reported.

109
Portal Hypertension

Elevated pressures in the portal venous system can be a consequence of prehepatic conditions, intrahepatic conditions, and posthepatic abnormalities. Intrinsic obstruction to intrahepatic portal venous flow leads to portal hypertension. Portal venous pressures greater than 12 mm Hg or hepatic wedge pressures 5 mm Hg greater than the inferior vena cava pressure define portal hypertension. Causes of this condition can be organized into prehepatic, posthepatic, and hepatic etiologies. Intrahepatic disease is responsible for most cases of splenic hypertension. The most frequent hepatic causes of portal hypertension include alcoholic cirrhosis and viral hepatitis. Portal hypertension can be categorized additionally according to sinusoidal function. Alcoholic cirrhosis produces a postsinusoidal obstruction of portal flow, whereas viral hepatitis produces a sinusoidal obstruction. Other etiologies include schistosomiasis, hemochromatosis, Wilson's disease, fatty infiltration, increased arterial blood flow, intrahepatic fibrosis, and intrahepatic vascular obstruction. Prehepatic abnormalities include portal vein thrombus or stenosis. Posthepatic conditions include right-side heart failure, constrictive pericarditis, and hepatic vein obstruction (Budd-Chiari syndrome). Portal hypertension is an insidious process with symptomatology gradually progressing over time. Clinical manifestations can consist of abdominal pain and distension secondary to ascites. Sudden obstruction of venous blood flow in the portal system may manifest as an acute abdomen.

Recurring injury to liver parenchyma leads to lobular fibrosis and nodule formation. This may result in compression of the terminal hepatic venules and elevation of pressures in the hepatic sinusoids. Elevation of intrahepatic pressure is transmitted to the portal system due to the lack of intrinsic valves. Increased portal pressure creates shunts into the systemic venous system at areas where they share common capillary beds. Increased venous flow through these vessels can cause varices to develop where collateral circulation is increased, such as the cardioesophageal junction, where the coronary vein communicates with the esophageal veins; the azygos system and superior vena cava; the rectum where the superior hemorrhoidal veins drain into the inferior and middle hemorrhoidal veins and then to the inferior vena cava; the falciform ligament of the liver communicating with periumbilical veins that empty into the epigastric vessels (caput medusae); and in the retroperitoneum through the vein of Retzius, which communicates with mesenteric and peritoneal veins that drain into the inferior vena cava.

Approximately 50% of cirrhotic patients develop esophagogastric varices. Esophageal and gastric varices occur when the esophageal and gastric veins are distended with portal blood flow. The overlying submucosa begins to erode, exposing the thin-walled veins. Increased pressure in the dilated vessel of erosion by ulceration causes the vessel to bleed. Bleeding occurs in up to 30% of patients with the combination of cirrhosis and varices. Treatment for variceal bleeding begins with airway protection (intubation and mechanical ventilation if needed), volume resuscitation, coagulopathy correction, proton pump inhibitors, and prophylactic antibiotics. Octreotide is administered to decrease splanchnic blood flow along with vasopressin to cause vasoconstriction. Nitroglycerin is given with the vasopressin to counteract the drug effect.

Endoscopic therapy is performed in conjunction with pharmacologic treatment. Endoscopic interventions include sclerotherapy and band ligation. Balloon tamponade is an option when medical and endoscopic therapy has failed. In this technique a Sengstaken-Blakemore tube is inserted into the esophagus of an intubated patient. The tube contains a gastric and esophageal balloon. The gastric balloon is inflated when the tube is inserted to prevent dislodgement when traction is applied. The esophageal balloon applies direct pressure on the bleeding vessels, causing tamponade. The tube is placed on traction, and the esophageal and gastric ports are suctioned to prevent aspiration. The technique is 90% effective at stopping acute bleeding, although one-half of the patients re-bleed when the balloon is removed. Therefore, this method is used to allow time for planning of possible transjugular intrahepatic portosystemic shunts (TIPS) or definitive surgery. The balloon is left in place no longer than 24 hours to prevent complications of perforation, aspiration, and obstruction.

Transjugular intrahepatic portosystemic shunt is used as a means of portal decompression. In this technique, a portosystemic fistula is created from the hepatic vein through the liver parenchyma into a portal tributary. A stent is placed through the newly created fistula to maintain patency. The entire procedure is conducted through a percutaneous internal jugular vein access. The technique is effective for stopping acute bleeds as well as preventing re-bleeding. It is contraindicated for patients with right-side heart failure, polycystic liver disease, and occasionally portal vein thrombosis. Complications include an increased incidence of hepatic encephalopathy and shunt failure due to occlusion.

Surgical interventions consist of esophageal transection and portosystemic shunt operations. Esophageal transection has an associated mortality rate of 76% and a complication rate of 26% when used in the setting of acute bleeding; therefore, it is not recommended. In this technique, an end-to-end anastomosis stapler is used to create a full thickness transection of the esophagus, thus dividing the bleeding varices. Portosystemic shunts, however, have been shown to be effective in the acute setting.

The recurrence rate for variceal bleeding is as high as 70%. Prophylaxis is generally started by giving the patient a β-blocker, such as propranolol. Repeated endoscopy is performed with either sclerotherapy or band ligation every 6 to 12 months. Transjugular intrahepatic portosystemic shunt can be used to decompress the portal system while the patient awaits a liver transplant. Surgically created portosystemic shunts are the most reliable means of controlling the sequelae of portal hypertension. There are two types of shunts: nonselective and selective. The basic goal of these procedures is to reroute portal blood to the systemic circulation. Following these procedures, complications such as hepatic encephalopathy and increased liver dysfunction can occur. Nonselective shunts include end-to-side portacaval shunts (portal vein proximal ligation with distal anastomoses to the inferior vena cava), side-to-side portal shunts (side-to-side portal to inferior vena cava anastomoses), interposition mesocaval shunts, and proximal

splenorenal shunts (splenectomy, splenic vein to left renal vein anastomoses). Selective shunts include the distal splenorenal shunt (splenic vein anastomosed to left renal vein and ligation of collaterals).

Ascites is another potential complication of portal hypertension. It is generally encountered with advanced hepatic disease and is indicative of poor outcome. Liver failure and associated ascites stems from increased sinusoidal pressure and lymph production. Lymphatic production eventually overwhelms thoracic duct drainage and spills over into the abdominal cavity. Sodium retention is derived from intravascular volume depletion and excessive aldosterone secretion. Antidiuretic hormone, which inhibits the excretion of free water, is produced in excess as well. Elevated sodium level contributes to fluid retention and increased ascites. Ascites produces symptoms of abdominal distension, pain, and labored breathing. The constant tension transmitted onto the abdominal wall can also lead to umbilical and inguinal hernia formation. Spontaneous bacterial peritonitis is another serious complication. Fluid cytology revealing white blood counts of $500/mm^3$ are suggestive of the diagnosis. Cefotaxime or ciprofloxacin is considered the treatment of choice. Optimal control of ascites begins with medical management. Dietary sodium restriction to less than 2 g/day and water restriction to less than 1.5 L/day are implemented. Diuretic therapy consists of loop diuretics and aldosterone antagonists (i.e., spironolactone). Surgical management is limited to cases refractory to medical treatment. Large volume paracentesis can be used to manage ascites when diuretic therapy fails. Peritoneovenous shunts provide a means for ascites to be drained into the systemic circulation and thus avoid the large shifts in volume with diuresis and paracentesis. Complications from this procedure are severe (sepsis, disseminated intravascular coagulopathy, and thrombosis), and the 1-year mortality rate is estimated at 50%. Transjugular intrahepatic portosystemic shunt is another effective means of control in up to two-thirds of patients who fail medical management.

Hypersplenism can commonly be associated with portal hypertension. Splenomegaly and pancytopenia are common findings. Splenic sequestration of circulating cells and secretion of bone marrow inhibitors lead to pancytopenia. Splenectomy alone does not correct portal hypertension and eliminates the option of a distal splenorenal shunt. The presence of hypersplenism is not an indication for portal decompression. The combination of hypersplenism and bleeding varices is, however, an indication for a distal splenorenal shunt.

110
Acute Liver Failure

Liver failure is classified as primary or secondary based on the etiology. Primary liver failure, in general, stems from pre-existing, underlying hepatic disease. Many patients with liver failure have a previous history of liver dysfunction. In addition, they often have had consequences of liver dysfunction such as gastrointestinal bleeding or encephalopathy. An additional group of patients develops primary hepatic failure without pre-existing liver disease. These patients often have severe liver failure hallmarked by massive hepatocellular necrosis, encephalopathy, coagulopathy, cerebral edema, and coma. Secondary hepatic failure can occur in critically ill patients who are injured, have overwhelming infection, or have acute respiratory distress syndrome. The primary illness of the patient dictates the severity of liver dysfunction. Therefore, hepatic recovery depends on the treatment of the primary illness. Common manifestations of secondary hepatic failure include cholestasis, jaundice, impaired synthetic ability, and encephalopathy.

Risk factors for liver disease include alcohol use, intravenous drug use, risky sexual practices, blood transfusion before 1992, exposure to toxins, and family history. Liver failure occurs acutely or chronically. Acute liver failure has two major subclasses that are grouped according to the temporal relationship of symptom onset. Fulminant hepatic failure is composed of acute liver failure with encephalopathy that develops within 2 weeks of the onset of jaundice. Subfulminant hepatic failure is defined as acute liver failure with encephalopathy that manifests within 2 to 12 weeks of jaundice.

The key clinical manifestations of liver failure include jaundice, ascites, edema, encephalopathy, and muscle wasting. Physical examination of these patients may reveal palmar erythema, bitemporal muscle wasting, spider angiectasia, and blood vessel collateralization (i.e., caput medusae).

In contrast to chronic liver failure, fulminant hepatic failure has a unique set of complications. One of the most significant is cerebral edema, which occurs in 80% of cases. Elevations in intracranial pressure generally manifest clinically as decerebrate posturing, spastic rigidity, seizures, hypertension, hyperventilation, bradycardia, and decreased pupil response. Cerebral edema is monitored best by invasive measurement of intracranial pressure. Intracranial pressure monitors are catheters that are surgically placed in the epidural, subdural, or intraventricular space. Strict attention must be paid to correction of existing coagulopathies before catheter placement. Management goals include maintaining intracranial pressures below 15 mm Hg and maintaining cerebral perfusion pressures above 50 mm Hg. Management options include head elevation, hyperventilation ($PaCO_2$ 25 to 30 = mm Hg), sedation, mannitol, and barbiturate coma for refractory cases.

Acid–base disturbances along with electrolyte abnormalities are commonplace. Proper fluid management is instituted to prevent hypovolemia or hypervolemia that can increase cerebral edema and other complications. Acidosis is a common problem due to lactate production and decreased liver metabolism of lactate. Severe acidosis is treated by sodium bicarbonate administration. Acetate solutions can be administered as well.

Hypoglycemia can be associated with liver failure and can be potentially fatal in severe cases. An infusion of 50% dextrose solution followed by maintenance fluids with 10% dextrose is the usual course of action.

Renal failure accompanies fulminant hepatic failure in 55% of cases. Hypovolemia is the most common cause of renal failure. Treatment for renal failure involves providing adequate volume resuscitation to maintain adequate urine output. Loop diuretics as well as renal dosages of dopamine can be used. Intravascular volume deficits can be corrected with blood products or albumin in the case of hypoalbuminemia.

Pulmonary edema, aspiration pneumonia, and acute respiratory distress syndrome are pulmonary complications that can frequently be associated with hepatic failure. Pulmonary complications are best managed by providing supportive therapy (i.e., supplemental oxygen and mechanical ventilation).

Infections can develop with hepatic failure. Common sources include the respiratory tract, the urinary tract, and indwelling intravenous catheters. Frequent isolated organisms include *Streptococcus, Staphylococcus,* and Gram-negative rods. An impaired immune process along with failure in other organ systems (i.e., respiratory, renal) predisposes a patient with hepatic failure to developing infection and sepsis. The presence of infection is a critical impedance to the treatment and management process, because it is a major contraindication to transplantation. Antibiotic prophylaxis is not routinely administered. However, aggressive management is warranted if signs of infection manifest. The typical workup includes blood, urine, and sputum cultures. Chest x-rays are required to evaluate for possible pneumonia. Broad-spectrum antibiotics with coverage for Gram-positive and Gram-negative organisms are begun after cultures are obtained. Antibiotic coverage is then tailored according to culture results. Antifungal therapy is started for positive fungal cultures or in the case of persistent fever (>5 days) despite antibiotic use.

The liver is responsible for the production of most of the factors involved in the clotting system. Therefore, coagulopathy is a common entity associated with liver failure. Dysfunctional platelets, splenic sequestration (splenomegaly), and depressed bone marrow production all contribute to impaired coagulation. Prolonged prothrombin time (PT) and international normalization ratio (INR) are the most common laboratory abnormalities detected (because of decreased factor II, VII, IX, and X levels). Coagulopathies may be overcome by frequent monitoring of the PT/INR ratio and the transfusion of fresh-frozen plasma to replenish clotting factors. In the case of thrombocytopenia (platelet count <50,000) or qualitative platelet defects (i.e., prolonged bleeding time), platelets can be transfused.

Most cases of fulminant hepatic failure are attributed to viral infection, drug reactions, or toxins. Hepatitis B virus (HBV) infection is associated with fulminant hepatic failure more often than are hepatitis A (HAV) or hepatitis C (HCV) viral infections. Hepatitis C virus infections are associated with subfulminant infections more often than fulminant infections. The hepatitis D virus (HDV) is an inactive virus that requires the presence of HBV particles to become virulent. Superinfections or co-infections with HDV and HBV are possible. Superinfections cause higher mortality rates and an increased incidence of liver failure.

Drug reactions are responsible for 35% of cases of hepatic failure. Acetaminophen is the causative agent in most cases. Problems with hepatic toxicity can arise from increasing the drug dosage, drug–drug interactions, and prolonged use of the drug. Other drugs that have been associated with hepatic toxicity include the anesthetic halothane, isoniazid, nonsteroidal anti-inflammatory drugs (NSAIDs), and antihistamines. Fulminant hepatic failure caused by halothane generally manifests within 2 weeks of receiving anesthesia and has a high mortality rate.

Mushroom poisoning, aflatoxins, and exposure to industrial toxins (e.g., carbon tetrachloride and trichloroethylene) are rare causes of hepatic failure. The clinical course of mushroom toxicity generally begins with vomiting and diarrhea. Mortality rates have been reported to be as high as 22%.

Medical management is the first line of treatment for hepatic failure. The success of medical therapy and ultimate prognosis depends on the extent of hepatic necrosis and the ability for hepatocyte regeneration. The most useful prognostic tool is the King's College criteria. These criteria were developed to predict the outcome of medical management and to assess the need for liver transplantation. According to these criteria, poor outcomes occur with medical management when one of the following three criteria is observed on initial presentation:

1. Initial acidosis (pH < 7.3)
2. Acetaminophen-induced disease with the following:
   - PT > 100 seconds or INR > 6.5
   - Serum creatinine level >3.4 = mg/dl
   - Hepatic encephalopathy (stage III–IV)
3. Nonacetaminophen-induced disease with the following:
   - Patients younger than 10 years or older than 40 years
   - Halothane-induced
   - Viral hepatitis (non-A or non-B)
   - Progression of jaundice to encephalopathy longer than 7 days
   - PT > 50 seconds or INR > 6.5 = mg/dl
   - Serum bilirubin >17.5 = mg/dl

The functional reserve of the liver can be ascertained through liver function testing. Common methods of testing include galactose clearance testing and arterial ketone body ratios.

Referral for liver transplantation evaluation is warranted for patients who are predicted to have poor medical outcomes. The evaluation is carried out within 12 to 24 hours and includes an extensive neurologic workup to rule out neurologic complications. The neurologic complications associated with increased intracranial pressure and cerebral edema are irreversible and are contraindications to transplantation. The King's College criteria provide early insight into the probability of successful medical management. Liver transplantation is considered when medical management alone is unsuccessful. The success of liver transplantation depends on proper patient selection. Referral for transplantation should be made before the development of multisystem organ failure, neurologic dysfunction, or sepsis.

Chronic liver disease is the result of prolonged and repetitive damage to the liver parenchyma. Multiple episodes of tissue injury are followed by regeneration and scar tissue formation (i.e., bridging fibrosis). This upsets the normal architecture of the hepatic parenchyma and also impairs function. Cirrhosis is defined as the irreversible alteration of nutrient exchange and hepatocyte metabolic and physiologic functions. Scar tissue created after repeated injury obstructs the normal flow of nutrients and metabolites between the sinusoids and the hepatocytes. Numerous complications result from chronic liver failure. They include portal hypertension, ascites, renal failure, coagulopathy, and encephalopathy. The complications and treatment of portal hypertension and chronic liver disease are discussed in Chapter 109.

111
Chronic Liver Failure

Repetitive damage to liver parenchyma leads to inflammation and disorganized regeneration of the hepatic lobules. Fibrosis and nodule formation cause compression of the terminal hepatic venules and elevation of pressures in the hepatic sinusoids. The intrahepatic increase of pressure limits the flow of portal blood into the liver and therefore increases the portal pressure. Complications of portal hypertension include ascites, increased collateral blood vessel flow, hepatic encephalopathy, hemorrhage, and hypersplenism. These topics are discussed in greater detail in Chapter 109.

Laboratory tests (Table 111.1) are used to assess the level of hepatic dysfunction. Often elevated liver transaminase and bilirubin levels will be discovered. Coagulopathy results from decreased synthetic function of the liver. This is evidenced by elevated prothrombin time and international normalized ratio. Hypersplenism can be evidenced by overall pancytopenia on complete blood count (white blood cell count <4,000 and platelet count >100,000). Electrolyte abnormalities include hyponatremia, hypokalemia, metabolic alkalosis, and azotemia.

Chronic liver disease adds risk to surgical procedures. Parenchymal blood flow and regulatory compensation mechanisms become altered by fibrosis from cirrhosis. Liver ischemia can result from stresses of surgery and anesthesia. The Child-Pugh classification system (Table 111.2) is used to stratify the risk of bleeding and mortality against the severity of disease.

Ascites is produced from several pathologic mechanisms. Sinusoidal hypertension results in transudate, which is collected by the lymphatic system. Increased hepatic lymphatic flow overcomes the drainage capability of the thoracic duct, and protein-rich lymphatic fluid accumulates in the abdomen. The ascitic fluid provides an osmotic gradient that draws fluid from the intestine. Decreased intravascular volume due to fluid shifts causes renal induced hyperaldosteronism with retention of sodium and water. Other contributing factors include salt retention and impaired clearance of free water (i.e., increased antidiuretic hormone).

Medical treatment is the first line for control of ascites. Fluid samples should be obtained via paracentesis to understand the nature of the ascites (chylous, malignant, or cardiac) and to rule out the possibility of bacterial peritonitis. Testing of ascitic fluid should include white blood cell count, total cell count, protein measurements (total and albumin), Gram stain, culture, glucose measurement, lactate dehydrogenase level, and amylase level. The serum albumin level is compared with the albumin measurement in the ascites in the serum–ascites albumin gradient. This test is used to help determine the cause of the ascites. Ascites secondary to portal hypertension produces a gradient greater than 1.1 g/dL. Ascites secondary to other causes creates a gradient less than 1.1 g/dL.

Low-sodium (1 to 2 g/day), high-carbohydrate diets are recommended. Restrictions in water intake to 1 to 1.5 L/day are implemented for patients with hyponatremia or increasing weight gain from fluid accumulation. Hyponatremia is a common electrolyte abnormality that can produce seizure activity in its severe form. Restriction of free water intake is used to slowly raise the serum sodium level. Rapid correction of sodium can produce osmotic fluid shifts and neurologic dysfunctions (i.e., central pontine demyelination). Diuretic therapies with aldosterone antagonists such as spironolactone are used. Furosemide and potassium supplementation are used as well. Large-volume paracentesis is used in some cases. Albumin is administered at 6 to 8 g/L of ascites removed to prevent drastic fluid shifts.

Transjugular intrahepatic portosystemic shunts (TIPS) are effective in resolving 80% of ascites cases that fail medical therapy. Peritoneovenous shunting is another method that provides a quick and durable treatment for ascites. Complications include disseminated intravascular coagulopathy (35%) and shunt occlusion (47%). Surgical portosystemic shunts are not recommended for ascites management.

TABLE 111.1. Laboratory tests used to assess levels of hepatic dysfunction.

Score	Ascites	Encephalopathy	Bilirubin = mg/dl level	Prothrombin time (prolonged seconds)	Albumin = g/dl level
1	None	None	<2	<4	<3.5
2	Controlled	Stage I–II	2–3	4–6	2.8–3.5
3	Moderate to severe	Stage III–IV	>3	>6	>2.8

Complications of ascites include spontaneous bacterial peritonitis (SBP) and hepatorenal syndrome. Spontaneous bacterial peritonitis is manifested as fever and abdominal pain. Bacterial culture and cell counts are performed with paracentesis fluid to make the diagnosis. Positive bacterial cultures, neutrophil counts exceeding 250/mm^3, and total bacterial counts greater than 500/mm^3 are indicative of infection. Low ascitic protein levels (<1.5/dL) predispose patients to SBP because of a lack of complement activity in the fluid. Enteric organisms are usually the cause of infection. Aggressive treatment with intravenous antibiotics is warranted. Empiric therapy consists of antibiotic coverage with a third-generation cephalosporin (i.e., cefotaxime) for 14 days or ciprofloxacin given over a 7-day course. Analysis of ascitic fluid is repeated 48 hours after implementing therapy. Prophylactic antibiotics are reserved for patients with low protein levels in the fluid and previous episodes of SBP and for patients awaiting liver transplantation.

Hepatorenal syndrome occurs in up to 55% of patients with chronic hepatic failure. The syndrome is characterized by oliguria, azotemia, and an elevation of the osmolarity ratio between the urine and the serum. Causative factors include decreased renal perfusion secondary to increased abdominal pressure, decreased intravascular volume, systemic vasodilation, and increased response of the renin–angiotensin system. These conditions culminate in renal vasoconstriction and impaired glomerular filtration. Tubular function and the renal parenchyma are unaltered, making this state of renal impairment reversible. Management focuses on adequate fluid resuscitation and on the use of vasodilators (e.g., dopamine, misoprostol) to counteract renal vasoconstriction. Other causes of renal failure include acute tubular necrosis, renal tubular acidosis, and interstitial nephritis. Acute tubular necrosis can be evidenced by abrupt rises in blood urea nitrogen and creatinine levels along with oliguria. Acute tubular necrosis impairs the concentration ability of the kidneys and causes sodium wasting. Urine sodium concentration is usually greater than 10 mEq/L in these patients.

Hepatic encephalopathy is a neuropsychiatric syndrome caused by systemic circulation of toxins, which are normally processed by the liver and absorbed by the intestine. Such toxins include ammonia, mercaptans, and γ-aminobutyric acid. Aromatic amino acids may be found in excess in the plasma. After crossing the blood–brain barrier, they begin to serve as precursors for the production of false neurotransmitters that then compete with true neurotransmitters such as dopamine and norepinephrine. Encephalopathy can be triggered by dehydration, increased protein intake, gastrointestinal bleeding, and sepsis. Clinical manifestations range from confusion to coma. Motor activity can be affected as well. Increased reflexes and confusion are characteristic of the early stages. Hypertonicity and rigidity can be seen during the intermediate stage and finally flaccidity in later stages. Medical treatment is the first step in management and is focused on reduction of nitrogen absorption from the gastrointestinal tract and decreasing ammonia production and increasing its metabolism. A diet low in protein and high in carbohydrates is suggested. Limiting episodes of gastrointestinal bleeding helps to prevent occurrences of encephalopathy. Antibiotics such as neomycin and kanamycin are not absorbed through the gastrointestinal tract. Therefore, they are effective at reducing bacterial numbers within the gut. Lactulose becomes oxalated into lactic and acetic acids by the gut flora. The acidic byproducts lower the pH in the colon and inhibit ammonia transport. Administering this cathartic may play a role in increased colonic emptying, thus decreasing the time for absorption.

Malnutrition is a common condition that occurs in the form of calorie as well as protein deficiencies. The poor synthetic function accompanied by advanced liver disease leads to impaired protein production. However, caution must be taken when administering protein to cirrhotic patients. High-protein supplementation can induce hepatic encephalopathy. Therefore, protein intake is generally restricted to 1 g/kg/day. Most calories for cirrhotic patients are supplied through carbohydrates. Enteral nutrition is favored over total parenteral nutrition when the option is available.

TABLE 111.2. The Child-Pugh classification system.

Class	Score	Mortality rate with hemorrhage
A	5–6 points	5%
B	7–9 points	25%
C	10–15 points	>50%

112
Hepatectomy

Advances made in modern hepatic surgery have facilitated safe resection of malignant and benign liver conditions. The perioperative mortality rate for experienced surgeons approaches about 5% in most cases. Segmental resections have become a popular technique for hepatic resection because it preserves hepatic function and allows better tumor clearance.

Wedge resections are preformed less often for two main reasons: increased rates of positive margins and hemorrhage. Positive margins often result from tumors fracturing away from the liver parenchyma during resection. Hemorrhage is a consequence of the inadequate ability to obtain control of vascular inflow and outflow. These limitations have decreased the number of wedge resections performed for surface tumors 2 cm or less.

The most common complications of hepatic resections are bleeding and biliary injury. In addition to improved intraoperative techniques, the risk of hemorrhage has been reduced by changes in fluid management by anesthesia. Blood loss is minimized by implementation of low central venous pressure anesthesia (<5 mm Hg) during tissue resection. The systolic blood pressure is maintained at 90 mm Hg as well. Placing the patient in the Trendelenburg position prevents air embolisms. Blood transfusions and volume expanders are reserved for instances of significant (>25% of blood volume) bleeding.

The inherent regenerative ability of the liver allows for up to 80% parenchymal resection in noncirrhotic patients. Postoperative liver dysfunction depends on the amount of functional liver tissue that remains after surgery. In general, normal liver function can be maintained in tissue resections of less than 50% of functional tissue. The altered regenerative ability in cirrhotic patients leaves them more susceptible to liver dysfunction postoperatively. Other complications include ascites, infection, hepatic failure, multisystem organ failure, and death.

The operative approach to resection is tailored to the condition to be treated. Resections for benign conditions are generally undertaken for symptoms or infection. As much normal liver tissue as possible should be left undisturbed. Techniques of minimal resection, such as enucleation, may be appropriate. A margin of normal tissue surrounding a neoplasm should be obtained.

The liver parenchyma may be transected in a number of different ways. The simplest techniques involve crushing the tissue with Kelly clamps and tying or clipping vascular or ductal structures. Vascular staplers can be used to transect tissue in areas where less precise dissection is needed. Fibrotic and cirrhotic hepatic tissue is more prone to fracturing and bleeding, making the resection more difficult. The procedure can be aided with thermal coagulation, ultrasonic dissection, or pressurized water dissection. Vascular control may be accomplished by the Pringle maneuver intermittently (every 5 to 15 minutes).

Liver resections are based on the segmental anatomy of the liver (discussed in Chapter 102). A right hepatectomy (right hepatic lobectomy) involves resection of segments V through VIII. An extended right hepatectomy (extended right lobectomy or right trisegmentectomy) includes the resection of segment IV as well.

Segments II through IV make up the left lobe. Therefore a resection of these segments results in a left hepatectomy (left hepatic lobectomy). An extended left hepatectomy (extended left lobectomy or left trisegmentectomy) includes the resection of lobes V and VII. A left lateral segmentectomy (sublobar) involves resection of segments II and III.

113
Biliary Physiology

The liver produces bile continuously and excretes it into the bile canaliculi. The normal adult produces 500 to 1,000 mL of bile daily. The secretion of bile is responsive to neurogenic, humoral, and chemical stimuli. Parasympathetic stimulation via the vagus nerve increases bile secretion, whereas sympathetic stimulation via splanchnic nerves decreases bile flow. Hydrochloric acid, partly digested proteins, and fatty acids in the duodenum stimulate the release of secretin from the duodenum that subsequently increases bile production and flow. Bile flows from the liver through to the hepatic ducts, into the common hepatic duct, through the common bile duct, and finally into the duodenum. With an intact sphincter of Oddi, bile flow is directed into the gallbladder.

Bile is mainly composed of water, electrolytes, bile salts, proteins, lipids, and bile pigments. Bile concentrations of sodium, potassium, calcium, and chloride are equal to plasma or extracellular fluid. The pH of hepatic bile is usually neutral or slightly alkaline but varies with diet; an increase in protein shifts the bile to a more acidic pH. The primary bile salts cholate and chenodeoxycholate are synthesized in the liver from cholesterol. They are conjugated there with taurine and glycine and act within the bile as anions (bile acids) that are balanced by sodium. Cholesterol and phospholipids from the liver are the principal lipids found in bile. The synthesis of phospholipids and cholesterol by the liver is in part regulated by bile acids. Bile color is due to the pigment bilirubin diglucuronide, a metabolic product from hemoglobin breakdown. In the intestine, bacteria convert it into urobilinogen, a small fraction of which is absorbed and secreted into the bile and may be secreted in urine.

Bile salts are excreted into the bile by the hepatocytes and aid in the digestion and absorption of fats in the intestines. Eighty percent of the conjugated bile acids are absorbed in the terminal ileum. The remainder is dehydroxylated (deconjugated) by gut bacteria, forming the secondary bile acids deoxycholate and lithocholate. These are absorbed in the colon, transported to the liver, con-

jugated, and secreted into the bile. Eventually, about 95% of the bile acid pool is reabsorbed and returned via the portal venous system to the liver. Five percent is excreted in the stool, leaving the relatively small amount of bile acids to have maximum effect.

The gallbladder, the bile ducts, and the sphincter of Oddi act together to store and regulate bile flow. The gallbladder's main function is to concentrate and store hepatic bile and deliver bile into the duodenum in response to a meal. In the fasting state, 80% of bile is stored in the gallbladder. This storage is due to the absorptive capacity of the gallbladder. It rapidly absorbs sodium, chloride, and water against significant concentration gradients, concentrating the bile 10-fold and leading to a marked change in bile composition. This rapid absorption is one mechanism that prevents a rise in pressure within the biliary system under normal circumstances. Gradual relaxation and emptying of the gallbladder during the fasting period also plays a role in maintaining a relatively low intraluminal pressure in the biliary tree.

The gallbladder's epithelial cells secrete two important products: glycoproteins and hydrogen ions. Glycoproteins are believed to protect the mucosa from the lytic action of bile and to facilitate the passage of bile through the cystic duct. Hydrogen ions transported in the lumen lead to a decrease in the gallbladder bile pH. The acidification promotes calcium solubility, thereby preventing its precipitation as calcium salts.

Gallbladder filling is facilitated by tonic contraction of the sphincter of Oddi, which creates a pressure gradient between the bile ducts and the gallbladder. During fasting the gallbladder does not simply fill passively. In association with phase II of the interdigestive migrating myenteric motor complex in the gut, the gallbladder repeatedly empties small volumes of bile into the duodenum. This process is mediated in part by the hormone motilin. In response to a meal, the gallbladder empties by a coordinated motor response of gallbladder contraction and sphincter of Oddi relaxation. One of the main stimuli to gallbladder emptying is the hormone cholecystokinin (CCK), which is released endogenously from the duodenal mucosa in response to a meal. When stimulated by eating, the gallbladder empties 50% to 70% of its contents within 30 to 40 minutes. Over the following 60 to 90 minutes the gallbladder gradually refills, correlated with a reduced CCK level. Defects in the motor activity of the gallbladder are thought to play a role in cholesterol nucleation and gallstone formation.

The vagus nerve stimulates contraction of the gallbladder, and splanchnic sympathetic stimulation is inhibitory to its motor activity. Parasympathomimetic drugs contract the gallbladder, whereas atropine leads to relaxation. Neurally mediated reflexes link the sphincter of Oddi with the gallbladder, stomach, and duodenum to coordinate the flow of bile into the duodenum. Antral distention of the stomach causes both gallbladder contraction and relaxation of the sphincter of Oddi.

Hormonal receptors are located on the smooth muscles, vessels, nerves, and epithelium of the gallbladder. Cholecystokinin is released into the bloodstream by acid, fat, and amino acids in the duodenum. Cholecystokinin acts directly on smooth muscle receptors of the gallbladder and stimulates gallbladder contraction. It also relaxes the terminal bile duct, the sphincter of Oddi, and the duodenum. Cholecystokinin stimulation of the gall-

bladder and the biliary tree also is mediated by cholinergic vagal neurons. Vasoactive intestinal peptide (VIP) inhibits contraction and causes gallbladder relaxation. Somatostatin and its analogues are potent inhibitors of gallbladder contraction. Other hormones such as substance P and enkephalin affect gallbladder motility; however, the physiologic role is unclear.

The sphincter of Oddi regulates flow of bile (and pancreatic juice) into the duodenum, prevents the regurgitation of duodenal contents into the biliary tree, and diverts bile into the gallbladder. It is a complex structure that is functionally independent of the duodenal musculature and creates a high-pressure zone between the bile duct and the duodenum. The sphincter of Oddi is 4 to 6mm in length and has a basal resting pressure of about 13mm Hg above the duodenal pressure. On manometry, the sphincter shows phasic contractions with a frequency of about four per minute and an amplitude of 120 to 140mm Hg. The sphincter primarily controls the regulation of bile flow. Relaxation occurs with a rise in CCK level, leading to diminished amplitude of phasic contractions and reduced basal pressure, thereby allowing increased flow of bile into the duodenum. During fasting, the sphincter of Oddi activity is coordinated with the periodic partial gallbladder emptying and an increase in bile flow that occurs during phase III of the migrating myoelectric complexes.

114
Biliary Tract Infections

Acute infections of the biliary tract are called *acute cholangitis*. The characteristic manifestations include fever, right upper quadrant abdominal pain, and jaundice. Infections can be mild or can produce septicemia. Severe forms manifest with a pentad of symptoms, including fever, jaundice, abdominal pain, mental status changes, and hypotension (Reynolds' pentad). Gallstone-induced cholangitis carries a mortality rate of 2% to 5%.

Two factors play an important role in the development of cholangitis: biliary obstruction and a heavy concentration of biliary bacteria. Obstruction of the biliary system increases bacteria within the system. Common organisms isolated from bile cultures include *Escherichia coli, Klebsiella*, enterococci, *Proteus, Pseudomonas, Bacteroides*, and *Clostridium*. Elevated intraductal pressures are key to the development of bacterial infection and bacteremia. The high pressures in the ductal system promote systemic bacteremia through reflux in hepatic sinusoids and the venous and lymphatic system associated with the bile ducts. Common problems that can lead to cholangitis include choledocholithiasis, strictures, cholangiocarcinoma, and preampullary cancers. There is a 4% to 7% associated risk of cholangitis with endoscopic retrograde cholangiopancreatography (ERCP) or percutaneous transhepatic cholangiography (PTC). Common laboratory abnormalities include leukocytosis, elevated liver function test, and hyperbilirubinemia. Ultrasound, computed tomography, and magnetic resonance imaging are used to evaluate for biliary dilatation, masses in the pancreas, or choledocholithiasis.

Antibiotics are the first line of treatment. Patients with mild biliary tract infections are treated with oral antibiotics as outpatients. Severe cases require intensive care unit admission, intravenous fluid resuscitation, and intravenous antibiotics tailored toward the commonly found organisms. Approximately 85% of patients respond to initial medical management. Patients who show no improvement within the first 24 hours require prompt biliary decompression. This is accomplished by either PTC or ERCP. Patients with proximally located strictures or patients with biliary-enteric anastomosis strictures are more amenable to the percutaneous approach. Obstructions caused by common duct stones or lesion near the ampulla require endoscopic intervention. Endoscopic therapy provides the ability to perform sphincterotomies, stenting, stone removal, and dilations. Surgical treatment is reserved for patients who have failed percutaneous or endoscopic intervention. Common duct exploration with T-tube placement to allow for drainage and decompression is the procedure of choice. The chance for successful treatment is less for patients with malignant causes of cholangitis. Hepatic abscesses should be suspected in all patients who are refractory to treatment. The recurrence rate of cholangitis is higher for patients whose gallbladder is not removed (25%). Interval cholecystectomies are performed 6 to 12 weeks after the resolution of infection.

115
Biliary Dyskinesia

Biliary dysmotility can manifest with symptoms similar to biliary colic. Dyskinesia is described as altered tone of the sphincter of Oddi, discoordinated contraction of the biliary ducts, and decreased emptying of the biliary system. Patients with biliary dyskinesia are often found to have no gallstones during evaluation. There are a variety of disorders that can be responsible. They are often overlooked until evaluation fails to reveal common causes for biliary colic. The biliary tract including the gallbladder is powered by longitudinal and circumferential smooth muscle cells. Cholecystokinin (CCK) is released in response to a meal, which stimulates contraction of the gallbladder and relaxation of the sphincter of Oddi. Abnormalities can be found in the gallbladder, the sphincter of Oddi, and at the ampulla of Vater.

Papillary stenosis is secondary to glandular hyperplasia or inflammation of the ampulla of Vater. Patients often have abdominal pain (right upper quadrant or epigastric), elevated liver function enzyme levels, common bile duct dilation, delayed egress of contrast material during cholangiography, and increased pressure at the sphincter of Oddi. The evaluation is completed with either endoscopic retrograde cholangiopancreatography (ERCP) or magnetic resonance cholangiogram (MRCP) and biliary manometry, if available. Cholescintigraphy (hepatobiliary iminodiacetic acid [HIDA] scan) shows decreased flow from the hepatic ducts to the duodenum. Treatment includes sphincterotomy via endoscopic or surgical treatment.

Hyperkinesia of the gallbladder is secondary to abnormal gallbladder contractility demonstrated after stimulation. This is generally evaluated via HIDA scan and CCK provocation. A normal study shows 55% to 75% of the gallbladder emptying in response to continuous CCK infusion. Delayed gallbladder emptying may be evident on HIDA scan as well as pain associated with gallbladder contraction. Gallbladder dyskinesia is a difficult diagnosis to make. Even when it is evident in a patient with biliary colic symptoms, it still may not be the source of the pain. Cholecystectomy may be offered to the patient with the understanding that the procedure may not resolve the pain. Delayed gallbladder emptying may have a positive predictive value of symptom relief after cholecystectomy.

Sphincter of Oddi dyskinesia can be caused by sphincter spasm, hypertonicity, and altered coordination of contractions. The diagnosis is usually one of exclusion. Medical therapy is the first line of treatment, consisting of nitrites and anticholinergics. Failing this, surgical or endoscopic sphincterotomy is warranted.

116
Benign Biliary Strictures

Benign biliary strictures can result from a number of conditions, including chronic pancreatitis, primary sclerosing cholangitis, acute cholangitis, several autoimmune diseases, and trauma. Most benign strictures occur iatrogenically because of bile duct injury during laparoscopic cholecystectomy. Early recognition of injury either intraoperatively or within the postoperative period avoids long-term complications. Late recognition of injury can lead to complications such as cholangitis, biliary cirrhosis, and portal hypertension. Bile duct injuries occur in 1 of 120 laparoscopic cholecystectomies (0.85%). Major bile duct injuries occur in about 0.55%, with bile leaks or minor injuries occurring in 0.3% of cases. Factors that influence the occurrence of laparoscopic bile duct injuries include surgical experience, chronic inflammation, infection (cholangitis), poor exposure, bleeding, and obesity. Routine operative cholangiography has been suggested to decrease the rate of biliary duct injuries. Cholangiography aids in defining the biliary anatomy. Good surgical technique with complete exposure of the structures in the triangle of Calot is important. Twenty-five percent of major ductal injuries manifest intraoperatively with bile leakage, as an abnormality identified on cholangiogram, or as late recognition of the anatomy. The remaining 75% manifest at variable times. Symptoms of pain, fever, and/or mild hyperbilirubinemia (2.5 mg/dL) are common for bilomas or bile peritonitis. Cystic duct stump leaks, a transection of the right hepatic duct, and laceration of the common bile duct are common injuries associated with biloma. The diagnosis of bile leakage should be suspected for any patient complaining of continued right upper quadrant pain or anorexia after cholecystectomy. Injuries that occlude the common hepatic or common bile duct manifest with jaundice with or without abdominal pain. Late presentations occur occasionally, with cholangitis or cirrhosis.

Percutaneous drainage is used for cystic leaks to drain intra-abdominal fluid collections. Persistent biliary drainage through the catheter signifies an ongoing leak.

Isotopic (hepatobiliary iminodiacetic acid [HIDA]) scans are used to ensure the diagnosis. A sinogram conducted through the percutaneous drain may reveal the biliary anatomy. Endoscopic retrograde cholangiopancreatography (ERCP) is used in cases without an active leak. Percutaneous transhepatic cholangiography can help diagnose strictures and can also be used to place decompressive stents in proximal lesions. Partial transection injuries identified during the initial operation can be treated with placement of a T-tube.

Evaluation begins with a computed tomography (CT) scan of the abdomen or ultrasound. Key findings include intrahepatic and extrahepatic ductal dilatation. These studies can also help determine the location and extent of injury.

Primary repair is optimal for minor lesions. A T-tube is placed either proximally or distally to stent the lesion. Ducts less than 3 mm tend to drain only one segment of the liver. These ducts can be ligated safely in most cases. Ducts greater than 3 mm can drain more than one segment and must be repaired. Major ductal injuries such as transections fare better if the injury is recognized and repair is made during the initial operation. Injuries that are identified during the postoperative period are treated initially with percutaneously placed transhepatic catheters to allow for decompression. Time is allowed for the acute inflammation to subside (6 to 8 weeks), and then patients undergo exploration and operative repair.

The standard of care for repair is the creation of an anastomosis between the duct and the intestinal tract. Duct-to-duct repairs are avoided because of their tendency for stricture. The most common procedures are Roux-en-Y hepaticojejunostomy or Roux-en-Y choledochojejunostomy. Injuries located at the right and left hepatic bifurcation require a bilateral hepaticojejunostomy. Cholangitis, abscesses, bile leakage, hemobilia and restenosis are common postoperative complications. Restenosis occurs in up to two-thirds of patients.

Strictures located at or above the hepatic duct bifurcation have less successful repairs compared with strictures below the duct bifurcation. Percutaneous procedures such as balloon dilation and stenting are less successful compared with surgery.

Noniatrogenic bile duct injuries are typically caused by nonpenetrating trauma. Penetrating trauma also causes isolated common bile duct injury, but it usually causes injury to the porta hepatis as well. The combination of common bile duct injury and hepatic artery injury can cause ischemia and stricture of the common bile duct. Severe episodes of acute pancreatitis and chronic pancreatitis can produce benign biliary strictures. The strictures are located in the intrapancreatic segment of the common bile duct. Strictures associated with acute pancreatitis tend to be self-limited. Chronic pancreatitis due to alcohol use is characterized by extensive fibrosis that leads to stricture. In addition, compression from a nearby pseudocyst can cause a mass effect that leads to stricture of the common bile duct.

Clinical manifestations include jaundice with or without pain. The diagnosis can be made using magnetic resonance cholangiopancreatography (MRCP), ERCP, or CT. Endoscopic retrograde cholangiopancreatography provides the opportunity to obtain biopsy specimens to rule out malignancy. Benign strictures must be differentiated from malignant causes. Chronic inflammation of the gland provides the setting for cancer development. The diagnosis of cancer is made with endoscopic ultrasound along with fine-needle aspiration or core-needle biopsies. In addition, laboratory tests for the tumor marker CA 19.9 should be performed.

Treatment for biliary strictures depends on the underlying cause. For isolated strictures, the treatment of choice is a Roux-en-Y hepaticojejunostomy. Strictures due to compression from a pseudocyst require drainage of the cyst and confirmation of duct patency postoperatively (MRCP, ERCP). Cases involving severe pancreatic scarring require excision of the surrounding scar. This can be accomplished by a Frey or Beger procedure. A biliary enteric anastomosis is done with the addition of a Puestow procedure. Whipple procedures are used to resect the stricture and surrounding scar in cases of intractable pain or when cancer is the suspected etiology. Stenting should be avoided to prevent complications of stent obstruction by clotting.

Gallstones lead to biliary strictures by causing repeated bouts of cholangitis or stone ulceration. As a result, strictures tend to form near the lower end of the bile duct (i.e., papillary stenosis). The first line of treatment is endoscopic sphincterotomy. Strictures that fail sphincterotomy must undergo an enteric anastomosis (Roux-en-Y hepaticojejunostomy). Mirizzi's syndrome is due to a large stone in the gallbladder or cystic duct compressing the common bile duct.

Sclerosing cholangitis is an idiopathic disease that frequently occurs in patients with ulcerative colitis. This disease causes multiple intrahepatic and extrahepatic biliary strictures. Malignancy can develop and can be difficult to diagnose. Strictures located in the larger bile ducts are treated endoscopically. Strictures in the bifurcation must be resected. Orthotopic liver transplantation may be indicated when end-stage liver disease appears or when cancer is suspected.

117
Choledochal Cysts

Choledochal cysts are congenital dilations of the biliary tract. They can be intrahepatic, extrahepatic, or both. They occur very rarely and most often in childhood. Part of the problem has been attributed to the associated anatomic variation of the pancreatic and biliary ducts called *anomalous pancreatobiliary duct junction*. This is characterized by the premature connection of the pancreatic duct and bile duct approximately 1 cm proximal to the ampulla of Vater. This creates a common passage for pancreatic secretions to reflux into the biliary system. The results are increased biliary pressures and inflammation of the biliary tree. The disorder is classified according to the Alonso-Lej system (Table 117.1).

Right upper quadrant pain, jaundice, and abdominal mass are the most common presenting symptoms. Adults are seen less often with abdominal pain and jaundice. In contrast, children are more likely to present with symptoms akin to biliary colic (right upper quadrant abdominal pain and jaundice). Other possible manifestations include cholangitis and pancreatitis. Complications of choledocholithiasis, stricture, and stenosis can also occur. The risk of cholangiocarcinoma increases with long-standing disease.

Laboratory values of patients with choledochal cysts are often nonspecific. Ultrasound or computed tomography can be used to help make the diagnosis; however, cholangiography by either magnetic resonance cholangiopancreatography (MRCP) or endoscopic retrograde cholangiopancreatography (ERCP) is needed to plan for surgery.

Optimal surgical management includes cyst resection, cholecystectomy, and drainage via Roux-en-Y hepaticojejunostomy. Internal drainage via cystenterostomy is not recommended because of the propensity for fibrosis and scarring as well as the increased risk of adenocarcinoma in the retained cyst. Hepatic lobectomy is an option for intrahepatic cysts confined to one hepatic lobe. Bilobar disease often has a high rate of intrahepatic stone formation. Long-term stent placement may facilitate stone removal. For complicated cases with diffuse disease, liver transplantation may be the only viable option.

TABLE 117.1. Alonso-Lej classification system.

Type	Characteristics	Rate of occurrence
I	Fusiform dilation of the common bile duct (CBD)	50%
II	Saccular diverticulum of the extrahepatic duct	<10%
III	Intraduodenal dilation (choledochocele)	<10%
IV	Intra- and extrahepatic dilations	35%
V	Multiple intrahepatic dilations (Caroli's disease)	<10%

118
Gallbladder Carcinoma

Gallbladder carcinoma occurs mostly in elderly patients, and 70% of cases are associated with cholelithiasis. The incidence of gallbladder cancer is increased seven times in persons with gallstones and chronic cholecystitis. Male to female ratio is 1:2. There is also an association with primary sclerosing cholangitis, choledochal cysts, and porcelain gallbladder. Gallbladder carcinoma is discovered incidentally in 1 in every 100 elective cholecystectomies.

The vast majority of tumors are adenocarcinomas. The histologic structure varies from scirrhous (60%), to papillary (25%), to mucoid (15%). Lymphatic metastasis occurs through the cystic duct node of Calot to the common duct lymph nodes. Nodal disease of the porta hepatis can cause common duct obstruction resulting in jaundice. Liver metastasis occurs with direct invasion through the gallbladder bed and venous drainage into the liver. Adjacent organ involvement includes the duodenum, colon, and stomach. At the time of diagnosis, only 25% of these cancers are localized to the gallbladder wall.

Right upper quadrant pain similar to biliary colic is the most common presenting symptom. Other symptoms include anorexia, jaundice, weight loss, and an abdominal mass. Chronic cholecystitis is the presenting syndrome in 45% of patients, followed by acute cholecystitis and malignant biliary obstruction. Because of the nonspecific nature of these symptoms, less than 20% of gallbladder cancers are diagnosed preoperatively.

Laboratory tests are often normal unless jaundice is present. Ultrasound is often the first radiographic test ordered. Common findings that may be indicative of gallbladder cancer are the presence of a heterogeneous mass replacing the gallbladder lumen or an asymmetric thickening of the gallbladder wall. A mass replacing the gallbladder or extending to adjacent organs may be visible on computed tomography. Magnetic resonance cholangiopancreatography (MRCP) is a noninvasive modality that allows for complete evaluation of the biliary, hepatic, and pancreatic parenchyma and can detect nodal involvement as well.

Surgical intervention is the only effective therapy. Radiotherapy and chemotherapy have not been shown to improve survival. The appropriate operative procedure depends on the pathologic stage of the tumor. Tumors that are confined to the muscular layer (TNM classification T1) are often recognized after routine cholecystectomy. For these tumors, a simple cholecystectomy is adequate provided there is no bile spillage during the procedure. Bile spillage is associated with poor survival in locally advanced disease. For advanced local disease (stage II/III), a radical cholecystectomy, which includes en bloc wedge resection of an adjacent 3 to 5 cm of normal liver and lymphadenectomy of nodal tissue in the hepatoduodenal ligament, is recommended. Resection of liver segments IVB and V are recommended for larger tumors to ensure negative margins. Whenever possible, a staging laparoscopy should precede attempted resection because of the high incidence of undetected hepatic or peritoneal metastasis. Palliative therapy may be the appropriate option for stage IV or unresectable tumors. Gallbladder carcinoma is often discovered incidentally after laparoscopic cholecystectomy for presumed benign disease. As stated earlier, simple cholecystectomy is adequate for T1 disease. Stage II/III disease will require re-exploration with radical resection and excision of previous laparoscopic port sites.

Overall, gallbladder carcinoma has a 5-year survival rate of less than 5% and a median survival of 6 months. Survival is mainly governed by pathologic stage. Cancers limited to the submucosa have an excellent prognosis. Muscularis invasion increases the rate of recurrence after resection. The 10-year survival rate for a localized lesion after simple cholecystectomy is 100%. The 5-year survival rate following resection of T2 and T3 tumors without nodal disease is 50%. Node positivity in the latter group has shown dismal survival rates.

119
Pancreatic Anatomy

The pancreas is a retroperitoneal organ situated transversely between the level of the twelfth thoracic and second lumbar vertebrae. The borders of the pancreas are the duodenum on the right, the spleen on the left, the omental bursa superiorly, the transverse mesocolon anteriorly, and the greater peritoneal sac inferiorly. The pancreas is divided into four regions: the head/uncinate process, the neck, the body, and the tail. The head of the pancreas fits within the medial border of the c-loop of the duodenum, and the uncinate process is an extension of the head of the pancreas that passes posterior to the superior mesenteric artery and anterior to the aorta. The neck of the pancreas is roughly 2 cm long, with the right margin defined by the origin of the anterosuperior pancreaticoduodenal artery. Anterosuperior to the neck is the pylorus, and posterior to the neck is the confluence of the superior mesenteric and splenic veins into the portal vein. The body of the pancreas lies anterior to the left aspect of the aorta, the splenic vein, and the left kidney and renal vessels. The superior leaflet of the transverse mesocolon covers the anterior surface of the body. The tail of the pancreas is relatively mobile compared with the other divisions and projects into the splenic hilum. The tip reaches the hilus in 50% of cases, lies below in 42%, and is above the hilus in 8% of cases.

The pancreas develops from two separate outpouchings of the duodenum during the fourth week of gestation. The more ventral bud is the hepatic diverticulum, which will form the liver, gallbladder, bile ducts, and head/uncinate process of the pancreas. The dorsal pancreatic bud is the second, more proximal, diverticulum, and it develops into the neck, body, and tail of the pancreas. During the fifth week of gestation, the ventral bud rotates clockwise around the duodenum to lie medial to the newly formed c-loop of the duodenum, and the ventral pancreas now lies inferior and slightly posterior to the dorsal pancreas. If this rotation is abnormal, an annular pancreas develops in which a band of normal pancreatic tissue encircles the second portion of the duodenum and can cause varying degrees of duodenal obstruction. The two segments of pancreas then fuse by the beginning of the sixth week of gestation. Failure of this fusion of the two pancreatic buds can lead to pancreas divisum, a condition in which the pancreas is two structurally distinct organs that drain separately. This is of little clinical significance, although it can lead to an increased incidence of pancreatitis.

Usually, there are two ducts draining the pancreas. This is the result of the pancreas developing originally as two separate structures. During the fusion process of the ventral and dorsal pancreatic buds, the ducts draining each also fuse together. In the mature pancreas, the main pancreatic duct (duct of Wirsung) originates in the tip of the tail and passes through the body and neck and then curves inferiorly through the head where it joins with the common bile duct from the ampulla of Vater, which drains into the duodenum through the major duodenal papilla. The minor or accessory pancreatic duct (duct of Santorini) tends to have a much more variable course and presence. The duct extends from the main pancreatic duct in the neck region of the pancreas to the minor duodenal papilla, which drains into the duodenum proximal to the major papilla. This duct drains the anterosuperior portion of the pancreatic head into either the main duct or the duodenum directly through the minor papilla.

The blood supply for the pancreas comes from both the celiac trunk and the superior mesenteric artery. The head of the pancreas receives its blood supply from two pancreaticoduodenal arcades, which lie in the anterior and posterior aspects of the head of the pancreas where it abuts the c-loop of the duodenum. The anterior and posterior superior pancreaticoduodenal arteries arise from the gastroduodenal artery, which is a branch of the common hepatic artery from the celiac trunk. The anterior and posterior superior arcades anastomose with the anterior and posterior inferior pancreaticoduodenal arteries arising from the superior mesenteric artery. The splenic artery, which is another branch of the celiac trunk, courses along the superior border of the pancreas and supplies blood to the neck, body, and tail of the pancreas. The first branch of the splenic artery is the dorsal pancreatic artery, which goes on to form the transverse pancreatic artery that courses through the inferior portion of the body and tail of the pancreas. This artery frequently has a branch that anastomoses with the posterior pancreaticoduodenal arcade. The great pancreatic artery comes off of the splenic artery around the junction of the body and tail of the pancreas, and it courses inferiorly to anastomose with the inferior pancreatic artery.

Venous drainage of the pancreas largely follows the arterial supply. All drainage eventually enters the portal vein, which is located posterior to the neck of the pancreas. The head of the pancreas is drained by the four pancreaticoduodenal veins. The anterior superior pancreaticoduodenal vein joins the right gastroepiploic vein to form the gastrocolic vein, which in turn drains into the superior mesenteric vein. The posterior superior pancreaticoduodenal vein drains directly into the portal vein. The anterior and posterior inferior pancreaticoduodenal veins enter the superior mesenteric vein. Veins that confluence into two venous channels, the splenic vein superiorly and the transverse pancreatic vein, drain the neck, body, and tail of the pancreas inferiorly.

There are five main collecting trunks and lymph node groups responsible for lymphatic drainage of the pancreas. The superior nodes are located along the superior border of the pancreas. The inferior nodes, responsible for draining the lower half of the head and body of the pancreas, are located along the inferior margin of the pancreas. The anterior and posterior nodes drain mostly the head of the pancreas. Finally, the splenic nodes, located near the hilum of the spleen, drain the tail of the pancreas.

The pancreas is innervated with both sympathetic and parasympathetic nervous systems. The sympathetic is from the splanchnic nerves, and the parasympathetic supply is via the celiac division of the posterior vagal trunk. The nerves arising from these sources travel in parallel with blood vessels to reach their destinations within the pancreas.

120
Pancreatic Anomalies

Annular Pancreas

An annular pancreas is a rare malformation in which a band of pancreatic tissue surrounds the descending portion of the duodenum with smooth continuation to the head of the pancreas. The incidence of annular pancreas is reported as 3 in 20,000 autopsies. The pancreatic tissue of the annulus is histologically normal and contains both acini and islets. The most widely accepted theory for the development of annular pancreas is that of fixation of the tip of the ventral pancreatic primordium to the duodenal wall before rotation during the fifth week of gestation. With subsequent growth, this results in fusion of this ventral tip with the dorsal primordium on the far side encircling the duodenum. Seventy-five percent of infants with annular pancreas have other anomalies. Duodenal stenosis or atresia occurs at the site of the annulus in about 40%, and trisomy 21 (Down's syndrome) is present in about 15% to 25%. Other anomalies include intestinal malrotation, tracheoesophageal fistula, and congenital heart defects.

Two-thirds of persons with annular pancreas remain asymptomatic for life. Infants with annular pancreas who are symptomatic often manifest in the first days of life with duodenal obstruction. Partial obstruction of the duodenum associated with annular pancreas may present later in childhood. Presentation of annular pancreas may also be delayed until adulthood.

The diagnosis of annular pancreas has traditionally been made at the time of surgical exploration for duodenal obstruction, with or without a preoperative upper gastrointestinal contrast study. Radiographic imaging plays a prominent role in diagnosing annular pancreas. Imaging modalities include ultrasound, computed tomography, and magnetic resonance imaging. The definitive diagnosis of annular pancreas is often made with endoscopic retrograde cholangiopancreatography (ERCP).

The treatment of annular pancreas is based on symptoms. No therapy is indicated for asymptomatic cases. The most common indication for operative therapy for infants and children with annular pancreas is associated with duodenal stenosis or obstruction. The operation of choice for duodenal obstruction associated with annular pancreas is duodenoduodenostomy. This procedure bypasses the obstructing lesion by creating an anastomosis between the side of the dilated proximal duodenum and the side of the decompressed distal duodenum.

Annular pancreas, especially in adults, is also associated with acute and chronic pancreatitis. The treatment of patients with pancreatitis associated with annular pancreas should be initially nonoperative. Pancreaticojejunostomy drainage, with or without duodenoduodenostomy, has also been used with success to treat chronic pancreatitis associated with annular pancreas. In some cases, pancreaticoduodenectomy has also been successful in treating chronic pancreatitis associated with annular pancreas.

Pancreas Divisum

Pancreas divisum is the most common congenital anomaly of the pancreas. It is a congenital anatomic abnormality that results from the failure of normal fusion of the dorsal and ventral pancreatic ducts. The presence of two completely separate pancreatic ducts, called *type 1 pancreatic divisum*, occurs in 4% to 14% of autopsy studies and in 2% to 7% of patients undergoing ERCP. Significant numbers of patients with "pancreas divisum" (5% to 23%) have only a dorsal duct, with no evidence of a ventral duct of Wirsung. This anatomic variant has been called *type 2 divisum*. A third variation (*type 3*) is having a dominant dorsal duct with only a small, narrow filamentous connection between the dorsal and ventral ducts. Common to all variants of pancreas divisum is that all or most pancreatic secretion flows through the accessory papilla. Pancreas divisum is not necessarily abnormal. The clinical relevance of pancreas divisum continues to be debated. A clear association between pancreas divisum and pancreatitis has not been proved. However, a growing body of evidence suggests that pancreas divisum plays a direct role in pancreatitis.

Three conditions have symptoms related to pancreas divisum: (1) acute recurrent pancreatitis, (2) chronic pancreatitis, and (3) chronic upper abdominal pain. The incidence of pancreas divisum rises to 25% for patients with acute recurrent pancreatitis, suggesting an association between the two conditions. An explanation of pancreatitis associated with pancreas divisum is the finding that the accessory papilla, through which the bulk of pancreatic flow occurs in this anomaly, is narrowed compared with the normal main pancreatic duct of the ventral pancreas. If the orifice of the accessory papilla is stenotic or too small to handle the flow of pancreatic juice, obstructive pancreatitis or pancreatic pain can result.

Endoscopic retrograde cholangiopancreatography is required to establish the diagnosis of pancreas divisum. Visualization of both major and minor papillae and two separate ductal systems or a complete absence of the duct of Wirsung is required for the definitive diagnosis of pancreas divisum. Magnetic resonance cholangio-pancreatography (MRCP) can also be used as a diagnostic tool. Determining the physiologic relevance of pancreas divisum has also been proposed by using intravenous secretin stimulation of pancreatic secretions during real-time ultrasound imaging of the pancreatic ducts. Functional stenosis of the accessory papilla with secretion-induced proximal ductal dilation is thought to be characteristic of clinically significant pancreas divisum.

All other causes of pancreatitis should be excluded before surgical or endoscopic intervention for symptomatic pancreas divisum. The efficacy of endoscopic dorsal duct stenting and/or sphincterotomy has been evaluated for treating patients with acute recurrent pancreatitis, chronic pancreatitis, and chronic abdominal pain syndrome associated with pancreas divisum. Short-term improvement of symptoms occurs in patients with acute recurrent pancreatitis; however, complication rates have been relatively high (15%), and the long-term success of stenting has not been satisfactory. The outcomes for patients with chronic pancreatitis treated by endoscopy are less satisfactory, with only 30% of patients showing improvement.

Operative dorsal duct sphincterotomy, with or without sphincteroplasty, is the preferred surgical treatment for patients, including children, with pancreas divisum and recurrent acute pancreatitis with documented hyperamylasemia. The operation is performed through a transverse duodenotomy opposite the ampulla of Vater. The accessory papilla is identified and dilated, and a sphincterotomy is performed to the level of the circular fibers of the duodenal muscularis. Concomitant cholecystectomy and sphincteroplasty of the ampulla of Vater and the ventral pancreatic duct orifice are also advocated by some surgeons. In the unusual patient with chronic pancreatitis attributed to pancreas divisum, a longitudinal pancreaticojejunostomy (Puestow procedure) should be constructed to the dilated dorsal pancreatic duct.

121
Pancreatic Physiology

The exocrine pancreas accounts for about 85% of pancreatic mass; extracellular matrix, about 10%; blood vessels and major ducts, about 4%; whereas endocrine tissue comprises only 2% of the gland. The endocrine and exocrine components are coordinated by a regulatory feedback system for digestive enzymes and hormone secretion. This complex system regulates the type of digestion and its rate and the processing and distribution of absorbed nutrients. This coordination is facilitated by the proximity of the islets and exocrine pancreas, specific islet hormone receptors, pancreatic acinar cell membranes, and the islet–acinar portal blood system. Although patients can live without a pancreas when insulin and digestive enzyme replacement is given, the loss of islet–acinar coordination leads to digestive dysfunction. About 20% of normal pancreas is required to prevent insufficiency.

Exocrine Pancreas

The pancreas secretes 500 to 800 mL/day of alkaline isosmotic pancreatic juice. Pancreatic juice is a combination of acinar cell and duct cell secretions. The acinar cells are pyramid shaped, with apices containing many enzyme-containing zymogen granules. The acinar cells secrete amylase, proteases, and lipases. Individual acinar cells secrete all types of enzymes, unlike the endocrine pancreas, where islet cells specialize in the secretion of one hormone type. However, the ratio of the different enzymes released is adjusted to the composition of digested food. About 40 acinar cells are arranged into a spherical acinus. Centroacinar cells are located near the center of the acinus and are responsible for fluid and electrolyte secretion. The acinar cells release pancreatic enzymes into the acinus lumen and combine with the water and HCO_3^- secretions of the centroacinar cells. The pancreatic juice then travels into small intercalated ducts. Several small intercalated ducts join to form an interlob-

ular duct. Interlobular duct cells contribute fluid and electrolytes. Interlobular ducts join to form approximately 20 secondary ducts that empty into the main pancreatic duct. Destruction of the branching ductal tree from recurrent inflammation, scarring, and deposition of stones eventually contributes to destruction of the exocrine pancreas and insufficiency.

Centroacinar cells contain the enzyme carbonic anhydrase, which is required for HCO_3^- secretion. The amount of HCO_3^- secreted varies directly with the pancreatic secretory rate. Cl^- secretion is inversely related to HCO_3^- secretion such that the sum is constant. In contrast, Na^+ and K^+ concentrations are kept constant throughout the spectrum of secretory rates. Secretin is released from duodenal mucosal cells in response to acidic chyme from the stomach and is the major stimulant for HCO_3^- secretion to buffer the acidic fluid entering the duodenum. Cholecystokinin also stimulates HCO_3^- secretion to a lesser extent but mainly potentiates secretin-stimulated HCO_3^- secretion. Gastrin and acetylcholine, both gastric acid secretion agonists, are also weak HCO_3^- secretion stimulants. Truncal vagotomy causes a reduction in bicarbonate and fluid secretion. The endocrine pancreas also influences the adjacent exocrine pancreatic secretions. Somatostatin, pancreatic polypeptide, and glucagon are all thought to inhibit exocrine secretion.

Pancreatic amylase and lipase are the only enzymes secreted in their active forms. Amylase completes the digestive process begun by salivary amylase by hydrolyzing starch and glycogen to glucose, maltose, maltotriose, and dextrins, which are moved across the brush border of the intestinal epithelial cells by active transport. Pancreatic lipase hydrolyzes triglycerides to 2-monoglyceride and fatty acid. Pancreatic colipase binds to lipase to increase its activity. Pancreatic phospholipase A_2 is secreted as a proenzyme, activated by trypsin, and hydrolyzes phospholipids but requires bile salts for its action like all lipases. Carboxylic ester hydrolase and cholesterol esterase hydrolyze neutral lipid substrates, such as esters of cholesterol, fat-soluble vitamins, and triglycerides. The hydrolyzed fat is then packaged into micelles for transport into the intestinal epithelial cells, where fatty acids are reassembled and packaged inside chylomicrons for transport through the lymphatic system into the bloodstream.

Protein hydrolysis in the stomach yields peptides that enter the intestine and stimulate intestinal endocrine cells to release cholecystokinin-releasing peptide (CCK-RP), cholecystokinin (CCK), and secretin, which stimulate the pancreas to secrete enzymes and HCO_3^- into the intestine. The proteolytic enzymes are secreted as proenzymes that require activation. Trypsinogen is converted to its active form, trypsin, by enterokinase produced by the duodenal mucosal cells. Trypsin then activates the other proteolytic enzymes. Trypsinogen activation in the pancreas is prevented by the presence of inhibitors secreted by the acinar cells (pancreatic secretory trypsin inhibitor [PSTI]). This inhibition ensures that pancreatic enzymes remain inactive until activated only in the duodenum. Chymotrypsinogen is activated by chymotrypsin. Elastase, carboxypeptidases A and B, and phospholipase are also activated by trypsin. Trypsin, chymotrypsin, and elastase cleave bonds between amino acids within peptides, and carboxypeptidases A and B cleave amino acids at the end of peptide chains. Individual amino acids and small dipeptides are then actively transported into the intestinal epithelial cells.

Endocrine Pancreas

There are approximately 1 million islets of Langerhans in the normal adult pancreas. They vary greatly in size from 40 to 900 μm. Larger islets are closer to the major arterioles, and smaller islets are deeper in the parenchyma. Most islets contain 3,000 to 4,000 cells of four major types: α-cells secrete glucagon, β-cells secrete insulin, δ-cells secrete somatostatin, and PP cells secrete pancreatic polypeptide.

Glucagon is a 29-amino-acid, single-chain peptide that stimulates hepatic glycogenolysis and gluconeogenesis and antagonizes insulin's effects through its hyperglycemic action. Glucose is the primary regulator of glucagon secretion. Glucagon release is stimulated by arginine and alanine. Insulin and somatostatin inhibit glucagon secretion in a paracrine fashion within the islet. The same neural impulses that regulate insulin secretion also regulate glucagon secretion so that the two hormones work together in a balance of actions to maintain glucose levels. Cholinergic and β-sympathetic fibers stimulate glucagon release, while α-sympathetic fibers inhibit glucagon release.

Insulin is a 56-amino-acid peptide composed of an α- and a β-chain joined by two disulfide bridges and a connecting peptide, or C-peptide. Proinsulin is made in the endoplasmic reticulum and transported to the Golgi complex, where it is packaged into granules and the C-peptide is cleaved off. There are two phases of insulin secretion. Phase 1 lasts 5 minutes after glucose challenge and stored insulin is released. Phase 2 is longer lasting because of sustained release from ongoing insulin production. Insulin synthesis is regulated by plasma glucose levels, neural signals, paracrine influence of other islet cells, and it is also influenced by plasma levels of arginine, lysine, leucine, and free fatty acids. Glucagon, gastric inhibitory polypeptide, glucacon-like peptide 1, and CCK stimulate insulin release, while somatostatin, amylin, and pancreastatin inhibit insulin release. Cholinergic fibers and β-sympathetic fibers stimulate insulin release, while α-sympathetic fibers inhibit insulin secretion.

Insulin inhibits hepatic glucose production and facilitates glucose transport into cells, thereby reducing plasma glucose levels. Insulin also inhibits glycogenolysis, fatty acid breakdown, and ketone formation and stimulates protein synthesis. There is considerable functional reserve capacity for insulin secretion. About 80% of the pancreas can be resected without the patient becoming diabetic if the remaining tissue is normal. For patients with chronic pancreatitis or other conditions in which much of the gland is diseased, resection of a smaller fraction of the pancreas can result in diabetes. Insulin receptors are dimeric, tyrosine kinase–containing transmembrane proteins that are located on all cells. Insulin deficiency (type I diabetes) results in an overexpression or up-regulation of insulin receptors, which causes an enhanced sensitivity to insulin. Type II diabetes is associated with a down-regulation of insulin receptors and relative hyperinsulinemia, with resulting insulin resistance.

Somatostatin is a peptide with a wide anatomic distribution found in neurons, the pancreas, gut, and other tissues. One gene encodes for a common precursor that is differentially processed to generate tissue-specific amounts of two bioactive products, somatostatin-14 and somatostatin-28. These peptides inhibit endocrine and exocrine secretions and affect neurotransmission, gastrointestinal and biliary motility, intestinal absorption, vascular tone, and cell proliferation. Endocrine release of somatostatin occurs during a meal predominantly stimulated by intraluminal fat. Acidification of the gastric and duodenal mucosa also releases somatostatin in isolated perfused organ preparations. Acetylcholine from the cholinergic neurons inhibits somatostatin release.

Pancreatic polypeptide (PP) is a 36-amino-acid, straight-chain peptide. Protein is the most potent enteral stimulator of PP release, closely followed by fat, whereas glucose has a weaker effect. Hypoglycemia strongly stimulates PP secretion through cholinergic stimulation. Phenylalanine, tryptophan, and fatty acids in the duodenum stimulate PP release, probably by inducing CCK and secretin release. Vagal stimulation of the pancreas is the most important regulator of PP secretion. Pancreatic polypeptide inhibits bile secretion, gallbladder contraction, and secretion by the exocrine pancreas. Studies suggest that the most important role of PP is in glucose regulation through its regulation of hepatic insulin receptor gene expression.

There are a number of other peptide products of the islet cells, including amylin and pancreastatin, as well as neuropeptides such as VIP, galanin, and serotonin. Amylin or islet amyloid polypeptide (IAPP) is a 37-amino-acid polypeptide expressed by the pancreatic β-cells, where it is stored along with insulin in secretory granules. The function of IAPP seems to be the modulation or counterregulation of insulin secretion and function. Pancreastatin is a recently discovered pancreatic islet peptide product that inhibits insulin, and possibly somatostatin release, and augments glucagon release. In addition to this effect on the endocrine pancreas, pancreastatin inhibits pancreatic exocrine secretion.

Intra-islet Regulation

The β-cells are located in the central portion of each islet and comprise approximately 70% of the total islet cell mass. These other cell types are located in the periphery: δ-cells are least plentiful at about 5%, α-cells about 10%, and PP cells about 15%. Control of islet secretion is complex and involves an interplay of neural signals, blood flow patterns, and autocrine, paracrine, and hormonal feedback loops. Although the islets account for about 2% of the pancreatic mass, they receive 20% to 30% of pancreatic arteriolar flow. Most of the exocrine pancreas blood supply comes from the pancreatic arterial flow; however, blood draining from the islet capillaries then perfuses the exocrine pancreas.

Acinar cells perfused with venous blood from the islets allow the endocrine pancreas to influence the exocrine pancreas. For example, insulin release, stimulated by high levels of carbohydrates in an ingested meal, promotes an amylase-rich exocrine secretion, which preferentially provides for digestion of starches and sugars. The peptide products of individual islet cells affect neighboring islet cells in a paracrine fashion. For example, somatostatin inhibits insulin secretion from the β-cells, glucagon secretion from the α-cells, and pancreatic polypeptide secretion from the PP cells. Islet hormone secretion is also regulated by endocrine feedback mechanisms. Insulin secretion is extremely sensitive to small increments in arterial insulin concentration.

122
Acute and Chronic Pancreatitis

Pancreatitis is defined as acute or chronic. Acute pancreatitis is associated with the abrupt onset of symptoms that dissipate once the attack resolves. Chronic pancreatitis occurs as multiple acute attacks. The most common causes of pancreatitis are gallstone disease and alcohol abuse. Other causes include pancreatitis induced by drugs, pancreatic duct obstruction, hereditary factors, trauma, and idiopathic causes. The development of acute pancreatitis is often associated with the passage of gallstones through the biliopancreatic tract. The mechanism by which this takes place has been debated. A common theory is that obstruction of the biliopancreatic tract results in a brief outflow obstruction, which causes bile reflux through the tract. The bile reflux in turn causes inflammation in the pancreas. Newer studies, however, have shown stone passage to result in pancreatitis without direct evidence of bile reflux through the pancreatic duct. The latest line of thought implicates pancreatic ductal obstruction and ductal hypertension with stone passage as the cause of acute pancreatitis. Injury to pancreatic acinar cells leads to intracellular activation of digestive enzymes such as trypsinogen. An inflammatory response within the pancreas then ensues. Circulating proinflammatory cytokines cause major systemic changes in the body. With severe attacks, capillary leak syndrome may develop, leading to fluid sequestration in areas such as the lungs.

The cause of chronic pancreatitis is most often alcohol abuse. This occurs more often in men, and patients generally report an extensive history of alcohol abuse. The popular theory behind chronic pancreatitis is that it is the result of multiple and repeated subclinical episodes of acute inflammation. The repeated episodes of inflammation eventually lead to pancreatic necrosis and fibrosis. Over time, the accumulated tissue loss leads to loss of endocrine and exocrine function. The nature of alcohol injury has been attributed to a number of mechanisms that include free radical production in the pancreas, induced hypertriglyceridemia, and direct pancreatic acinar injury.

Clinical signs associated with acute and chronic pancreatitis are similar. It is often difficult to distinguish the two entities without knowledge of previous attacks. Common symptoms include epigastric abdominal pain, nausea, and vomiting. The pain is often described as sharp and radiates to the mid-back. Patients may report partial relief of pain with sitting up and leaning forward. Fever, tachycardia, shortness of breath, and hypotension can also be associated with an acute episode. Fluid losses from capillary leak syndrome and repeated emesis result in hypovolemia and hypotension. Abdominal distension with tympani and absent bowel sounds suggest an associated ileus. Patients with severe pancreatitis may also show signs of retroperitoneal hemorrhage in the form of flank ecchymoses (Grey Turner's sign) and periumbilical ecchymoses (Cullen's sign). Chest radiographs may show a pleural effusion and occasionally evidence of adult respiratory distress syndrome in severe cases.

Amylase and lipase levels are often elevated. The rise in the two pancreatic enzymes occurs in parallel; however, the amylase level may return to baseline before the lipase level. Prolonged amylase elevation (>1 week) may be a clue to the presence of pancreatic abscess, pseudocyst, or ascites. Leukocytosis with a left shift is common. Hypovolemia may manifest itself as elevations of hematocrit and hemoglobin levels. This is confirmed by a simultaneous elevation of blood urea nitrogen level and a creatinine ratio of 20:1. Endocrine dysfunction is indicated by elevated serum glucose level. Hypoalbuminemia and hypocalcemia can also be present; however, a decrease in ionized calcium in the setting of severe pancreatitis has a poor prognosis.

Imaging studies are helpful for determining the extent of the disease and for evaluating possible complications. Chest radiographs may reveal pleural effusions (commonly on the left side) and basilar atelectasis. Abdominal plain films may show paralytic ileus. In the case of chronic pancreatitis, calcified intraductal protein plugs may appear as pancreatic calcifications. Computed

TABLE 122.1. Ranson's criteria for nongallstone pancreatitis.

Admission	Initial 48 hours
Age >55 years	Hematocrit decrease >10
WBC >16 k	BUN increase >5 mg/100 mL
Serum glucose >200 mg/100 mL	Calcium <8 mg/100 mL
AST >250 U/100 mL	Base deficit >4 mEq/L
LDH >350 IU/L	pO_2 < 60 mm Hg
	Fluid loss >6 L

tomography is useful in evaluating the degree of pancreatic edema, necrosis, and fluid collection. The magnitude of an episode of pancreatitis is determined during the first 48 hours. A clinical scoring system known as Ranson's criteria (Tables 122.1 and 122.2) was devised to determine the severity and prognosis of an attack.

Patients with fewer than three criteria are categorized as having a mild attack. The mortality rate associated with less than three criteria is less than 1%. However, the morbidity and mortality rates rise as more criteria are associated with the attack. If a patient meets three to four criteria, the mortality rate approaches 15%. When seven or more criteria are met, the mortality rate is as high as 90%.

The treatment of acute pancreatitis is aimed at limiting progression and alleviating symptoms. In the acute setting, hypovolemia should be addressed by aggressive volume resuscitation. Complications such as adult respiratory distress syndrome may hamper the resuscitation efforts. In such cases, a Swan Ganz catheter proves useful. Electrolyte abnormalities are common because of poor nutritional status and frequent emesis. Electrolyte replacement is mandatory, especially for decreased ionized calcium level. Nausea and vomiting can be alleviated with nasogastric decompression. Studies have shown a benefit to administering prophylactic antibiotics to patients with severe pancreatitis. Patients are given parenteral nutrition via a central venous catheter. Proton pump inhibitors or H_2-blockers are used for prophylaxis against the formation of stress ulcers. Good pulmonary toilet and pain control have a role in preventing pulmonary complications.

With pancreatitis caused by gallstones, surgery should be delayed until resolution of the attack. The benefit of

TABLE 122.2. Ranson's criteria for gallstone pancreatitis.

Admission	Initial 48 hours
Age >70 years	Hematocrit decrease >10
WBC >18 k	BUN increase >2 mg/100 mL
Serum glucose >220 mg/100 mL	Calcium <8 mg/100 mL
AST >250 U/100 mL	Base deficit >5 mEq/L
LDH >40 IU/L	Fluid sequestration >4 L

endoscopic duct clearance in the early stages of gallstone pancreatitis has been debated. In mild pancreatitis, duct clearance can be delayed, because most cases resolve spontaneously. In the case of severe pancreatitis, there is no clear evidence of its merit.

Complications of pancreatitis include fluid collections, abscesses, ascites, fistulas, false aneurysms, splenic vein thrombosis, necrosis, and pseudocysts. The consensus is that sterile pancreatic and peri-pancreatic fluid collections should be treated conservatively. The conditions eventually resolve, and, therefore, surgical intervention may simply complicate matters. In the case of infected fluid collections, intravenous antibiotic therapy in combination with percutaneous drainage is necessary. Infected pancreatic necrosis is less likely to respond to antibiotic therapy alone or in conjunction with percutaneous drainage. Surgical debridement of all necrotic tissue with antibiotics provides the optimal therapy in this case.

Pancreatic pseudocysts result from communication of the pancreatic duct system into a cystic cavity created by localized inflammation. Pseudocysts lack an epithelial lining and therefore are not true cysts. They generally contain high levels of pancreatic enzymes, and persistent elevation of amylase or lipase can be a clue to their existence. Intervention is only necessary in pseudocysts that are symptomatic or continue to enlarge. Large pseudocysts (greater than 6 cm) are more likely to be symptomatic due to mass effect and encroachment onto adjacent organs or vessels. Some common complications include early satiety, gastric outlet obstruction, obstructive jaundice, pseudoaneurysm, and hemorrhage. There are many treatment options for Pseudocysts, including internal and external drainage, endoscopic drainage, laparoscopic drainage, and open laparotomy. External drainage increases the risk of infection and external pancreatic fistula; therefore, it is generally reserved for patients who are poor surgical candidates. The treatment of a pseudocyst is directed by its anatomic make up. Pseudocysts that are directly adjacent to the stomach or duodenum may be effectively treated by endoscopic cystogastrostomy or cystoduodenostomy. Patients with pseudocysts at the head of the pancreas may be amenable to transpapillary stent placement via endoscopic retrograde cholangiopancreatography. Surgical drainage consists of cystogastrostomy, Roux-en-Y cyst jejunostomy, or cyst duodenostomy. Pancreatic ascites and pleural fistulas can be treated conservatively in up to 60% of patients. Endoscopic therapy includes sphincterotomy and stenting. Surgical options include partial pancreatectomy or Roux-en-Y drainage. Splenic vein thrombosis responds to splenectomy when left-side portal hypertension, gastroesophageal varices, and bleeding develop.

123
Pancreatic Pseudocysts

The pancreatic pseudocyst is a common complication of pancreatitis. Unlike true cysts, pseudocysts do not have an epithelial lining. Local inflammation of surrounding membranes and organs results in a cavity that limits the escape of pancreatic fluid from the damaged pancreas. The encapsulated fluid collection can be found in the pancreas itself or more commonly in the lesser sac. The fluid contained in the cyst consists of high concentrations of pancreatic enzymes that fail to reabsorb. In the case of chronic pancreatitis, pseudocysts can form from the aggregation of dilations within the pancreatic duct. These ducts eventually enlarge and lose their epithelial lining, forming the pseudocyst.

Pseudocyst development usually manifests as protracted disease (5 to 7 days) or clinical deterioration in a patient with acute pancreatitis. Persistent elevation of amylase level and leukocytosis may occur as well. For a patient with chronic pancreatitis, symptoms of compression (abdominal pain, nausea, vomiting) may be clues to its presence. The best imaging studies for diagnosing a pseudocyst are computed tomography and ultrasound. Computed tomography is particularly useful in defining the cyst and pancreatic anatomy, information that is helpful for planning a drainage procedure. Endoscopic retrograde cholangiopancreatography (ERCP) can be used when there are signs of obstructive jaundice. With ERCP, cystic compression of the common bile duct can be differentiated from stricture. Endoscopic retrograde cholangiopancreatography is usually timed within 24 hours of cyst drainage because of the possibility of bacterial introduction into the cyst.

Complications of pseudocysts include infection, rupture, and hemorrhage. Infected pseudocysts may manifest with fever and leukocytosis. Percutaneous drainage with computed tomography or ultrasound guidance is useful in identifying the source of infection. Resolution of the infection may occur with percutaneous drainage and antibiotic therapy. Free rupture of a pseudocyst can occur into the peritoneum or into the gastrointestinal tract. Free rupture manifests as acute peritonitis and requires prompt surgical intervention. Abdominal washout and external drainage should be performed. Rupture into the gastrointestinal tract may go unrecognized and, in some cases, aids in the drainage of the cyst. Surgical intervention is required only when septicemia ensues. Hemorrhage into a pseudocyst may occur as it erodes into an adjacent blood vessel such as the splenic or gastroduodenal artery. Initial management should incorporate angiography along with selective embolization. Patients in extremis may require prompt surgical intervention consisting of excision of the cyst and bleeding vessel.

Nonoperative treatment is successful in some cases. It consists of percutaneous drainage via a small-diameter catheter, which is placed with computed tomography or ultrasound guidance. This technique is contraindicated in cases of free rupture of the pseudocyst, cyst hemorrhage, when malignancy is suspected, or when adjacent structures prevent safe placement of the catheter.

Surgical interventions for pseudocyst include excision, internal drainage, and external drainage. Generally operative treatment is delayed until maturation of the cyst occurs. In the case of acute pancreatitis, it may take 4 to 6 weeks for the cyst wall to become thick enough to hold sutures. In contrast, cysts associated with chronic pancreatitis are considered mature at the time of diagnosis. No treatment is necessary for asymptomatic mature pseudocysts less than 5 cm in diameter. Close observation with ultrasound every 3 to 6 months should be conducted. Surgery is indicated for cysts that are symptomatic, enlarging, and infected. External drainage is an option mostly reserved for patients who are critically ill and poor operative risks. It is also used for cysts that have not reached maturity and are unable to support an anastomosis. During this procedure, a large-bore drainage catheter is placed in the cyst lumen and brought through the abdominal wall. This procedure is complicated by pancreatic fistula in 20% of patients and by recurrent cyst formation. Excision of the cyst is appropriate for pseudocysts localized to the tail of the pancreas with the remainder of the gland being free of disease.

Internal drainage is the technique of choice whenever possible. The three techniques that are commonly used are cystogastrostomy, cystoduodenostomy, and Roux-en-Y cystojejunostomy. Cystogastrostomy is preferred when the cyst wall lies in close approximation to the stomach. The technique can be done using an endoscopic, laparoscopic, or open approach. Cysts located near the head of the organ may be more amenable to cystoduodenostomy. The Roux-en-Y technique is suitable for cysts in a variety of locations. It is important to biopsy a portion of the pseudocyst to rule out malignant causes such as cystadenoma or cystadenocarcinoma. A malignant process should be suspected if the cyst appears to be septated or calcified. Also the presence of a cyst in a patient with no history of pancreatitis should raise suspicion of malignancy.

124
Pancreatic Adenocarcinoma

Pancreatic cancer is more common in men than in women and more common among blacks than whites. Most cases occur in persons between 60 and 80 years of age. Known risk factors include a history of chronic pancreatitis and cigarette smoking. The incidence of diabetes mellitus is greater in patients with pancreatic cancer, but the relationship between diabetes and pancreatic cancer is debated. Some consider diabetes a risk factor for pancreatic cancer, while others argue that diabetes may be a manifestation of the cancer. The incidence of pancreatic cancer is greater in families with hereditary nonpolyposis colon cancer (HNPCC), with familial breast cancer (associated with the *BRCA-2* mutation), with Peutz-Jeghers syndrome, with ataxia telangiectasia, and with the familial atypical multiple mole melanoma (FAMMM) syndrome. Even in the absence of one of these familial cancer syndromes, individuals with a family history of pancreatic cancer have an increased risk of developing pancreatic cancer.

Several genetic abnormalities that are associated with pancreatic cancers include activation of oncogenes, inactivation of tumor suppressor genes, and excessive expression of growth factors. Most pancreatic cancers demonstrate mutations of the K-*ras* oncogene. K-*ras* plays a key role in regulating cellular growth. Its activation is a guanosine triphosphate (GTP)–dependent event, terminated by GTP hydrolysis. Oncogenic point mutations of K-*ras* interfere with the termination event, resulting in permanent activation of K-*ras* and a continuous transmission of growth signal to the nucleus. Mutation of the *p53* tumor suppressor gene is the most common genetic event in all human cancers and is detected in 75% of pancreatic cancers. This gene plays an important role in regulating the cell cycle, DNA synthesis and repair, apoptosis, and cell differentiation. Several growth factors are often up-regulated in pancreatic cancer. The most commonly observed is the epidermal growth factor (EGF) receptor family.

Ductal adenocarcinoma accounts for up to 90% of all pancreatic neoplasms. Most adenocarcinomas arise in the pancreatic head or uncinate process. At the time of diagnosis, they are usually larger than 3 cm in diameter with nodal and distant metastases. Tumors originating in the body or tail of the pancreas are often larger and more likely to have spread before their detection. An area of chronic pancreatitis often surrounds the tumor, presumably because of tumor-induced obstruction of adjacent ducts. Perineural growth of the tumor is highly characteristic of this cancer and may account for the tendency of pancreatic cancer to extend into a neighboring neural plexus leading to abdominal and back pain.

The nature of symptoms is determined by the location of the tumor. Symptoms include unexplained episodes of pancreatitis, painless jaundice, nausea, vomiting, and weight loss. Lesions in the head of the pancreas cause bile duct, duodenal, or pancreatic duct obstruction. With further spread, patients have upper abdominal and back pain due to peripancreatic nerve plexus involvement. Ascites develops when peritoneal carcinomatosis or portal vein occlusion occurs. Tumors arising in the neck, body, or tail of the pancreas usually do not lead to jaundice or gastric outlet obstruction, and symptoms may be limited to weight loss and vague upper abdominal pain. New-onset diabetes mellitus is occasionally the first symptom of pancreatic cancer. This can be mediated by a factor released from the tumor that either inhibits insulin release from islets or induces peripheral insulin resistance. Migratory thrombophlebitis (Trousseau's syndrome) can be associated with pancreatic cancer. It is probably a paraneoplastic phenomenon that results from a tumor-induced hypercoagulable state. The physical findings in patients with pancreatic cancer depend on the extent of the disease. Metastatic liver nodules and supraclavicular lymphadenopathy ("Virchow's node") may be palpable. Distal common bile duct obstruction caused by the tumor often leads to bile duct and gallbladder distention. Thus, a palpable gallbladder in a patient with painless jaundice (i.e., Courvoisier's sign) should suggest a periampullary neoplasm. Pancreatic head lesions frequently cause elevated bilirubin and alkaline phosphatase levels. The two most widely used pancreatic cancer serum markers are carcinoembryonic antigen and the carbohydrate antigen CA 19.9. Both are frequently elevated in patients with advanced disease, but, unfortunately, the circulating levels of these tumor markers are often normal in patients with early tumors. Therefore, using these tumor markers to screen patients has not been useful. CA 19.9 can also be elevated in patients with cholangitis and jaundice due to other causes.

For jaundiced patients the initial imaging study is usually an abdominal ultrasound examination. It may reveal a pancreatic mass with extrahepatic ductal dilation in the absence of biliary tract stones. Ultrasound is usually followed by helical contrast-enhanced computed tomography (CT). Helical CT, with phased imaging for visualization of the pancreas and major peripancreatic vessels, is the most widely used method of evaluating tumor resectability. Circumferential encasement, invasion, or occlusion of the portal vein/superior mesenteric vein and/or the superior mesenteric artery is generally considered to be a sign of unresectability, although resection is still technically possible if only the venous structures are involved. Other CT changes indicating unresectability include extension beyond the pancreatic capsule and into the retroperitoneum, involvement of neural or nodal structures surrounding the origin of either the celiac axis or superior mesenteric artery, and extension of the tumor along the hepatoduodenal ligament. There have been recent claims that endoscopic ultrasound provides staging information that is superior to that obtained by CT. However, endoscopic ultrasound is operator dependent. Although the sensitivity and specificity of magnetic resonance imaging appear to equal those of CT, CT is currently more widely employed. Endoscopic retrograde cholangiopancreatography (ERCP) can be particularly helpful for evaluating patients with obstructive jaundice without a detectable mass on CT. It can identify stones or other nonmalignant causes of obstructive jaundice, define the location of the bile duct obstruction, and identify ampullary or periampullary lesions. The role of ERCP in the management of patients with a mass detected on CT is more controversial, because a malignant lesion cannot be entirely excluded by ERCP and resection is indicated, regardless of the ERCP findings.

Biopsy to confirm the presence and identify the type of cancer is usually required before chemoradiation therapy of unresectable pancreatic tumors or neoadjuvant treatment of resectable tumors. Percutaneous biopsy, performed with either CT or ultrasound guidance, or transduodenal biopsy, performed with endoscopic ultrasound guidance, is routinely employed in these situations. Controversy surrounds the issue of whether all patients with potentially resectable tumors should undergo preoperative biopsy. A biopsy specimen might yield false-negative results, and, at least theoretically, transcutaneous biopsy might promote intraperitoneal dissemination of the tumor. Therefore, routine preoperative biopsy for confirmation of the diagnosis in the management of patients with potentially resectable lesions is not usually recommended. However, if this policy of not performing preoperative biopsy is followed, 5% to 10% of patients undergoing resection for suspected cancer will be found to have benign lesions.

The role of staging laparoscopy in pancreatic cancer is debated. Proponents claim that 20% to 40% of patients believed to have stage I or II disease have unrecognized small metastases to peritoneal surfaces and that the metastases can be laparoscopically detected, thus preventing a needless laparotomy. With modern imaging techniques, few patients with pancreatic head tumors are deemed unresectable at operation merely because they are found to have metastases that might have been found by laparoscopy. More commonly, unappreciated vascular involvement is the operative finding that prevents resection, and, for these patients, benefit can still be provided by a bilioenteric and possibly a gastroenteric bypass. Laparoscopy is more appropriate in the case of body or tail lesions, because, with left-side lesions, neither obstructive jaundice nor gastric outlet obstruction is likely to develop and therefore there is no role for surgical bypass for these patients.

Tumors of the head, neck, and uncinate process are generally resected by pancreaticoduodenectomy, with or without preservation of the pylorus. The two procedures yield similar survival rates and have similar morbidity rates. The pylorus-preserving operation is technically easier and faster, but it may be associated with a higher incidence of and more prolonged delayed gastric emptying. Long-term survival, when the operation is performed for ductal adenocarcinoma, is unusual. Five-year survival rates of 15% to 20% have been reported from some medical centers, but rates of 10% to 15% are more common, and most of the patients who survive for 5 years die during the subsequent 5 years. A number of factors affect the survival rate. The most influential is the presence of tumor at the resection margin.

Most body and tail cancers have already metastasized to distant sites or extended locally by the time of diagnosis. Splenic vein involvement or occlusion is not uncommon and is not considered a sign of nonresectability. On the other hand, involvement of the splenic/superior mesenteric vein confluence generally precludes resection. Resection involves a distal pancreatectomy with splenectomy. Only 10% of cancers involving the tail or body of the pancreas are resectable at the time of diagnosis. The 5-year survival rate for patients who are deemed resectable is somewhat lower than that for patients with resectable cancer of the pancreatic head (8% to 14%).

Establishing the diagnosis and relieving symptoms of jaundice, gastric outlet obstruction, and pain are the goals of palliative treatment. Tissue diagnosis can usually be made by CT- or ultrasound-guided percutaneous fine-needle aspiration. Decompression of the obstructed biliary tract can be achieved using either an endoscopic or a percutaneous-transhepatic approach. At the time of ERCP, a transpapillary stent is placed across the obstructed segment of bile duct. Plastic or expandable metal stents can be used, but metal stents give more complete and more long-lasting relief of jaundice. Plastic stents can become obstructed by tumor or debris, and, as a result, they must be changed every 2 to 3 months. The percutaneous-transhepatic approach to duct decompression is usually reserved for patients in whom a stent cannot be placed endoscopically. Pancreatic tumors can extend into and obstruct the duodenum, leading to gastric outlet obstruction. Many patients can be palliated by endoscopic placement of expandable endoluminal metal stents into the duodenum. For lesions that are not amenable to stents, surgical gastrojejunostomy may be required. Most patients can be adequately treated with orally or transcutaneously administered analgesics. Narcotic medications may be required. When or if this fails, percutaneous CT-guided or endoscopic ultrasound–guided celiac plexus block can be helpful.

Symptoms of unresectable pancreatic cancer can mostly be relieved by nonsurgical means. Surgical palliation is used for patients who are undergoing laparotomy for anticipated resectable disease that is determined unresectable at the time of surgery. In this situation, biliary tract decompression can be achieved by creating either a cholecystojejunostomy or a choledochojejunostomy. The former is most appropriate for patients with nondilated ducts in whom the cystic duct–common bile duct junction is far from the pancreatic tumor. Choledo-

chojejunostomy, on the other hand, should be performed when the tumor is close to or at the cystic duct–common bile duct junction and the bile duct is dilated. Either a loop or a Roux-en-Y segment of jejunum can be used with similar results. Duodenal obstruction can be managed by creation of a side-to-side gastrojejunostomy in which an antecolic jejunal loop is anastomosed to the posterior wall of the gastric antrum. Duodenal obstruction, even in advanced pancreatic cancer, occurs in less than 25% of patients, and therefore controversy surrounds whether a prophylactic gastrojejunostomy should be performed before gastric outlet obstruction develops. Gastrojejunostomy can cause delayed gastric emptying and result in symptoms identical to duodenal obstruction. Therefore, gastrojejunostomy is performed selectively in patients whose tumors are locally advanced but without distant metastases, because they have an expected survival of 8 to 12 months. On the other hand, prophylactic gastrojejunostomy is not advocated for patients with distant metastasis, because their expected survival is only 3 to 6 months and they are less likely to develop duodenal obstruction prior to death. Palliation of pain can be achieved intraoperatively by injecting alcohol into the celiac plexus.

Different protocols for chemoradiation treatment of unresectable pancreatic cancer have been reported. Patients undergoing resection may also benefit from adjuvant chemoradiation therapy. The combination of 5-fluorouracil with radiation therapy has been reported to increase the 2-year survival rate from 18% to 43% for patients with tumor-free resection margins. This approach has been widely employed. In addition, it is claimed that up to 15% of selected patients with locally advanced lesions deemed to be unresectable can be made resectable by administration of chemoradiation therapy.

125
The Spleen

The spleen lies in the posterior left upper quadrant adjacent to the greater curvature of the stomach, the tail of the pancreas, the splenic flexure of the colon, and the left kidney. The parietal peritoneum surrounds the spleen, creating reflections of peritoneum known as the *suspensory ligaments*. The entire surface of the spleen is enveloped by a fibrous capsule that extends into the splenic parenchyma itself. As it enters the splenic tissue, the fibrous tissue forms a network of branching trabeculae that create compartments in the splenic tissue. The primary arterial supply to the spleen is the splenic artery. The splenic artery is torturous in shape and gives off several vessels, including the short gastric, pancreatic branches, and the left gastroepiploic artery.

The splenic artery terminates into several terminal branches in the splenorenal ligament. These terminal branches enter the hilum of the spleen where they course through the parenchyma along the trabeculae. The two functional tissues in the spleen are the white pulp (lymphatic tissue) and red pulp. The splenic arterioles exit the trabeculae and enter the white pulp. At this point, their outer adventitial layer is replaced by a lymphatic sheath that is contiguous with the white pulp. The arterioles shed the lymphatic sheath at the interface of the white pulp and red pulp, called the *marginal zone*. The red pulp is composed of splenic sinusoids and sinuses along with splenic cords. The splenic sinusoids drain into splenic veins in the red pulp. The splenic vein travels a course similar to the arterial system. The venous system coalesces into five vessels in the splenorenal ligament that ultimately join together to form the splenic vein. The splenic vein courses posterior to the artery behind the pancreas. The superior mesenteric vein and the splenic vein connect to form the portal vein at the neck of the pancreas.

The spleen shares the responsibility of hematopoiesis during initial fetal development. The spleen continues to serve in this capacity until the fifth month of gestation. For the remainder of its life, the spleen functions to filter the blood and provide immune protection. The filtering mechanism of the spleen works in the following way. Blood is brought to the spleen through the splenic arterioles. In the spleen, the circulating blood is passed through the mesh-like endoreticular system. The cellular components of the blood must be able to traverse the numerous pores lining the splenic sinusoids. The cells that do not pass through are phagocytized by splenic macrophages. Red blood cells that have reached the end of their life span are rigid and are incapable of traversing the splenic sinusoids without being entrapped. The spleen removes these senile cells from the circulation. The spleen also removes diseased red cells (malaria) and bacteria that evaded the host's immune defenses. The spleen is also responsible for the maturation and maintenance of red blood cells. Immature red blood cells lose their nuclei and have surface features corrected (i.e., removal of spurs or pits).

Hereditary anemic conditions can be accentuated by the filtration of blood through the spleen. Splenic tissue often traps abnormal red cells caused by sickle cell, thalassemia, and hereditary spherocytosis. Anemia, splenomegaly, and even splenic infarction can occur due to splenic filtration in these disease states. Antibody-mediated cellular destruction occurs in the spleen in autoimmune hemolytic anemia and idiopathic thrombocytopenic purpura (ITP). Antibodies specific to either red blood cell or platelet cell membranes bind to the cells and trigger phagocytosis in the spleen.

The spleen serves an immunologic function by augmenting the complement system. The spleen performs this function through its large phagocytic capacity and through the production of properdin and tuftsin. Properdin is a molecule that activates the alternative complement pathway. Tuftsin is a molecule that increases the phagocytic activity of polymorphonuclear neutrophil leukocytes (PMNs) and macrophages. Tuftsin is cleaved from the heavy chain of immunoglobulin G, the majority of which happens in the spleen.

Splenectomy and Associated Conditions

Immune or idiopathic thrombocytopenia purpura is characterized by a low platelet count and normal bone marrow. The diagnosis is one of exclusion. Idiopathic thrombocytopenia purpura develops because of antibody-mediated platelet destruction. Immunoglobulin G auto antibodies bind to specific antigens on the platelet cell membrane. The platelets coated with the auto antibodies are phagocytized in the reticuloendothelial system. Biopsy examination of the bone marrow shows normal megakaryocytes. The disease occurs more frequently in women just as other autoimmune diseases. Most women are affected before the fourth decade. In the pediatric population, males and females are equally affected. The onset of illness occurs suddenly, with remission occurring spontaneously in most children (80%). Clinical manifestations include purpura, epistaxis, and mucosal bleeding (gingival). Additional less common bleeding occurrences are gastrointestinal bleeding, intracranial bleeding, and hematuria.

Treatment is tailored to the severity of disease. Observation is recommended for patients who are asymptomatic or whose platelet counts range from 30,000 to 50,000. Bleeding complications are less likely to occur with counts greater than 50,000. Medical therapy (i.e., prednisone) is initiated for patients with platelet counts less than 20,000 or at less than 50,000 for patients at risk of bleeding. More than 60% of patients respond with increased platelet counts. Treatment generally requires 1 to 3 weeks to take effect. Intravenous immunoglobulin is used as a treatment adjunct to prepare for surgery (splenectomy) or for labor. Patients typically respond within 3 days. Splenectomy is reserved for severe cases of ITP that are refractory to medical therapy or for patients who are experiencing severe side effects from medical therapy. Splenectomy produces complete remission of disease in over 60% of cases. Pregnant women in the second trimester who have failed medical therapy and have appropriately low platelet counts (10,000 to 30,000) are also eligible for splenectomy. Splenectomy is not suggested when platelet counts are above 50,000. Splenic sequestration is a positive predictor of the success of splenectomy.

[111]Indium-labeled platelet scintigraphy may allow the surgeon to better delineate the location of platelet destruction (hepatic or splenic) and therefore predict the success of splenectomy. Patients with splenic sequestration have an 87% to 93% response rate to splenectomy as opposed to 7% to 30% of patients with hepatic sequestration. An increase in platelet count occurs within the first 10 days after splenectomy. Platelet counts of 150,000 by postoperative day 3 and 500,000 by postoperative day 10 are indicative of long-term success. Patients who fail to respond to splenectomy are given steroid therapy with or without immune modulating agents (cyclophosphamide, azathioprine). Failure of splenectomy may be caused by the presence of an accessory spleen, which is a remnant of functioning splenic tissue overlooked at the time of splenectomy. An accessory spleen is identified by [111]indium-labeled platelet scintigraphy or the absence of asplenic morphology on peripheral blood smears (Howell-Jolly bodies, Heinz bodies). Patients with an accessory spleen who continue to be symptomatic should have the accessory spleen removed.

Hereditary spherocytosis is an autosomal dominant condition characterized by a deficit in a red blood cell cytoskeletal protein called *spectrin*. The protein deficiency results in rigidity of the red cell membrane, increased osmotic fragility, and spherical morphology. The rigidity of the erythrocytes makes them less able to traverse the splenic sinusoids without becoming entrapped. Common clinical features include anemia, splenomegaly, and jaundice. Spherocytes on peripheral blood smears, elevated reticulocyte counts, elevated osmotic fragility, and a negative Comb's test confirm the diagnosis. Splenectomy reduces the amount of hemolysis and lessens the severity of anemia. The procedure is recommended for patients more than 4 years of age (to allow adequate time to develop immune function). Ultrasound of the right upper quadrant is recommended to evaluate for gallstones. If gallstones are found, a cholecystectomy is recommended at the same time as splenectomy.

Enzymatic deficiencies in red blood cells such as glucose-6-phosphate dehydrogenase deficiency (X-linked recessive) and pyruvate kinase (autosomal recessive) deficiency can result in hemolytic anemia. Pyruvate kinase deficiency manifests with abnormal glucose metabolism, decreased cell flexibility, and hemolysis. Splenomegaly is caused by erythrocyte entrapment. Splenectomy decreases the rate of hemolysis and decreases the need for blood transfusions. Glucose-6-phosphate dehydrogenase deficiency results in hemolysis after exposure to particular chemicals or drugs. Splenectomy is seldom recommended for this disease.

Splenectomy is indicated for complications of thalassemia and sickle cell disease. The complications include hypersplenism, acute splenic sequestration crisis, and splenic abscess. Acute splenic sequestration crisis causes rapid splenomegaly and abdominal pain and requires multiple blood transfusions. Hypersplenism is associated with anemia, thrombocytopenia, and leucopenia. Splenic abscess manifests with fever, leukocytosis, abdominal pain, and splenomegaly. *Salmonella* and *Enterobacter* are common isolates from splenic abscesses.

In the past, the treatment of Hodgkin's disease required a staging laparotomy with splenectomy. Staging laparotomies were used to assess the extent of disease present below the diaphragm. Improvements in radiographic imaging (computed tomography and positron emission tomography scans) have decreased the use of operative staging for Hodgkin's disease. Patients who have intra-abdominal disease now undergo systemic chemotherapy. Radiation therapy is a viable option for early-stage Hodgkin's disease as well. Staging laparotomies with splenectomy are reserved for early-stage disease when the pathologic information provided will influence the outcome of therapy. Non-Hodgkin's lymphoma is the most common primary neoplasm of the spleen. Approximately 50% to 80% of patients with non-Hodgkin's lymphoma have disease involvement of the spleen. Manifestations include splenomegaly, abdominal pain, fullness, and early satiety due to mass effect on the stomach. Splenectomy is indicated for patients with hypersplenism and associated pancytopenia.

Splenectomy is recommended for parasitic cysts of the spleen. Spillage of cyst contents can precipitate an anaphylactic reaction. Alternatively, echinococcal cysts of the spleen can be injected with hypertonic saline, ethanol, or silver nitrate solution.

Splenic pseudocysts are often caused by trauma. Pseudocysts are not true cysts, because they lack an epithelial lining. Focal areas of calcification can be detected in 50% of cases. The decision to perform a splenectomy is based on the size of the cyst and the symptoms. Cysts smaller than 4 cm in diameter are usually asymptomatic and resolve spontaneously. Large symptomatic cysts are treated by partial or complete splenectomy. Alternatively, unilocular cysts can be drained percutaneously.

Splenic abscesses occur rarely but can be potentially fatal (80% in immunocompromised patients and up to 20% in patients with normal immune function). Most cases are the result of hematogenous spread from other locations of infection (endocarditis, osteomyelitis, and intravenous drug use). Conditions such as neoplasms, trauma, hemoglobinopathies, polycythemia, acquired immunodeficiency syndrome, and urinary tract infections can precipitate splenic abscesses. Direct spread of infection from locations such as the pancreas, the colon, and the kidney is also possible. Commonly isolated organisms include *Staphylococcus*, *Streptococcus*, *Enterococcus*, *Mycobacterium*, *Actinomyces*, and *Candida* in immunocompromised individuals. Symptoms are usually nonspecific and include vague abdominal pain, fever, and occasionally pleuritic chest pain. Abscesses are usually unilocular in adults and multilocular in children. Unilocular abscesses are often amenable to percutaneous drainage along with intravenous antibiotics. Success rates are reported between 75% and 90%. Splenectomy is indicated for multiloculated abscesses and failed attempts at percutaneous drainage. Drains are placed in the left upper quadrant at the time of surgery, and intravenous antibiotics are continued.

Various leukemias (chronic lymphocytic leukemia, hairy cell leukemia, and chronic myelogenous leukemia) are complicated by hypersplenism or splenomegaly. Splenectomy is offered to these patients as a palliation of symptoms.

Wandering Spleen

The condition known as *wandering spleen* is caused by the absence of suspensory ligaments to fix the spleen in place. The defect is thought to arise from a congenital malformation or can be caused by abdominal wall laxity and multiparity. An unusually long vascular pedicle becomes predisposed to tension or torsion. Patients are usually asymptomatic, but severe pain can accompany torsion of the splenic vessels because of congestion, ischemia, and infarction. Computed tomography scan with intravenous contrast is used to confirm the diagnosis. Common findings include whirling of the vascular pedicle and the absence of splenic enhancement. Wandering spleen can be treated with splenopexy or splenectomy.

Complications of Splenectomy

Thrombocytosis occurs in patients who have undergone splenectomy, most often for myeloproliferative conditions such as polycythemia vera and chronic myelocytic leukemia. Complications manifest with hemorrhagic or embolic events (especially pulmonary embolism). Overwhelming postsplenectomy infection is a serious complication. Fatalities occur in 1 of 800 patients. Infection often occurs more than 2 years after splenectomy but can occur at any time. Symptoms begin with a prodromal phase of fever, chills, sore throat, malaise, myalgias, and vomiting. Clinical deterioration develops rapidly to sepsis, shock, disseminated intravascular clotting, respiratory distress, decreased mental status, coma, and death. Mortality rate approaches 50% to 70% even with intensive medical care and antibiotics. The most commonly responsible organism is *Streptococcus pneumoniae* (50% to 90%). Other culprits include *Haemophilus influenzae*, *Neisseria meningitidis*, *Salmonella*, and *Capnocytophaga canimorsus*.

Vaccinations against encapsulated organisms such as type B *Haemophilus, Meningococcus*, and *Pneumococcus* are recommended 2 weeks before a planned splenectomy. Patients who undergo emergent splenectomies for trauma should be vaccinated before hospital discharge.

Penicillin is often administered in the pediatric population as a form of prophylaxis. Many patients are given oral antibiotics (i.e., amoxicillin) to be taken for all febrile illnesses.

126
Abdominal Wall Hernias

Rectus diastasis is caused by attenuation of the linea alba. The transversalis fascia remains intact, preventing herniation. A noticeable bulge may be produced when the patient strains due to protrusion of that anterior abdominal wall. Reassurance of the benign nature of this condition is all that is necessary.

Epigastric hernias form between the xiphoid process and the umbilicus. The lesions occur at sites of penetration of the linea alba by nerves and vessels. The openings may allow the protrusion of preperitoneal fat or peritoneum into the subcutaneous space. Herniation of preperitoneal contents can generate pain that is out of proportion to the size of the lesion because of pressure placed on the nerves that traverse the opening. Multiple lesions occur in one of five patients. The defects are repaired by simple primary closure.

Spigelian hernias are small defects (<2 cm) that occur in the region of the semilunar line. The lesions are nonpalpable in most cases and manifest as a localized area of pain. Most lesions appear at or below the arcuate line where the posterior rectus fascia terminates. The hernia sac protrudes through the defect but remains below the fascia of the external oblique in an interparietal position. Diagnosis is confirmed by computed tomography scan. Small defects are repaired by primary closure of the transverse abdominis and internal oblique fascia; large defects can require prosthetic mesh.

The umbilicus is a common site for hernia. Congenital umbilical hernias are very common. African Americans are eight times more likely to have congenital umbilical hernias than whites. By 2 years of age most will have closed. Umbilical hernias occurring after 5 years of age warrant operative closure. Complications of incarceration and strangulation are rare in the pediatric population. Umbilical hernias in adults are often acquired lesions. They occur more often in women and in circumstances of increased abdominal pressure (e.g., obesity, pregnancy, ascites). Rupture or strangulation of an umbilical hernia is a rare occurrence, but it can occur in the setting of chronic ascites. Peritonitis and death can result from acute rupture of an umbilical hernia. Surgical repair is indicated for symptomatic hernias, large defects, thinning overlying skin, and uncontrollable ascites. Defects less than 3 cm are repaired primarily. Defects greater than 3 cm are repaired with prosthetic material. Large defects may be better repaired by laparoscopic means.

Ventral/incisional hernias result from inadequate healing of a previous abdominal midline incision. Factors such as undue tension on the wound, wound infections, increased intra-abdominal pressure, obesity, malnutrition, advanced age, and drugs (e.g., steroids, chemotherapy, immunosuppressants) are all contributors to poor wound healing and hernia formation. Large defects may cause difficulties in abdominal wall closure after laparotomy. Retracted abdominal musculature, intestinal edema, and venous stasis all contribute to loss of domain. Small defects (<4 cm) can be repaired with primary closure. Defects greater than 4 cm should have prosthetic mesh placed. Recurrence rates for primary closure are approximately 10% to 50%. Prosthetic mesh is placed one of three ways: onlay patch (mesh placed on top of primarily closed fascia), interposed between the fascial defects, or placed between tissue planes. Hernia repairs can be conducted through an open laparotomy or laparoscopically. Massive defects are closed with the aid of serial abdominal insufflations to obtain more domain.

Obturator hernias are protrusions of intraperitoneal contents through the obturator canal. The canal is created by the union of the pubis and the ischium. Normally, the canal is covered by a membrane, which is penetrated by the obturator nerve and vessels. Herniation into the canal can cause impingement of the obturator nerve (producing pain on the medial aspect of the thigh (Howship-Romberg sign) or incarceration and strangulation. Fifty percent of patients experience a complete or partial bowel obstruction. The diagnosis can be made using an abdominal computed tomography scan. The repair is done either openly or laparoscopically through a posterior approach. During the procedure, the hernia sac is reduced along with removal of preperitoneal fat. The canal is closed primarily or with mesh.

Lumbar hernias are caused by congenital or acquired defects in the lumbar area of the posterior abdominal wall. Most defects occur in the superior lumbar triangle (bordered by the twelfth rib, paraspinal muscles, and internal oblique muscle). Lumbar hernias in the inferior triangle (bordered by the iliac crest, latissimus dorsi, and external oblique) occur less often. The defect develops as the lumbodorsal fascia becomes weaker, allowing the protrusion of preperitoneal fat and hernia sac. Incarceration is a rare event. Primary repair is made difficult by the bony land marks bordering the defects. Therefore, most repairs involve prosthetic mesh placement.

Sciatic hernias occur vary infrequently. The diagnosis is difficult to make because of the rarity of the hernia and because they are often asymptomatic until intestinal obstruction occurs. Patient often complain of an uncomfortable mass in the gluteal or intragluteal area that may progressively enlarge. Sciatic hernias rarely produce sciatic neuralgia. In cases of suspected bowel involvement, a transperitoneal approach is required to reduce the hernia and inspect the bowel. Prosthetic mesh repair is usually preferred over primary repair. A transgluteal approach is appropriate for reducible hernia with uncompromised bowel. The patient is placed in the prone position. An incision is created from the greater trochanter over the top of the mass. The gluteus maximus is opened, and the sac is visualized. The muscle edges of the defect are repaired primarily with interrupted sutures, or prosthetic mesh is affixed to the defect.

Congenital or acquired defects of the pelvic diaphragm can result in perineal hernias. These are large but very uncommon defects that occur after abdominoperineal resection or perineal prostatectomy. Older, multiparous women are primarily affected. Symptoms are usually related to protrusion of a mass. Sitting or standing accentuates the bulging effect through the defect. The hernia is often identified on physical examination. These hernias are repaired through an abdominal incision, with reduction of the hernia sac and primary closure of the defect. Mesh is placed when needed.

Hernias that develop between the layers of the abdominal wall are called *interparietal hernias*. These are rare defects that are often associated with previous incisions. A Spigelian hernia is an example of an interparietal hernia. Abdominal computed tomography is often useful for making the diagnosis. As with other hernias, large defects require mesh. The separation of components technique may be useful when mesh cannot be placed.

127
Morbid Obesity

Morbid obesity is defined as a body mass index (BMI) $>40\,\text{m/kg}^2$. Patients with a BMI $>35\,\text{m/kg}^2$ and obesity-related comorbidities are also considered morbidly obese. It is estimated that more than 20% of the U.S. population is obese (BMI >30). Americans spend more than $30 billion annually in weight loss aids, and the annual direct cost of treating obesity-related disease exceeds $50 billion. Furthermore, there are more than 400,000 obesity-related deaths annually in the United States. Obesity may soon eclipse smoking as the leading preventable cause of premature death.

Treatment options for obesity include dietary modification, exercise, medications, and surgery. Orlistat (Xenical®) and sibutramine (Meridia®) are two FDA-approved medications often used to treat obesity. Orlistat is a pancreatic lipase inhibitor that blocks absorption of triglycerides. Sibutramine is an appetite suppressant that inhibits serotonin and norepinephrine uptake. Unfortunately, medical treatment of obesity is plagued by low long-term success rates.

Although more invasive, weight loss (bariatric) surgery yields much higher rates of long-term weight loss. Bariatric procedures are designed to restrict caloric intake and/or promote malabsorption, thus reducing caloric absorption. In the United States, the two most common bariatric procedures are Roux-en-Y gastric bypass (gastric bypass) and adjustable gastric banding (the Lap-Band®).

Gastric bypass was initially described in the 1960s and combines elements of restriction and malabsorption. The upper stomach is divided and separated to create a 30- to 60-cc gastric pouch. The remainder of the stomach, the so-called remnant, is defunctionalized. The jejunum is then divided 30 to 60 cm distal to the ligament of Treitz, and a 100- to 150-cm Roux limb is created. This Roux limb is positioned in an antecolic/antegastric or retrocolic/retrogastric fashion. The gastrojejunostomy can be constructed with a circular end-to-end anastomosis stapler, linear stapler, or a hand-sewn technique.

Overall, perioperative mortality rate is less than 1%. Early, life-threatening, postoperative complications include anastomotic leak, staple line failure of the remnant, pulmonary embolism, and intra abdominal infection. Relative ischemia in the gastric pouch, coupled with inherent Roux limb tension and technical difficulty in construction, lead to a greater incidence of leaks at the gastrojejunostomy compared with the jejunojejunostomy. The early signs of an anastomotic leak can be very subtle. Patients may manifest tachycardia, tachypnea, increased pain, fever, and/or leukocytosis. An upper gastrointestinal contrast study or computed tomographic scan can aid in the diagnosis. Treatment of an anastomotic leak usually requires laparotomy, abdominal washout, and placement of drains. Edematous, friable tissue may preclude definitive repair of the perforation. In this situation, establishment of a controlled fistula with drains should be the goal. Placement of a gastrostomy tube in the remnant provides long-term nutritional access to the alimentary tract.

Long-term outcomes after gastric bypass are encouraging. Patients typically lose 50% to 75% of their excess weight and more than 70% have improvement or resolution of comorbidities such as type 2 diabetes mellitus, hypertension, hyperlipidemia, and sleep apnea. Clinically significant malabsorption (hypoalbuminemia and liver failure) following gastric bypass is rare. However, bypass of the duodenum, proximal jejunum, and most of the stomach reduces absorption of calcium, iron, and vitamin B_{12}. Thus, many patients require life-long vitamin and mineral supplementation. Long-term complications of gastric bypass include anastomotic ulcer and stricture, small bowel obstruction, cholelithiasis, incisional hernia, and chronic nausea and vomiting. Anastomotic strictures are usually amenable to endoscopic dilation, and re-operation is rarely required. Compared with traditional "open" gastric bypass, laparoscopic gastric bypass has significantly reduced wound complications such as infection and incisional hernia. Rapid weight loss after gastric bypass surgery increases the risk of developing cholelithiasis, and many surgeons have recommended postoperative Actigall to reduce this risk. Choledo-cholithiasis poses a unique therapeutic dilemma, because the duodenum and ampulla are not accessible to standard upper endoscopy and endoscopic retrograde cholangiopancreatography (ERCP). Therapeutic options for obstructive jaundice from choledocholithiasis include percutaneous transhepatic cholangiography, common bile duct exploration, and intraoperative ERCP via the defunctionalized gastric remnant. The lack of endoscopic access to most of the stomach and duodenum also complicates the diagnosis and management of peptic ulcer disease (bleeding, perforation, and obstruction) and neoplasms.

Adjustable gastric banding (AGB) is a relatively new bariatric procedure. The most common AGB device in the United States is the Lap-Band®, which received FDA approval in 2001, although it has been used in Europe for more than 10 years. The Lap-Band consists of an inflatable silicone band that is placed just distal to the gastroesophageal junction. The band is connected to a subcutaneous port. The volume of the band is adjusted by percutaneous injection of saline into the port device. Adjustable gastric banding is a purely restrictive procedure that limits caloric ingestion.

Weight loss following AGB is more gradual and typically occurs over about 3 years. This is in contrast to gastric bypass, which yields weight loss over 12 to 18 months. Some experienced medical centers have reported loss of 50% to 75% of excess weight, which is comparable with gastric bypass. One of the primary advantages of AGB is that there is no intestinal anastomosis. This eliminates the risk of anastomotic leak, malabsorption, and problems related to lack of endoscopic access to the foregut. Most patients do not require postoperative vitamin or mineral supplements. Experienced surgeons can complete the procedure in less than an hour in an outpatient setting.

Compared with gastric bypass, perioperative complications such as bleeding, infection, anastomotic leak, and cardiopulmonary morbidity are fewer with AGB. However, there is a paucity of long-term outcome data (>10 years) for AGB. Successful weight loss following AGB depends on band adjustments to maintain the restrictive effect. The average patient will require three to six band adjustments in the first year after surgery. These adjustments, which involve injecting saline into the subcutaneous port, are often performed under fluoroscopy to better assess the restriction to flow through the band. One of the more serious complications of AGB is band slippage. This occurs when the stomach inferior to the band slides superiorly through the band. This can rotate the band, creating a proximal gastric obstruction and/or gastric ischemia. Once the diagnosis is confirmed with an upper gastrointestinal contrast study, emergent surgical intervention is required to reduce or remove the band. Other major complications of AGB include band erosion, catheter/port malfunction, and infection. Overall, 10% to 15% of patients require re-operation for complications related to their band. Patients who fail ABG are candidates for Roux-en-Y gastric bypass.

128
Physiologic Effects of Laparoscopy

In the last decade there has been a tremendous growth in the field of laparoscopic surgery. The success of laparoscopic cholecystectomy has driven improvements in equipment and surgical skill that have made numerous procedures amenable to the laparoscopic approach. Patients realize the benefits of minimally invasive surgery and now actively seek surgical treatment for diseases that they would not have previously considered.

Although laparoscopy has been shown to cause fewer untoward effects than traditional open surgery, there are specific physiologic changes that occur during laparoscopic surgery. The insufflation of carbon dioxide gas into the peritoneal cavity, preperitoneal space, or retroperitoneal space increases intra-abdominal pressure and causes impaired ventilation, decreased venous return, circulatory depression, decreased renal perfusion, and increased intracranial pressure. These physiologic changes can make intraoperative management of patients more challenging; however, benefits are derived postoperatively. Decreased pain, earlier return to ambulation, and an attenuated stress response are associated with decreased postoperative complications and a quicker return to full activity. However, the benefits of laparoscopy depend on its relative effects during and after the procedure, so not all patients may be suitable candidates for laparoscopic surgery. A description of the effects of laparoscopy on pulmonary, cardiac, immune function, and other organ systems follows.

The establishment of pneumoperitoneum causes increased intra-abdominal volume and pressure. This impedes diaphragmatic excursion and causes increased peak airway pressures, decreased pulmonary compliance and vital capacity, decreased functional residual capacity, and increased alveolar dead space. Additionally, anesthetics and positive pressure ventilation cause shunting and alveolar collapse. Initially, pneumoperitoneum may improve shunting by increasing airway pressure and creating intrinsic positive end-expiratory pressure, thereby keeping alveoli open and improving oxygenation. This is a short-lived effect and is no longer a factor within 30 minutes of beginning the procedure.

The use of carbon dioxide to create pneumoperitoneum increases the delivery of CO_2 to the lungs by up to 50%. This leads to increased end tidal CO_2 and may produce an acidosis if CO_2 exchange across alveoli is impaired. Patients at particular risk for this are those with high metabolic and cellular respiratory rates, such as those in septic shock.

Patients with chronic obstructive pulmonary disease are also at high risk for developing acidosis due to large ventilatory dead space. Other patients with poor cardiac output and impaired local regional blood flow are also at risk for developing acidosis with pneumoperitoneum. Close monitoring of end tidal CO_2 and arterial blood gas measurements are paramount for these high-risk patients if they are to undergo laparoscopic procedures.

Although the direct effects of pneumoperitoneum generally cause a decline in pulmonary function during surgery, postoperatively patients generally have less pain and subsequently less pulmonary embarrassment. Compared with patients receiving open surgery, patients who undergo laparoscopic procedures have superior results on pulmonary function testing. These benefits translate into a lower incidence of atelectasis and improved oxygenation postoperatively.

Similar to the pulmonary consequences of laparoscopy, the physiologic changes in the cardiovascular system are due to the increased intra-abdominal pressure. Pneumoperitoneum increases the central venous pressure (CVP), pulmonary capillary wedge pressure (PCWP), mean arterial pressure (MAP), and systemic vascular resistance. Patients with cardiac diseases tolerate these effects poorly. The increased preload augments cardiac output, but the increased afterload counteracts this effect. The net effect is increased cardiac work. Interestingly, although wedge pressure, a marker of preload, increases with pneumoperitoneum, studies have shown that the resultant increase in intra-abdominal pressure decreases venous return. Increased pressure on the vena cava, which occurs with pneumoperitoneum, is believed to be the primary reason for this effect. Optimizing patients' volume status before surgery minimizes this effect.

Positioning also has unique effects on circulatory physiology in patients undergoing surgery. Trendelenburg's position increases intrathoracic pressures, CVP, PCWP, and MAP. This results in increased cardiac work. Reverse Trendelenburg's positioning causes reductions in cardiac output by decreasing preload and may cause hypotension.

Additionally, the effects of carbon dioxide itself have a physiologic impact. Carbon dioxide absorption causes arteriolar dilation, myocardial depression, and decreased blood pressures. These effects are somewhat counterbalanced by a sympathetic response. The specific roles of catecholamines, the renin–angiotensin system, and vasopressin are unclear; however, they may be involved in the reduced diuresis and blood pressure elevations that can occur during long laparoscopic operations.

The effects of laparoscopy on the coagulation system may be considered with reference to Virchow's triad. Hypercoagulability is linked to three distinct physiologic abnormalities: (1) endothelial injury, (2) stasis, and (3) increased viscosity or abnormalities in circulating blood components. Pneumoperitoneum causes decreased venous return and leads to venous stasis. However, tissue trauma is less with laparoscopic surgery. The effects of laparoscopy on coagulation factors are less pronounced than with open surgery. Studies have shown a greater increase in D-dimer level after open surgery. Antithrombin III and protein C levels have also been shown to decrease to a lesser extent after laparoscopic procedures. The net effect of these factors may translate into a slight decrease in risk for thromboembolic disease; however, deep venous thrombosis prophylaxis is still indicated for laparoscopic procedures.

In general, surgical procedures are immunosuppressive, but laparoscopic procedures appear to be less so. Studies have shown that open surgery causes more immunosuppression as assessed by delayed-type hypersensitivity reactions and by the more pronounced reduction of lymphocytes and natural killer cells postoperatively. C-reactive protein, one of the most extensively studied markers of inflammation, is significantly lower after laparoscopic procedures compared with open procedures. However, this difference is not significant when laparoscopic procedures are compared with minilaparotomy. This suggests that the amount of abdominal wall trauma influences the degree of immunosuppression. Another point of controversy involves tumor implantation at port sites following laparoscopy for oncologic procedures. There are conflicting data regarding this point, but recent studies suggest that this is not significantly different from the incidence of tumor implantation at wound sites after open surgery. Currently, there are many oncologic procedures performed laparoscopically with excellent results.

Other miscellaneous effects include increased intracranial pressures and a quicker return to bowel function postoperatively. The increased intracranial pressure seen with laparoscopy is likely twofold. The vasoactive properties of CO_2 cause an increase in cerebral blood flow, and pneumoperitoneum is associated with increased CVP. The quick return to bowel function associated with laparoscopic procedures may be due to the reduced surgical trauma. The reduced trauma results in less sympathetic activity and thus less inhibition of gastrointestinal motility.

Part XIII
Vascular System

129
Vascular Anatomy of the Lower Extremities

The external iliac artery becomes the common femoral artery after passing under the inguinal ligament. The common femoral artery and vein are enveloped by the femoral sheath. Scarpa's triangle is defined by the adductor longus muscle medially, the Sartorious muscle laterally, and by the inguinal ligament superiorly. The femoral vessels and nerves are in the following orientation lateral to medial: femoral nerve, femoral artery, femoral vein, and lymphatics (NAVeL). The common femoral artery gives off several branches that include the superficial epigastric artery, the superficial circumflex artery, and the superficial and deep external pudendal arteries. The fossa ovalis is a medial opening in the fascia lata where the saphenous vein enters the femoral triangle. Approximately 4 cm below the inguinal ligament, the common femoral artery splits into the superficial femoral artery and the profunda (deep femoral artery). The profunda courses medially and posteriorly to the femur, giving rise to medial and lateral femoral circumflex arteries and perforating branches to supply the muscles of the flexor compartment and the femur. An important junction is created between the geniculate arteries of the knee and the descending branch of the lateral femoral circumflex artery. This creates a source of collateral blood flow when the superficial femoral artery is occluded.

The superficial femoral artery continues inferiorly through the adductor canal (Hunter's canal) after the origin of the profunda. Hunter's canal begins at the apex of the femoral triangle. It is bordered by the vastus medialis on the anterolateral aspect, the adductor longus muscle on the posterior border, and by the Sartorious muscle superiorly. Hunter's canal contains the superficial femoral artery, the saphenous nerve, and the nerve to the vastus medialis. The saphenous nerve departs the canal through the adductor hiatus to join the saphenous vein, traveling toward the medial ankle and foot.

The adductor hiatus marks the end of the superficial femoral artery and the beginning of the popliteal artery. The popliteal artery travels inferiorly between the femoral condyles and deep to the soleus muscle. As the popliteal artery courses through the popliteal fossa, it gives multiple branches of geniculate arteries (superior lateral and medial geniculate arteries, inferior lateral and medial geniculate arteries). The popliteal vein lies posterolateral to the artery in the adductor hiatus, dorsal to the artery behind the knee, and then moves medial to the artery inferiorly. The small saphenous vein joins the popliteal vein in the popliteal fossa.

Approximately 3 cm below the knee, the popliteal artery bifurcates into the anterior tibial artery and the tibioperoneal trunk. The anterior tibial artery exits the deep posterior compartment through the interosseous membrane and enters the anterior compartment medial to the fibula. Here it is joined by the deep peroneal nerve and continues to travel through the anterior compartment toward the dorsum of the foot.

The dorsalis pedis artery begins as a continuation of the anterior tibial artery beginning anterior to the ankle joint. The dorsalis pedis artery traverses the dorsum of the foot in between the tendons of the extensor hallucis longus and the extensor digitorum longus. The dorsalis pedis has named branches, including the tarsal arteries (medial and lateral), the arcuate artery, and the first dorsal metatarsal artery. The metatarsal arteries (second, third, and fourth) arise from the arcuate artery. The dorsalis pedis artery terminates as the deep plantar artery and joins the plantar arch on the sole of the foot.

The tibioperoneal trunk travels in the deep posterior compartment approximately 3 cm distally and then divides into the posterior tibial artery and the peroneal artery. The posterior tibial artery travels along with the tibial nerve in a medial course toward the medial malleolus. The peroneal artery travels in a lateral direction toward the ankle medial to the fibula. It terminates in branches to the ankle and the heel. The posterior tibial artery passes posterior to the medial malleolus and terminates into the medial and lateral plantar arteries. The plantar arch is formed from a communication between the deep plantar artery and the lateral plantar artery.

130
Noninvasive Vascular Testing

Atherosclerotic disease produces alterations in blood flow and perfusion downstream from the lesions. Noninvasive vascular testing is used to evaluate these pathologic changes. Through a series of physiologic measurements, vascular lesions can be mapped and observed over time.

Vascular pressure measurements are used to delineate the severity and location of atherosclerotic disease in the lower extremity. The most common test is the ankle–brachial index (ABI). This is an objective way to document the severity of disease. The test uses a blood pressure cuff and Doppler ultrasound to determine the systolic pressure in the ankle and in the arm. A normal ankle–brachial ratio is 0.9 to1; signs of ischemia such as claudication begin in patients with indices of 0.5 to 0.7, and indices of 0.4 and below are indicative of rest pain and severe ischemia. The index is also used for postoperative follow up and detection of graft failure. Erroneous readings can occur in patients with diabetes and renal failure because of arterial calcifications and decreased collapsibility of the vessels.

Segmental pressures provide greater detail concerning the disease involvement of the arteries of the lower extremity. The technique involves placing pneumatic cuffs at intervals along the lower extremity (upper thigh, lower thigh, calf, and ankle). Systems have been developed that automatically inflate and deflate the cuffs. Arterial pulses are detected using a Doppler ultrasound probe. Upper thigh systolic pressures are greater than brachial systolic pressures in normal people. Aortoiliac disease causes decreases in upper thigh pressures below that of the brachial causing a ratio <1. Pressure gradients of 30 mm Hg or more indicate occlusions between segments.

Limb plethysmography augments segmental pressures. This technique involves the measurement of limb volume changes during the cardiac cycle. Pulse volume recordings (PVRs) are measured through segmentally placed air plethysmograph cuffs. The contour and amplitude of the waveforms are evaluated to determine the presence of upstream lesions. Transmetatarsal waveforms are helpful for diabetic patients, because there is less influence from arterial calcification.

Digital pressure readings are helpful for patients with disease confined to the digital arteries (Raynaud's disease). Digital measurements are obtained with smaller cuffs and photoplethysmography probes. These tests help predict the success for healing ulcers and for amputations. Pressures greater than 30 mm Hg imply the potential for successful healing. In contrast, measurements below 10 mm Hg imply a poor healing potential.

Treadmill testing is used to differentiate between patients with true claudication and patients with neurogenic causes for lower extremity pain. A subset of patients has complaints consistent with claudication but has a normal examination of pulses at rest. Treadmill exercise provides a good way of eliciting and quantifying the claudication symptoms.

The measurement of tissue oxygen tension (tcO_2) is another way to evaluate the adequacy of tissue perfusion. The technique involves the transcutaneous measurement of oxygen tension through segmentally arranged polarographic electrodes on the skin. The general locations include the torso, thigh, calf, and dorsum of the foot. This test is also used to evaluate patients who have diabetes, because it is not affected by arterial wall calcification. Normal patients demonstrate measurements of 50 to 60 mm Hg in the foot. Measurements of 40 mm Hg or more imply good healing potential. In contrast, measurements less than 10 mm Hg imply potential failure to heal.

Doppler ultrasound provides information concerning the severity of disease. It is used to detect pulses that are not perceivable with palpation. Duplex ultrasound is used to identify the location of the occlusion and to evaluate previous bypasses for patency. This form of ultrasound uses B-mode two-dimensional images with the Doppler measurement of blood flow. The Doppler aspect involves measuring shifts in frequency that are directly correlated to blood flow. A visual color scale is applied that signifies the velocity of the blood flow. Hemodynamically significant lesions can be demonstrated by high peak velocities (peak systolic velocity >300 cm/sec), elevated velocity (lesion velocity/upstream velocity >3.5) ratios, or through low velocities (<40 cm/sec). The results of Doppler ultrasound may indicate the need for further diagnostic testing such as angiography.

131
Acute Limb Ischemia

Acute limb ischemia causes high morbidity and mortality rates. Even with many recent technical advances, the estimated mortality rate approaches 25%, with an amputation rate of 20%. Acute limb ischemia is caused by thrombosis, embolism, or trauma. The condition can manifest acutely or develop gradually. Slow progression to arterial occlusion has a more favorable prognosis due to the development of collateral blood flow. The most common presenting complaints are rest pain, claudication, paresthesias, and cyanosis. The signs and symptoms of limb ischemia have been classically described as the six Ps: pain, pallor, poikilothermia, pulselessness, paresthesias, and paralysis. The end result of untreated disease is irreversible tissue damage and necrosis. Pathologic changes can be histologically detected after only 4 hours of ischemia. Irreversible tissue damage develops after 6 hours.

The degree of leg ischemia can be grouped into one of three major categories (Table 131.1). The pathophysiology of ischemic tissue damage plays out over three progressive stages. The first stage is hallmarked by continued growth of the arterial thrombus until all collateral vessels are occluded. The second stage includes tissue edema and fluid accumulation leading to elevated compartmental pressures. The elevated pressures cause a compression of the local vessels and further impairment of blood flow. The third stage involves narrowing and obstruction of the microvascular system due to edema. Occlusion at this level causes irreversible tissue ischemia. Additional injury takes place once the tissue is reperfused. Free radicals such as superoxide and hydroxyl radicals are responsible for the damage known as *reperfusion injury*. Reperfusion is also associated with the release of toxic metabolites (lactic acid, potassium, thromboxane, and myoglobin) into the systemic circulation. These substances can cause cardiac arrhythmia, renal failure, and metabolic acidosis.

Atherosclerotic plaques are composed of a soft central core of necrotic cellular elements (red blood cells, hemosiderin, and lipid-laden macrophages) and lipid material. The central core is covered by a fibrous cap composed of collagen, glycosaminoglycans, smooth muscle cells, and fibroblasts. Vascular smooth muscle cells, fibroblasts, collagen, and scattered calcifications make up the rest of the plaque. External mechanical forces act on the fibrous cap (the weakest portion of the plaque), causing rupture of the plaque. Inflammatory cells present at the borders of the necrotic core and the fibrous cap release degradative enzymes and cytokines that cause the plaque to destabilize. The central core is the most thrombogenic portion of the plaque. Vessel occlusion due to progressive growth of the plaque occurs once the central core is exposed. The most common sites for plaque formation are the distal aorta, the iliac arteries, the popliteal bifurcation, and the femoral artery at the adductor canal.

Previous bypass grafts can ultimately succumb to thrombosis. Autologous vein grafts develop areas of thrombosis at the anastomosis due to intimal hyperplasia or at areas where fibrotic valves are present. Prosthetic grafts tend to develop thrombus or become kinked as they cross a joint, causing alteration in blood flow.

Sudden-onset ischemia is most often due to an arterial embolic event. Embolic material becomes lodged at distal arterial bifurcations as the caliber of the vessels becomes smaller. An embolic event should be suspected when a patient with a previous history of cardiac arrhythmias has a sudden onset of limb ischemia.

In addition to thrombosis, emboli, and trauma, there are less common causes for acute limb ischemia. Shock and sepsis can cause acute impairment of lower extremity blood flow due to profound hypoperfusion. Vasoactive drugs such as cocaine can cause severe vasoconstriction and vessel spasm to the point of producing lower limb ischemia. Vascular inflammatory conditions such as Takayasu's arteritis are rare causes of ischemia. Hypercoagulable states can cause arterial thrombus formation and ischemia.

TABLE 131.1. The three major categories of leg ischemia.

Category	Description	Collaterals	Reversible	Treatment
I	Viable tissue	Abundant	Yes	Revascularization
II	Threatened viability		Yes	Revascularization
III	Permanent neuromuscular damage		No	Amputation

Evaluation

History and physical examination are paramount to obtaining the diagnosis. During the history taking, information concerning cardiac arrhythmias (atrial fibrillation) and other comorbidities must be obtained (hypertension, diabetes, coronary artery disease, cerebral vascular accidents, and tobacco use). Details concerning the onset of symptoms and whether symptoms occur unilaterally or bilaterally are important. The physical examination includes a thorough vascular examination with emphasis on the following:

- Auscultation for detection of bruits (e.g., carotid artery, abdominal aorta)
- Palpation and comparison of extremity pulses
- Complete skin inspection for evidence of infection or necrosis

Doppler ultrasound provides helpful information concerning the level of disease and severity. Doppler ultrasound is used to detect pulses that are not identified by palpation. Ankle–brachial indices (ABIs) provide an objective way to determine the severity of disease. This test uses a blood pressure cuff and Doppler ultrasound to determine the systolic pressure in the ankle and in the arm. A normal ankle–brachial ratio is 0.9 to 1. Signs of ischemia such as claudication begin to appear in patients with indices of 0.6. Indices of 0.4 and below are indicative of rest pain and severe ischemia. Doppler ultrasound is used to obtain segmental pressure measurement. Readings are taken with a blood pressure cuff below the knee, above the knee, and on the thigh. Proximal occlusions are detected when pressure decreases by 30 mm Hg between two adjacent levels. Duplex ultrasound is used to identify the location of the occlusion and to evaluate previous bypasses for patency.

Contrast angiography is still the most accurate method for identifying occlusive lesions. Preoperative arteriograms are obtained in most cases to plan for possible intervention. The arteriogram is generally done by accessing the contralateral vessel, which is distal to the obstruction. This enables the safe administration of thrombolytic therapy without causing bleeding at the catheter insertion site. In the case of bilateral iliac occlusions, the brachial artery may be used as an access point. Diagnostic images are used for the suprarenal abdominal aorta, the iliac vessels, and infrainguinal vessels down to the level of the feet. Patients with renal failure or contrast allergy may be imaged using carbon dioxide injections. Signs indicative of an embolic etiology include thrombus localized to an arterial bifurcation, multiple arterial beds showing filling defects, and the normal appearance of adjacent and contralateral vascular structures.

Treatment

Localized embolic lesions are amenable to embolectomy. Thrombotic lesions may be treated with thrombectomy, bypass grafting, or bypass revision if a bypass is present. In the past, delayed operative intervention was recommended along with interim high-dose heparin therapy when possible to avoid early graft failure and perioperative mortality. Current limb salvage procedures have a 70% to 80% success rate and a perioperative mortality rate of 15%. In the past, failed bypass grafts were treated with graft thrombectomy and patch angioplasty. The current trend is graft replacement rather than revision.

Medical therapy for acute limb ischemia is predominantly the intra-arterial use of thrombolytic agents (streptokinase, urokinase, recombinant tissue plasminogen activator, and reteplase). Current techniques use specialized catheters with several side ports to administer thrombolytic agents over the length of the thrombus. The catheters are positioned in the thrombus and allow the introduction of infusion guidewires, which increases the effective length of thrombolytic administration. Standard doses include Urokinase 4,000 IU/min for 4 hours with reduction of the dose to 2,000 IU/min until clot resolution. Operative repair to correct the causative lesion may be needed after successful thrombolysis. In some instances, percutaneous techniques such as balloon angioplasty and stenting may be accomplished. Systemic anticoagulation is required once thrombolytic therapy is ended. Patients with severe ischemia can benefit from thrombolytic therapy by avoiding the cardiopulmonary complications associated with surgery and the increased perioperative mortality.

132
Chronic Lower Extremity Ischemia

Chronic lower limb ischemia involves the gradual decrease in tissue oxygenation and perfusion due to vascular disease. The most frequently observed causes include atherosclerosis, thromboangiitis obliterans, vasculitis, trauma, popliteal artery entrapment, and popliteal cystic adventitial disease. Atherosclerosis is the most common underlying cause of chronic lower limb ischemia. Comorbidities such as diabetes, hypertension, hypercholesterolemia, and tobacco use play significant roles in the progression of atherosclerosis. Risk factors have an additive effect. Patients with diabetes have an increased risk of tissue loss caused by peripheral neuropathy, small vessel occlusions, and impaired wound healing. Amputations are required for up to 34% of diabetic patients compared with only 8% for nondiabetic persons. Buerger's disease (thromboangiitis obliterans) causes chronic inflammation of neurovascular bundles in the hands and feet, which ultimately cause arterial and venous thrombosis. The distal nature of this disease makes it resistant to revascularization attempts. Smoking plays an important role in the propagation of the disease; therefore, smoking cessation helps to improve the condition. Arterial entrapment and cystic adventitial disease are conditions that primarily affect younger persons. Traumatic injuries to arterial structures may be overlooked initially but give rise to ischemic disease over time.

Collateralization is a common occurrence with chronic ischemic disease. Collateral vessels are not newly formed vessels but are existing vessels that increase in size as an occlusion develops. These vessels originate from the branches of large- and medium-sized arteries. Collateral beds are divided into three functional units: stem arteries, mid-zone arteries, and re-entry arteries. When collateral development takes place at the same rate as the progression of stenosis, symptomatology becomes less apparent. Sudden occlusions prevent the adequate development of collateral flow to compensate. Collateral blood flow can become impaired by extension of atherosclerosis to the communicating portions of the collateral bed (i.e., stem arteries and re-entry vessels).

There are two basic classifications of lower limb ischemia that are based on severity of disease. Functional ischemia encompasses ischemic disease that is not apparent at rest but becomes noticeable with the onset of physical activity. This level of disease allows enough blood flow to maintain the resting state but is unable to increase blood supply when the demand rises. Functional disease may limit physical activity but imposes little threat of limb loss. The amputation rate for patients with functional disease is 5% to 7%. The most classic example is claudication. Claudication develops when arterial supply is less than the metabolic demand of active muscle, causing a cramping sensation in the muscle mass. The most common area is the calf muscle, which becomes symptomatic with femoral artery disease. Aortoiliac disease can cause claudication of the buttocks and thigh muscles. Common characteristics of claudication include pain experienced in an active muscle group, reproducibility of pain (walking 100 feet), and cessation of pain with rest.

Modification of risk factors (smoking cessation, diabetes and hypertension control, proper diet) aids in stabilizing the disease and provides improvement in more than 50% of patients. Exercises such as walking programs require the patient to walk until the claudication symptoms are elicited. The patient must record the distance traveled and at what point symptoms begin. The goal is to walk further each day to build tolerance to hypoxia in the muscles. Antiplatelet therapies such as pentoxifylline and clopidogrel have been used with some success. Objective findings for functional disease are identified by stress testing (treadmill exercise). Surgical intervention is reserved for lifestyle-altering disease. From 20% to 30% of patients are eligible for operative intervention for progression of disease. Vascular reconstructions are not taken lightly for this patient group. A failed arterial bypass puts the patient's limb at risk for ischemia and loss. Therefore, a risk/benefit ratio must be established and the patient appropriately counseled.

Critical limb ischemia is characterized by tissue loss (ulcerations, gangrene) or ischemic rest pain. Ischemic rest pain is restricted to the foot (dorsal surface involving the metatarsal heads and toes) and is relieved by placing the foot in a dependent position. Patients often complain of being awakened from sleep by the pain and having to dangle the foot over the bed to find relief. Rest pain is often associated with ischemic changes in the skin, including hair loss, muscle wasting, thin skin, and thickened nails. Rest pain is the consequence of blood flow that is inadequate to meet the metabolic needs at the resting state. The condition usually progresses to tissue loss when left untreated. Approximately 20% of these patients require amputation. Vascular reconstruction is indicated for patients with a reasonable operative risk with localized disease amenable to endarterectomy or bypass procedure.

The evaluation of lower extremity ischemia begins with a battery of noninvasive tests, which include Doppler ultrasound, ankle–brachial indices (ABIs), and segmental plethysmography. Erroneously high ABI readings occur in patients with diabetes or renal failure because of vessels stiffened by calcific medial sclerosis. Treadmill exercise is a good way to illicit ischemic symptoms in asymptomatic patients who have a normal exam at rest. Repeated ABIs and Doppler ultrasound may reveal ischemic signs in these patients after exercise.

Angiography is reserved for patients who are to undergo an intervention. The arteriogram is generally performed by accessing the contralateral vessel that is distal to the location of the obstruction. Diagnostic radiologic studies include images of the suprarenal abdominal aorta, the iliac vessels, and infrainguinal vessels down to the level of the feet. Patients with renal failure or contrast allergy can be imaged using carbon dioxide injections. The pressure gradient across a lesion can be measured by obtaining pull-back pressures. This involves measuring proximal and distal to the level of the obstruction. Differences greater than 15 mm Hg between arterial segments indicate a hemodynamically important lesion. Pressure gradients may not be present in a lesion during the resting state but can be elicited with the administration of a vasodilator. Noninvasive tests (magnetic resonance angiography, duplex ultrasound) can be used in place of angiography when angiography is contraindicated.

Proper patient selection is paramount to the success of any vascular intervention. Surgical therapies are reserved for patients with lifestyle-altering claudication and patients with critical limb ischemia (rest pain or tissue loss). Many patients with aortoiliac occlusive disease respond to conservative management such as risk factor modification. Percutaneous transluminal angioplasty (PTA) is successful for aortoiliac occlusions. The outpatient procedure uses local anesthetic and has a low morbidity rate. Percutaneous transluminal angioplasty is indicated for aortoiliac stenosis or short segment occlusions. Stenting can be undertaken when PTA is inadequate. Success rates of PTA are as much as 80% for 5 years. External iliac procedures are less successful, with patency rates of 50% to 60% for 5 years. Surgical options include aortoiliac thromboendarterectomy, aortobifemoral bypass, axillofemoral bypass, iliofemoral bypass, and femorofemoral bypass.

Infrainguinal occlusive disease is the most common form of chronic lower extremity ischemic disease. Patients present with claudication due to superficial femoral disease or with rest pain due to multisegmental disease. Arteriograms to visualize the anatomy are obtained for patients who undergo intervention. Some isolated lesions are amenable to PTA; however, most patients have more complex disease. Percutaneous transluminal angioplasty is limited by small vessel size, diffuse disease, and impaired runoff. Stents are useful for femoral and popliteal lesions. Advancements in stent technology have produced more flexible stents as well as drug-eluting stents. Adequate inflow proximal to the level of disease is paramount to graft survival. Concomitant aortoiliac disease must be treated before therapeutic treatments to distal lesions are made. Autologous vein grafts are the conduit of choice for creating arterial bypasses below the knee. The ipsilateral greater saphenous vein is the conduit vessel of choice. Above the knee arterial bypasses use prosthetic materials (i.e., Dacron®, polytetrafluoroethylene) with patency rates comparable to using autologous vein.

Creating an infrainguinal arterial bypass involves using the greater saphenous vein oriented in a reverse direction. The direction of the vein is reversed to prevent blood flow obstruction by the valves in the lumen of the vein. Patency rates for this procedure are 75% to 85% over 5 years. Limb salvage can be achieved in 90% of cases.

In situ saphenous vein bypasses use the greater saphenous vein as a conduit, leaving it in its natural position as opposed to removing it and reversing its direction. The technique relies on the disruption of the internal valves using a valvulotome. Arteriovenous fistulas are avoided by ligation of greater saphenous side branches. The advantages of this technique over traditional methods include preservation of the endothelium and vasa vasorum and improved size match at the venous to arterial anastomoses. Patency rates are reported to be 80% at 5 years, and limb salvage rates range between 84% and 90%.

Technical considerations important to graft survival include ensuring adequate blood inflow and outflow and avoiding small vessel anastomoses when possible. Some surgeons recommend the construction of multiple sequential distal anastomoses to improve runoff instead of a small single anastomosis.

133
Lower Extremity Venous Insufficiency

The veins of the lower extremity are separated into three types: superficial, deep, and perforating. The deep veins of the lower extremity accompany the major arteries and include the superficial femoral vein, common femoral vein, and external iliac vein. The main superficial veins are the greater and lesser saphenous running on the medial and lateral lower extremity, respectively. Perforator veins connect the superficial and deep systems, promoting flow of blood from the superficial vessels to the deep veins, except in the foot, where the opposite is true. The major structural difference when comparing veins and arteries is the presence of valves promoting forward flow of blood through the veins. The number of valves decreases as veins become more proximal. Blood is returned to the heart by pressure changes from diaphragmatic excursion and extremity muscle contraction, with healthy valves preventing backward flow. Incompetence of venous valves and reflux at the saphenofemoral junction are the major contributors to venous insufficiency leading to superficial varicosities in the lower extremity and ulcer formation at the medial malleolus.

Risk factors for the development of venous insufficiency and the related complications include family history, female gender, advanced age, prolonged standing, and a history of venous thrombosis of the lower extremity veins or inferior vena cava. Alterations in collagen and elastin are thought to contribute on a molecular level. Steroid hormones play a major role in venous disease in females, as both progesterone and estrogen cause venous smooth muscle dilatation. Incompetence of the valves causes reflux of blood into the superficial veins and a resultant increase in pressure. The increased pressure over time leads to tortuosity, dilatation, and subsequent varicosities.

Patients with venous insufficiency complain of pain and swelling of the lower extremity and can experience ulceration in prolonged, untreated disease with perforator incompetence. The symptoms are usually worse at night and after prolonged standing and are relieved with compression and/or elevation and rest. Making the diagnosis begins with a thorough physical examination, which includes direct visualization of the superficial varicosities, edema, ulcerations, and other characteristic pigmentation related to venous insufficiency. Historical physical examination techniques to evaluate the competence of the perforators and the saphenofemoral junction have been replaced or at least supplemented with ultrasonography. Duplex ultrasonography is a noninvasive, accurate way to identify venous thromboembolisms and venous insufficiency. It is able to discriminate between perforator incompetence and saphenofemoral reflux. Plethysmography is used in conjunction with ultrasound and quantifies limb volume increases caused by perforator and valvular incompetence, offering a measure of the severity of disease without providing etiologic information.

Therapeutic interventions for venous insufficiency, varicosities, and ulceration vary with the severity of the disease as well as the degree of patient concern. Indications for intervention include bleeding, thrombophlebitis, ulceration, discomfort, swelling, and concerns about cosmesis. Discomfort and swelling after prolonged standing and sitting are treated with elevation and compression stockings. Superficial varicosities are treated with sclerotherapy or operative excision based on size. Sclerotherapy is indicated for varices less than 3 mm and is performed in the outpatient setting. A sclerosing agent is injected and pressure is applied, which leads to scarring and obliteration of the offending vessel. If saphenofemoral reflux is identified and/or varices larger than 3 mm are present, operative intervention is indicated. Saphenofemoral reflux is treated with stripping of the greater saphenous vein from the saphenofemoral junction to the knee, and below the knee if varices are present in the lower leg. Laser and radiofrequency ablation are a minimally invasive means of greater saphenous stripping, but they are not indicated when the vein is 12 mm or larger. With these techniques, the vein is accessed by endovascular means and ablated from within. Stab avulsions are used to remove varices too large for sclerosant therapy in conjunction with saphenous stripping.

Ulcerations caused by chronic venous insufficiency occur at the medial malleolus and are initially treated with local wound care and compression dressings changed weekly. Healing usually occurs after several months. Once resolved, compression hose are required for life to prevent a recurrence. Chronic nonhealing ulcers and relapses may require an operation to identify and ligate the incompetent perforators. Previously, this was a difficult surgery, requiring large incisions and extensive dissection to ensure adequate removal of the incompetent perforators. Ultrasound has improved the accuracy of identifying the incompetent perforators, allowing a directed approach to ligation. Additionally, endoscopic techniques have led to subfascial endoscopic perforator surgery (SEPS), which allows the surgeon to insufflate and explore subfascially with the aid of an endoscope, identifying and ligating the perforators through much smaller incisions. This technique is very useful in operations above the knee but is much more difficult to apply below the knee in the tighter confines of the lower leg. A combination approach is probably best using open techniques to ligate the perforators in the lower leg not accessible with the endoscope. Venous reconstruction and valvuloplasty are a rarely used option that can be considered for severe cases. Valvuloplasty is best used for large, floppy incompetent valves from primary venous insufficiency, which differ from the fibrotic valves that develop after venous thrombosis and are not amenable to this approach. Venous valve transplantation from the deep femoral, saphenous, or axillary veins has also been described.

The control of venous incompetence with greater saphenous stripping or ablation for superficial varicosities and perforator ligation for chronic ulcerations are initially successful. However, long-term results suffer because of neovascularization, recanalization, and patient noncompliance. The most difficult aspect of treating venous insufficiency is its chronic nature, requiring lifetime compression stockings, which are often uncomfortable for the patient and discarded after successful interventions, leading to recurrent disease.

134
Arterial Aneurysms

Arterial aneurysms are abnormal enlargements of arterial segments at least 1.5 times larger than the normal diameter. The most common arteries affected are the aorta and the iliac, femoral, and popliteal arteries. Complications of aneurysmal disease include rupture (aortic aneurysms) and thromboembolic events (popliteal aneurysms). Aneurysms occur in two basic forms, fusiform and saccular. Fusiform aneurysms display uniform enlargement of the arterial wall. In contrast, saccular aneurysms involve only a portion of the arterial wall. Arterial aneurysms are more prevalent in the elderly population; however, young patients with connective tissue defects (Marfan's and Ehlers-Danlos syndromes) can be affected as well. The most common etiology is atherosclerotic disease. Other causes include infection (mycotic aneurysm), aortic dissection, arteriovenous fistulas, and poststenotic dilatation.

The development of an arterial aneurysm is a multifactorial process. On histologic examination, the aneurysm walls display attenuation of the media and adventitia. Genetic defects such as type III collagen deficiencies, fibrillin defects (Marfan's syndrome), and procollagen type III defects (Ehlers-Danlos type IV) occur in some individuals. Increased activity of proteolytic enzymes in the arterial wall (elastase and matrix metalloproteinases) is a part of the pathogenesis. The risk factors for atherosclerosis and for arterial aneurysms are identical, as are some elements of their pathologic features. Therefore, atherosclerosis commonly coexists with aneurysmal disease. In atherosclerosis, remodeling of the media layer occurs beneath the plaque. This process is similar to the process in aneurysm formation.

Aortic Aneurysm

Aortic aneurysms are most often located within the abdomen. They are characterized by their location in relation to the renal arteries. Most abdominal aortic aneurysms are located below the origin of the renal arteries, with a short segment of normal artery in between. Forty percent of infrarenal aneurysms have synchronous aneurysms in other segments of the aorta. In 40% of cases, the aneurysm extends to the iliac arteries. In juxtarenal aneurysms, the aortic dilatation occurs at the level of the renal arteries. Suprarenal aneurysms occur above the renal arteries. The male to female ratio is 8:1. The average age of patients with this condition is 75 years. Important risk factors include smoking, hypertension, family history, and atherosclerotic disease. When left untreated, abdominal aortic aneurysms continue to enlarge and rupture. Rupture is a serious and often fatal complication, with an overall mortality rate between 78% and 94%. The diameter of the aneurysm is directly proportional to the risk of rupture (4 to 5 cm, 1% to 3%/year; 5 to 7 cm, 11%/year; and >7 cm, 20%/year). Hypertension, chronic obstructive pulmonary disease (COPD), and female gender are factors that are associated with an increased risk of rupture. Aneurysms have been shown to enlarge at an average rate of 0.4 cm per year.

Thoracic aortic aneurysms are less prevalent than their abdominal counterparts. Multisegmental disease occurs in up to 25% of cases. In addition, 44% of these cases also have an infrarenal component. Thoracic aneurysms may be the result of arterial wall degeneration (Marfan's syndrome) or dissection. Aneurysms occur in the ascending aorta, the aortic arch, and the descending aorta. Aortic dissections and aneurysms located in the ascending aorta or aortic arch have a poor prognosis. Expansion rates vary according to location and etiology. Aneurysms involving the arch expand at a rate of 0.56 cm per year. Aneurysms of the descending aorta expand at a rate of 0.42 cm per year. Aortic dissections expand more rapidly; 95% eventually rupture.

Thoracoabdominal aneurysms are caused by atherosclerosis, dissection, and degenerative disease. Four subtypes of this aneurysm have been described. Type I involves aneurysmal disease of the thoracic and abdominal aorta above the level of the renal arteries. Type II disease consists of aneurysms extending through the descending aorta and the abdominal aorta below the renal vessels. Type III disease incorporates a small portion of the descending aorta and the abdominal aorta below the renal vessels. Type IV disease involves the majority of the abdominal aorta.

Rupture of an aortic aneurysm is a potentially fatal event. Ruptures occur in the retroperitoneum or in the peritoneal cavity. Intraperitoneal ruptures are caused by disruption of the anterior portion of the aneurysm wall. This condition is marked by hypovolemic shock and high mortality rate. Ruptures into the retroperitoneum are the result of posterior disruptions of the aneurysm. Clinical manifestations include back pain, abdominal pain, syncope, and diaphoresis. When these symptoms are accompanied by chest pain, the patient may be erroneously diagnosed with a myocardial infarction.

Many aneurysms are asymptomatic, with most (80%) diagnosed incidentally on routine imaging. However, some clinical manifestations include vague abdominal or back pain. Severe pain radiating to the back in conjunction with a tender pulsatile mass are ominous signs of impending rupture. The diagnosis of abdominal aortic aneurysms can be inhibited by body habitus; however, thin patients with large aneurysms may have an expanding pulsatile mass on physical examination. Radiographic imaging is the most reliable way to identify an aneurysm. Plain films of the abdomen may reveal an egg shell calcification of the aorta. The most useful test is abdominal ultrasound. This modality is accurate, reproducible, and correlates well with measurements taken with computed tomography. The low cost and noninvasive nature of the test make it useful for the follow up of aneurysmal disease. Limitations are encountered with visualization of tributaries of the aorta, including the renal and iliac arteries. Computed tomography provides more detail of these areas and therefore is needed for preoperative planning. Computed tomography scans delineate the aortic anatomy and vessel anomalies (renal artery stenosis and iliac aneurysms). Magnetic resonance angiography is useful for the evaluation as well. Computed tomography is beginning to overtake arteriography as the imaging modality of choice. Arteriography is still instrumental in delineating aortic dissections and intimal tears before surgery.

Preoperative cardiac testing (electrocardiogram, dobutamine echocardiogram, cardiac myoview, or multiple gated acquisition scan) is paramount for planning surgical intervention. Fifty percent of patients with aortic aneurysms have coronary artery disease also. The risk of perioperative fatality from myocardial infarction is about 5%. Important coronary artery disease should be treated (revascularization or catheterization) before a planned aneurysm intervention. Other conditions such as COPD should be evaluated and medically treated also.

An aneurysm larger than 6 cm should be treated surgically. Patients with an aneurysm measuring 4 to 5 cm are considered for surgical repair if the growth rate exceeds 0.5 cm in 6 months. Prompt surgical repair is warranted for aneurysms that are rapidly expanding, are tender, and cause back pain. Embolization originating from the aneurysm is another indication for repair. Open surgical repair can be accomplished transperitoneally (midline incision) or retroperitoneally (oblique flank incision). The 5-year survival rate for aneurysm repair is about 67%.

Endovascular repairs are a suitable approach for high-risk patients with a limited life expectancy. This technique involves cannulization of the femoral artery to introduce the endovascular prosthetic graft. From 2 to 3 cm of nonaneurysmal artery is required below the renal arteries to anchor the graft. Only patients without tortuous aortas are eligible for graft placement. The endovascular graft affixes to the infrarenal neck and the iliac arteries via self-expanding or balloon-expandable stents. The advantages include avoiding an abdominal incision and the morbidity of an open repair. Complications common to endovascular repairs include endoleak (incomplete exclusion of the aneurysm), migration of the graft, limb occlusion, and late rupture.

The techniques of surgical repair for thoracic and thoracoabdominal aneurysms vary depending on location and etiology. Degenerative aneurysms require replacement of the aortic root and valves along with the conduit. The coronary arteries require re-implantation or bypass. A median sternotomy is required for the repair of the ascending aorta. Aneurysms of the descending aorta are approached through a posterolateral thoracotomy. A thoracoabdominal incision is required to repair a thoracoabdominal aneurysm.

Preoperative evaluation and perioperative treatment of comorbidities (coronary artery disease and COPD) have decreased the mortality rate of open aneurysm repair to 5% to 10%. The most common complications of open repair are myocardial infarction, renal failure, and pneumonia. Bleeding is a potential complication that arises from technical complications of the anastomosis, coagulopathy, or venous injuries. Rare complications include lower limb ischemia, paraplegia, sexual dysfunction, and colonic ischemia. Colonic ischemia occurs in approximately 1% of cases. This condition is hallmarked by abdominal pain, bloody diarrhea, distended abdomen, and leukocytosis. An important finding on sigmoidoscopy is mucosal sloughing. Colonic ischemia carries a mortality rate ranging from 50% to 90%, depending on whether full thickness necrosis and gangrene occur. Surgical management involves colon resection with the creation of a colostomy. Lower limb ischemia can be caused by emboli showering distally into the limb or from thrombosis of the graft itself. Pseudoaneurysm, graft thrombosis, and graft infection are late-occurring complications.

Femoral and Popliteal Aneurysms

Popliteal aneurysms comprise 70% of all peripheral aneurysms. Femoral arteries are the second most common peripheral aneurysm. Most of these lesions occur in men, with 50% being bilateral. Aortic aneurysms occur in conjunction with femoral (75%) and popliteal (33%) aneurysms. Most of these types of aneurysms are asymptomatic. Distal embolization is a frequent complication, producing distal ischemia, with 25% requiring amputation. Rupture is a rare complication, occurring in less than 15% of cases.

The diagnosis is made with a physical examination or with duplex ultrasound. Angiography is used to delineate the extent of the disease as well as to evaluate the patency of runoff vessels. Indications for treatment include embolus, thrombosis, limb ischemia, and transverse diameters greater than 2 cm (popliteal aneurysms) and 2.5 cm (femoral aneurysms). Prosthetic grafts are used to repair femoral aneurysms, and the greater saphenous vein is the preferred conduit for popliteal aneurysms. With thrombosis, thrombectomy or thrombolytic therapy may be needed to establish distal flow. Patency and limb salvage rates have been reported between 59% and 85 % and 70% and 80%, respectively.

135
Peripheral Artery Aneurysms

Aneurysms of the lower extremity occur most often in the popliteal arteries, followed by the iliac and femoral arteries. The majority of peripheral aneurysms are degenerative, although traumatic, poststenotic, dissecting, mycotic, and anastomotic aneurysms occur as well. Degenerative peripheral aneurysms are associated with aneurysms elsewhere at least 50% of the time, including abdominal aortic aneurysms (AAAs) or aneurysms of other peripheral arteries. Unlike AAAs, for which rupture is the primary concern, aneurysms of the lower extremity are more likely to cause occlusive symptoms related to thrombosis or distal embolization. Ten percent of femoral aneurysms and 25% of popliteal aneurysms are associated with emboli, and about 40% of popliteal aneurysms are associated with thrombosis. Outcomes are significantly worse for patients with symptoms of ischemia. Amputations are needed by one-fourth of patients with symptomatic popliteal aneurysms.

Fifty percent of patients with popliteal aneurysms have bilateral disease, and one-fourth have an associated AAA. Untreated popliteal aneurysms can cause significant ischemia in the lower leg due to thrombosis and distal embolization. Continued expansion rarely leads to rupture but often causes compressive symptoms behind the knee. The diagnosis of popliteal aneurysms may begin with palpation of a pulsatile (or nonpulsatile) mass behind the knee on physical examination; however, imaging studies are required for confirmation and adequate assessment. Duplex ultrasonography is the most appropriate initial study because of its convenience and noninvasive nature, allowing assessment of size, flow, and possible thrombus. Additionally, computed tomography are noninvasive methods to assess the size and character of these lesions. If treatment is required, angiography is vital to assess outflow to the distal leg and to plan the appropriate intervention, especially in the case of chronic embolization.

Operative repair is based on ligation of the aneurysm to prevent continued distal embolization and bypass using autogenous vein (usually reversed saphenous). The approach can be medial or posterior, and the conduit is anastomosed proximally to the distal superficial femoral artery or proximal popliteal artery where the caliber of the vessel appears normal. The distal target is typically the distal popliteal artery, but the tibioperoneal trunk or other distal vessels can be used depending on the available outflow. Long-term patency is excellent for asymptomatic patients; however, limb salvage is less than 75% when patients present with ischemic symptoms.

Endovascular repair with covered stents is an option for poor operative candidates; however, long-term results are not available. Open repair remains the procedure of choice for reasonable operative candidates.

Iliac artery aneurysms are usually associated with AAA and rarely occur in isolation. Most iliac aneurysms are located in the common iliac arteries, with only 10% occurring in the internal iliac arteries. The external iliac arteries are rarely aneurysmal. Iliac aneurysms are not usually identified on physical examination, although an internal iliac aneurysm may be palpated as a pulsatile mass on rectal examination. Aneurysms greater than 3 cm require repair, and the operative approach depends on the condition of the contralateral iliac artery. If both iliac arteries are affected, the usual approach is aortic replacement with aortobiiliac or aortobifemoral anastomosis. Unilateral aneurysms can be approached via a peritoneal or retroperitoneal approach. The conduit of choice for both techniques is synthetic, either expanded polytetrafluoroethylene (ePTFE) or Dacron®.

Degenerative aneurysms of the femoral artery are exceedingly rare; however, aneurysmal disease of the femoral arteries is increasing due to iatrogenic complications. The femoral artery is the most common vessel accessed for angiographic procedures, and this causes an increasing number of injuries. The femoral artery is also a common location for vascular anastomoses, leaving the potential for pseudoaneurysm formation as well. Diagnosing femoral artery aneurysms may begin with patient complaints of groin pain or a mass in the groin or even acute hemorrhage after a surgical or endovascular procedure. Ultrasonography is a useful diagnostic tool. Compression is often therapeutic for pseudoaneurysms after percutaneous interventions. Operative repair is required for symptomatic, degenerative aneurysms greater than 2.5 cm and pseudoaneurysms related to an anastomosis. Postintervention pseudoaneurysms require repair if compression fails to control expansion and/or bleeding.

Arteries of the upper extremity are less likely to develop aneurysms than arteries of the lower extremity. Aneurysms of the lower extremities are also associated with aneurysms elsewhere, most often the subclavian artery. Distal ischemia is the most common symptom; however, cerebral ischemia is the most dire and occurs due to embolization through the vertebral or carotid arteries. Ligation of the subclavian artery proximally and bypass with autologous vein is the treatment of choice. Associated thoracic outlet syndrome should be considered with aneurysms of the distal subclavian artery. If present, resection of the clavicle or rib should be considered along with bypass. Proximal subclavian lesions generally require median sternotomy for adequate access. Endovascular exclusion with covered stents provides a less invasive treatment.

The most important characteristic to remember with all degenerative peripheral aneurysms is their frequent association with aneurysms elsewhere. Screening ultrasonography or other screening methods should be considered for all patients with peripheral arterial aneurysms. Open repair with ligation or resection and bypass is the primary treatment modality; however, endovascular techniques are increasingly used and may become the primary treatment when long-term follow-up data are available.

136
Visceral Aneurysms

An aneurysm is defined as a dilation of an artery to more than 1.5 times its normal diameter. Aneurysms occur in any artery but are most common in the abdominal aorta, thoracic aorta, cerebral vessels, iliac, popliteal, and femoral arteries. Visceral aneurysms are much less common; however, when present, they warrant careful evaluation and treatment. The risk of all aneurysms is rupture, which occurs when the pressure in the vessel exceeds the wall tension. Aneurysms are classified based on shape, wall constituents, and etiology. The shape of aneurysms is fusiform (the vessel is diffusely dilated) or saccular (only one wall of the vessel is dilated). The wall constituents determine if it is a true aneurysm or a pseudoaneurysm. A true aneurysm has a wall composed of all layers of the arterial wall while pseudoaneurysms have an adjacent structure forming a portion of the wall. The etiology of an aneurysm is dissection (due to internal damage and hypertension), mycosis (infection), or trauma.

Hepatic artery aneurysms account for approximately 20% of splanchnic arterial aneurysms. They tend to be asymptomatic but can rupture and cause life-threatening hemorrhage. Most hepatic artery aneurysms are due to atherosclerosis; however, some are due to trauma, iatrogenic injury, or, very rarely, mycosis. Traumatic and iatrogenic etiologies tend to cause pseudoaneurysms. Although symptoms are rare, they can include vague right upper quadrant or epigastric pain. If the aneurysm erodes into the portal vein, symptoms of portal hypertension develop. If the erosion is into the biliary tree, Quincke's triad of jaundice, biliary colic, and hemobilia can occur.

Because most hepatic artery aneurysms are asymptomatic, they tend to be incidental findings on computed tomography (CT) scan. If, however, an aneurysm is suspected, many imaging modalities are used. Plain abdominal radiograph or an upper gastrointestinal series can demonstrate a rimmed calcification in the right upper quadrant or a smooth filling defect in the duodenum.

Ultrasound, CT scan with contrast, or magnetic resonance imaging (MRI) are effective in providing a diagnosis. The gold standard for evaluation is selective angiography, because it defines the location and identifies collateral pathways.

All extrahepatic aneurysms greater than 2 cm and pseudoaneurysms greater than 1 cm should be treated. The location of the hepatic artery aneurysm determines the treatment options to a large extent. Extrahepatic lesions require surgical treatment. Hepatic artery aneurysms of the common hepatic artery are ligated and excised, because the liver still receives collateral flow from the pancreaticoduodenal and gastroduodenal arteries. Before ligation, the segment to be excised should be temporarily clamped and the liver observed for color changes. Intraoperative Doppler is also useful to confirm adequate arterial blood flow. If inadequate collateral flow is observed or if the patient is low risk, vascular reconstruction with reversed saphenous vein grafts should be performed. Extrahepatic aneurysms of the proper hepatic artery require vascular reconstruction to prevent hepatic ischemia. Intrahepatic arterial aneurysms are usually treated with transcatheter, selective embolization, which avoids morbid hepatic lobectomies and, because of its precision, limits hepatic devascularization. Patients require follow-up imaging after embolization, because aneurysm recurrence and recanalization are possible.

Splenic artery aneurysms are often diagnosed because of the improved quality and increased use of vascular imaging studies. Overall, splenic artery aneurysms account for about 60% of visceral aneurysms. The patients at high risk for splenic artery aneurysms are multiparous women and patients with liver disease causing portal hypertension and splenomegaly. Women are four times more likely than men to have a splenic artery aneurysm. The hormone relaxin, released during pregnancy, is believed to weaken the arterial wall. This, along with the increased intravascular volume, portal congestion, and pre-existing fibrodysplasia, promote aneurysm formation in pregnant women. The splenic artery is also the most common visceral artery to develop a pseudoaneurysm. Splenic pseudoaneurysms are associated with penetrating trauma and pancreatitis. With pancreatitis, the elastase and other digestive pancreatic enzymes act directly on the vessel wall. These pseudoaneurysms tend to be very fragile and are more likely to rupture.

Like most visceral aneurysms, splenic artery aneurysms are usually asymptomatic. The most common symptoms are vague epigastric and left upper quadrant pain. Evaluation should include an abdominal plain film, which usually demonstrates a calcified ring in the left upper quadrant. Computed tomography scan and angiography are used to confirm the diagnosis and delineate the location and size. Rupture of a splenic artery aneurysm manifests with sudden left upper quadrant pain and signs of hypovolemia. Some patients temporarily stabilize. This phenomenon is called *double rupture*, and it is caused by tamponade of the initial aneurysmal bleed into the lesser sac followed by an inevitable flooding into the peritoneal cavity.

Women of childbearing age with a known splenic artery aneurysm should undergo elective repair. If the aneurysm is symptomatic or ruptured, emergent repair is needed. There are several options for surgical repair. A simple proximal and distal ligation without reconstruction can be used for proximal aneurysms. Other options are splenectomy, aneurysm exclusion with vascular reconstruction to allow for splenic salvage, or percutaneous embolization with a coil or gel foam.

Renal artery aneurysms are rare in the general population; however, patients with hypertension or fibromuscular disease of the renal artery have higher rates. Renal artery aneurysms tend to be slightly more common in women and occur most often in the right renal artery (except in pregnant women for whom the left renal artery is more commonly affected). Most renal artery aneurysms are saccular and are located at the first or second bifurcation of the renal artery. The risk of rupture is fairly low. The exception to this is in pregnant women where rupture is more common, especially in the third trimester. Ruptured renal artery aneurysms in pregnant women have a 70% maternal mortality rate and a 100% fetal mortality rate. For this reason, women with known renal artery aneurysms who are planning pregnancy should undergo prophylactic repair.

Treatment options for renal artery aneurysms are observation, transcatheter occlusion, or surgical repair. Observation involves life-long CT scan with contrast, careful blood pressure monitoring, and education regarding symptoms of rupture including flank pain or hematuria. Observation is not an option for renal artery aneurysms greater than 2.5 cm, renovascular hypertension with lateralizing serum renin levels, symptomatic aneurysms, documented expansion, renal embolization, or young women planning to become pregnant. Transcatheter occlusion is used for intraparenchymal lesions and high-risk surgical patients. Surgical treatment is with aneurysmectomy and arteriorrhaphy for saccular lesions or ligation and bypass for fusiform lesions.

137
Renovascular Hypertension

Renal occlusive disease is the cause of hypertension in less than 5% of all hypertensive patients. The etiologies of renovascular hypertension include atherosclerosis, fibromuscular dysplasia, Takayasu's arteritis, radiation vasculitis, neurofibromatosis, and thromboembolism. The diagnosis is more prevalent in patients with severe hypertension (diastolic pressure <115), refractory hypertension, new-onset hypertension in patients younger than 20 years of age, and hypertension in females younger than 50 years of age. Therefore, these constitute the situations when the physician should be alert to the diagnosis of renovascular hypertension.

Reduced blood flow to the kidney is the inciting event in the pathophysiology of renovascular hypertension. A stenosis of greater than 60% of the diameter of the renal artery is necessary to significantly impact renal perfusion. The drop in mean arterial pressure is then detected by baroreceptors in the afferent renal arterioles, stimulating renin secretion from the juxtaglomerular apparatus. Renin from the renal vein converts angiotensinogen from the liver to angiotensin I. In the lungs, angiotensin I is converted to angiotensin II by angiotensin-converting enzyme (ACE). Angiotensin II is a potent vasoconstrictor of vascular smooth muscle. In addition to vasoconstriction, angiotensin II stimulates the release of aldosterone from the adrenal cortex. Aldosterone causes the conservation of salt and water by the kidneys, resulting in increased extracellular volume. The combination of vasoconstriction and increased extracellular volume results in hypertension. Unilateral disease enhances renin secretion from the affected kidney while reducing secretion from the normal kidney. The normal kidney becomes exposed to hypertension, causing increased glomerular filtration. The increased workload placed on the normal kidney over time can lead to nephrosclerosis. Bilateral disease results in overall renal hypoperfusion with decreased creatinine clearance and, in time, azotemia.

Pathologically, atherosclerosis is responsible for about 90% of renovascular hypertension. It is present more commonly in men than in women. The plaque begins in the aorta and continues into the renal arteries, resulting in stenosis of the orifice. Lesions occur bilaterally in 50% of patients. The proximal one-third of the renal artery is generally affected, sparing the remainder of the vessel. Atherosclerotic plaques may fracture, hemorrhage, and embolize into the kidney parenchyma, causing infarction.

Fibromuscular dysplasia is the second most common etiology. Three types of fibromuscular dysplasia are differentiated by the portion of the arterial wall affected. Medial wall fibroplasia is found in 85% of dysplastic lesions. Women between the ages of 25 and 45 years are predominantly affected. The lesion can be single or multiple, giving a "string of lakes" appearance. Bilateral disease is present in 70% of cases. Premedial fibroplasia causes 10% of dysplastic lesions and is present almost exclusively in women. Five percent of lesions can be attributed to intimal fibroplasia. Children and young adults are more commonly affected by this form.

As previously mentioned, the diagnosis should be considered for pediatric hypertensive patients, young women, patients refractory to medical therapy, and patients with coexisting atherosclerosis. In particular, patients with hypertensive crisis, left heart failure, and flash pulmonary edema have an increased incidence of the disease. A dramatic response to ACE inhibitor therapy may also be a clue to renovascular disease. The diagnosis can be confirmed with physiologic or anatomic tests. Physiologic tests consist of selective renin sampling, split renal function testing, intravenous pyelography, and radionucleotide tests. Selective renin sampling and split renal function testing are cumbersome and impractical. In pyelograph and radionucleotide tests, the diagnosis is based on demonstrating asymmetric renal function. Findings of intravenous pyelography include delayed appearance of contrast dye in the affected kidney along with decreased kidney size and delayed concentration of contrast in the collecting system. Radionucleotide studies are used to evaluate renal perfusion and excretory function. In renovascular occlusive disease, angiotensin II causes vasoconstriction of the efferent arterioles. This compensatory mechanism creates a back pressure on the kidney that in turn helps increase glomerular filtration. Administration of an ACE inhibitor ameliorates this effect, reducing the glomerular filtration rate (GFR). A renal scan is conducted before and after administration of an ACE inhibitor. A decrease in GFR suggests the presence of renovascular occlusion.

Anatomic tests include renal ultrasound, magnetic resonance imaging (MRI), and arteriography. Doppler ultrasound can reveal decreased renal size as well as reduced perfusion of the affected kidney. Tardus parvus is an effect seen with greater than 60% stenosis in which the flow waveform distal to the stenosis is delayed or diminutive. Magnetic resonance imaging is a good tool to evaluate the arterial anatomy. Angiography is both diagnostic and therapeutic when combined with percutaneous techniques. Initial investigation usually begins with noninvasive studies such as ultrasound and MRI. If the diagnosis is suggested with noninvasive studies then angiography along with percutaneous intervention (i.e. angioplasty, stenting) are indicated.

The initial treatment consists primarily of medical therapy. This includes β-blockers, diuretics, vasodilators, and ACE inhibitors. More aggressive treatment is indicated for patients who take two to three antihypertensive drugs requiring increasing dosages. Long-term success rates of percutaneous intervention for fibromuscular dysplasia are equivalent to surgical therapy. The success rate for angioplasty is best for fibromuscular disease. The rate of restenosis approaches only 10%, with most remaining amenable to repeated angioplasty. Balloon angioplasty is particularly effective for fibromuscular dysplasia and for certain atherosclerotic lesions. Atherosclerotic lesions occurring at the vessel orifice are less amenable to angioplasty. Surgical correction ranges from endarterectomy to kidney removal with reimplantation. Ostial lesions respond well to transaortic endarterectomy. Arterial bypasses with autologous or prosthetic material to the proximal aorta or iliac artery can be effective for occlusive lesions. The use of autologous vein rather than artery is encouraged in bypasses for children. The innate distensibility of vein allows it to dilate with time. Extra-anatomic bypasses to the splenic or hepatic arteries avoid the morbidity of aortic cross clamping in patients who may not tolerate it. The size of the affected kidney has prognostic value for the success of revascularization. Kidneys 7 to 8 cm in size tend to recover better than kidneys smaller than 6 cm.

Surgical correction is most effective for children and for ostial lesions. The cure rate for children ranges from 70% to 85%. Among atherosclerotic patients one-third are cured by surgery and one-half have some improvement in their hypertension.

138
Cerebrovascular Disease

Stroke is the third leading cause of death, causing 1 of every 15 deaths in the United States. In the United States as a whole, stroke is more prevalent among elderly men and African Americans. In the southeastern United States, stroke is 1.4 times more likely to occur than in any other region of the country. Twenty-five percent of victims die within 1 year of having a stroke. Serious disabilities resulting from stokes include hemiparesis, immobilization, aphasia, and depression. Stroke victims comprise one-half of all patients hospitalized with acute neurologic diseases.

Major risk factors for stroke include hypertension, smoking, sickle cell disease, transient ischemic attack (TIA), asymptomatic carotid stenosis, and cardiac diseases (e.g., atrial fibrillation, endocarditis, mitral stenosis, and recent, severe myocardial infarction). The most important treatable risk factor for stoke is hypertension. The relative risk for stroke in patients who have hypertension (systolic blood pressure <160 mm Hg or diastolic blood pressure >95 mm Hg) is four times that of normotensive patients. Control of hypertensive disease would produce a 38% decrease in all strokes and a 40% decrease in fatal strokes.

Common clinical manifestations include TIAs, amaurosis fugax, reversible ischemic neurologic deficits (RIND), or stroke. Transient ischemic attacks are defined as brief episodes of ischemia causing a transient focal neurologic deficit. Episodes usually last about 2 to 15 minutes and have a rapid onset. The hallmarks of TIAs include multiple attacks without persistent deficit and return to baseline within 24 hours. Attacks of the left carotid system manifest with motor dysfunction, loss of vision in the left eye (amaurosis fugax), sensory symptoms (numbness, paresthesias of the right upper/lower extremity and/or face), and aphasia. Transient ischemic attacks of the right carotid can produce similar symptoms on the right side, except that aphasia occurs only in individuals with dominant right hemispheres for speech. With a RIND, signs and symptoms last less than 48 hours, and the patient is left with no or subtle neurologic deficit. Amaurosis fugax is characterized as a transient loss of vision in one eye. The onset is usually sudden, and symptoms can last for several minutes. Patients often report a visual sensation of a window shade being pulled over their eye. When the entire central retinal artery is transiently occluded, patients complain of almost complete loss of vision in the eye.

Atrial fibrillation is the most powerful and treatable cardiac precursor of stroke. Atrial fibrillation is the etiology of almost one half of all cardiogenic emboli leading to stroke. Anticoagulation therapy (i.e., Coumadin®) decreases the stoke risk by as much as 68%. Smoking doubles the relative risk for ischemic stroke with a reduction of risk once smoking is stopped. Heavy alcohol use raises the risk of stroke due to brain hemorrhage.

One of the leading causes of ischemic stroke is atherosclerotic disease. The carotid bifurcations are the usual source of emboli. Strokes are caused in three basic ways: embolization of atherosclerotic and thrombotic material, thrombosis with occlusion, and stenosis leading to hypoperfusion. Other possible sources of cerebral emboli include atherosclerosis of the aortic arch and small-vessel atherosclerosis (lipohyalinosis) causing occlusion of small penetrating brain arteries leading to subcortical or lacunar infarcts. Thirty percent of ischemic strokes are cryptogenic, meaning that no cause can be identified for them.

Atherosclerotic plaques form along the outer wall of the carotid sinus as seen in postmortem specimens, on angiograms of carotid stenosis, and in carotid endarterectomies. Turbulent fluid-flow patterns along the outer wall of the sinus and low wall shear stress promote atherosclerosis development. Decreased flow in these areas leads to prolonged exposure to lipids, white blood cells, platelets, and coagulation factors.

Atherosclerotic plaques are composed of a soft central core of necrotic cellular elements (red blood cells, hemosiderin, and lipid-laden macrophages) and lipid material.

The central core is covered by a fibrous cap composed of collagen, glycosaminoglycans, smooth muscle cells, and fibroblasts. Vascular smooth muscle cells, fibroblasts, collagen, and scattered calcifications make up the rest of the plaque. External mechanical forces act on the fibrous cap (the weakest portion of the plaque), causing rupture of the plaque. Inflammatory cells present at the borders of the necrotic core and at the fibrous cap release degradative enzymes and cytokines, which cause the plaque to destabilize also. Symptoms of TIA, amaurosis fugax, and stroke occur once the plaque becomes unstable and disrupts, releasing the contents of the central core into circulation. In addition, blood can dissect into the interior of the plaque once it has ruptured and cause the plaque to expand. The ruptured plaque leaves behind a deep ulcer. The ulcer's surface promotes thrombogenesis. Emboli follow a predictable pattern of distribution based on the laminar flow patterns of blood and their location of origin. Emboli originating at the carotid bifurcation tend to follow a path into the ophthalmic and middle cerebral arteries. Emboli originating from the cardiac circulation are found equally distributed throughout the brain.

Evaluation begins with an evaluation for carotid artery occlusive disease. Duplex ultrasonography is the preferred method of noninvasive testing to determine the severity and location of carotid occlusive disease. Computed tomography or MRI scans are used as adjuncts to rule out the presence of intracranial lesions. Arteriography is useful to further delineate the degree of stenosis and to evaluate for proximal atherosclerotic disease involving the aortic arch, intracranial vascular disease, and other arterial diseases (e.g., fibromuscular dysplasia). If the carotid arterial system cannot be identified as the source, then the workup must be completed with echocardiogram, coagulopathy workup, brain imaging, and arteriography to exclude other possible sources.

Medical treatment begins with antiplatelet therapy consisting of aspirin or clopidogrel bisulfate therapy started at the time of diagnosis. Tight control of hypertension and diabetes is warranted as well.

Carotid endarterectomy is indicated for symptomatic patients with carotid stenosis of 50% or greater and for patients who continue to have symptoms despite medical therapy. The risk of operation often outweighs the benefits for asymptomatic patients. Therefore, carotid endarterectomy is offered only to asymptomatic patients who have a good operative risk and advanced stenosis (60% to 99% stenosis). Symptomatic patients are much more likely to experience stroke or death when treated only medically. The procedure is typically delayed for 4 to 6 weeks for patients diagnosed with acute stroke to avoid converting a bland infarct into a hemorrhagic infarct. However, recent studies have shown that early carotid endarterectomy for severe carotid stenosis after a minimal stroke can be done with results similar to delayed procedures. Delayed surgery may expose this subset of patients to recurrent stroke. Patients suffering severe neurologic deficits after stoke are not candidates for operation unless there is substantial improvement in their clinical condition.

Coexisting coronary artery disease is prevalent in one-fourth to one-third of patients diagnosed with atherosclerotic carotid stenosis. For patients with symptomatic, high-grade carotid lesions and stable coronary disease, a staged approach consisting of carotid endarterectomy followed by coronary artery bypass grafting is reasonable. For patients with unstable coronary artery disease, carotid endarterectomy can take place at least 2 weeks after coronary artery bypass grafting.

139
Acute Mesenteric Ischemia

Mesenteric ischemia is caused by inadequate blood supply to the intestine or colon. The condition ranges from transient bowel dysfunction to tissue necrosis and transmural gangrene.

Deprivation of oxygen and nutrients results in ischemic injury to the intestine. The mesenteric anatomy has a network of rich collateral flow. Collateral blood flow opens when a major blood vessel is occluded. Collateral flow remains present as long as the pressure in the vascular bed is below the systemic pressure. Several hours of ischemia causes vasoconstriction in the obstructed vascular bed. This in turn raises the pressure above the systemic pressure and decreases the collateral flow. The vasoconstrictive state can be irreversible if allowed to persist for a significant amount of time. This explains the progressive nature of bowel ischemia that occurs even after correction of the underlying cause. Ischemic damage is produced during the hypoxic period and during the reperfusion period. Oxygen free radicals are responsible for the injury of reperfusion.

Intestinal ischemia can be acute or chronic. Acute intestinal ischemia often results in decreased intestinal viability and generally is caused by arterial disease. Examples of arterial causes for acute mesenteric ischemia include superior mesenteric artery embolism (50%), nonocclusive mesenteric ischemia (25%), superior mesenteric artery thrombosis (10%), and focal segmental ischemia. Chronic disease occurs most often in older patients with associated atherosclerotic disease of the mesenteric arteries. Acute occlusion is generally more damaging than the chronic form because of the lack of time allowed for enlargement of collateral vessels.

Acute mesenteric artery occlusion is most often caused by cardiogenic embolus of the superior mesenteric artery. The occlusion usually occurs distal to the origin of the artery. Diagnosing intestinal ischemia requires careful observation. Patients are generally more than 50 years of age and have several comorbidities, such as congestive heart failure, cardiac arrhythmias, myocardial infarction, and hypotension. Typically, patients present with a sudden onset of abdominal pain without impressive physical findings. The diagnosis of superior mesenteric artery embolism may be suggested by sudden severe abdominal pain and rapid evacuation of the bowels. In the absence of abdominal pain, abdominal distension and gastrointestinal bleeding may be the only clue to the diagnosis. Abdominal distension is often the first sign of intestinal infarction. In 75% of patients, occult blood is identified in the stool. The diagnosis of mesenteric ischemia must be made in a timely fashion. This requires an awareness of the patients most at risk for this condition.

Laboratory studies often show leukocytosis and metabolic acidosis in advanced cases with bowel gangrene. Abdominal plain films may show fluid-filled bowel loops with bowel wall edema. Duplex ultrasound can aid in the identification of portal and superior mesenteric vein thrombosis. Computed tomography has been useful in detecting arterial and venous thromboses and evidence of ischemic bowel. Findings indicating ischemia include bowel wall thickening, bowel dilation, and engorged mesenteric veins. Intramural gas or portal venous gas is observed with advanced bowel ischemia. Arteriography is critical in determining the cause and location of the lesion. Selective angiography along with papaverine infusion (vasodilator) is the mainstay of diagnosis and treatment for both occlusive and nonocclusive forms. Papaverine is administered into the obstructed vascular bed to minimize the vasoconstrictive response to hypoxia. Liberal use of mesenteric angiography is the key to early diagnosis of acute mesenteric ischemia.

Initial treatment includes aggressive resuscitation, abdominal plain films, and angiography along with intra-arterial vasodilator therapy. Broad-spectrum antibiotics are administered because of the likelihood of positive blood cultures, possibly caused by bacterial translocation through the compromised bowel wall. The decision to undergo exploratory laparotomy is based on clinical evidence of impending bowel ischemia. It is important to make the diagnosis before the onset of intestinal necrosis. The mortality rate approaches 90% after intestinal gangrene has developed. The goal of laparotomy is to restore arterial flow and to inspect the viability of the intestine. Embolectomy, thrombectomy, and arterial bypass are techniques used to restore blood flow. Nonviable intestine should be resected and reanastomosed primarily when possible. When the viability of bowel segments is questionable, a second look operation should be scheduled within 12 to 24 hours. Intra-arterial vasodilator therapy can be instituted operatively and continued 12 to 24 hours postoperatively. Anticoagulation in this disease condition is controversial. Complications include intestinal or intraperitoneal hemorrhage. Thrombolytic therapy has been used in some patients with success. The likelihood of successful therapy increases when symptoms have been present for less than 12 hours and when only a partial occlusion is present.

140
The Diabetic Foot

Neuropathy is the most common condition leading to the development of diabetic foot ulcers. Neuropathy is an independent risk factor for the future development of ulcerations. Neuropathy can be present in varying degrees involving somatic and autonomic sensations. The loss of sensation increases the likelihood of inadvertent and unrecognized limb injury. Patients lose the protective sensation of pain, heat, and pressure, thereby exposing the limb to injury. Severe neuropathy may develop into a claw foot or Charcot degeneration because of intrinsic muscle wasting and midfoot bone destruction, respectively. Autonomic dysfunction manifests as decreased sweating and vasodilation. This causes the foot to become warm and dry, predisposing it to skin breakdown and infection. Bony deformities and abnormal pressure may result in impaired microcirculation and ulcer formation. Microvascular and macrovascular vessel diseases produce ischemia in the limb that impairs healing.

The evaluation of diabetic foot conditions starts with a thorough history and physical examination. When acquiring information from the patient, it is important to gain a sense of existing vascular insufficiency. A history of previous nonhealing ulcers on the ipsilateral limb may suggest underlying vascular insufficiency. There may be a history of similar lesions on the contralateral limb as well. Symptoms such as rest pain and claudication are common with vascular insufficiency but may not manifest in the diabetic patient because of peripheral neuropathy. Smoking and high cholesterol level are risk factors for diabetic foot conditions. Systemic effects of infection may manifest as fever and chills but are not always seen in diabetic patients. Hyperglycemia is a sensitive indicator of ongoing infection. A history of increased blood glucose levels requiring higher doses of insulin can often be elicited.

Physical examination involves a thorough inspection of the skin, web spaces, and nail beds. Ulcers are generally located on the plantar surfaces over the metatarsal heads or on the heel. Heavily encrusted areas over ulcerations should be debrided to determine the extent of the wound. Sterile probing of the wound may reveal undrained areas of infection or exposed bone. Cultures of purulence or abscesses should be taken to help direct antibiotic therapy. Signs of infection include erythema, edema, tenderness, crepitance, and purulent drainage. Fever, chills, tachycardia, hypotension, and sepsis may indicate undrained infection. Untreated infections can spread throughout the remainder of the limb.

The Wagner classification system grades diabetic ulcers according to the extent of injury (Table 140.1). An important screening tool for diabetic patients is sensory assessment. A useful test is the Semmes-Weinstein monofilament test for sensorimotor neuropathy. In this test, a 5.07-mm diameter monofilament is pressed against the skin. Failure to detect the stimulus equates to an increased risk of developing ulcers.

A thorough vascular examination should be included in the physical examination. Peripheral pulses should be assessed via direct palpation or with ultrasound when pulses are not palpable. The nature of wounds may also provide clues to the nature of the vascular supply. Characteristics that follow arterial insufficiency include dry flaking skin, loss of hair, pallor with elevation of the limb, distal ulcerations, the absence of granulation tissue on wounds, and the absence of bleeding during debridement. Noninvasive studies may be helpful in accessing vascular insufficiently. Measurements of transcutaneous oximetry have proved to be reliable in predicting the ability to heal a wound. Doppler waveforms and pulsed volume recordings may be obtained. Ankle–brachial indices may be inaccurate due to the stiffness of calcified arteries that can occur with diabetes. The combination of absent pulses and significant tissue damage is an indication to proceed with arteriography. For diabetic patients with pre-existing renal disease, arteriography techniques may be modified by giving nonionic contrast material, adequate hydration, and kidney-protecting agents (N-acetylcysteine, bicarbonate).

TABLE 140.1. The Wagner classification grades of diabetic ulcers.

Grade	Characteristic of ulcer
0	Intact skin with bony deformities
1	Superficial local ulcer
2	Deep ulcer exposing tendon, bone, ligament, or joint
3	Osteomyelitis or abscess
4	Gangrene involving toes and forefoot
5	Gangrene involving the entire foot

Debridement of nonviable tissue is the first step in treatment of diabetic foot wounds. Adequate debridement consists of excision to the level of freshly bleeding tissue. Abscess cavities should be promptly incised and drained with cultures repeated at the time of surgery. Local wound care involves keeping the tissue moist and applying wetness to wet saline dressings. Other modalities such as enzymatic debridement, growth factors, and hyperbaric oxygen may provide little additional improvement.

The empiric therapy for diabetic foot infections can be directed with an understanding of the microbiology involved. Superficial wounds are generally seeded with aerobic Gram-positive organisms such as *Staphylococcus aureus* or *Streptococcus*. First-generation cephalosporins are usually adequate treatment for these infections. Infections of deep ulcerations are generally polymicrobial in nature. These include Gram-positive cocci along with Gram-negative bacilli (i.e., *Escherichia coli, Klebsiella, Enterobacter, Proteus,* and *Pseudomonas*) and anaerobic species (i.e., *Bacteroides* and *Peptostreptococcus*). Infections of this nature can be life threatening, requiring hospitalization, intravenous broad-spectrum antibiotics, intravenous fluid resuscitation, electrolyte correction, and tight glycemic control. Effective antibiotic combinations include clindamycin plus a fluoroquinolone or late-generation cephalosporin or clindamycin plus an antipseudomonal agent. Antibiotic therapy is continued until cellulitis resolves. Imaging studies such as magnetic resonance imaging are useful in evaluating the extent of disease and the presence of abscesses or osteomyelitis. Patients in extremis should be appropriately resuscitated and then undergo amputation of the septic source. Wounds are generally left to heal, if possible, by secondary intention with possible revision once the patient has recovered. Osteomyelitis is treated with surgical debridement (i.e., amputation) along with antibiotics.

Plans for possible revascularization should be formulated while the infection and wounds are being treated. All noninvasive and invasive studies can be performed during this time. Possible interventions include angioplasty, stenting, and surgical bypasses.

141
Chronic Venous Insufficiency

Chronic venous insufficiency is a condition that develops from elevated pressures in the venous system. The causes range from congenital malformations to trauma and deep venous thrombosis. Whatever the cause, venous hypertension and valvular dysfunction lead to venous stasis. The failure of the valve allows the reverse flow of venous blood through the system. The weight of the blood column is transmitted through the venous system in a linear fashion called *hydrostatic pressure*. This venous hypertension leads to the formation of newer, weaker capillaries that allows the extravasation of proteins.

Muscular contraction during ambulation or exercise produces increased venous pressure within the deep system. Valvular dysfunction of the perforating veins may allow the dynamic pressures that develop in the deep venous system to transmit to the superficial system. Over time, the increased venous pressures lead to dilation and tortuosity of the superficial veins, forming varicosities. Clinical manifestations include leg edema, warmth, heaviness, fatigue, and pain. Symptoms may be relieved with bed rest and extremity elevation.

Venous stasis ulcers are a complication of long-term disease. These ulcers are generally positioned superior to the medial malleolus and have an irregular shape. The ulcers occur secondary to venous obstruction and increased venous pressures, creating increased capillary permeability and extravasation of fluid and exudates. Endothelial damage resulting from venous hypertension causes inflammation. The extravasated proteins accumulate around the capillaries, creating pericapillary cuffing. Brawny edema results from the accumulation of proteinaceous deposits. The exchange of nutrients from the circulation to the surrounding tissue is impaired, leading to atrophy of the overlying skin and ulcer formation.

The diagnosis of chronic venous insufficiency is made by physical examination and is confirmed with Doppler ultrasound. Ultrasound is conducted with the patient standing to stimulate reflux and evaluate valve function. The study is enhanced by applying external compression with pneumatic cuffs. In addition, ultrasound can identify thrombosis and obstruction.

Chronic venous insufficiency is generally treated nonoperatively. The mainstay of management consists of external compression, bed rest, and extremity elevation. External compression is the key component to preventing the development of edema and skin ulceration. The mechanism by which this works has been debated. Popular beliefs include improved microcirculation, increased subcutaneous tissue pressure preventing capillary leak, and reduced ambulatory venous pressure. Venous ulcerations are treated with a combination of compressive dressings and local wound care. The dressings are impregnated with a mixture of calamine, zinc oxide, sorbitol, glycerin, and magnesium aluminum silicate (Unna's boot). These dressings are normally changed weekly. Ulcers heal within 2 months on average. Cellulitis can be treated with antibiotics. Dermatitis generally responds to topical steroid preparations. Patients are fitted with compression stockings once the ulcers heal. The stockings are worn for life during the day when the patient is ambulatory.

Surgical management is reserved for patients with severe symptoms and recurrent ulcers despite optimal medical therapy. Management options include phlebectomy, radiofrequency ablation, perforator vein ligation, valvuloplasty, and venous reconstruction. Sclerotherapy is a means of ablation that is effective for varicosities approximately 1 mm in size. The venectasia is injected the with dilute sclerosant solutions (0.2% sodium tetradecyl or hypertonic saline). Pressure dressings are applied for 1 to 3 days. From 2 to 3 weeks after the initial injection, the lesions are incised to allow the collected blood to drain, and a second pressure dressing is applied.

Phlebectomy is accomplished by creating small stab incisions at the areas of varicosities. The vessels are brought out through the incisions and ligated. Vein stripping is added to this procedure when the valves of the greater or lesser saphenous veins are compromised. Radiofrequency ablation is a fairly novel technique that uses a radiofrequency ultrasound probe to destroy the saphenous vein from within the lumen. Direct valvular repair is another technique, but the option is not viable for patients who have post-thrombotic disease. Post-thrombotic valve disease has been treated with venous transposition grafts with fair results. Total venous obstructions may be treated with venous bypass procedures.

142
Vascular Trauma

Vascular trauma differs significantly from elective vascular surgery primarily because of the injured patient's physiology. A peripheral vascular injury may be only one component of life-threatening injuries affecting many body systems and should be prioritized accordingly. The patterns of injury differ according to mechanism. Blunt injuries result in vessel wall contusion, pseudoaneurysm formation, and thrombosis. Low-velocity injuries and stab wounds can result in vessel lacerations with little surrounding damage, and high-velocity injuries (>2,500 fps) can result in complete transection with extensive surrounding damage to musculoskeletal and soft tissue structures.

Signs of injury are either hard or soft signs. Hard signs include expanding hematoma, palpable thrill or audible bruit, absent pulses, massive external hemorrhage, or symptoms of ischemia (the 5 Ps: pain, pallor, paresthesia, poikilothermia, paralysis). Hard signs require evaluation with angiography, exploration, or both. Soft signs include small stable hematoma, unexplained hypotension, injury to an adjacent nerve, history of hemorrhage at the injury scene that is absent on later evaluation, and proximity of penetrating wounds to a major vessel. The treatment of soft signs is debated. Arteriography is the standard diagnostic measure in the evaluation of vascular injury, although other modalities (magnetic resonance arteriography [MRA], computed tomography arteriography [CTA], duplex sonography) are used in specific circumstances.

Repair Choices

The anatomy of the injury and the physiology of the patient determine the level of repair necessary. The choices for repair technique include ligation, lateral or direct repair, patch angioplasty, resection and reanastomosis, resection with interposition graft, and shunt procedures. The contralateral saphenous vein is the preferred conduit for peripheral injury, whereas polytetrafluoroethylene (PTFE) may be used for injuries above the groin. The complexity of repair should be inversely proportional to the patient's physiologic status. Proximal and distal control is essential to clearly examine the anatomy of injury and to ensure proper repair technique. This may be performed with atraumatic clamps, vessel loops, compression, and intravascular catheters.

Special Circumstances

Cervical Injuries

Unstable patients with cervical injury should be explored expeditiously. Stable patients require evaluation according to the zone of injury. Zones I and III require angiography; zone II has historically required exploration, although some cases can be treated nonoperatively. External carotid and jugular venous injuries can be ligated. Blunt injury can manifest with hemispheric deficit in the absence of brain injury and is treated with anticoagulation as the clinical situation permits.

Thoracic Injuries

A unique challenge to thoracic vascular injury is exposure, because specific operative approaches afford exposure of limited vessels. If possible, preoperative angiography is crucial to planning the operative approach. Pseudoaneurysm from blunt thoracic aortic injury most often occurs distal to the left subclavian artery, distal to the ligamentum arteriosum. The gold standard for diagnosis for this injury is aortography, although other modalities may be required (chest x-ray or CTA for screening, transesophageal echo [TEE] if the patient cannot undergo arteriography). Repair can be delayed until the patient is stabilized and is often performed using a prosthetic graft with full intraoperative anticoagulation.

Abdominal Injuries

Most venous injuries are either ligated (including the portal vein and inferior vena cava) or packed. Direct repair sometimes results in thrombosis. Celiac axis, inferior mesenteric artery (IMA), and internal iliac arteries usually can be ligated without adverse sequelae. Exposure and proximal control is essential and is accomplished by medial visceral rotation and aortic cross-clamping at the diaphragmatic hiatus. Iliac vein bifurcation injuries require division of the common iliac artery for exposure. Polytetrafluoroethylene can be used with minimal intestinal spillage; however, gross fecal soilage requires ligation and extra-anatomic reconstruction. For retroperitoneal hematomas caused by penetrating trauma, exploration is mandatory, whereas with blunt trauma only central hematomas and lateral, expanding hematomas are explored.

Peripheral Injuries

Physical examination is useful to identify pulse or ankle–brachial index (ABI) discrepancies that require arteriography. Proximity injuries without hard signs of injury do not mandate evaluation. Venous injuries (including popliteal vein injury) can be ligated with impunity. Primary repairs are done if feasible but frequently thrombose. Common femoral artery/superficial femoral artery (CFA/SFA) injuries may require PTFE reconstruction, even in a contaminated field. Popliteal injuries cause limb loss more often than any other peripheral vessel and can require bypass or interposition graft. Arteriography is mandatory in the setting of posterior knee dislocation to rule out associated popliteal injury. Infrageniculate injuries can be ligated provided that at least one tibial artery is uninjured. The brachial artery is the peripheral vessel most often injured and can require interposition graft. Radial or ulnar artery injuries can be ligated provided the palmar arch is intact and/or there are no symptoms of hand ischemia.

Combined Injuries

Combined orthopedic and vascular injuries require careful planning of operative management. An extremity that is not clinically ischemic should undergo orthopedic repair followed by vascular repair. If the extremity is ischemic, a shunt is placed before orthopedic stabilization. Mangled extremities often require amputation. If there is a question regarding the viability of a mangled extremity, this is best addressed in conjunction with orthopedic consultation. The use of prosthetic grafts in contaminated fields is debated but occasionally is necessary. The principle of soft tissue coverage is imperative to prevent late complications not only for prosthetic repairs but also for autogenous repairs. Extra-anatomic bypass should be considered in a contaminated field.

Fasciotomy is often required to relieve or prevent compartment syndrome in peripheral injuries. Risk factors for compartment syndrome include combined venous/arterial injury, prolonged ischemia time, and extensive musculoskeletal and soft tissue injury. Calf fasciotomy is most often needed and is accomplished through generous medial and lateral incisions to decompress anterior, lateral, and deep/superficial compartments.

Ultrasound is useful to access minor injuries, because many regress with time. Injuries that progress to pseudoaneurysm or traumatic arteriovenous (AV) fistula require intervention.

Anticoagulation is frequently contraindicated for acutely injured patients and is not mandatory either intraoperatively or postoperatively. Anticoagulation is, however, the mainstay of treatment for blunt cervical vascular injuries. Antiplatelet therapy is useful postoperatively as a measure to prevent graft thrombosis.

Catheter embolectomy is an essential adjunct to peripheral arterial repair, because the physiology of acute injury includes spasm and thrombosis formation. Completion arteriography is required if a palpable pulse cannot be obtained following reconstruction.

Vascular repair in the trauma setting must take into account the overall physiologic status of the patient with temporizing measures (shunt, ligation, packing) used for patients in extremis. Complex repairs are best reserved for stable patients.

143
The Lymphatic System

The lymphatic system is responsible for the collection of the body's interstitial fluid and returning it to the venous system. Approximately 2 to 4 liters of interstitial fluid is transported each day. In addition to transporting lymph fluid, the lymphatic system is also responsible for immunogenic filtering of the fluid through lymph nodes and the transport of macromolecules (chylomicrons, proteins). Lymphatic capillaries are dispersed throughout the body. Lymphatic capillaries have large openings that allow the passage of lymphocytes, erythrocytes, and bacteria. The lymphatic capillaries empty into transporting vessels, which periodically connect to lymph nodes. Lymphatic vessels are morphologically similar to blood vessels in that they possess an adventitia, media with smooth muscle, and intima.

The lymph nodes are small, bean-shaped structures surrounded by a capsule. Multiple afferent collecting channels deliver lymph into the lymph node. Lymphatic fluid can exit only via a single efferent channel. The inner aspect of the lymph node, which is composed of cortical and medullary sinuses, filters the lymphatic fluid. Lymphocytes dominate the cortical areas, and plasma cells and macrophages inhabit the medulla.

The cisterna chyli forms from the union of the lower extremity and visceral lymphatic channels. The cisterna chyli is renamed the thoracic duct after it traverses the diaphragm. The thoracic duct courses to the right and anterior to the vertebral column. Along the way it receives drainage from the intercostals and thoracic visceral collecting vessels. At the level of T5, the thoracic duct crosses to the left side of the thorax. The thoracic duct empties into the venous system at the left subclavian vein. The lymphatic drainage of the right upper extremity, head, and neck collect into the right subclavian vein by way of the right lymphatic duct.

Lymphatic fluid is propelled primarily through the system through peristaltic contractions of the lymphatic vessels. Additional movement is provided through muscular contractions, increased intra-abdominal pressures

from straining, and pressure changes in the thoracic cavity with breathing. Interstitial fluid is created from filtering of plasma fluid across the capillaries' semipermeable membrane. The movement of fluid between the intravascular space and the interstitial space depends on the hydrostatic and osmotic pressures in these two spaces.

Edema is caused by excess interstitial fluid production or decreased elimination. Several processes produce interstitial fluid accumulation. Increased permeability of the capillary membrane allows more fluid to enter the interstitial space. Obstructions on the venous limb of the capillary bed increase the hydrostatic pressure in the vascular system. This limits the absorption of fluid and causes its accumulation. Finally, defects intrinsic to the lymphatic system such as fibrosis, hypoplasia, and obstruction limit the transport of interstitial fluid, causing it to accumulate.

Lymphedema is the accumulation of excess interstitial fluid due to impaired lymphatic flow. This condition exists in two basic forms, primary and secondary. Primary lymphedemas include lymphedema congenita, Milroy's disease, lymphedema praecox, and lymphedema tarda. The most common form is lymphedema praecox, which comprises 80% of cases. This condition manifests with edema beginning in puberty. Lymphedema congenita is a severe form of disease present at birth. Edema involves the lower extremities and the right side most often. Twenty-five percent of cases involve bilateral disease. Milroy's disease is a hereditary form of lymphedema. In this type, edema occurs from the knee to the dorsum of the foot along with lymphatic abnormalities (cystic hygromas, pulmonary and intestinal lymphangiectasia). Lymphedema tarda exhibits delayed presentation (20 to 30 years of age). Lymphedema varies in severity. Early disease includes pitting edema of soft tissues and typically involves the distal portions of the lower extremity, including the dorsum of the foot and toes. Severe and prolonged disease causes fibrosis of the underlying tissues, imparting a hard texture. The overlying skin becomes hypertrophic and hyperkeratotic, similar to eczema. The impaired lymphatic flow also impairs the local host immune response, leaving the affected limb susceptible to spontaneous episodes of bacterial cellulitis hallmarked by fever, pain, and inflammation. Secondary lymphedema is attributed to neoplastic infiltration (prostate cancer, lymphoma), surgical excision of lymphatic tissue (axillary nodal dissection), or fibrosis secondary to inflammation (infection or radiation).

Radiographic evaluations of lymphedema can be invasive or noninvasive. Lymphangiography is an invasive form of lymphatic imaging. The technique provides detailed images of the lymphatic system using subcutaneous injections of vital dyes that are taken up by the lymphatic vessels. A surgical incision is created, and the marked lymphatic vessels are exposed and cannulized. Contrast (ethiodized oil) is injected into the lymphatic system, and a series of radiographs are obtained over 24 hours. Findings indicative of lymphedema include hypoplasia (small vessels and few in number) and hyperplasia (due to lymphatic obstruction producing numerous dilated channels). Lymphoscintigraphy is a noninvasive way to image the lymphatic system. This technique involves the injection of technetium-labeled colloid into the subcutaneous tissues. The radioisotope is taken up by the lymphatic system and examined with a special gamma camera. This technique has the advantage of being noninvasive but produces images with less resolution than lymphangiography; however, the diagnosis of lymphedema can still be confirmed in most cases. Magnetic resonance imaging is another method used to evaluate the lymphatic system. It can be used to image lymph nodes, vessels, and surrounding tissues.

Conservative treatment for lymphedema is sufficient for most patients. Key features of this type of therapy include strict attention to skin hygiene, elevation, and protection from injury. Elevation is efficacious for early disease, when tissues are soft. External compression stockings can be custom-made for patients with a pressure gradient from the toe to the groin. These devices are effective in the early stages of disease when swelling is minimal to moderate. Advanced disease (woody and indurated tissues) may respond to pneumatic mechanical compression devices or to specialized massages. Pharmacologic therapy involves the administration of benzopyrene to decrease edema caused by protein accumulation.

Surgical therapy is composed of three different techniques. The first involves the complete excision of fibrotic subcutaneous tissues. The wound is then covered with a split thickness skin graft or with staged advancements of skin flaps. The second technique involves transferring a pedicle of lymphatic-containing tissue. Tissues that have been used for pedicle creation include omentum, defunctionalized bowel, and de-epithelialized skin. This technique attempts to spontaneously form connections with the defective lymphatics; however, it has not proved to be very successful. The third final technique involves creating lymphovenous fistulas or vein grafts to bypass dysfunctional lymphatic segments.

Lymphatic Tumors

Lymphangiomas are benign malformations of the lymphatic vessels. Greater than 50% are evident at the time of birth. These indolent lesions can invade local tissue, although progression to true malignancy is a rare occurrence. Lymphangiomas manifest in one of three forms: lymphangioma simplex, cavernous lymphangioma, and cystic hygroma.

Cystic hygromas are lymphatic cysts lined by an epithelial layer. They are often located on the head or in the axilla. Surgical resection is the treatment of choice.

Lymphangioma simplex is a lesion composed of capillary-sized lymphatic vessels. In contrast, cavernous lymphangiomas are derived from dilated lymphatic channels enclosed in a fibrous capsule. Lymphangiosarcoma is a malignancy that develops in extremities affected by lymphedema. The neoplasm occurs rarely but is nonetheless very aggressive and has a high mortality rate.

Chylous Ascites

Specialized lymphatics of the small intestine (lacteals) are responsible for the collection and transportation of digested fat (chyle). Chyle is normally routed through the lacteals to the cisterna chyli and finally to the thoracic duct. An obstruction to its normal route of transportation leads to the development of fistulas in the peritoneal, thoracic, or pericardial cavities. A reduced fat diet (medium-chain triglyceride diet) decreases chyle formation and decreases volume through the fistula. Primary closure of the fistula is required if dietary changes are ineffective. Spontaneous chylous ascites in an elderly patient is an indication of occult malignancy.

Part XIV
Endocrine System

144
Thyroid and Parathyroid Anatomy

Thyroid Gland

The thyroid gland originates from cells of endodermal origin as a midline diverticulum in the floor of the pharynx. The cells descend in the neck and develop into the bilobed thyroid gland. The site of origin in the buccal cavity is marked by the foramen cecum at the base of the tongue. The path of descent becomes the thyroglossal duct, which later undergoes involution. The calcitonin-producing C-cells of the thyroid gland originate from the neural crest. These cells are the only component of the thyroid gland that is not endodermal in origin.

A thyroglossal duct cyst and fistula are developmental anomalies that result from failure of the complete involution of the thyroglossal duct. Thyroglossal duct cysts are midline structures that can be found anywhere from the base of the tongue to the suprasternal notch. Most develop in early childhood or infancy as a mass immediately beneath the hyoid bone. Thyroglossal fistula is a result of chronic infection and drainage of a thyroglossal duct cyst. Failure of thyroid descent may also result in lingual thyroid. In most cases, this is the only thyroid tissue. Airway obstruction or dysphagia can be caused by enlargement of the lingual thyroid tissue. Lingual thyroid growth can be suppressed with thyroxine therapy or ablated with radioactive iodine.

Thyroid tissue located in the lateral neck used to be called *lateral aberrant thyroid tissue* and was explained as an embryologic anomaly. This concept has been disproved, and it is now thought that thyroid tissue found in the lateral neck may be metastatic deposits from well-differentiated thyroid carcinoma.

The thyroid gland lies next to the thyroid cartilage, anterior and lateral to the junction of the larynx and trachea. The gland encircles about 75% of the diameter of the junction of the larynx and the trachea. The two lateral lobes are joined at the midline by an isthmus, which lies anterior to or below the cricoid cartilage. The pyramidal lobe is the most distal portion of the thyroglossal duct and, in the adult, can be a prominent structure. A thin layer of fascia surrounds the thyroid. This is part of the fascial layer, which invests the trachea, and is separate from the thyroid capsule. This fascia coalesces with the thyroid capsule posteriorly and laterally to form a suspensory ligament, called the *ligament of Berry*. The ligament of Berry has important surgical implications because of its relation to the recurrent laryngeal nerve.

On the right side, the recurrent laryngeal nerve separates from the vagus as it crosses the subclavian artery, passing posteriorly and ascending in a lateral position to the trachea along the tracheoesophageal groove. The right recurrent laryngeal nerve can usually be found no further than 1 cm lateral to or in the tracheoesophageal groove at the level of the lower border of the thyroid. As it ascends to the midportion of the thyroid, however, the nerve assumes its position within the tracheoesophageal groove. At this location, the nerve might divide into one, two, or more branches as it enters into the first or second ring of the trachea, with the most important branch disappearing beneath the inferior border of the cricothyroid muscle. The nerve can usually be found immediately anterior or posterior to a main arterial trunk of the inferior thyroid artery at this level. Unusually, a nonrecurrent right laryngeal nerve can arise directly from the vagus and course directly medially into the larynx. This nonrecurrent anatomy is found in 0.5% to 1.5% of patients.

On the left side, the recurrent laryngeal nerve separates from the vagus as the nerve traverses over the arch of the aorta. The left recurrent laryngeal nerve then passes inferiorly and medially to the aorta and begins to ascend toward the larynx, finding its way into the tracheoesophageal groove as it ascends to the level of the lower lobe of the thyroid. Both recurrent laryngeal nerves are consistently located in the tracheoesophageal groove when they are within 2.5 cm of their entrance into the larynx. These nerves pass either inferiorly or posteriorly to an arterial branch of the inferior thyroid artery and eventually enter the larynx at the level of the cricothyroid articulation on the caudal border of the cricothyroid muscle. Here the nerve is immediately adjacent to the superior parathyroid, the inferior thyroid artery, and the most posterior aspect of the thyroid. Great care is needed in surgical dissection in this area because the nerve is essentially tethered as it dives beneath the cricothyroid muscle and can be placed on stretch by overly vigorous dissection.

The motor function of the recurrent laryngeal nerve is abduction of the vocal cords from the midline. Damage to a recurrent laryngeal nerve results in paralysis of the vocal cord on the side affected. Such damage might result in a cord that remains in a medial position or just lateral to the midline. A normal voice, albeit weakened, can occur if the remaining functioning contralateral cord is able to approximate the paralyzed cord. If the vocal cord remains paralyzed in an abducted position and closure cannot occur, a severely impaired voice and ineffective cough can be the result. If recurrent laryngeal nerves are damaged bilaterally, complete loss of voice or airway obstruction requiring emergency intubation and tracheostomy may be necessary.

The superior laryngeal nerve originates from the vagus nerve at the base of the skull and descends toward the superior pole of the thyroid along the internal carotid artery. At the level of the hyoid, it divides into two branches. The larger internal branch has sensory function and enters the thyrohyoid membrane, where it innervates the larynx. The smaller external branch continues to travel along the lateral surface of the inferior pharyngeal constrictor muscle and usually descends anteriorly and medially along with the superior thyroid artery. Within 1 cm of the superior thyroid artery's entrance into the thyroid capsule, the nerve usually takes a medial course and enters into the cricothyroid muscle. During a thyroid lobectomy, the external branch is not usually seen, because it has already entered the inferior pharyngeal muscle fascia. This nerve is at risk of being severed or entrapped if superior pole vessels are ligated at too great a distance above the superior pole of the thyroid. Damage to the external branch can cause a severe loss in quality of voice or voice strength. Although this may not be as clinically devastating as recurrent laryngeal nerve damage, it is extremely bothersome to patients whose occupation demands good voice quality.

The thyroid gland is supplied by four main arteries, two superior and two inferior. The superior thyroid artery is the first branch of the external carotid artery, and it enters the superior pole of the thyroid at its apex. Care must be taken when securing the superior thyroid artery to prevent injury to the external laryngeal nerve. The inferior thyroid artery is a branch of the thyrocervical trunk. This artery ascends into the neck on either side behind the carotid sheath and then arches medially and enters the thyroid gland posteriorly. There is no direct arterial supply to the thyroid at the inferior boundaries, because most of these vascular structures are venous. An occasional inferior arterial supply occurs from a thyroidea inferior mesenteric artery, which arises directly from the innominate artery or the aorta.

The recurrent laryngeal nerve is usually directly adjacent to the inferior thyroid artery within 1 cm of its entrance into the larynx. Careful dissection of the artery in this case is essential and cannot be completed until knowledge of the position of the recurrent laryngeal nerve is gained. The inferior thyroid artery nearly always supplies both the superior and inferior parathyroid glands, and care must be taken when evaluating the parathyroids after inferior thyroid artery division.

Three pairs of venous systems drain the thyroid. Superior venous drainage is immediately adjacent to the superior arteries and joins the internal jugular vein at the level of the carotid bifurcation. The middle thyroid veins exist in more than half of patients and course immediately laterally into the internal jugular vein. The two or three inferior thyroid veins descend directly from the lower pole of the gland into the innominate and brachiocephalic veins.

Lymphatic channels occur immediately beneath the capsule of the thyroid and drain through numerous lymphatic channels into the regional lymph nodes. These regional lymph nodes exist in a pretracheal position immediately superior to the isthmus, paratracheal nodes, tracheoesophageal groove lymph nodes, mediastinal nodes in the anterior and superior position, jugular lymph nodes in the upper, middle, and lower distribution, and retropharyngeal and esophageal lymph nodes. Papillary carcinoma of the thyroid is often associated with adjacent nodal metastasis. Medullary carcinoma has a strong predilection for metastatic lymphatic involvement, usually in the central compartment (the space between the internal jugular veins). For this reason, central-compartment lymph node dissection is indicated at the time of total thyroidectomy for medullary carcinoma.

Parathyroid Glands

The superior parathyroid glands arise from branchial pouch IV, and the inferior parathyroids arise from branchial pouch III. The glands are intimately associated with the derivatives of their respective pouches—the inferior glands with the thymus and the superior glands with the lateral thyroid component (later to become the tubercle of Zuckerkandl). As the thymus descends, the inferior glands also migrate caudally and settle near the lower pole of the thyroid. Migration is variable. At one extreme, the ectopic glands can be high in the carotid sheath, or, at the other, they can be deep in the mediastinum. The inferior glands are more likely to be found in an ectopic location than are the superior glands.

Rarely, a parathyroid becomes completely enclosed in the thyroid parenchyma (typically an inferior gland).

When the superior portion of the thyroid lobe is dissected and rolled medially, an area containing fat beneath the encasing fascia is visible. The superior parathyroid gland nearly always lies within the fat beneath the thyroid sheath in this location. The inferior parathyroid gland can also be in the thyroid sheath on the posterior aspect of the lower portion of the lobe and, like the superior gland, is usually encased in a small amount of fat. The position of the inferior parathyroid is more variable, however, and can be along the branches of the inferior thyroid vein lateral or inferior to the lowermost portion of the thyroid lobe. Because of the similar consistency and color of the parathyroids and the fat that surrounds them, parathy-roids in both positions are most efficiently sought by following the smaller branches of the inferior thyroid artery into the parathyroid substance.

The superior and inferior parathyroid glands have a single end artery, which supplies them medially from the inferior thyroid artery. If the main trunk of the inferior thyroid artery is sacrificed for dissection, both parathy-roids on that side can be devascularized, because there is no collateral blood supply to maintain viability. Careful dissection should attempt to divide only the branches of the inferior thyroid entering the thyroid capsule during excision. With careful technique, it is possible to maintain good vascular supply to the superior and inferior parathyroid even when a total thyroidectomy is performed.

145
Thyroid Physiology

The thyroid plays a key role in regulating metabolism for the rest of the body. The hormones generated by the thyroid are thyroxine (T4), triiodothyronine (T3), and calcitonin. The functional unit of the thyroid gland is the thyroid follicle. It is composed of a single layer of cuboidal-shaped thyroid follicular cells with colloid protein deposited in the center. During development, neural crest–derived C-cells migrate into the thyroid gland adjacent to the thyroid follicles. The C-cells produce the hormone calcitonin, which is involved in calcium metabolism. Thyroid hormones exert their actions in peripheral cells by interacting with nuclear thyroid hormone receptors. In this way, the hormone's effects are mediated by regulating gene expression. Thyroid hormones are involved with the regulation of oxygen consumption, lipid and carbohydrate metabolism, growth, and maturation.

The essential element of thyroid hormone is iodine. Iodine is converted to iodide and absorbed in the gut. From the bloodstream, iodide enters the thyroid follicular cell via secondary active transport. Iodide is important not only for thyroid hormone synthesis but also for normal function of the thyroid gland. Once inside the thyroid gland, iodide is oxidized and coupled to tyrosine molecules by the enzyme thyroid peroxidase. Two conformations can be created from this reaction, monoiodotyrosine (MIT) and diiodotyrosine (DIT). These molecules are then coupled to one another to form either T4 (two DIT moieties coupled together) or T3 (one MIT plus one DIT). Both molecules are bound to a glycoprotein called *thyroglobulin* and stored in the follicular center as colloid. When the time comes for thyroid hormone secretion, multiple pseudopodia descend from the apical surface of the follicular cell, scooping out colloid material. The thyroid hormones become unbound from thyroglobulin through hydrolysis. Thyroid hormone diffuses into the circulation by crossing the basement membrane.

Once in the circulation, thyroid hormones bind to plasma proteins (i.e., thyroxine-binding globulin) or remain free. Most T4 binds to plasma proteins, and most T3 is unbound. The free fraction of thyroid hormone is physiologically active, which explains why T3 is more active than T4 and has a shorter half life. In addition, peripheral T4 can be converted to the more active T3 in the plasma or in the liver.

Calcitonin is secreted by parafollicular C-cells within the thyroid gland. This hormone inhibits calcium absorption by osteoclasts and thereby lowers serum calcium levels. Calcitonin secretion is stimulated by high levels of serum calcium.

Thyroid hormone secretion is regulated by the hypothalamic–pituitary axis. Thyroid-stimulating hormone (TSH) acts as a growth factor and stimulates thyroid hormone release. Thyroid-stimulating hormone encourages thyroid cell growth and differentiation, increases iodine uptake and organification, and stimulates the release of T3 and T4. The release of TSH is stimulated by thyrotropin-releasing hormone (TRH) produced from the paraventricular nucleus of the hypothalamus. Increased circulating levels of thyroid hormone impose a negative feedback on TSH release as well a TRH. Other stimulators of thyroid hormone include catecholamines and human chorionic gonadotropin (hCG). Glucocorticoids have a depressant effect on TSH secretion.

A number of drug classes have been developed that are effective in treating thyroid dysfunction. The thioamides include PTU (propylthiouracil) and methimazole. Their mechanisms of action include inhibition of the oxidation of inorganic iodine and also blocking the coupling of iodotyrosine moieties. Propylthiouracil has the added effect of blocking peripheral conversion of T4 to T3. Methimazole is longer acting and can cross the placenta; therefore, it should be avoided in pregnancy. Both drugs have a 1% chance of causing agranulocytosis. Supplemental iodine has been given as treatment for hyperthyroidism. Its effect is exerted through inhibition of thyroid hormone release. Steroids can lower thyroid hormone production by suppressing TSH release from the anterior pituitary and by blocking the peripheral conversion of T4 to T3. β-Blockers blunt the catecholamine-mediated stimulation of thyroid hormone release.

The most important test for evaluating thyroid function is a serum TSH. In hypothyroidism, TSH levels are increased; in hyperthyroidism, they are decreased. This can be very useful for distinguishing between hypothyroidism and euthyroid states. Patients with no clinical signs of hyperthyroidism can still have a depressed TSH level, which suggests hyperthyroidism. Initial screening should also include total and free T4 levels.

Radioactive iodine uptake has been useful for assessing gland activity. Oral ^{123}I is given, and the amount of uptake is determined using radioscintigraphy. Normal uptake is 15% to 30% within 24 hours.

Pituitary insufficiency can be detected with TRH stimulation tests. The normal response to TRH administration should be an increase in TSH. Patients with pituitary insufficiency are unable to produce this response. Patients with primary hypothyroidism (excess TSH) have an exaggerated response to TRH administration, with increased TSH release. The T3 suppression test is used to evaluate for hyperthyroidism. Exogenous T3 is given for 1 week to 10 days. The exogenous T3 causes a depression in TSH. In a normally functioning gland, this results in less thyroid hormone production, which is reflected in a decrease in radioactive iodine uptake. A hyperfunctioning thyroid gland can continue to produce hormone despite the drop in TSH. This is reflected in continued increase in radioactive iodine uptake.

146
Hyperthyroidism

Hyperthyroidism results from a state of elevated circulating thyroid hormone. There are several causes of the condition. The elevated levels of thyroid hormone can be caused by hormone overproduction, release from glandular destruction, or exogenous administration. The most common causes are Grave's disease and toxic nodular goiter. Other less common causes include molar pregnancy, thyrotoxicosis factitia, thyroiditis, drug-induced thyrotoxicosis (caused by lithium or amiodarone), thyroid-stimulating hormone (TSH)–secreting pituitary tumor, and iodine ingestion. Common manifestations of hyperthyroidism include a goiter, tachycardia, tremor, nervousness, diaphoresis, heat intolerance, palpitations, arrhythmias (atrial fibrillation), weight loss, and fatigue. Untreated disease can cause death from thyroid storm, heart failure, or severe wasting. Thyroid storm is a life-threatening complication of untreated or undertreated hyperthyroidism. The symptoms appear abruptly and are often precipitated by the stress of trauma, infection, surgery, pulmonary embolism, diabetic ketoacidosis, and labor. The most obvious signs are high fever, mental status changes, and tachycardia. Hypotension, cardiovascular collapse, and shock are events that can lead to death.

Grave's disease is an autoimmune condition that stems from antibody stimulation of TSH receptors. The disease is chronic in nature, with many relapses and remissions. Stimulation of the TSH receptors causes increased synthesis and secretion of thyroid hormone. Other features that follow the condition include exophthalmos and pretibial myxedema. Exophthalmos is characterized by lid lag, stare, lid retraction, and proptosis. It is thought to originate from separate antibodies directed against certain ocular structures such as the extraocular muscles. The severity of exophthalmus varies from mild forms to diplopia and vision loss. Pretibial myxedema is an associated affliction of the skin characterized by nonpitting edema on the pretibial surfaces. Infiltration of a proteinaceous substance produces the edema. The lesions are often pruritic and red and then turn brawny in later stages. These manifestations can appear at any time during the course of Grave's disease. Other autoimmune-related diseases may also be present, including vitiligo, insulin-dependent diabetes, pernicious anemia, and collagen vascular diseases.

Plummer's disease (toxic nodular goiter) is another common cause of thyrotoxicosis. In general, the symptoms associated with Plummer's disease are less severe than with Grave's disease. This condition occurs more often in elderly patients and is hallmarked by single or multiple hyperfunctioning thyroid nodules.

Elevated thyroid hormones can be present without increased thyroid gland activity. Inflammatory conditions such as thyroiditis can cause a destruction of glandular tissue, which releases excess triiodothyronine (T3) and thyroxine (T4) into the blood. Metastatic thyroid cancers and other tumors such as struma ovarii cause the ectopic production of thyroid hormone.

Human chorionic gonadotropin is a potential thyroid gland stimulator. Elevated levels occur in conditions such as molar pregnancy, choriocarcinoma, and hyperemesis gravidarum.

Drugs such as lithium, amiodarone, and interferon-α have been reported to cause hyperthyroidism. Iodine excess can result from taking drugs containing iodine, the administration of iodine contrast materials, and ingestion. Excess iodine results in increased synthesis and secretion of thyroid hormone.

The evaluation of hyperthyroidism includes a thorough history and physical examination with inquiry into medications and family history. Serum TSH should be measured first. Thyroid-stimulating hormone is generally depressed unless there is a pituitary tumor producing excess TSH. The next step is to measure serum free T4 level, which is elevated in most cases. If this is normal, free T3 level should be measured. Radioactive iodine ^{123}I-uptake studies will determine if the thyroid gland itself is hyperfunctioning.

Effective treatment of hyperthyroidism includes medication, radioablation, and thyroidectomy. Several classes of drugs are effective in treating thyroid dysfunction. The thioamides include propylthiouracil (PTU) and methimazole. Their mechanisms of action include inhibition of the oxidation of inorganic iodine and blocking the coupling of iodotyrosine moieties. Propylthiouracil has the added effect of blocking peripheral conversion of T4 to T3. Methimazole is longer acting and can cross the placenta; therefore, it should be avoided during pregnancy. Both drugs have a 1% chance of causing agranulocytosis. β-Blockers, such as propranolol, blunt the catecholamine-mediated stimulation of thyroid hormone release. Steroids can lower thyroid hormone production by suppressing TSH release from the anterior pituitary as well as blocking the peripheral conversion of T4 to T3.

Radioactive ablation (^{131}I) has proved safe and effective for the treatment of hyperthyroidism. It has now become the treatment of choice for Grave's disease and toxic nodular goiter. This treatment is recommended for patients over the age of 40 years with recurrent hyperthyroidism and for patients who are poor surgical risks.

It is contraindicated for young children, pregnant women, and women who wish to become pregnant.

Indications for subtotal thyroidectomy include large multinodular goiters, malignant thyroid nodules, pregnant patients, children, patients noncompliant to medical therapy, and patients with ophthalmopathy. Before surgery, patients are given antithyroid medications such as PTU to induce a euthyroid state. Lugol's solution is given 2 weeks prior to surgery. The purpose of this is to prevent thyroid storm and to limit the vascularity of the thyroid gland. A similar regimen is given to patients who are hyperthyroid and require other types of emergent surgery. Before surgery it is important to administer propranolol to minimize the catecholamine effects and Lugol's solution to prevent the release of thyroid hormone. Propylthiouracil decreases the production as well as the peripheral conversion of T4 to T3. Subtotal thyroidectomy corrects the hyperthyroidism and helps with cosmesis by removing the goiter. Usually all but about 5 g of thyroid tissue is removed to avoid hypothyroidism. The mortality rate associated with the procedure is very low, less than 0.1%, and the risk of recurrent nerve injury is less than 2%.

147
Thyroid Nodules

Most thyroid nodules are composed of benign collections of colloid or adenomas. Solitary nodules of the thyroid are present in only 4% of the population. The evaluation of a thyroid nodule is aimed at ruling out thyroid cancer. The greatest risk factors for thyroid cancer are a personal history of low-dose head and neck radiation and a family history of thyroid cancer. Low-dose radiation (<2,000 rad) has been used in the past as therapy for a variety of conditions (e.g., acne, hemangiomas, ringworm, adenoids, enlarged thymus, and Hodgkin's lymphoma). The risk of thyroid cancer increases to 40% in patients with a thyroid nodule and a history of such radiation. Medullary thyroid cancer can be passed along by autosomal dominant inheritance. The familial form accounts for 25% of thyroid cancers (e.g., familial medullary thyroid cancer, multiple endocrine neoplasia [MEN] types 2a and 2b). The familial form is associated with a *RET* point mutation. Malignancy is more likely to occur in younger patients and in men.

Characteristics of malignant disease include hard, fixed lesions that are attached to surrounding structures such as the trachea or strap muscles. Malignancy occurs in about 15% of solitary lesions. In contrast, multinodular lesions are less likely to be malignant. The presence of palpable cervical lymphadenopathy suggests metastasis and therefore malignancy. Rapid enlargement of the nodule along with symptoms of invasion (hoarseness due to vocal cord paralysis) and compression (stridor, dyspnea, or dysphagia) are indications for possible malignancy.

The evaluation begins with a physical examination to determine whether the nodule is solitary or multiple. Cervical lymphadenopathy may be detected as well as possible deviations of the trachea. Fine-needle aspiration (FNA) is the first test employed. Results of FNA are classified as benign, intermediate (suspicious for malignancy), malignant, or nondiagnostic. Approximately 65% of biopsy specimens are benign, with malignant diagnoses comprising 5%. The technique is limited in certain instances. Patients with previous head and neck radiation or familial thyroid cancer tend to have multifocal disease, which makes FNA less reliable. The differentiation between follicular adenoma and follicular carcinoma cannot be made without evidence of capsular or vascular invasion. This is not possible with FNA.

Ultrasound is useful for evaluating nonpalpable lesions and lymphadenopathy and for distinguishing cystic from solid lesions. It is also used in the follow-up evaluation of patients with benign disease. Computed tomography and magnetic resonance imaging are used to detect the involvement of adjacent structures as well as to evaluate large lesions or substernal lesions. Magnetic resonance imaging is better at differentiating ongoing disease from post-treatment fibrosis.

Radionucleotide imaging is used to evaluate the functional activity of a nodule and to confirm its location. In this test, radioactive iodine (^{123}I) is administered. Nodules are defined as hot or cold depending on the amount of radioactive substrate that they take up. Cold nodules have less uptake of ^{123}I than the surrounding tissue. Approximately 85% of nodules are determined to be cold and have a 25% risk of being malignant. Hot nodules take up more ^{123}I than the surrounding tissue. These lesions comprise only 5% of cases and have a 1% risk of malignancy.

Thyroid function tests are not a part of the routine evaluation. Most thyroid cancers are found in euthyroid patients; therefore, laboratory tests are of little value. However, hyperthyroidism with a thyroid nodule is associated with a lower risk of malignancy. Serum thyroglobulin levels are measured to assess patients during nonoperative treatment or after total thyroidectomy. Serum calcitonin level measurements are useful for patients with a family history of medullary thyroid cancer or MEN 2.

Conservative treatment is recommended for thyroid nodules identified as benign by FNA. Ultrasound evaluation is conducted to establish a size baseline. A baseline thyroglobulin level is obtained as well. Thyroid-stimulating hormone (TSH) suppression is effective in size reduction in 50% of cases. This involves the administration of thyroxine to cause a negative feedback inhibition of TSH from the pituitary. Thyroidectomy is only indicated for nodules that are refractory to TSH suppression, continue to enlarge, or begin to produce symptoms.

Thyroid cysts are treated with aspiration of the cyst. Several aspirations may be needed. Thyroid lobectomy is indicated for cysts that require more than three aspirations, cysts that are 4 cm or greater, and cysts with complex features.

A patient who has symptoms of compression or invasion, a rapidly expanding lesion, or lymphadenopathy should undergo a thyroid lobectomy. Patients with a thyroid nodule confirmed to be thyroid cancer should have a total thyroidectomy.

148
Thyroiditis

The term *thyroiditis* describes a diverse group of disorders that result in inflammation of the thyroid gland. The etiology ranges from autoimmune to infectious. Endocrine dysfunction of the thyroid gland may be associated with the disorder, and it could result in hypothyroidism or hyperthyroidism.

The infectious variety of thyroiditis can be acute or chronic. The usual route of spread is through hematogenous seeding into the gland. Common microbial agents include *Staphylococcus, Pneumococcus, Salmonella,* mycobacteria, fungi, and *Pneumocystis* organisms. Congenital abnormalities of the thyroid gland such as thyroglossal duct fistula, immunocompromised states, and underlying autoimmune disorders may render an individual more susceptible to infection. The classic clinical presentation is sudden onset of neck pain associated with fever. Pain on swallowing that radiates to the ear is also characteristic. Ultrasound evaluation may reveal abscess within the thyroid. Needle aspiration and culture may aid in isolating the causative organism. The infectious variety is generally treated with antibiotics directed against the causative organism.

Hashimoto's thyroiditis is the most common cause of hypothyroidism. It is named after a physician who described it in 1912. It is an autoimmune disorder that gradually leads to destruction of the thyroid gland. Like most of the thyroid disorders, the disease is more prevalent in women and typically affects patients between the ages of 45 and 65 years. In adolescents, 40% of goiters are from autoimmune thyroiditis. Patients with Hashimoto's thyroiditis have an increased risk of developing other forms of autoimmune disorders, such as type 1 diabetes, lupus, myasthenia gravis, and Sjögren's syndrome. In Hashimoto's thyroiditis, the immune system reacts against various thyroid antigens. The pathologic hallmark of the disease is the gradual depletion of thyroid epithelial cells and replacement with mononuclear cell infiltration. Fibrosis of the gland is characteristic as well. Destruction of the thyroid cells takes place through combined cell- and antibody-mediated pathways. Antithyroid-stimulating hormone receptor, antithyroglobulin, and antithyroid peroxidase antibodies are often detected. Pathologic characteristics include diffuse glandular enlargement, extensive parenchymal infiltration with mononuclear cells, and atrophic thyroid follicles. Characteristic eosinophilic, granular epithelial cells are found lining the atrophic follicles called *Hürthle cells*. Fibrosis may also be present in Hashimoto's thyroiditis, but, in contrast to Riedel's thyroiditis, it does not extend beyond the capsule of the thyroid gland into the surrounding structures.

Approximately 20% of patients with Hashimoto's thyroiditis present with signs and symptoms of hypothyroidism; a few patients present with hyperthyroidism (hashitoxicosis). Most patients are euthyroid when the diagnosis is made. The most common presenting symptom is tightness in the throat, often associated with a painless, nontender enlargement of the thyroid gland. Rapid enlargement of the thyroid gland should raise suspicion of thyroid lymphoma or carcinoma. Palpation usually demonstrates a diffusely enlarged, firm thyroid gland. Usually the pyramidal lobe is enlarged. In early cases of Hashimoto's thyroiditis, patients may present with a transient rise in serum thyroid hormone levels; however, as the disease progresses, the serum thyroid-stimulating hormone (TSH) level rises as serum thyroxine (T4) and triiodothyronine (T3) levels fall. The diagnosis is confirmed by the presence of circulating antithyroid antibodies. These antibodies are directed against the membrane-bound enzyme involved in thyroid hormone synthesis, thyroid peroxidase (TPO), formerly called *antimitochondrial antibodies*, in almost 100% of patients and against thyroglobulin in about 50% of patients. Fine-needle aspiration of the thyroid gland occasionally is useful in confirming the diagnosis of Hashimoto's thyroiditis or for patients in whom malignancy is suspected.

In the absence of compressive symptoms, patients demonstrating goiter, with or without evidence of hypothyroidism, are best treated with thyroid hormone. Thyroid goiter size is usually reduced with thyroxine treatment. Surgical intervention is indicated for patients complaining of obstructive symptoms, for cosmetically unacceptable goiters, or when thyroid cancer other than lymphoma is found on needle aspiration. Thyroxine therapy with long-term follow-up monitoring of TSH levels is recommended.

Subacute thyroiditis, also called *granulomatous thyroiditis* or *De Quervain thyroiditis*, is a less common variant of thyroiditis. It is thought to be caused by viral infection. Again, the disorder affects mostly women aged 30 to 50 years. A preceding history of upper respiratory infection is common for most patients. Associations have been reported with mumps, measles, coxsackievirus, and adenovirus. In the pathogenesis of the disease, it is speculated that viral-induced tissue damage of the thyroid gland releases an antigen. As a result, cytotoxic T lymphocytes react to the antigen, leading to thyroid follicular cell destruction. The presentation of the disease can be insidious or sudden, characterized by neck pain, fever, fatigue, malaise, myalgia, and anorexia. Some patients complain of the symptoms of thyrotoxicosis, including palpitations, sweating, and heat intolerance, which are caused by the release of thyroid hormones from disrupted follicles in the inflamed thyroid gland. Palpation of the thyroid gland may show a tender, firm gland with mild unilateral or bilateral enlargement. Laboratory tests usually demonstrate an elevated erythrocyte sedimentation rate (ESR) associated with a neutrophilia. Thyroid function tests often reveal elevated levels of thyroid hormones (T4 and T3) with suppression of TSH. However, as the disease resolves, thyroid hormone levels return to normal. In contrast to Graves' disease, radioiodine uptake in the acute stage of the disease is low. This is because the released thyroid hormone, a result of inflammation, suppresses the serum TSH concentration.

Treatment with nonsteroidal anti-inflammatory drugs (NSAIDs) for pain relief is all that is required in most cases of subacute thyroiditis. In the early stages of the disease, the use of β-blocking agents may be useful for alleviating the thyrotoxic symptoms. For severe cases, it may be necessary to prescribe steroids for short periods. Prednisone 40 mg once daily for 1 to 2 weeks, followed by a gradual reduction of the dose, is recommended for such cases.

Subacute lymphocytic thyroiditis, also called *painless thyroiditis*, is a rare form of thyroiditis occurring in postpartum women. The exact cause is unknown; however, evidence suggests an autoimmune etiology due to the presence of antithyroglobulin and antithyroid peroxidase antibodies. Clinically, patients may present with palpitations, tachycardia, tremor, weakness, and fatigue. Unlike the previously discussed forms, this variant does not present with localized pain in the neck. Symptoms may take 1 to 2 weeks to develop and then last 2 to 8 weeks before disappearing. Laboratory tests reveal elevated T3 and T4 levels with decreased TSH level. Histologically, there can be minimal gland enlargement with lymphocytic infiltration within the thyroid parenchyma.

Riedel's thyroiditis is rare and occurs mainly in middle-aged women. The chief element of the disease is marked fibrosis of the thyroid gland along with adjacent structures. Fibrosis in other areas of the body, such as the retroperitoneum, can occur as well. The onset is insidious, causing symptoms of compression to adjacent structures, including the trachea, esophagus, and recurrent laryngeal nerve. The thyroid usually appears asymmetrically enlarged and hard. This can be easily confused with carcinoma. Hypothyroidism can be associated with Riedel's thyroiditis, but this is rather unusual. Surgical resection may be required to prevent encroachment of the trachea or esophagus. Treatment consists of thyroid hormone replacement for cases associated with hypothyroidism.

149
Thyroid Malignancies

Most thyroid neoplasms consist of well-differentiated follicular cell–derived tumors (e.g., papillary thyroid carcinoma, follicular cell thyroid carcinoma, and Hürthle cell carcinoma). Medullary thyroid cancers arise from the parafollicular cells, which are of neural crest origin. Anaplastic thyroid cancer is a very rare but aggressive malignancy, which has few treatment options and a poor prognosis. Most thyroid malignancies occur in patients who are euthyroid. Only 2% of thyroid malignancies are associated with hyperthyroidism.

Papillary Carcinoma

The most common thyroid malignancy is papillary thyroid carcinoma (70% to 80% of cases). The lesion occurs predominantly in young women (<40 years old). The risk of thyroid cancer development increases with radiation exposure (therapeutic or environmental).

The typical microscopic finding is papillary structures composed of follicular cells. The cells have characteristic intranuclear inclusion bodies and cellular grooving. Psammoma bodies are calcified cells that result from sloughing of papillary structures. Psammoma bodies are pathognomonic for papillary thyroid carcinoma. Subtypes of papillary carcinoma exist but are rarely seen (<1% of papillary carcinomas). These include columnar, insular, and tall cell variants. These lesions tend to be more aggressive in behavior and occur in older persons.

The most common manifestation is a painless solitary mass. Evaluation generally consists of ultrasound to determine whether the mass is solid or cystic and to search for other nodules. Solid lesions that are identified in the thyroid and palpable lymph nodes should undergo biopsy by fine-needle aspiration (FNA). This is a reliable means of evaluation, because the diagnosis can be made based on the cellular architecture of the individual cells.

Individual cases of papillary thyroid carcinoma are ranked as low risk or high risk based on the patient's age,

metastasis, extent of primary lesion, and tumor size (characteristics included in the AMES/AGES classification system; Table 149.1). Low-risk lesions have a more favorable prognosis following surgical resection (5- to 10-year survival rates of >90%). Recurrence rates for low-risk lesions are approximately 5% to 11% compared with 48% for high-risk lesions. The mortality rate for low-risk lesions is 0.07% to 5% compared with 48% for high-risk lesions.

The mainstay of treatment is surgical resection. The degree of resection depends on the size of the tumor and on the patient's age and radiation exposure. Lymph node metastasis is more prevalent in the younger group. In fact, lymph node involvement occurs in as many as 90% of patients aged 15 years or younger with papillary thyroid carcinoma. Total thyroidectomy plus lymph node dissection is recommended for this group of patients. Older patients with a history of neck irradiation have an increased incidence of multifocal disease and a higher incidence of thyroid cancer arising elsewhere in the gland. Therefore, total thyroidectomy is recommended for these patients. Lesions less than 1 cm without palpable lymphadenopathy require only a thyroid lobectomy and isthmusectomy. Recurrence rates are reported to be <5% in these cases, with a mortality rate of 0.1%. Lesions less than 2 cm occurring in patients between ages 15 and 40 years can be treated with a lobectomy plus isthmusectomy, when the lesion involves only one lobe, or by total thyroidectomy. The advantages of total thyroidectomy include a lower incidence of local recurrence, improved efficacy of postoperative ^{131}I ablation, and avoidance of reoperation and the associated complications with recurrence. Total thyroidectomy is recommended for lesions <2 cm. A modified radical neck dissection must be added to any of the above procedures when palpable lymphadenopathy is present.

Adjunct therapies for well-differentiated thyroid carcinomas include radioiodine remnant ablation, supple-

TABLE 149.1. AMES/AGES tumor classification system.

	Low risk	High risk
Age	<40 years	>40 years
Sex	Female	Male
Extent of tumor	No local extension or capsular invasion. Lesion confined to thyroid	Invasion of capsule or extension beyond thyroid
Metastasis	None	Regional, distant
Tumor size	<2 cm	>4 cm
Histologic grade	Well differentiated	Poorly differentiated

mental thyroid hormone, and radioiodine therapy. Radioiodine remnant ablation involves the administration of low-dose ^{131}I to destroy microscopic remnants of disease. This therapy is indicated for lesions >1.5 cm, cases associated with lymph node metastasis, invasive follicular cell thyroid cancer, and Hürthle cell cancer. Patients are placed on a 2 μg/kg dose of thyroid hormone after ablation therapy. Supplemental thyroid hormone acts to suppress thyroid-stimulating hormone (TSH), which promotes tumor growth, invasion, and angiogenesis.

Recurrent disease is evaluated using ultrasound or computed tomography (CT) scan of the neck. Distant metastasis can be detected using chest x-ray, radioactive iodine scans, or CT. Serum levels of thyroglobulin are monitored during the postoperative period. Completion thyroidectomy should be undertaken for residual thyroid tissue. Lymphadenectomy is done for recurrence within regional or local lymph node groups. Distant metastases and lymphatic metastases can also be treated with high-dose ^{131}I therapy.

Follicular Carcinoma

Follicular thyroid cancer predominantly affects older women. The neoplasm develops from thyroid epithelium. Clinically, patients seek medical attention for a painless solitary thyroid nodule or a rapidly growing nodule in a pre-existing multinodular goiter. Lymphatic involvement and multifocal disease are rare with these lesions (10%), in contrast to papillary carcinoma. However, follicular carcinoma is capable of hematogenous spread to the lungs and bones. Histologic evaluation shows follicular cell invasion of the capsule, the lymphatic system, and vasculature. Lesions that do not show invasion of the above structures are simply follicular adenomas and not carcinomas. Follicular carcinoma is classified into two forms: minimally invasive and widely invasive.

Ultrasound is used to determine both the size of the lesion and if multifocal disease is present. Radioactive iodine scans will demonstrate a cold hypofunctioning nodule. Computed tomography or magnetic resonance imaging (MRI) can evaluate for possible local extension of the tumor. Fine-needle aspiration obtains tissue for cytologic evaluation. The diagnosis of follicular thyroid cancer is made by looking only at the histologic architecture of the tissue and demonstrating invasion of the capsule or lymphatics. In this case, FNA can determine only that the lesion is composed of a follicular neoplasm and not that the lesion is invasive. Intraoperative frozen sections tend to be inadequate also.

Surgical resection is the primary form of treatment. Lesions >2 cm that are contained in one lobe are amenable to thyroid lobectomy plus isthmusectomy. Lesions >4 cm are malignant in 50% of cases. These lesions require a total thyroidectomy. Lymph node dissections are only required if there is palpable lymphadenopathy. Radioablative ^{131}I therapy is used postoperatively as an adjunct. Serum thyroglobulin levels are measured postoperatively to monitor for recurrences. The situation may arise where the final pathologic diagnosis determines the lesion to be an invasive follicular carcinoma. Completion thyroidectomy may be needed in addition to radioiodine ablation.

Hürthle Cell Carcinoma

Hürthle cell carcinoma is a variant of follicular thyroid cancer. The lesions contain a large number of oxyphilic cells. Hürthle cell tumors differ from follicular cell tumors in that they have a higher rate of regional lymph node recurrence. Fine-needle aspiration is inadequate when attempting to make the diagnosis just as in follicular cell carcinoma. The treatment for Hürthle cell lesions is the same as for follicular cell cancer.

Medullary Carcinoma

Medullary thyroid cancer develops from the parafollicular C-cells that originate from neural crest cells. These tumors produce calcitonin but do not cause hypocalcemia. The tumors may exist in either sporadic forms (75%) or familial forms (25%; multiple endocrine neoplasia [MEN] 2a or 2b). Sporadic lesions are generally limited to one lobe of the thyroid, whereas hereditary forms tend to involve both lobes and are often associated with C-cell hyperplasia. Sporadic forms may present as a palpable mass or as an elevation of calcitonin levels. Fine-needle aspiration and demonstration of elevated calcitonin levels are used to make the diagnosis. Screening should be done to rule out the possibility of pheochromocytoma using 24-hour urine collection for catecholamines. Screening should also include evaluation for hyperparathyroidism and genetic evaluations for *ret* proto-oncogene mutations.

Sporadic lesions are treated with total thyroidectomy with central lymph node dissection. Modified radical neck dissections are indicated when cervical nodal groups are clinically involved with disease. Adjunct radioiodine ablation therapy is not used for these lesions. Patients are monitored postoperatively for recurrence by measuring basal and stimulated calcitonin levels. Elevated calcitonin levels may indicate the presence of distant metastasis (bones, lungs, liver) or local recurrence. Ultrasound of the neck is used to evaluate for local recurrence.

Anaplastic Carcinoma

Anaplastic thyroid cancer comprises 2% to 6% of thyroid cancers. These cancers are the most aggressive of thyroid cancers. They arise *de novo* or from a well-differentiated lesion. The 5-year survival rate is estimated at 3.6%, with a median survival rate of 4 months. These tumors manifest most often as a rapidly expanding thyroid mass in an older patient (60 years). Tumor necrosis may cause areas of fluctuance. Most tumors are >5 cm by the time the diagnosis is made. Symptoms of hoarseness, dyspnea, dysphagia, and neck pain are common because of direct invasion into surrounding structures. Superior vena cava syndrome is another possible presentation. The diagnosis is made primarily through FNA showing giant cells with intranuclear cytoplasmic invaginations.

No single form of adequate therapy exists. Many medical centers combine surgical resection, radiation, and chemotherapy. These combination treatments may improve local disease control but have no effect on long-term survival. Complete surgical excision is often difficult to accomplish because of local invasion into the surrounding tissues. Short-term survival may be improved with partial resection, but without improvement of long-term survival. The only beneficial surgical procedure is a palliative tracheostomy, used when external tracheal compression occurs.

Lymphoma

Primary thyroid lymphoma makes up <1% of thyroid cancers. Non-Hodgkin's B cell lymphoma is the most common type. Often there is association with Hashimoto's thyroiditis (70 to 80 times greater than in the normal population). Patients are usually women in the seventh decade of life. The common presentations are a rapidly enlarging neck mass, hoarseness, dysphagia, and fever. On physical examination, the mass is firm to palpation and may demonstrate unilateral or bilateral involvement. Ultrasound examination may reveal a pseudocystic pattern. Tissue diagnosis is achieved with FNA. Core needle biopsies are implemented when FNA fails to provide the diagnosis. Computed tomography or MRI of the neck, chest, and abdomen evaluates spread beyond the thyroid.

The treatment of choice is a combination of radiation therapy along with chemotherapy (CHOP—cyclophosphamide, doxorubicin, vincristine, and prednisone). Thyroidectomy is seldom needed.

150
Calcium Physiology

Calcium is one of the essential elements of the body. Calcium plays a principal role in bone structure, the excitation of plasma membranes, the activity of plasma enzymes, and the function of extracellular and intracellular signaling molecules (e.g., calmodulin, protein kinase C). The average adult body contains approximately 1 to 2 kg of calcium. Most is stored in bone and teeth (99%), and the remainder is present in soft tissues and in the extracellular space (1%). Plasma calcium is bound to plasma proteins (albumin) 40% of the time. The remainder is bound to plasma anions (10%) or is in a free ionized form (50%). The plasma distribution of calcium is affected by protein concentrations and the pH. Intracellular Ca^{2+} is found within the endoplasmic reticulum and mitochondria. Active transport mechanisms (i.e., Ca^{2+} ATPase pumps and NA^+/Ca^{2+} ion exchangers) maintain low intracellular levels of Ca^{2+}, creating a gradient across the plasma membrane. The daily dietary intake of Ca^{2+} is estimated at 600 to 800 mg per day. The intestine absorbs about 25% of the daily dietary intake. Ten percent of absorption is accomplished passively; the remainder is done by active transport mediated by $1\alpha,25(OH)_2$ D, an active vitamin D metabolite. Intestinal absorption can be increased in conditions such as low dietary intake, rapid growth, pregnancy, and lactation.

The ionized form of Ca^{2+} (iCa^{2+}) is biologically active and is regulated by extracellular iCa^{2+}, parathyroid hormone (PTH), vitamin D, and calcitonin. These mediators act on the kidneys, the intestine, and the bone to effect changes in serum iCa^{2+} levels. Low iCa^{2+} levels stimulate the increase of parathyroid cell size and numbers. Upregulation of parathyroid synthesis takes place in addition to the increased release of preformed hormone. Parathyroid hormone has direct and indirect effects on the kidneys, bone, and intestine. It stimulates increased Ca^{2+} ion reabsorption in the distal tubules of the kidney. It also stimulates the activity of $25(OH)D_3$ 1α-hydroxylase, the enzyme responsible for $1\alpha,25(OH)_2$ D synthesis.

Other actions include the decrease of phosphate and bicarbonate reabsorption. Parathyroid hormone has indirect effects on the intestine, which are mediated through $1\alpha,25(OH)_2$ D. $1\alpha,25(OH)_2$ D stimulates the intestinal absorption of dietary calcium. Parathyroid hormone stimulates osteoclast activity and inhibits osteoblast activity leading to bone resorption in excess of bone formation. Calcitonin is secreted by the parafollicular C-cells of the thyroid gland. Calcitonin has the ability to inhibit osteoclasts and bone resorption but does not play a significant role in the regulation of calcium. Vitamin D is synthesized from 7-dehydrocholesterol in the epidermis. The reaction is catalyzed by ultraviolet rays. From there the product $25(OH)D$ is converted to its active form ($1\alpha,25[OH]_2$ D) in the proximal tubules of the kidney. $1\alpha,25(OH)_2$ D, better known as *calcitriol*, works in a manner similar to other steroid hormones by binding to intracellular receptors.

Hypercalcemia

Hypercalcemia is defined as an abnormal increase in serum ionized calcium levels. Primary hyperparathyroidism is the most common cause of hypercalcemia. The effect is mediated through elevations in PTH as well as $1\alpha,25(OH)_2$ D, causing increased Ca^{2+} resorption from the bone and decreased elimination through the kidney. Malignancy is the primary cause of hypercalcemia in the hospitalized patient. The effect is caused by lytic lesions in the bone causing destruction and the release of calcium stores and through paraneoplastic syndromes. Other causes include immobilization, vitamin D excess, renal failure, and milk-alkali syndrome.

Gastrointestinal manifestations consist of anorexia, constipation, peptic ulcer disease, pancreatitis, and gallstones. Depression, lethargy, and seizures are all neurologic symptoms that can accompany hyperparathyroidism. Severe cases can manifest with coma or death.

Neuromuscular weakness and fatigue are also common complaints. Cardiovascular changes include hypertension and calcification of the aortic or mitral valves. Renal symptoms consist of increased urinary frequency, nocturia, and polydipsia. These effects are caused by the antagonism of antidiuretic hormone by hypercalcemia. Nephrolithiasis with formation of calcium oxalate or calcium phosphate stones frequently occurs. In addition, nephrocalcinosis, which involves calcification of the renal parenchyma, also occurs.

Parathyroid hormone measurements are obtained from the patient's serum to determine if the condition is due to hyperparathyroidism. Serum ionized Ca^{2+} levels, serum phosphate levels, and urinary Ca^{2+} levels are obtained. Blood urea nitrogen and creatinine levels can reveal underlying renal dysfunction. If the PTH level is elevated, the patient should be questioned about possible links to hereditary forms of hyperparathyroidism (i.e., multiple endocrine neoplasia syndromes). If the PTH is low, then other non-PTH–mediated causes for hypercalcemia should be investigated (history, physical examination, and radiographs).

The initial management for hypercalcemia involves medical treatment aimed to increase the elimination of calcium. Administration of isotonic saline along with loop diuretics is usually the first step taken. Patients who fail to respond to diuresis may require bone resorption–inhibiting agents such as bisphosphonates (i.e., pamidronate and zoledronic acid), calcitonin, mithramycin, and gallium nitrate. Cases caused by vitamin D excess may respond to glucocorticoids.

Hypocalcemia

Hypocalcemia is defined as abnormally decreased serum iCa^{2+} levels. Low Ca^{2+} levels alter transmembrane depolarization and ultimately result in central nervous system dysfunction. Clinical manifestations include distal extremity paresthesias, perioral numbness, and muscle spasms. Facial muscle spasm caused by percussion of the facial nerve is Chvostek's sign. Trousseau's sign is defined as carpopedal spasm caused after inflation of a blood pressure cuff above the brachial artery. Cardiac involvement is demonstrated by a prolonged QT interval that can lead to ventricular fibrillation or heart block.

There are numerous causes for hypocalcemia. Iatrogenic causes include parathyroid or thyroid surgery, citrate overload through the infusion of blood products, and phosphate overload from phosphate-containing drugs (e.g., enemas). Vitamin D deficiencies from malabsorption or liver disease can cause hypocalcemia as well. Hypocalcemia is seen in a constellation of biochemical abnormalities that go along with tumor lysis syndrome. Hypocalcemia is treated medically with administration of supplemental Ca^{2+} and vitamin D.

151
Hyperparathyroidism

Hyperparathyroidism is divided into three major classes (primary, secondary, and tertiary) based on the etiology. Central to all forms of hyperparathyroidism is the hypersecretion of parathyroid hormone (PTH). Parathyroid hormone is produced from the chief cells of the parathyroid gland. Parathyroid regulates the serum calcium level, and secretion is directed by the serum phosphorous and calcium levels. Elevated phosphorous level stimulates PTH production. Likewise, decreased serum calcium level causes stimulation of PTH.

Clinical manifestations involve derangements in the musculoskeletal system, urinary tract, gastrointestinal tract, central nervous system, and cardiac system. Skeletal manifestations involve bone pain, pathologic fractures, and osteoporosis. Elevated PTH causes increased osteoclast activity and calcium resorption of bone. Morphologic changes in the bone occur, such as thin trabeculae that resemble osteoporosis and fibrosis of the bone marrow with hemorrhage and cyst formation (osteitis fibrosa cystica). Brown tumors of hyperparathyroidism are composed of giant cells, osteoclasts, and hemorrhage. Renal symptoms consist of increased urinary frequency, nocturia, and polydipsia. Nephrolithiasis with formation of calcium oxalate or calcium phosphate stones frequently occurs. In addition, nephrocalcinosis, which involves calcification of the renal parenchyma, also occurs. Gastrointestinal manifestations consist of constipation, peptic ulcer disease, pancreatitis, and gallstones. Depression, lethargy, and seizures are all neurologic symptoms that can accompany hyperparathyroidism. Neuromuscular weakness and fatigue are also common complaints. Cardiovascular changes include hypertension and calcification of the aortic or mitral valves.

Primary Hyperparathyroidism

Primary hyperparathyroidism can be caused by parathyroid adenoma (~80%), primary hyperplasia (~15%), and parathyroid carcinoma (~5%). Sporadic forms are more prevalent than familial forms (e.g., multiple endocrine neoplasia [MEN] types 1 and 2 and familial hypocalciuric hypercalcemia). Primary hyperparathyroidism can present as an elevated serum calcium level that is noted during routine testing of an asymptomatic patient. The most common manifestation is a rise in the ionized serum calcium level. Primary hyperparathyroidism is the most common reason for calcium elevation in asymptomatic patients, whereas malignancy is the most common cause of symptomatic hypercalcemia. Evaluation involves measurement of serum ionized calcium and PTH. Other biochemical abnormalities are serum phosphate decrease or increase (with renal failure), hyperchloremic metabolic acidosis (due to renal bicarbonate wasting), and increased alkaline phosphatase. Osteopenia is evaluated by dual energy x-ray absorption scanning of the hip, lumbar spine, and forearm.

Parathyroid adenomas are the most common cause of primary hyperparathyroidism. The lesions are typically solitary, encapsulated, circumscribed nodules that weigh up to 5 g. The weight of a normal parathyroid is less than 50 mg. Chief cells make up the majority of the gland, and adipose tissue is decreased. Parathyroid hyperplasia occurs sporadically or in association with the MEN syndromes. Multiglandular hyperplasia is most common. Cell hyperplasia with a decrease in stromal fat can be seen histologically.

Carcinoma of the parathyroid comprises less than 5% of primary hyperparathyroidism cases. Cytologicparathyroid adenoma and carcinoma have the same appearance. Cytology samples fail to demonstrate tissue invasion, which is needed to confirm the diagnosis. Physically the lesions are well-circumscribed nodules that weigh as much as 10 g. Parathyroid carcinoma presents with more severe symptoms at an earlier age. Clinical symptoms include dehydration, nausea, vomiting, polyuria, and weight loss. A palpable neck mass is present in 50% of cases. Complete surgical resection offers the only chance for cure. Disease recurs in one third of patients and is treated by re-exploration and resection. Distant metastasis occurs in up to one third of patients.

Secondary and Tertiary Hyperparathyroidism

Chronic stimulation of normal parathyroid glands leads to hyperplasia of the glands and secondary hyperparathyroidism. The most common cause is chronic renal failure; other causes include decrease dietary intake of calcium, steatorrhea, and vitamin D deficiency. Chronic renal failure causes hyperparathyroidism by two mechanisms. First, renal failure causes hyperphosphatemia due to decreased phosphate excretion. Excess phosphate levels cause a decrease in serum calcium, which in turn stimulates PTH secretion. The second method involves decreased vitamin D production due to decreased 1α-hydroxylase associated with renal failure. Vitamin D deficiency reduces intestinal absorption of calcium. Tertiary disease is the consequence of long-standing overstimulation that results in altered feedback inhibition of the parathyroid cells. In this situation, PTH is secreted independent of the serum calcium concentration.

Medical management is aimed at resuscitation to correct dehydration, promote renal excretion of calcium, inhibit bone resorption, and correct the underlying pathology when possible. Normal saline is administered to correct dehydration and increase urine output. Loop diuretics such as furosemide are a given to promote diuresis and excretion of calcium. Medications such as calcitonin prevent calcium resorption from bone. Bisphosphonates directly inhibit osteoclast activity and therefore prevent bone resorption. Secondary hyperparathyroidism is controlled through the use of oral calcium and 1,25-D_3 supplementation. Dietary changes and the administration of oral phosphate binders (calcium acetate) are used to treat hyperphosphatemia.

Surgical Management

Symptomatic disease provides a clear indication for parathyroidectomy. Asymptomatic patients are generally followed and treated medically. Medical surveillance involves serum calcium measurement at 6-month intervals along with yearly bone mineral density evaluation. Indications for parathyroidectomy for asymptomatic patients include hypercalcemia in excess of 1 mg/dL above the upper limit of normal, hypercalciuria in excess of 400 mg/day, reduction of creatinine clearance 30% from normal, decreased bone mineral density, patients less than 50 years of age, and inability to comply with medical surveillance.

The standard procedure for surgical management involves an open parathyroidectomy through a transcervical incision. Preoperative localization studies are optional. The success rate without such studies is as high as 95% with a less than 2% rate of complications. The standard procedure is a bilateral neck exploration that can be conducted through general or locoregional anesthesia. Complete exploration involves the identification of all four glands. The four parathyroid glands are usually found in close relation to the thyroid gland. They can generally be identified on the posterolateral surface of the upper and inferior lobes. The superior parathyroid glands can typically be seen in close approximation with the posterior aspect of the middle and upper thirds of the thyroid gland. The position of the lower parathyroid glands is more variable; however, they are usually located anterior to the recurrent laryngeal nerves within 2 cm of the lower pole of the thyroid gland. The thyrothymic ligament is a thin area of tissue that connects the thyroid gland inferiorly with the thymus. This is another normal location for the inferior parathyroid glands.

Ectopic positions of the superior glands include the tracheoesophageal groove and also inferior to the inferior parathyroid glands. Other ectopic locations include the posterior or middle mediastinum. Ectopic positioning of the inferior glands is more common and more widely distributed than with superior glands. Thymic tissue is a common location for ectopic inferior glands. Ectopic sites range from an intrathymic parathyroid gland located in the anterosuperior mediastinum to an undescended inferior parathyroid gland (parathymus) located superior to the superior parathyroid gland. Undescended inferior glands are identified at the angle of the mandible anterior to the carotid artery. Some may even be found at the base of the skull.

The definitive surgical treatment depends on the disease pattern of the parathyroid glands. Single-gland enlargement may be a single adenoma. In this case, simple resection of the solitary enlarged gland is curative for most patients. Disease that consists of multiglandular enlargement can be approached in two ways. The standard method is to conduct a subtotal parathyroidectomy removing 3.5 glands. The incidence of postoperative hypocalcemia and permanent hypoparathyroidism is 0% to 16% and 4% to 5%, respectively. Patients with familial causes of hyperparathyroidism show a higher incidence of recurrent disease. The second method involves total parathyroidectomy with autotransplantation. This method involves selecting a portion of the parathyroid tissue for implantation. The selected tissue is diced into approximately 25 pieces to increase its surface area. Approximately 75 mg of the autograft is implanted into a muscle compartment (generally the forearm of the nondominant hand). The remainder of the parathyroid tissue is cryopreserved. This method is preferred over the subtotal method, because it allows for easier re-exploration and resection of the parathyroid tissue if postoperative hypercalcemia occurs. Postoperative hypocalcemia can be addressed by transplanting additional parathyroid tissue from the cryopreserved supply.

Operative treatment for secondary and tertiary disease is indicated by the failure of medical therapy and by the appearance of symptoms. In particular, the development of calciphylaxis and soft tissue calcifications are clear indications for parathyroidectomy. The surgical options are almost identical to those for multiglandular parathyroid disease described earlier. The only addition is complete cervical thymectomy to address supernumerary parathyroid glands that are associated with secondary and tertiary diseases (15% to 20%).

Minimally invasive variations of parathyroidectomy aim at reducing the amount of dissection involved in the surgical exploration. These techniques rely on preoperative localization studies and intraoperative biochemical detection of cure. Studies such as sestamibi scintigraphy or cervical ultrasound are used preoperatively to locate the lesion. Before the procedure, a baseline serum PTH measurement is obtained. The limited dissection is conducted based on preoperative localization studies to identify the suspected lesion. A second baseline measurement of PTH is obtained immediately before the gland is excised. A third PTH measurement is obtained 10 minutes following resection. A PTH level drop of 50% is indicative of adenoma removal.

152
Adrenal Physiology

The adrenal glands are responsible for the production of glucocorticoids (cortisol), mineralocorticoids (aldosterone), and androgens (estrogen, estradiol, progesterone, testosterone, dehydroepiandrosterone [DHEA]). The glands are located in the retroperitoneum at the upper pole of the kidneys. The glands are pyramidal shaped and are composed of an outer cortex and an inner medulla. The blood supply to the adrenal glands is derived from three sources: the inferior phrenic artery, the aorta, and the renal artery. Venous drainage from the right adrenal gland is accomplished by a central vein, which connects to the vena cava. The left adrenal gland drains directly into the left renal vein. The innervation of the adrenal gland is principally by preganglionic sympathetic fibers to the adrenal medulla. There is no known innervation to the adrenal cortex.

The adrenal cortex is composed of three distinct areas: the zona glomerulosa, the zona fasciculata, and the zona reticularis. The middle zona fasciculata comprises about 75% of the adrenal cortex. The cells in this zone are large with numerous lipid bodies. The reticularis is a small compact layer that has small compact cells. The zona fasciculata and reticularis synthesize glucocorticoids and androgens, whereas mineralocorticoids are produced in the zona glomerulosa. The adrenal medulla synthesizes catecholamines.

Each zone of the adrenal gland contains a cadre of specific enzymes responsible for the production of glucocorticoids, mineralocorticoids, or adrenal androgens. The job of synthesizing each specific steroid subtype is divided among the three zones of the cortex (glomerulosa, mineralocorticoids; fasciculata, glucocorticoids; reticularis, androgens). Steroid hormones are derived from cholesterol, which is gathered from plasma or synthesized in the adrenal cortex using acetyl coenzyme A.

The number of carbon atoms differs between the types of steroid produced (estrogens, 18 carbon atoms; androgens, 19 carbon atoms; and glucocorticoids, 21 carbon atoms). The common precursor (δ5-pregnenolone) is created from cholesterol in the adrenal mitochondria by an inner membrane enzyme known as CYP11A1.

δ5-Pregnenolone is the basic building block for all of the steroid hormones. After being produced in the mitochondria, δ5-pregnenolone is shuttled to the smooth endoplasmic reticulum where it can enter three different biochemical pathways. One of the key enzymes (17α-hydroxylase) responsible for cortisol and androgen production is present only in the inner zones of the cortex (zona fasciculata and zona reticularis). Glucocorticoids are produced by the zona fasciculata under the influence of adrenocorticotropic hormone (ACTH). 17α-Hydroxylase is required for synthesis of the precursors of cortisol and androgens 17-hydroxypregnenolone and 17-hydroxyprogesterone. This enzyme is absent in the zona glomerulosa, restricting the production of cortisol and androgens to the zonae fasciculata and reticularis.

Glucocorticoids

Glucocorticoid production is primarily under the influence of ACTH. Adrenocorticotropic hormone secretion follows a circadian rhythm in which levels are highest in the morning (5 a.m. to 9 a.m.) and decrease throughout the day, reaching the lowest levels during the evening (6 p.m. to midnight). Cortisol is bound to corticosteroid-binding globulin approximately 75% of the time. The remainder is either in a free form (10%) or bound to albumin (15%).

Steroid hormones exert their effects by altering the expression of specific genes. Steroid molecules bind to steroid receptors in the cytoplasm of the target cell. The steroid–receptor complex travels to the nucleus and binds to DNA, activating the transcription of specific genes. Cortisol plays an important role in many areas of peripheral metabolism. It plays an important role in the processing of protein, carbohydrates, and fat. To summarize, cortisol causes the mobilization of glucose (increased gluconeogenesis and decreased peripheral uptake) by stimulating glucagon and antagonizing insulin. This causes an elevation in blood glucose levels. Cortisol effectively decreases the production of protein and increases the breakdown of lipids. This increases the amount of raw materials delivered to the liver for gluconeogenesis. Cortisol regulates the intravascular volume by preventing the migration of free water into the cells, decreasing the permeability of capillaries, and stimulating angiotensinogen and inhibiting of prostaglandins. In addition, glucocorticoids have anti-inflammatory properties. Cortisol impairs interleukin-2 synthesis and effectively limits lymphocyte activation and migration.

Mineralocorticoids

The chief mineralocorticoid produced by the adrenal gland is aldosterone. Aldosterone synthesis and secretion are primarily influenced by the renin–angiotensin system, to a lesser extent by the serum K^+ level, and to an even lesser extent by ACTH. The outer portion of the adrenal cortex (zona glomerulosa) is responsible for the production of aldosterone.

The renin–angiotensin system works in the following way. Reduced blood flow to the kidney is the inciting event. Decreases in mean arterial pressure or depressions in serum Na^+ levels are detected by baroreceptors and chemoreceptors in the afferent renal arterioles. These two changes stimulate the secretion of renin from the juxtaglomerular apparatus. Renin from the renal vein converts angiotensinogen from the liver to angiotensin I. In the lungs, angiotensin I is converted to angiotensin II by angiotensin-converting enzyme (ACE). Angiotensin II is a potent vasoconstrictor of vascular smooth muscle. In addition to vasoconstriction, it also stimulates the release of aldosterone from the adrenal cortex. In turn, aldosterone causes the conservation of salt and water by the kidneys, resulting in increased extracellular volume. Increases in serum K^+ result in increased secretion of aldosterone. Similarly, decreases in serum K^+ result in decreased aldosterone secretion.

Adrenal Androgens

Androgen production from the adrenal glands comprises more than 50% of circulating androgens in the premenopausal female and only a small percentage in the male. Most androgens in the male are produced in the testicles. The adrenal gland produces three types of androgens; DHEA, DHEA sulfate, and testosterone. The secretion of adrenal androgens is stimulated by ACTH. The production of adrenal androgens depends on the activity of 3β-hydroxysteroid dehydrogenase (3β-HSD) and 17α-hydroxylase. Enzymes such as 3β-HSD and aromatase convert DHEA into active androgens or estrogens in peripheral tissues.

Adrenal Medullary Hormones

The cells in the adrenal medulla are responsible for the production and excretion of catecholamines. The chromaffin cells within the adrenal medulla take up the amino acid tyrosine and convert it to either norepinephrine or epinephrine. Newly formed catecholamines are stored within electron-dense granules along with adenosine triphosphate and other neuropeptides. The sympathetic nervous system is the primary stimulator of catecholamine release. Preganglionic sympathetic fibers terminate within the adrenal medulla. From there, acetylcholine is released from the synaptic end, stimulating the release of catecholamines from the adrenal medulla. Stresses such as exercise, hypoglycemia, trauma, and shock are common stimulants that lead to the release of catecholamines. Epinephrine and norepinephrine are released into the systemic blood system to interact with distal target cells. While in the circulation, the hormones are bound to albumin and other serum proteins. Their actions are mediated by interaction with membrane-bound adrenergic receptors. Adrenergic receptors are transmembrane proteins that are coupled to a class of intracellular-signaling molecules known as G-proteins. The receptors can be grouped into α- or β-subtypes. The varied subtypes of adrenergic receptors give rise to the different actions of catecholamines on specific tissues. The basic action of each receptor subtype is explained in Table 152.1.

Common physiologic responses to catecholamines include (1) vasoconstriction, (2) bronchial dilation, (3) lipolysis, (4) elevated metabolic rate (oxygen consumption, heat production, and muscle breakdown), (5) pupillary dilation, and (6) inhibition of gastrointestinal function and motor activity.

TABLE 152.1. The basic action of each receptor subtype.

Receptor	Agonist	Action	Tissue response
α_1	Epinephrine (E)/ norepinephrine (NE)	Increased Ca^{2+}	Increases contraction in vascular smooth muscle, increases heart rate, contracts the radial muscle of the eye, sphincter contraction in the gastrointestinal (GI) system
α_2	E/NE	Decreased cyclic adenosine monophosphate (cAMP)	Peripheral: regulates arterial and venous vascular tone, inhibits NE release, relaxes smooth muscle of the GI tract
β_1	E/NE	Increased CAMP	↑Cardiac contractility and rate, lipolysis in adipocytes, release of renin from kidney
β_2	E	Increased cAMP	Relaxes smooth muscle, vasodilation, bronchodilation, relaxation of bladder and uterus, stimulates liver gluconeogenesis and glycogenolysis
β_3			Lipolysis

153
Cushing's Syndrome

Glucocorticoid excess is responsible for Cushing's syndrome, which is most commonly caused by iatrogenic means. Other causes are classified as either adrenocorticotropic hormone (ACTH) dependent (pituitary or ectopic) or ACTH independent (primary adrenal). The clinical manifestations characteristic of the syndrome include truncal obesity, plethora, striae, proximal muscle weakness, buffalo hump, osteopenia, and hypertension. When Cushing's syndrome occurs in combination with systemic malignancy, patients exhibit mainly catabolic features. Features such as cachexia, hypokalemia, hypertension, and edema dominate the clinical picture.

Adrenocorticotropic hormone–dependent disease is derived from the pituitary or from an ectopic source. When the source of the syndrome stems from excess ACTH production from the pituitary, it is called *Cushing's disease*. Cushing's disease is the cause of up to 80% of all noniatrogenic cases. Ectopic sources arise from neoplasms outside the pituitary and account for only 10% of cases. Lung cancers, such as small cell and bronchial carcinoid, are generally the culprits. Other sources include medullary thyroid cancer, pheochromocytoma, and pancreatic islet tumors. Adrenocorticotropic hormone–independent causes include adrenal adenoma, adrenal cancer, and adrenal micronodular dysplasia. Adrenal adenomas are generally smaller than 4 cm in diameter and occur unilaterally. Most secrete only one hormone. In contrast, adrenal carcinomas tend to be large (>6 cm), unilateral, and are capable of secreting multiple hormones. Adenocarcinoma is distinguished from adenoma based on the size of the lesion, the types of hormones secreted, and the presence of metastasis. The hallmark of micronodular dysplasia is the presence of small multiple nodules that may be found bilaterally.

Findings are generally dramatic, but in subclinical cases the diagnosis may not be as apparent. When making the diagnosis, the first thing to establish is the presence of elevated cortisol level. This is best done by measuring a 24-hour free urinary cortisol level. The second issue is distinguishing between ACTH-dependent and ACTH-independent etiologies. There are several methods to accomplish this. A low-dose dexamethasone test can be useful to evaluate patients with incidental adrenalomas and subclinical disease. In this test, a low dose of dexamethasone is given at night, and a serum cortisol sample is drawn approximately 9 hours later. For a normal individual, the plasma cortisol level should be less than 3 to 5 µg/dL. Patients with Cushing's syndrome fail to suppress cortisol production. High-dose dexamethasone testing is done to distinguish between primary pituitary processes and ectopic causes. The theory behind the test is that primary pituitary causes will have some suppression when a high dose of dexamethasone is given. Plasma ACTH levels are useful to evaluate when trying to differentiate between dependent and independent causes.

Adrenal neoplasms secrete high levels of cortisol, which in turn suppress the level of ACTH from the pituitary through negative feedback. Pituitary tumors and ectopic sources generally cause high levels of ACTH.

The corticotropin-releasing hormone stimulation test is useful to evaluate pituitary versus ectopic causes. In this test, patients with a primary adrenal source show a small rise in ACTH. Patients with a pituitary source have an exaggerated response to exogenous ACTH; whereas ectopic sources should not cause a change. The source of ACTH secretion can also be determined by sampling venous blood from the inferior petrosal sinuses. Blood from the pituitary is drained back into the systemic circulation by way of the inferior petrosal sinuses into the internal jugular veins. During this test, catheters are inserted into the sinuses from femoral vein access. A simultaneous measurement of ACTH is taken from a peripheral venous site. A ratio between the inferior petrosal sinus ACTH and the peripheral blood is calculated. A ratio of 3:1 is indicative of Cushing's disease. A ratio of 1:8 is suggestive of an ectopic tumor. Corticotropin-releasing hormone is given to increase the sensitivity of the test.

Once the biochemical tests are complete, radiographic imaging is employed to localize the causative lesion. Magnetic resonance imaging (MRI) with gadolinium is helpful for visualizing pituitary tumors. Computed tomography or MRI can be used to evaluate possible chest lesions or adrenal masses.

The definitive treatment for pituitary microadenomas is transphenoidal resection. Cure rates approach 95% with this procedure. The recurrence rate is less than 5%, and half of these are amenable to repeated resection. Occasionally bilateral adrenalectomy may be required for failed transphenoidal resections.

Small unilateral adrenal lesions without metastasis should be resected by open or laparoscopic adrenalectomy. Large lesions should be approached through transabdominal laparotomy along with abdominal exploration and liver biopsy. Bilateral adrenalectomy is the treatment of choice for bilateral micronodular adrenal hyperplasia. Ectopic lesions should be excised when possible. Ketoconazole can be given for adrenal blockade when the source cannot be established or in the case of widespread metastasis.

154
Hyperaldosteronism

Aldosterone is a mineralocorticoid produced and secreted by the adrenal cortex. The function of the hormone is to regulate the exchange of sodium for potassium and hydrogen ions in the distal tubules of the kidney. The result of sodium retention produces an increase in fluid volume and blood pressure. Under normal circumstances aldosterone is under the control of the renin–angiotensin system. In the case of hyperaldosteronism, excess aldosterone results in hypernatremia, hypokalemia, and hypertension. Typical symptoms include malaise, muscle weakness, polyuria, polydipsia, cramps, and paresthesias. Hypertension may be severe and persist despite medical treatment. Diastolic hypertension may be more prevalent than systolic.

Causes of hyperaldosteronism are grouped into primary and secondary causes. The hallmark of primary hyperaldosteronism is that it occurs independent of the renin–angiotensin system. Examples include adrenal adenoma (aldosteronoma), idiopathic adrenocortical hyperplasia, and adrenocortical carcinoma. Secondary causes include renal vascular disease and cirrhosis with associated hypovolemia.

Hyperaldosteronism should be suspected in any hypertensive patient with concomitant hypokalemia. A key feature of primary hyperaldosteronism is elevated aldosterone with decreased renin levels. Secondary hyperaldosteronism is characterized by an increase in aldosterone as well as renin. A series of screening tests will help to confirm the diagnosis. All antihypertensive and diuretic medications must be stopped prior to evaluation. The first test done should be a 24-hour urinary potassium measurement. Patients with primary hyperaldosteronism have high levels of urinary potassium ($>30\,mEq/24\,hr$). In addition, a ratio of plasma aldosterone and renin must be obtained. A ratio of 30 or more is confirmatory. Captopril can be given to reduce plasma aldosterone levels. However, it has no effect on primary hyperaldosteronism.

After confirming the diagnosis of primary hyperaldosteronism, the differentiation must be made between aldosteronoma, idiopathic hyperplasia, and adrenal carcinoma. Computed tomography can be used to identify most aldosteronomas 1 cm or greater. Findings suggestive of primary hyperaldosteronism include an adenoma in one gland and atrophy of the contralateral gland. For lesions greater than 3 cm, adrenocortical carcinoma should be suspected.

Nuclear medicine tests such as an iodocholesterol scan can be used as an adjunct to computed tomography. The tests should demonstrate which glands are hyperfunctioning by showing the increased uptake of radioactive material. In the case of idiopathic hyperplasia, both glands will show increased activity. A more invasive approach involves selective sampling of adrenal veins for aldosterone. An aldosteronoma will increase secretion of aldosterone in response to adrenocorticotropic hormone administration. The unilateral increase in aldosterone level suggests the presence of an aldosteronoma. Bilateral elevation suggests idiopathic adrenal hyperplasia.

Surgical resection is the treatment of choice for aldosteronoma. Most are small benign lesions amenable to laparoscopic resection. Idiopathic adrenal hyperplasia is best treated medically. Spironolactone and potassium-sparing diuretics such as amiloride have proven to be effective.

155
Pheochromocytoma

Pheochromocytomas are catecholamine-producing tumors derived from chromaffin cells. The tumors are primarily located in the adrenal medulla (90%) but can also occur outside the adrenal gland. The rule of 10s is used to characterize the disease (10% bilateral, 10% extra-adrenal, 10% in children, 10% familial, and 10% malignant). The hallmarks of presentation include hypertension, severe headaches, palpitations, and diaphoresis. The symptoms often occur episodically due to episodic release of catecholamines.

Hypertension may be sustained, paroxysmal, or absent in some patients. Cardiovascular changes are caused by increased vascular resistance mediated by increased sympathetic tone. Decreased intravascular volume often accompanies the cardiovascular changes, which can manifest as orthostatic hypotension. Other associated symptoms include anxiety, flushing, pallor, nausea, and tremors. Complications of pheochromocytoma include dilated cardiomyopathy, myocardial infarction, arrhythmias, stroke, and decreased gastrointestinal transit. Hypertensive crisis is a potentially life-threatening complication. Pheochromocytomas can be of hereditary or sporadic origin; most are of the sporadic form. Familial forms are associated with hereditary diseases such as multiple endocrine neoplasia type 2 (MEN 2), von Hippel-Lindau disease, and von Recklinghausen's neurofibromatosis. Familial pheochromocytomas occur bilaterally more often than sporadic cases.

Extra-adrenal pheochromocytomas, also called *functional paragangliomas*, can occur in sympathetic ganglia anywhere from the neck to the bladder. The most common extra-adrenal site is the organ of Zuckerkandl. Norepinephrine is the predominant catecholamine secreted by these tumors because of their lack of the enzyme phenyl ethanolamine N-methyl transferase (PMNT).

Overall, pheochromocytoma is a rare cause of hypertension, accounting for less than 1% of hypertensive cases. Therefore, evaluation is indicated when hypertension is associated with headaches, palpitations, and diaphoresis. It is also indicated for cases refractory to medical therapy, for cases associated with incidentalomas, for hypertensive crises precipitated by anesthesia, surgery, or ionic contrast administration, or for a family history of pheochromocytoma, MEN 2, neurofibromatosis, von Hippel-Lindau disease, or labile blood pressure.

Biochemical testing is the mainstay of evaluation. Testing consists of 24-hour urine collection for measurement of catecholamines, metanephrines, and vanillylmandelic acid (VMA). Plasma measurements of catecholamines and metanephrines can be done as well. Computed tomography (CT) or magnetic resonance imaging (MRI) is useful for locating the lesion after biochemical tests have confirmed the diagnosis. Computed tomography can detect lesions 1 cm or greater. Contrast agents are not needed and should be avoided to prevent hypertensive emergency. Magnetic resonance imaging may provide more specificity than CT. Nuclear medicine studies such as ^{131}I-metaiodobenzylguanidine (^{131}I-MIBG) scans or octreotide scans can aid in localizing extra-adrenal disease. ^{131}I-Metaiodobenzylguanidine works on the premise that uptake into chromaffin tissues will reveal the site of the tumor. Iodine preparations administered before and after testing prevent thyroid uptake. Octreotide labeled with ^{111}In-D-phe1-octreotide binds to somatostatin receptors within the tumor. This modality can detect extra-adrenal disease as well as metastasis. Positron emission tomography scans with 6-^{18}F-fluorodopamine have been used recently.

Surgical resection is the treatment of choice. Adrenalectomy can be accomplished through a transabdominal incision (for bilateral tumors) or a flank incision or laparoscopically. Control of hypertension is essential before a surgical procedure is undertaken. Preoperative medical treatment helps to prevent hypertensive crisis during the procedure. α-Adrenergic blockade is the first step. This is generally done with phenoxybenzamine given 1 week before surgery. β-Blockade is indicated only for patients experiencing arrhythmias or tachycardia with α-blockade. α-Blockade must precede β-blockade to avoid unopposed α-receptor stimulation causing increased blood pressure. Fluid resuscitation is necessary to correct intravascular volume depletion associated with the disease. Postoperative complications include hypotension and hypoglycemia (caused by rebound hyperinsulinemia).

Malignant pheochromocytomas are difficult to distinguish from benign disease. Malignant risk factors include sporadic type, female patients, extra-adrenal disease, and the presence of direct local invasion.

The mainstays of treatment for malignant disease include surgical resection or debulking when complete resection is not possible. Symptoms can be palliated with adrenergic blockade (α and β). Chemotherapy alone is of little help. Better results may be achieved when combined with ^{131}I-MIBG ablation therapy. Selective embolization may be useful in nonresectable cases.

When pheochromocytoma is associated with pregnancy, there is a 50% mortality rate for both mother and fetus. Adrenalectomy before 24 weeks of gestation is preferred, because the risk of spontaneous abortion is low. Medical treatment must always precede surgery. Medical therapy is the first line of treatment for pregnancies past 24 weeks. Cesarean section is preformed at delivery followed by adrenalectomy after recovery.

156
Adrenal Incidentalomas

An incidentaloma is an unsuspected adrenal mass that is discovered during a routine examination. The prevalence of incidentalomas is rising because of improvements in and increased use of abdominal imaging methods. They are identified on about 2% of abdominal computed tomography scans (CTs) and in 9% of autopsies. The incidence also increases with age.

The investigation of these masses should include evaluation for hormonal activity and possible malignancy. The differential diagnosis includes cortical adenoma, pheochromocytoma, cortisol-producing adenoma, aldosteronoma, myelolipomas, adrenal cysts, metastatic cancer, and adenocarcinoma.

Most incidentalomas are nonfunctioning cortical adenomas. These are smooth, well-encapsulated, homogenous-appearing lesions.

Hormonally active lesions can be caused by pheochromocytoma, a cortisol-producing adenoma, or an aldosteronoma. Pheochromocytoma should be ruled out before an invasive procedure is done. This avoids stimulating an inadvertent hypertensive crisis in these patients. Occasionally an incidentaloma can represent a case of subclinical hypercortisolism, also known as *Cushing's syndrome*. Biochemical testing shows increased cortisol production, but these patients lack the overt signs of the syndrome. Aldosteronoma is very rarely associated with incidentalomas. However, the diagnosis should be considered for a patient who has hypertension and hypokalemia.

Adrenocortical carcinomas are large, irregularly shaped lesions. Up to 50% are hormonally active. Calcification, necrosis, hemorrhage, local invasion, and lymphatic involvement can occur. The risk of malignancy increases in lesions 6 cm or larger. Primary cancers from other locations such as breast, lung, melanoma, lymphoma, and renal cell cancer can metastasize to the adrenal gland.

The evaluation of incidentalomas includes radiographic imaging and biochemical testing. Pheochromocytoma is investigated using plasma metanephrine measurements or 24-hour urinary collection for catecholamines and metanephrines. Cushing's syndrome is evaluated by low-dose dexamethasone suppression testing and is confirmed by 24-hour free urinary cortisol and plasma adrenocorticotropic hormone. A screening test for hyperaldosteronism is administered only to patients with hypertension and hypokalemia. The test is composed of measuring plasma aldosterone and renin levels. A plasma aldosterone to plasma renin ratio of greater than 20 indicates hyperaldosteronism. A finding of elevated 24-hour urine cortisol levels secures the diagnosis.

Computed tomography and magnetic resonance imaging (MRI) are the standard radiographic modalities used for evaluation. Abdominal CT imaging can often differentiate the possible causes and assess the risk of carcinoma. Magnetic resonance imaging can be used when CT results are equivocal. The malignant nature of a lesion can be determined by evaluating lipid content and signal intensity. Fine-needle aspiration is generally reserved for metastatic lesions, when having the diagnosis will change the course of treatment for the primary cancer. Fine-needle aspiration is performed only after pheochromocytoma has been excluded.

Nonfunctioning adrenal cortical adenomas that measure less than 4 cm in diameter can be safely observed. An abdominal CT or MRI study should be performed 4 months after the initial studies and then again 1 year later. Evaluation for hormonal activity should be repeated 1 year after initial testing.

Adrenalectomy is indicated for lesions 6 cm in diameter or greater, for hormonally active lesions, and for intermediate-sized lesions that are enlarging during observation. Benign-appearing, nonfunctional lesions measuring 4 to 5 cm can be resected or observed.

157
Multiple Endocrine Neoplasia Syndromes

The multiple endocrine neoplasia (MEN) syndromes are a group of familial diseases characterized by neoplasms of multiple endocrine tissues. The syndromes arise from genetic mutations of tumor suppressor and proto-oncogenes. Tumors are benign or malignant in nature. Tumors associated with MEN syndromes tend to behave different from the same tumors that arise sporadically. The MEN tumors tend to occur at an earlier age, are multifocal, are preceded by states of tissue hyperplasia, are more aggressive, and have a higher recurrence rate. Lesions can appear in several endocrine tissues simultaneously or over different time periods. The syndromes include MEN 1 (parathyroid hyperplasia, duodenal and pancreatic tumors, and pituitary adenomas), MEN 2a (medullary thyroid carcinoma [MTC], pheochromocytomas, parathyroid hyperplasia), MEN 2b (MTC, pheochromocytomas, mucosal neuromas, and Marfan characteristics), and non-MEN familial MTC.

The gene for MEN has been identified on chromosome 11q13. The gene product is a tumor suppressor gene named *menin* that is located in the nucleus. Protein normally functions to inhibit transcription of specific genes. A variety of mutations result in the alteration of the menin protein and loss of tumor suppressor function. Multiple endocrine neoplasia I follows an autosomal dominant mode of inheritance with 100% penetrance but variable expression. Therefore, each patient affected will display some but not all of the traits that define the syndrome. The neoplasms involved with MEN 1 include parathyroid hyperplasia (90% to 97% of cases), duodenal or pancreatic tumors (30% to 80% of cases), and pituitary adenoma (15% to 50% of cases).

Hyperparathyroidism is generally the first abnormality to present in the syndrome. Hypercalcemia is the prominent clinical manifestation associated with nephrolithiasis, nephrocalcinosis, and osteopenia. Compared with its sporadic counterparts, MEN 1–associated hyperparathyroidism occurs at an earlier age, produces a milder hypercalcemia, and produces hyperplasia in all four glands.

Evaluation includes measurement of serum calcium and parathyroid hormone levels. Patients are treated with open parathyroidectomy with removal of 3.5 glands or all four with re-implantation into the forearm. Partial thymectomy is performed in addition to removing ectopic parathyroid tissue.

The second most common element of MEN 1 is pancreatic or duodenal neuroendocrine tumor development. Neoplastic changes tend to be multifocal evidenced by diffuse islet cell hyperplasia and microadenoma development. The most common neuroendocrine neoplasm is the gastrinoma. MEN 1–associated gastrinoma is typically malignant and is located in the wall of the duodenum or in the head of the pancreas. The lesions are usually small and therefore are difficult to locate with computed tomography (CT) or angiography. Endoscopic ultrasound is a useful modality for locating the lesions. Symptoms include abdominal pain, secretory diarrhea, weight loss, and reflux. Surgical resection is advocated to remove the tumor and prevent metastases. Pancreaticoduodenectomy with extensive regional lymphadenectomy offers the best chance for cure.

Insulinoma is the second most common pancreatic neuroendocrine tumor associated with MEN 1. The tumors cause increased production of endogenous insulin, resulting in hypoglycemia, diaphoresis, dizziness, confusion, or syncope. The lesions are small, uniformly dispersed throughout the pancreas, and carry only a 10% chance of malignancy. Evaluation consists of a 72-hour fasting test with demonstration of hypoglycemia, and elevated insulin as well as C-peptide levels. Insulinomas can be located by selective catheterization of arteries feeding into the pancreas and measurement of insulin production from the hepatic vein. Intraoperative palpation is another method. Small lesions can be enucleated, and multiple lesions may require partial pancreatectomy. Metastasis from malignant tumors can be treated with streptozocin, along with hypoglycemic control with octreotide or diazoxide.

Pituitary adenoma is another component of MEN 1. The most common lesion is the prolactin-secreting adenoma. Symptoms are produced by mass effect (compression on the optic chiasm, causing visual field defects) or elevated prolactin secretion. Hypopituitarism can also occur secondary to compression of normal areas of the pituitary by the adenoma. Clinical manifestations of amenorrhea and galactorrhea occur in women, whereas hypogonadism usually occurs in men. Pituitary adenomas are treated either with surgical ablation or radiation. Dopamine agonists such as bromocriptine can be used to suppress prolactin secretion.

Multiple endocrine neoplasia type 2 syndromes are divided into three subtypes, MEN 2a, MEN 2b, and familial non-MEN MTC. The MEN 2 syndromes are passed on by autosomal dominant inheritance. Mutations in the *RET* proto-oncogene on chromosome 10 are responsible for the syndrome. All patients affected by MEN 2 develop MTC because of the complete penetrance of the disease. The other components of MEN 2 demonstrate incomplete penetrance; therefore, not every patient displays these neoplasms.

Multiple endocrine neoplasia 2a is characterized by MTC, pheochromocytoma, and hyperparathyroidism. Type 2b is characterized by MTC, pheochromocytomas, mucosal neuromas, and a Marfan appearance (long limbs with short bodies). Mucosal neuromas consist of thick nonencapsulated bundles of nerves located in the tongue, gingiva, oral mucosa, vocal cords, nose, and conjunctiva. Intestinal disorders (large colon, pseudo-obstruction) may arise from ganglioneuromas present in the myenteric and submucosal plexus.

The MTC of MEN 2 is bilateral and multifocal. Medullary thyroid carcinoma arises from parafollicular C-cells found within the thyroid gland. The C-cells are responsible for calcitonin production. Hyperplasia of the C-cells is the precursor lesion to MEN 2 MTC. Medullary thyroid carcinoma associated with MEN 2b can manifest in infancy and is the most aggressive form of MTC. Affected patients demonstrate elevated calcitonin levels. Many patients present with a palpable neck mass. Metastasis to regional lymph nodes is common by the time of presentation. Up to 70% of patients presenting with a palpable neck mass have lymphatic metastasis. Therefore, early diagnosis before calcitonin levels are elevated is important. Prognosis is affected by the stage of the tumor at diagnosis. Early diagnosis offers the best chance for a cure. Metastasis is also accomplished through direct invasion of surrounding structures. Invasion into the recurrent laryngeal nerve, jugular vein, and carotid arteries can be indicated by hoarseness, dysphagia, bleeding, or arterial stenosis. Medullary thyroid carcinoma can metastasize to the breast, liver, bone, or lung. The diagnostic workup includes calcitonin measurement and fine-needle aspiration. Elevated carcinoembryonic antigen (CEA) can

occur also. Persistent hypercalcitonin levels after thyroidectomy plus lymph node dissection indicates metastasis. Multiple endocrine neoplasia–related MTC represents 25% of all cases of MTC. Therefore, genetic testing is advocated for any patient diagnosed with MTC. Inquiries into family history as well as personal history of symptoms of hypercalcemia and catecholamine excess should be made. First-degree relatives of a patient testing positive for the *ret* mutation should undergo genetic screening.

Pheochromocytomas are neoplasms that are derived from adrenal medulla or chromaffin cells. Neoplastic changes in these cells cause overproduction and secretion of catecholamines. Clinical manifestations include headache, hypertension, palpitations, tremors, and anxiety. Certain stress can trigger hypertensive crises and cardiovascular collapse that lead to death. On rare occasions (10%), pheochromocytoma occurs before MTC. Lesions typically begin as diffuse hyperplasia that develops into nodules characteristic of pheochromocytoma (>1 cm). When associated with MEN 2, lesions tend to be bilateral and multifocal. Malignancy and extra-adrenal lesions are rarely encountered, which contrasts with sporadic pheochromocytomas. Screening for a synchronous pheochromocytoma should be done before attempting thyroid surgery for MTC. Perioperative α-adrenergic blockade should be instituted for patients who have pheochromocytoma. Testing and treatment for pheochromocytoma is discussed in Chapter 155.

Hyperparathyroidism in MEN 2 is limited to the MEN 2a subtype. Multiglandular hyperplasia results in hypercalcemia and its associated symptoms (i.e., kidney stones, altered mental status, and osteopenia), similar to hyperparathyroidism seen in MEN 1. Enlarged parathyroid glands may be apparent at the time of thyroidectomy for MTC.

Familial, non-MEN MTC occurs in the absence of the other endocrine neoplasms associated with MEN 2. Familial MTC is characterized by an indolent course with later presentation in age. Clinical symptoms may not be apparent.

Surgical treatment is the mainstay of MTC management. Radioactive iodine ablation is of no use, because the C-cells do not take up the radioactive isotope. Total thyroidectomy along with central node dissection is indicated for patients with MEN-associated MTC lacking a palpable neck mass. Total parathyroidectomy with autotransplantation is generally done simultaneously because of the inability to spare the parathyroid glands during thyroidectomy. Patients with a palpable neck mass and MEN-associated MTC should undergo total thyroidectomy, total parathyroidectomy with autotransplantation, and radical lymph node dissection. Recurrent disease is indicated by an elevated calcitonin level. Chemotherapy and radiation show no benefit, leaving reoperation as the only viable option.

Part XV
Surgical Specialties

158
Pelvic Inflammatory Disease

Pelvic inflammatory disease (PID) affects young, sexually active females. In the United States, about 8% of all women reported that they have received treatment for PID at some point. Although PID is mostly treated medically, it has the potential to result in significant surgical complications and long-term morbidity. The acute infection often results in pelvic adhesions, with the potential for long-term infertility and chronic pelvic pain. Infertility is seen in about 10% of patients, and 3% or more experience ectopic gestation.

Pelvic inflammatory disease is a polymicrobial inflammatory condition that results from the ascension of microorganisms from the cervix and vagina to the upper genital tract and the peritoneal cavity. Most cases of PID are considered to be the sequelae of the sexually transmitted pathogens *Chlamydia trachomatis* and *Neisseria gonorrhoeae*. The ascent of these organisms from the lower to the upper genital tract is the most common antecedent of PID. However, *Bacteroides* and genital mycoplasmas frequently accompany *C. trachomatis* and *N. gonorrhoeae* in the upper genital tract. Several risk factors for PID have been identified. These include young age (less than 20 years), multiple sexual partners, nulliparity, and prior history of PID. Adolescents tend to have ectopy, which exposes a large zone of the columnar epithelium to the attachment of *C. trachomatis* and *N. gonorrhoeae*.

Pelvic inflammatory disease is a difficult diagnostic challenge in many cases. It should be suspected in patients presenting with fever, leukocytosis, lower abdominal pain, vaginal discharge, and adnexal tenderness on vaginal examination. Some patients, however, have minimal or absent symptomatology, particularly in the presence of a chlamydial infection. The lack of symptoms does not preclude PID and tubal damage. The variable presentation of PID has lead to the formulation of certain diagnostic criteria that include a combination of all three major findings (lower abdominal tenderness, cervical motion tenderness, and bilateral adnexal tenderness) and one of the minor findings (fever higher than 38.3°C, mucopurulent cervicitis, elevated erythrocyte sedimentation rate or C-reactive protein, cervical infection with *C. trachomatis* or *N. gonorrhoeae*, or the presence of a pelvic mass on ultrasonography). However, it was determined that these criteria are too stringent and resulted in failing to offer treatment to many women who do not fulfill them. Currently, the Centers for Disease Control and Prevention recommends that "empiric treatment for PID should be initiated in sexually active young women and other women with a risk for sexually transmitted diseases if the following minimum criteria are present and no other cause for illness can be identified: uterine/adnexal tenderness or cervical motion tenderness."

One of the diagnoses often confused with PID is acute appendicitis. Right lower quadrant pain of shorter duration (less than 12 hours) is more consistent with appendicitis, whereas women with PID tend to have pain for at least 48 hours duration. Gastrointestinal symptoms including nausea and vomiting tend be more common with acute appendicitis than with PID. Subtle objective findings may exist that distinguish the two conditions. Cervical and adnexal tenderness is elicited more often with PID, although women with acute appendicitis often demonstrate these physical findings. Indeed, any intra-abdominal pathologic condition that results in peritoneal irritation may confuse the clinical picture.

Several laboratory studies have been evaluated as aids in making the diagnosis of PID. White cell count is non-specific and is elevated in less than 40% of patients with PID. Elevated levels of erythrocyte sedimentation rate and C-reactive protein have been found to have high specificity and sensitivity; however, their timely availability is inconsistent. The use of laparoscopy, pelvic ultrasonography, and pelvic computed tomography (CT) scanning may be helpful in confirming a diagnosis. When PID is present, laparoscopy confirms it by identifying tubal edema, erythema, and exudate. The presence of a tubo-ovarian abscess can be confirmed in this manner. Therefore, laparoscopy is considered the gold standard for the diagnosis of PID, and a low threshold for diagnostic laparoscopy should be maintained for patients who are ill and the diagnosis remains unclear. Various imaging techniques such as ultrasound and CT scanning can also confirm a pelvic abscess. Distinction between tubo-ovarian abscess (TOA) and tubo-ovarian complex (TOC) is possible with ultrasonography. Tubo-ovarian complex is an acute inflammatory pelvic mass composed of adherent, edematous infected pelvic structures in PID. Tubo-ovarian complex responds to medical treatment in more than 95% cases.

Once the diagnosis of PID is made, it should be decided whether hospitalization or outpatient therapy is appropriate. The indications for hospitalization are (1) inability to exclude surgical emergency (i.e., appendicitis), (2) pregnancy, (3) failure of patient to respond to outpatient therapy, (4) intolerance of oral regimen because of nausea and vomiting, (5) cases with tubo-ovarian abscess, and (6) immunocompromised hosts. Some specialists believe that all women with PID should be admitted to the hospital for more intensive care, which might preserve their fertility.

One of the following outpatient therapy combinations is recommended: cefoxitin 2.0 g intramuscularly with oral probenecid, or ceftriaxone 250 mg intramuscularly or equivalent cephalosporin, plus doxycycline 100 mg orally two times daily for 10 to 14 days. The first part of the therapy is aimed at *N. gonorrhoeae*. Because cefoxitin is active against the penicillinase-producing gonorrhea, this agent should be used when such strains occur. The doxycycline is added to cover *Chlamydia* either as a single pathogen or as a coexisting agent with *N. gonorrhoeae*. Follow-up evaluation of patients treated on an outpatient basis should be carried out within 48 to 72 hours. If there is no improvement in the patient, she should be admitted for intravenous antibiotics.

Recommendations for inpatient treatment include cefoxitin 2.0 g intravenously every 6 hours plus a loading dose of gentamicin 2.0 mg/kg intravenously, followed by a maintenance dose of 1.5 mg/kg intravenously every 8 hours. This regimen is continued for at least 48 hours after the patient shows clinical improvement. Doxycycline 100 mg orally twice daily is given after the patient is discharged from the hospital to complete a total of 10 to 14 days of therapy. An alternative regimen is clindamycin 900 mg intravenously every 8 hours plus a loading dose of gentamicin 2.0 mg/kg intravenously followed by a maintenance dose of 1.5 mg/kg intravenously every 8

hours. This regimen is continued for at least 48 hours after the patient improves. Following this, the patient is discharged on doxycycline 100 mg orally twice daily to complete a total of 10 to 14 days of therapy. If the creatinine level is elevated, an adjusted dose of gentamicin or one of the other recommended regimens is advised. The use of broad-spectrum antibiotics, which must include an antibiotic with anaerobic activity, will result in cures. Surgery becomes necessary under the following conditions: (1) the intraperitoneal rupture of a tubo-ovarian abscess, (2) the persistence of a pelvic abscess despite antibiotic therapy, and (3) uncertain diagnosis.

Historically, total abdominal hysterectomy with bilateral salpingo-oophorectomy was considered the procedure of choice when surgery for PID was required. The surgical approach to PID and TOA has become more conservative over the past 20 years. If surgery is indicated after failure of medical management, a conservative approach with drainage of TOA and removal of devitalized tissue is recommended. When the whole adnexa is involved, removal may be required. For young women whose reproductive goals have not been achieved, especially in the presence of unilateral disease, a unilateral salpingo-oophorectomy may be more appropriate than total hysterectomy with removal of both ovaries and fallopian tubes. Laparoscopy has also become an important asset in the operative management of TOA. Laparoscopic visualization of the pelvic structures allows definitive diagnosis of PID. Laparoscopy also allows aspiration of TOA and lysis of adhesions. Less invasive interventions have also become available for the treatment of TOA. Interventional radiologic techniques for percutaneous drainage of TOA are often used as the first line of therapy with excellent results. This approach has the clear advantage of avoiding anesthesia and surgery and preserving pelvic organs.

Rupture of a tubo-ovarian abscess is a true surgical emergency. It is most often associated with a sudden severe increase in abdominal pain and a shocklike state. Without surgical treatment, mortality rate approaches 100%. With prompt surgical intervention and intensive medical management, the mortality rate is less than 5%. The patient must be explored promptly through a large midline incision. Hysterectomy and oophorectomy are usually indicated. The operation can be technically difficult because of the distortion and edema due to the inflammatory process. At the conclusion of the procedure, the abdomen should be liberally irrigated. If the uterus is removed, the vaginal cuff should be left open for drainage.

159
The Pregnant Patient

Most indications for surgical intervention during pregnancy, such as acute appendicitis, symptomatic cholelithiasis, breast masses, or trauma, are unrelated to pregnancy itself. Altered maternal anatomy and physiology and the safety of the fetus are the issues to be considered by the surgeon. The presentation of surgical diseases in the pregnant patient may be atypical, and a standard evaluation may be unreliable due to pregnancy-associated changes in diagnostic tests or laboratory values. Physicians may also be more conservative in diagnostic evaluation and treatment. These factors can cause a delay in diagnosis and treatment, adversely affecting maternal and fetal outcomes.

Pregnancy causes several changes in coagulation and fibrinolysis. Platelets become more reactive. There is increased hepatic and endothelial cell synthesis of many procoagulant factors, and fibrinolytic activity is impaired. Overall, pregnancy is a hypercoagulable state, and the risk of thromboembolism doubles during pregnancy. Compression stockings should be used whenever surgical treatment is needed.

Anesthesia concerns during pregnancy include the safety of the mother and the fetus. The fetus may be exposed to the teratogenic effects of anesthetic agents, to the risk of preterm labor, and to the risk from changes in maternal physiology caused by anesthesia. The most profound effects on the fetus are related to the decreased uterine blood flow or decreased oxygen content of uterine blood. Unlike circulation to other vital organs, such as the brain, uterine circulation is not autoregulated. When treating maternal hypotension, vasopressors such as dopamine and epinephrine, while increasing the maternal systemic pressure, have little or no effect on uterine circulation. Other maneuvers, such as fluid bolus, Trendelenburg's position, compression stockings, or leg elevation, have a larger impact on increasing uterine blood flow. If vasopressors are necessary, ephedrine is the drug of choice, because it causes less uterine vasoconstriction than epinephrine or norepinephrine. Small doses of phenylephrine are also safe for use by pregnant women who are hypotensive.

In addition to the risks related to maternal hypoxia or hypotension, the risk of spontaneous abortion and teratogenesis related to anesthetic agents is of major concern. For a congenital defect to result, exposure to the teratogen must occur during the vulnerable differentiation stage of the affected organ system in the first trimester of human embryonic development. Therefore, delaying semielective surgical procedures until after the first trimester may reduce the risk of teratogenicity. During the second trimester, after organ system differentiation has occurred, there is almost no risk of anesthetic-induced malformation or spontaneous abortion. The physiologic changes associated with pregnancy have implications for anesthetic management. Pregnant women have decreased oxygen reserve and thus are subject to rapid development of hypoxia and hypercapnia with hypoventilation. This vulnerability becomes especially important during intubation and anesthesia. During intubation, pregnant women are also at increased risk for gastric aspiration due to the decreased gastroesophageal sphincter tone. Because of this increased risk of aspiration, nasogastric suction should be freely employed. The stomach should be emptied before emergency procedures and continually decompressed throughout the operation and the early postoperative period. The gravid uterus may press on the inferior vena cava, decreasing venous return and causing cardiac output to decrease by as much as 30%. Anesthesia can suppress the normal physiologic compensation for aortocaval compression, in which event hypotension can ensue. To maintain cardiac output, the pregnant patient should be placed in the left lateral decubitus position.

Consultation with the obstetrician is essential. Transvaginal ultrasound can be used when the surgical field involves the abdomen. Fetal heart rate monitoring for fetal status and tocometer monitoring for uterine activity should be performed before and after the procedure.

Monitoring consists of measuring uterine contractions with a tocometer, fetal heart rate with a Doppler transducer, and fetal movement and tone with ultrasonography. These measurements are good indicators of fetal health. Preoperative ultrasonography can also approximate gestational age when an accurate history cannot be obtained. Gestational age plays a pivotal role in all surgical decision making for a pregnant patient. Although the fetal heart rate can be heard 14 weeks after conception, it serves as an indicator of fetal oxygenation only after 26 weeks. Fetal heart rate abnormalities, such as absence of variability, late or variable decelerations, and bradycardia, are predictive of fetal distress.

Radiographic studies are useful diagnostic methods during pregnancy. The accepted maximum dose of ionizing radiation during the entire pregnancy is 5 rads (0.05 Gy). The fetus is at the highest risk from radiation exposure from the preimplantation period to approximately 15 weeks' gestation. Primary organogenesis occurs during this time, and the teratogenic effects of radiation, particularly to the developing central nervous system, are at their highest. Perinatal radiation exposure has also been associated with childhood leukemia and certain childhood malignancies. The radiation dose that has been associated with congenital malformation is >10 rads (0.1 Gy). Radiation exposure to the fetus from the more common radiology procedures is well below that threshold. Nonetheless, prudence on the part of the clinician is required to avoid unnecessary fetal exposure to ionizing radiation, especially during the first trimester and early second trimester when the risk from exposure is greatest. Magnetic resonance imaging (MRI) avoids exposure to ionizing radiation but poses an unknown risk to the fetus. Currently, MRI is not advised during the first trimester of pregnancy. Ultrasonography is routinely used by obstetricians during pregnancy. It is an alternative diagnostic tool when trying to avoid exposure to ionizing radiation.

If a surgical problem arises during pregnancy, the urgency of surgical treatment must be balanced against the risk that the treatment poses to the mother and the fetus. Urgent procedures, such as appendectomy, should be undertaken in a timely fashion. In such cases, the risks to both mother and fetus outweigh the risks of miscarriage and preterm labor. Semielective procedures are best done during the second trimester. In the first trimester, when organogenesis is ongoing, concerns arise about the teratogenic risks of medications and surgical interventions. During the first trimester, surgical procedures are associated with a miscarriage rate of 12%; during the second trimester, this rate falls to 0% to 5.6%. The incidence of preterm labor with surgical procedures is 5% in the second trimester but rises to 30% to 40% in the third trimester. Elective procedures should be delayed until 6 weeks after delivery. Even though surgical procedures have been associated with a greater incidence of preterm labor, especially in the third trimester, routine prophylactic use of tocolytics is not recommended. Tocolytics have several side effects and do not improve outcome when used prophylactically. They are best used to treat active uterine irritability. Terbutaline, magnesium, and indomethacin have been used in different studies with equivalent results. In general, for patients with postoperative contractions before 32 weeks, indomethacin would be a reasonable treatment, whereas terbutaline could be the first line treatment for patients at more than 32 weeks' gestation.

The incidence of preterm labor associated with nonobstetric surgery is related to both gestational age and the indication for surgery. The later in gestation the woman is, the higher the risk of preterm contractions or preterm labor. Intraperitoneal surgeries and disease processes with intraperitoneal inflammation are the most likely to have postoperative courses complicated by preterm contractions and preterm labor. A delay in treatment appears to increase the chance of preterm labor, likely related to the primary disease process. Laparoscopic and open techniques have an equal incidence of preterm labor.

The major concerns of laparoscopy during pregnancy include injury to the uterus, decreased uterine blood flow, fetal acidosis, and preterm labor from increased intra-abdominal pressure. The following guidelines for laparoscopic surgery during pregnancy are recommended:

1. Obstetric consultation should be obtained preoperatively.
2. When possible, operative intervention should be deferred until the second trimester, when fetal risk is lowest.
3. Pneumoperitoneum enhances lower extremity venous stasis already present in the gravid patient, and pregnancy induces a hypercoagulable state. Therefore, pneumatic compression devices should be used.
4. Fetal and uterine status, as well as maternal end-tidal CO_2 and/or arterial blood gases, should be monitored.
5. The uterus should be protected with a lead shield if intraoperative cholangiography is a possibility. Fluoroscopy should be used selectively.
6. Given the enlarged gravid uterus, abdominal access should be attained using an open technique.
7. Dependent positioning should be used to shift the uterus off the inferior vena cava.
8. Pneumoperitoneum pressures should be minimized to 8 to 12 mm Hg and not allowed to exceed 15 mm Hg.

Trocar placement in the pregnant patient should not differ radically from placement in the nonpregnant patient early in pregnancy. Later in pregnancy, as the gravid uterus enlarges superiorly, adjustments in trocar placement must be made to avoid uterine injury and to improve visualization. The camera port must be placed in a supraumbilical location, and the remaining ports are placed under direct camera visualization. Currently, the general tendency is to limit laparoscopic surgery for pregnant women to the first 28 weeks of gestation. Later in pregnancy, when the uterus is no longer confined within the pelvis and the lower abdomen, laparoscopic surgery becomes more difficult.

160
Ovarian Tumors

Ovarian carcinomas are divided into epithelial, germ cell, and stromal malignancies. Most cases of ovarian cancer are of the epithelial type. Most patients present with advanced disease, which is treated with surgical resection followed by platinum-based chemotherapy. Advances in chemotherapy brought improved survival, and understanding of genetic risk factors has permitted preventive strategies, such as bilateral salpingo-oophorectomy.

The median age of patients with ovarian cancer is 60 years. A strong family history of ovarian or breast cancer is the most important risk factor. Nulliparity is associated with an increased risk of ovarian cancer, whereas oral contraceptive use, pregnancy, and lactation are associated with a reduced risk. It appears that repeated stimulation of the epithelium of the ovarian surface, which occurs in the nulliparous state as a result of uninterrupted ovulation, may predispose the epithelium to malignant transformation. A strong family history of breast cancer, ovarian cancer, or both may be related to the presence of an inherited mutation in one of two tumor suppressor genes, *BRCA-1* and *BRCA-2*, located on chromosomes 17q and 13q, respectively. Their gene products are involved in DNA repair. Women with a germline mutation in *BRCA-1* have a lifetime risk of ovarian cancer that ranges from 16% to 44% and a lifetime risk of breast cancer that ranges from 56% to 87% Women with germline mutations in *BRCA-2* have a lifetime risk of breast cancer that is similar to that for carriers of the *BRCA-1* mutation, and their lifetime risk of ovarian cancer is approximately 10%.

A second familial disorder that carries with it an increased risk of ovarian cancer is referred to as the *Lynch II syndrome*. Affected families have a predominance of hereditary nonpolyposis colon cancer, often on the right side of the colon, and sometimes in association with other cancers, such as those of the endometrium, stomach, ovaries, or genitourinary tract. Women with a known germline mutation in *BRCA-1* or *BRCA-2* who have completed childbearing may reduce their risk of ovarian cancer by undergoing bilateral salpingo-oophorectomy. Prophylactic bilateral salpingo-oophorectomy in women with *BRCA-1* or *BRCA-2* germline mutations has also been reported to reduce the risk of breast cancer, presumably by decreasing levels of circulating estrogen and progesterone. Patients at high risk for ovarian cancer who decline to undergo prophylactic bilateral salpingo-oophorectomy should have screening that includes frequent pelvic examinations and measurement of serum CA 125 levels. Transvaginal pelvic ultrasonography should be considered. However, early ovarian cancer often evades such screening methods, and the effectiveness of screening for ovarian cancer in high-risk patients has not yet been demonstrated.

The symptoms of ovarian cancer are nonspecific and often suggest the presence of upper abdominal disease. Patients may report abdominal fullness, dyspepsia, or bloating as the result of increased abdominal pressure from ascites. Occasionally, patients with early-stage disease present with pelvic pain due to ovarian torsion, although most patients with early-stage disease are asymptomatic. Physical findings are diverse and typically include a palpable ovarian mass. Therefore, ovarian cancer should be considered for any premenopausal woman with an unexplained enlargement of the ovary or any postmenopausal woman with a palpable ovary.

If ovarian cancer is suspected, transvaginal ultrasonography is often performed. Transvaginal ultrasonography appears to be more sensitive than computed tomography scanning for the detection of pelvic masses. The finding of a complex ovarian cyst, defined by the presence of both solid and cystic components, is highly suggestive of cancer. Such cysts require surgery for definitive diagnosis. Percutaneous biopsy of complex cysts is to be avoided because of the risk of tumor spillage into the pelvic cavity. In contrast, simple ovarian cysts have smooth walls, are filled with fluid, and do not contain a solid component. These cysts are often benign and generally do not require surgical intervention. Careful follow up is recommended.

Although the serum CA 125 level is elevated in more than 80% of patients with advanced epithelial ovarian cancer, it is neither sufficiently sensitive nor specific to be diagnostic. Thus, measurement of the CA 125 level is not usually helpful in the preoperative evaluation of a complex ovarian cyst, and surgery is generally necessary for definitive diagnosis. However, a serum CA 125 level of more than 65 U/mL in a postmenopausal woman with an abdominal or pelvic mass should raise the possibility of ovarian cancer. The CA 125 level is also useful in assessing the patient's response to postoperative chemotherapy and in detecting early recurrence.

If ovarian cancer is suspected on physical examination and transvaginal ultrasonography, an exploratory laparotomy is indicated for histologic confirmation, staging, and tumor debulking. Histologic confirmation is necessary to rule out other causes of ovarian cyst. Many fluid-containing cystic tumors of the ovary are also accompanied by papillary projections and are called *papillary serous cystadenomas*. Because of epithelial variation in these tumors, it is often difficult to be sure where they fit in the spectrum of benign to malignant disease. A similar problem of malignant potential exists for the *mucinous cystadenoma*, which is a cystic tumor containing sticky, gelatinous material. These mucinous tumors are less likely to be malignant than the serous cystadenomas. It is not always possible to be sure by gross inspection whether cystic tumors with solid components are benign or malignant. It is usually necessary to excise the involved ovary completely, even though there is no definite evidence of malignancy. The malignant potential of the cystadenoma is then determined by histologic examination. Frozen-section examination of the tumor at the time of surgical intervention is necessary to determine the proper course of therapy for patients in the reproductive age group.

Surgical staging, performed during exploratory laparotomy, provides important information that can guide postoperative decision making, especially for early-stage disease. Tumor debulking or cytoreduction is an important component of surgery, because patients with residual tumor 1 cm or less in diameter have higher survival rates than those with more extensive residual disease. The standard surgical approach involves a vertical midline incision. Epithelial ovarian cancers disseminate along peritoneal surfaces and by lymphatic channels. The first site of spread is the pelvic peritoneum. Later the abdominal peritoneal surfaces and diaphragms are involved. The omentum is a common site for metastases, as are both the para-aortic and pelvic lymph nodes. Because the entire abdominal cavity is not accessible through a transverse pelvic incision, surgery for ovarian malignancies should

be performed through a full-length midline abdominal incision. The visceral and parietal surfaces are inspected for metastatic disease, and biopsy specimens are taken of suspicious areas. If ascites is present, it should be aspirated and heparinized. Cytologic evaluation for metastatic cells is performed. In the absence of ascites, peritoneal washings with balanced salt solution or lactated Ringer's solution are obtained from the pelvis, abdominal gutters, and subdiaphragmatic areas and sent for cytologic evaluation. A total abdominal hysterectomy and bilateral salpingo-oophorectomy are performed, along with omentectomy and biopsy of para-aortic lymph nodes.

Although initial surgery is almost always necessary in the treatment of suspected ovarian cancer, it is important to recognize two groups of patients for whom alternative approaches might be considered. The first group includes patients with a complex ovarian cyst and iron-deficiency anemia caused by occult gastrointestinal bleeding. Clinical suspicion of a Krukenberg's metastasis from a gastric or other gastrointestinal primary site should prompt an initial endoscopic evaluation before a definitive surgical procedure. The second group of patients includes those with suspected ovarian cancer who are poor surgical candidates. For these patients, the diagnosis is confirmed with biopsy, and chemotherapy is initiated. If the patient responds to treatment and becomes a better surgical candidate, debulking of the tumor can be attempted.

Women with low-grade early-stage cancers who have undergone appropriate surgical staging can be treated with surgery without adjuvant therapy. If the lesion is bilateral (stage IB), abdominal hysterectomy and bilateral salpingo-oophorectomy are sufficient. For the limited group of patients with unilateral low-grade lesions, fertility can be preserved by performing adnexectomy and staging biopsies without removing the uterus or contralateral adnexa. For all other patients, appropriate initial surgery includes bilateral salpingo-oophorectomy, abdominal hysterectomy if the uterus has not been removed, appropriate staging, and tumor resection. Most patients with epithelial ovarian cancer require postoperative adjuvant chemotherapy in an attempt to eradicate residual disease. Platinum-based adjuvant treatment can reduce the risk of relapse, resulting in a disease-free survival rate of approximately 80%. Platinum-based chemotherapy is associated with an overall survival advantage for high-risk patients with early-stage disease. Intravenous administration of taxane and platinum-based chemotherapy is the current standard of postoperative care for patients with advanced ovarian cancer.

Disease recurrence is a major problem for patients with advanced ovarian cancer. Recurrent disease is generally incurable, and palliation of symptoms is the goal of treatment. A common sign of relapse is a rise in the serum CA 125 level in the absence of symptoms and abnormalities on physical examination or computed tomography scanning. A marker-only relapse usually antedates the development of clinical recurrence. In most cases of advanced ovarian cancer, death is associated with bowel dysfunction or obstruction. Although invasion of the small bowel and colon is unusual, growth of the tumor adjacent to the bowel leads to mesenteric compromise and dysfunction with distention, nausea, and vomiting. When bowel obstruction occurs early in the clinical course of ovarian cancer, and particularly if it occurs before the administration of chemotherapy, surgical intervention is warranted and should be aggressive. Resection or bypass of the involved small bowel is indicated; colonic resection also may be indicated. It is important to perform adequate radiographic studies preoperatively so that obstructed small bowel is not decompressed into a compromised colon. When bowel obstruction occurs after chemotherapy, the prognosis is unfavorable. Surgery is often difficult because of extensive tumor. Laparotomy can be complicated by enteric injury or fistula. The best approach for these patients is the use of a percutaneous or endoscopically positioned gastrostomy tube and intravenous fluids or conservative nutritional support. Such a procedure may allow the patient to remain in a supportive home environment for a greater period of time.

Most women with epithelial cancers have stage III tumors at the time of diagnosis. Widespread peritoneal dissemination, omental involvement, and ascites are the rule in these cases. When advanced ovarian carcinoma is discovered at the time of exploratory celiotomy, there may be a tendency to limit surgery to a diagnostic biopsy. However, successful reduction of tumor volume to nodules 2 cm or less is possible in at least 50% of women with advanced ovarian cancer. Survival following chemotherapy is inversely related to the volume of residual disease at the time of primary surgery.

Most ovarian cancer is found on peritoneal surfaces and not invading viscera. Therefore, a retroperitoneal approach facilitates mobilization of the involved mesothelium. The lateral aspects of the paracolic gutters are incised and dissection carried medially to undermine tumor in these locations. Tumor nodules on anterior and posterior cul-de-sac peritoneum are resected by developing planes in the retroperitoneal spaces. Hysterectomy, adnexectomy, and omentectomy are performed. Disease on the right diaphragm may be resected by transecting the falciform ligament and retracting the liver inferiorly. If required to remove all remaining tumor, splenectomy and resection of small or large bowel may be needed.

161
Renal Physiology

The kidney has three major functions. First, it maintains fluid and electrolyte homeostasis. Second, it functions as an endocrine organ producing the active metabolite of vitamin D and erythropoietin. Third, the kidney is an organ of excretion for certain intermediate and end products of metabolism and for several drugs.

The kidney is the main organ of regulation of fluid and electrolyte balance. The kidney filters approximately 144 L of fluid daily. The renal tubules reabsorb back into the bloodstream 98% to 99.5% of this filtrate. In healthy humans excreting maximally concentrated urine, approximately 500 mg/day is required to excrete obligatory solutes. The kidney is also capable of removing approximately 20 L of solute-free water. Therefore, a healthy individual could receive as much as 20 L of water daily, excrete all of it, and not alter any water compartment in the body.

Concentration of the urine depends on the presence of antidiuretic hormone (ADH). Antidiuretic hormone is produced in the supraoptic nucleus of the hypothalamus and translocated to the posterior pituitary gland for storage and release. The regulation of ADH release is normally under the control of the osmolality of the extracellular fluid near the osmole receptors in the supraoptic and paraventricular nuclei of the hypothalamus. Antidiuretic hormone secretion is almost completely suppressed when plasma osmolality is less than 280 mOsm/kg water and is stimulated when osmolality exceeds 290 mOsm/kg water. Although the osmolality of the plasma is the major determinant of ADH release, ADH release can occur in response to other stimuli. Depletion of the intravascular volume and hypotension can result directly in release of ADH and in a resetting of the relationship between osmolality and plasma ADH concentration so that ADH is released despite lower osmolalities. Depletion of intravascular volume by 10% is sufficient to stimulate ADH release despite normal plasma osmolality. Similarly, hypotension causes ADH release despite a normal osmolality of the plasma and a normal intravascular volume. In addition, a variety of other stimuli, called "stressful" (pain and vomiting), can cause ADH release in the presence of normal plasma osmolality, volume status, and blood pressure. Ethanol inhibits ADH release because of inhibition of calcium channels in the pituitary. This reduction in ADH levels contributes to the diuretic effect seen with acute intoxication. Antidiuretic hormone binds to specific receptors on the basolateral membrane of the collecting duct cells. Adenylate cyclase is then activated, and cyclic adenosine monophosphate (cAMP) is produced. Cyclic AMP activates protein phosphatases, and further metabolic steps cause a change in the water permeability of cells of the collecting duct. The increase in the water permeability of the collecting duct allows the fluid within the lumen to come into osmotic equilibrium with the hypertonic medullary interstitium. Therefore, the maximum tonicity of the urine that can be achieved depends on a normal response by distal tubule cells to ADH and the tonicity of the medullary interstitial fluid.

Water and electrolyte balance are also under the control of the renin–angiotensin–aldosterone system. Renin, an enzyme produced by the kidney, is the rate-limiting step in this system. Its release is stimulated by an intrarenal baroreceptor mechanism by β-adrenergic stimulation and by changes in the delivery of sodium or chloride to the distal nephron. Renin causes the conversion of angiotensinogen, a precursor protein produced in the liver, to angiotensin I (AI). A second enzyme, angiotensin-converting enzyme, which is found in all vascular beds (particularly in the lung), catalyzes the conversion of AI to angiotensin AII. Angiotensin II causes vasoconstriction, elicits the production of aldosterone by the adrenal cortex, and inhibits further renin release. Aldosterone production and release by the adrenal cortex are also enhanced by hyperkalemia and negative sodium balance. Adrenocorticotropic hormone (ACTH) may play a permissive role in its production. The predominant action of aldosterone is to stimulate the reabsorption of sodium and secretion of potassium by the distal nephrons; it thus minimizes the amount of sodium that is excreted in the urine.

The kidney is the sole organ of excretion of sodium, and the urinary excretion of sodium matches the dietary intake. The urinary excretion of sodium is less than 1% of the filtered load. Sixty percent of filtered sodium is reabsorbed in the proximal convoluted tubule. The remaining is reabsorbed in the thick ascending limb of Henle's loop and the distal nephron. In the distal nephron, aldosterone enhances the rate of sodium reabsorption. With normal renal function, the urine can be rendered almost free of sodium. On the other hand, in conditions of excess intake of sodium, the kidney can excrete at least as much as intakes of several hundred milliequivalents per day.

The renal mechanism of handling potassium is different from that involved in sodium homeostasis. Unlike sodium, the urine cannot be rendered free of potassium. The renal responses to rapid alterations in potassium intake are slower than those for sodium. Rates of potassium ingestion and excretion can be increased progressively without change in the plasma or tissue concentration of potassium as long as such steep increases in intake occur during several days. Sudden and large increases in potassium intake can overwhelm the capacity of the kidney to excrete the load and the ability of other tissues to sequester potassium. The major regulatory site for potassium excretion is the distal nephron. In this segment, potassium is taken up across the basolateral membrane into the cell by the operation of the Na^+/K^+ ATPase pump. The main determinate for potassium excretion appears to be the concentration of potassium in the luminal fluid. When luminal flow is high, the secreted potassium is rapidly diluted, and the gradient for potassium secretion is maintained. In states of low flow, the cell-to-lumen potassium concentration gradient is decreased, and the rate of secretion is diminished. Thus, flow rate past the distal tubule is a major factor influencing the urinary excretion of potassium. Aldosterone increases the rate of potassium secretion by several mechanisms. It increases the permeability of the luminal membrane to potassium; enhances the rate of sodium reabsorption, rendering the tubule lumen more electronegative; and increases the activity of the Na^+/K^+ ATPase pump. The rate of aldosterone secretion is influenced by the plasma concentration of potassium. Increases in dietary intake of potassium can directly increase the secretion of aldosterone.

Renal Bicarbonate Processing

Cellular metabolism results in the formation of a number of nonvolatile acids. The rate of nonvolatile acid production is related to dietary protein intake and to the rate of endogenous protein catabolism. Daily nonvolatile acid production would consume the total body fluid buffering capacity in about 2 weeks were it not for the fact that the kidneys excrete nonvolatile acids and, in so doing, regenerate bicarbonate. Virtually all filtered bicarbonate is absorbed, together with sodium, by the proximal tubule. Apical membrane Na^+ exchange permits H^+ secretion into urine and Na^+ entry into cells, with subsequent absorption of sodium bicarbonate to blood. The rate of proximal bicarbonate reabsorption is modulated by the same effectors that regulate proximal sodium absorption. Among these, the extracellular fluid volume exerts a central effect. Volume contraction raises the rate of proximal tubular sodium bicarbonate reabsorption. Hypokalemia also increases the rate of bicarbonate reabsorption, presumably by raising the intracellular hydrogen ion concentration. This factor accounts for the fact that in hypokalemic, hypochloremic metabolic alkalosis associated with volume contraction, alkalosis can persist after volume deficits are restored. In these cases, correcting potassium deficits is required to correct the alkalosis.

In addition to reabsorbing all filtered bicarbonate, the kidneys excrete the daily acid load, derived mainly from sulfur-containing amino acids. The hydrogen ions that are excreted in the final urine are secreted mainly in the collecting tubules. This secretory process is facilitated by aldosterone and is inhibited by a trivial quantity of free hydrogen ions that lower the urine pH below the critical level of 4.0 to 4.5. This limitation is normally overcome by the presence of urinary buffers that combine with free hydrogen ions, thus permitting continued secretion of acid. The most important urinary buffer is ammonia, and it is the only buffer that can increase substantially in the presence of an acid load. Limitation of the capacity to generate adequate urinary ammonia usually leads to acidosis. The main site of ammonia production in the kidney is the proximal tubule.

Renin–Angiotensin Physiology

Renin is a proteolytic enzyme that is produced and stored in the granules of the juxtaglomerular cells surrounding the afferent arterioles of glomeruli in the kidney. Renin acts on the basic substrate angiotensinogen (a circulating α_2-globulin made in the liver) to form angiotensin I. Angiotensin I is then enzymatically transformed by angiotensin-converting enzyme (ACE), which is present in many tissues (particularly the pulmonary vascular endothelium), to the octapeptide angiotensin II. Angiotensin II is a potent pressor agent and exerts its action by a direct effect on arteriolar smooth muscle. In addition, angiotensin II stimulates production of aldosterone by the zona glomerulosa of the adrenal cortex.

The juxtaglomerular cells are specialized myoepithelial cells that cuff the afferent arterioles and act as pressure transducers, sensing renal perfusion pressure and corresponding changes in afferent arteriolar perfusion pressures. A reduction in circulating blood volume leads to a corresponding reduction in renal perfusion pressure and afferent arteriolar pressure. This change stimulates the juxtaglomerular cells to release renin into the renal circulation. This results in the formation of angiotensin I, which is converted in the kidney and peripherally to angiotensin II by ACE. Angiotensin II influences sodium homeostasis via two major mechanisms: it changes renal blood flow so as to maintain a constant glomerular filtration rate, thereby changing the filtration fraction of sodium, and it stimulates the adrenal cortex to release aldosterone. Increasing plasma levels of aldosterone enhance renal sodium retention and thus result in expansion of the extracellular fluid volume. A second control mechanism for renin release is centered in the macula densa cells, a group of distal convoluted tubular epithelial cells directly opposed to the juxtaglomerular cells. They may function as chemoreceptors, monitoring the sodium load presented to the distal tubule. Under conditions of increased delivery of filtered sodium to the macula densa, a signal is conveyed to decrease juxtaglomerular cell release of renin, thereby modulating the glomerular filtration rate and the filtered load of sodium.

162
Urologic Anatomy

The adrenal glands lie within the perirenal (Gerota's) fascia superomedial to the kidneys, buried within the perinephric fat. However, the adrenals are embryologically and functionally distinct and are physically separated from the kidneys by connective tissue septa and varying amounts of adipose tissue. Thus, in cases of renal ectopia, the adrenal gland is usually located close to its normal anatomic position and does not follow the kidney. Similarly, in cases of renal agenesis, the adrenal is typically present. The right gland assumes a more pyramidal shape and rests more superior to the upper pole of the right kidney. The left gland is more crescentic and rests more medial to the upper pole of the left kidney, or it may even lie directly on the renal vessels at the left renal hilum.

Each adrenal is a composite of two separate and functionally distinct glandular elements, cortex and medulla. The medulla, which forms the central core of each adrenal, consists of chromaffin cells derived from the neural crest and intimately related to the sympathetic nervous system. The cells of the medulla produce catecholamines, primarily epinephrine and norepinephrine, which are released directly into the bloodstream through an extensive venous drainage system. The adrenal cortex is mesodermally derived and completely surrounds and encases the medulla. Three cell layers are identified in the cortex. The outermost layer is the zona glomerulosa, which produces aldosterone in response to stimulation by the renin—angiotensin system. Centripetally located are the zona fasciculata and zona reticularis, which produce glucocorticoids and sex steroids, respectively. Unlike the zona glomerulosa, these latter functions are regulated by pituitary release of adrenocorticotropic hormone (ACTH).

The adrenals are very vascularized. The arterial supply is relatively symmetric bilaterally. Multiple small arteries supply each adrenal gland. The three major arterial sources for each gland are (1) superior branches from the inferior phrenic artery, (2) middle branches directly from the aorta, and (3) inferior branches from the ipsilateral renal artery. In contrast to the multiple arteries, usually a single large adrenal vein exits each gland from its hilum. On the right side, this vein is very short and enters directly into the inferior vena cava on its posterolateral aspect. The adrenal vein on the left is more elongated and is typically joined by the left inferior phrenic vein before entering the superior aspect of the left renal vein. The adrenal lymphatics in general exit the glands along the course of the venous drainage and eventually empty into para-aortic lymph nodes. The adrenal medulla receives greater autonomic innervation than any other organ in the body. Multiple preganglionic sympathetic fibers enter each adrenal along the course of the adrenal vein and synapse with chromaffin cells in the medulla. This rich sympathetic innervation of the medulla reaches the adrenal via the splanchnic nerves and celiac ganglion. In contrast, the adrenal cortex is believed to receive no innervation.

The kidneys lie in the retroperitoneum along the borders of the psoas muscle. Gerota's fascia forms an important anatomic barrier around the kidney and tends to contain pathologic processes originating from the kidney. Superiorly, Gerota's fascia fuses and tapers to disappear over the inferior diaphragmatic surface. Medially, Gerota's fascia extends across the midline and is contiguous with Gerota's fascia on the contralateral side, although the anterior and posterior leaves are generally fused and inseparable as they cross the great vessels. Inferiorly, Gerota's fascia remains an open potential space, containing the ureter and gonadal vessels on either side. The posterior relations of the kidneys to the abdominal wall musculature are relatively symmetric. The twelfth rib crosses the upper third of each kidney. Because the left kidney lies more cephalad than the right kidney, the eleventh rib lies directly posterior to the upper aspect of the left kidney and not the right kidney.

In contrast to the similarities of posterior anatomic relations in each kidney, the anterior relation of each kidney is significantly different. The right kidney lies behind the liver, and it is separated from the liver by reflection of the peritoneum, except for a small area of its upper pole, which comes into direct contact with the liver's retroperitoneal bare spot. The extension of parietal peritoneum that bridges between the perirenal fascia covering the upper pole of the right kidney and the posterior aspect of the liver is called the *hepatorenal ligament*. Excessive traction on this attachment or the hepatocolic ligament during right renal surgery can cause hepatic parenchymal tears. The duodenum is applied directly to the medial aspect and hilar structures of the right kidney. The hepatic flexure of the colon, which also is extraperitoneal, crosses the lower pole of the right kidney.

On the left, the retroperitoneal tail of the pancreas and the related splenic vessels are applied directly to the upper to middle portion and hilum of the kidney. Superior to the pancreatic tail, the left kidney is covered by peritoneum of the lesser sac and here is related to the posterior gastric wall. Below the pancreatic tail, the medial aspect of the kidney is covered by peritoneum of the greater sac and is related to the jejunum. The lower pole of the left kidney is crossed by the splenic flexure of the colon, generally in an extraperitoneal position. The spleen is separated from the upper lateral portion of the left kidney by peritoneal reflection. However, there is typically a peritoneal extension between the perirenal fascia covering the upper pole of the left kidney and the inferior splenic capsule, called the *splenorenal*, or *lienorenal*, ligament. Just as with the adjacent and often contiguous splenocolic ligamentous attachment, care must be taken not to exert undue tension on the splenorenal ligament during operative procedures on the left kidney to avoid inadvertent tearing of the spleen. Such tearing may necessitate splenectomy during left nephrectomy. Both splenocolic and splenorenal ligaments and the contralateral hepatocolic and hepatorenal ligaments are typically avascular and can be divided sharply with safety.

The renal artery and vein typically branch from the aorta and inferior vena cava, respectively, to supply each kidney. The renal vein is more anterior than the renal artery, whereas the urinary collecting system is the most posteriorly located structure of the renal hilum. The renal arteries and veins typically branch from the aorta and inferior vena cava at the level of the second lumbar vertebral body, below the level of the anterior takeoff of the superior mesenteric artery. The right renal artery passes behind the inferior vena cava in its course and is considerably longer than the left renal artery. The main renal artery typically divides into four or more segmental vessels. The renal arteries are end branch vessels and do not communicate with each other. This is in contrast to the renal venous system, which contains many intrarenal anastomoses. The right renal vein is short (2 to 4 cm) and enters the right lateral aspect of the inferior vena cava

directly, usually without receiving other venous branches. The left renal vein is generally three times the length of the right (6 to 10 cm) and must cross anterior to the aorta to reach the left lateral aspect of the inferior vena cava. Lateral to the aorta, the left renal vein typically receives the left adrenal vein superiorly, a lumbar vein posteriorly, and the left gonadal vein inferiorly.

The adult ureter is usually 25 to 30 cm long. The ureter is arbitrarily divided into segments for the purposes of surgical or radiographic demonstration. The "abdominal" ureter extends from the renal pelvis to the iliac vessels, and the "pelvic" ureter extends from the iliac vessels to the bladder. For radiographic purposes, the ureter is divided into three segments. The upper ureter is commonly described from the renal pelvis to the upper border of the sacrum, the middle ureter from the upper border to lower border of the sacrum, and the lower ureter from the lower border of the sacrum to the bladder, respectively. There are three areas of relative narrowing in the ureter that are of clinical importance: ureteropelvic junction, the point where the ureter crosses anterior to the iliac vessels, and the ureterovesical junction. Spontaneous passage of ureteral stones can be hampered at these areas of narrowing. The ureters lie on the psoas muscle and pass medially to the sacroiliac joints and cross the iliac vessels anteriorly. An important anatomic landmark for easy identification of the ureters is at the site where the ureters cross anterior to the iliac vessels. After crossing the iliac vessels, the ureters swing laterally near the ischial spines before passing medially to penetrate the base of the bladder. The ureteral blood supply originates from the renal, aortic, iliac, mesenteric, gonadal, vasal, and vesical arteries. Free intercommunication between these vessels permits extensive ureteral mobilization and transposition. Pain fibers refer stimuli to the T12 through L2 segments, whereas the autonomic innervation is associated with intrinsic parasympathetic motor and sympathetic vasomotor ganglia. The lymphatic drainage is to segmental periaortic and caval nodes. The ureter may be drawn medially in retroperitoneal fibrosis and laterally as a result of enlargement of periaortic lymph node involvement with tumor or an aortic aneurysm. It is essential to be aware of the course of the ureter during aortic and pelvic surgery and in difficult dissections of adjacent organs.

The cephalad portion of the bladder is attached to the anterior abdominal wall by the urachus, a fibrous remnant of the cloaca that attaches the bladder to the anterior abdominal wall. The obliterated umbilical artery in the medial umbilical fold serves as an important landmark for the surgeon. It may be traced to its origin from the internal iliac artery to locate the ureter, which lies on its medial side. The superior aspect of the bladder is covered by peritoneal reflection. Inferiorly, the bladder is attached to the pubic bone by dense condensations to the posterior aspect of the pubic bone, called the *puboprostatic ligaments* in males and *pubovesical ligaments* in females. The superior, middle, and inferior vesical arteries, which are branches of the hypogastric artery, are the major source of blood supply to the bladder. In females, additional branches from the vaginal and uterine arteries supply the bladder. The veins of the bladder coalesce into the vesicle plexus and drain into the internal iliac vein. The bulk of the lymphatic drainage passes to the external iliac lymph nodes. Some anterior and lateral drainage may go through the obturator and internal iliac nodes, whereas portions of the bladder base and trigone may drain into the internal and common iliac groups.

The prostate is a fibromuscular organ that lies just inferior to the bladder and contains the prostatic urethra. The prostate is supported anteriorly by the puboprostatic ligament and inferiorly by the urogenital diaphragm. The ejaculatory ducts exit in the posterior portion of the prostate across the verumontanum, a mound within the prostate gland. The prostate has a peripheral zone, a central zone, and a transitional zone, an anterior segment, and a preprostatic sphincteric zone. Benign prostatic hyperplasia develops from the periurethral glands at the site of the median or lateral lobes, whereas the posterior lobe is prone to cancer formation. The prostate is separated from the rectum by the two layers of Denonvilliers' fascia, serosal rudiments of the pouch of Douglas, which once extended to the urogenital diaphragm.

The arterial supply to the prostate is derived from the inferior vesical, internal pudendal, and middle rectal (hemorrhoidal) arteries. The veins from the prostate drain into the periprostatic plexus, which has connections with the deep dorsal vein of the penis and the internal iliac (hypogastric) veins. The neurovascular bundles responsible for erection are located near the posterolateral surface of the urethra and prostate gland. Special care in preserving these nerves is crucial to maintaining potency after radical prostatectomy.

The testis is an ovoid, firm scrotal organ that measures $4 \times 2.5 \times 2.5$ cm. The left testis commonly resides lower in the scrotum than the right. The testis is covered by a tough membrane, the tunica albuginea, except at its dorsal aspect, where the epididymis and vascular pedicle are attached. The epididymis is a crescent-shaped body that curves around the dorsal portion of the testis. The vas deferens is a 4-mm-thick walled, firm tubular structure that originates at the inferior pole of the epididymis and follows a cranial course with the spermatic vessels. The arterial blood supply to the testis and epididymis originates from the aorta just below the renal arteries. The left spermatic vein empties into the left renal vein, and the right spermatic vein empties directly into the inferior vena cava. The primary lymphatic drainage from the testis is to the periaortic nodes in the vicinity of the kidney.

The penis is composed of two corpora cavernosal bodies (responsible for erectile function of the penis) and one corpora spongiosum where the urethra courses through. Each corporal body is covered by tunica albuginea, and, collectively, all corporal bodies are covered by a thick layer of fascia. All corporal bodies are capped by the glans of the penis. The male urethra, which is approximately 20 cm long, is divided into four anatomic sections: prostatic, membranous, bulbous, and penile. The voluntary external urinary sphincter lies within the urogenital diaphragm and is an important anatomic landmark to preserve the function of the urinary sphincter after prostatic or urethral surgery. The female urethra is approximately 4 cm long and lies below the pubic symphysis and anterior to the vagina. The principal blood supply to the penis and urethra originates from the internal pudendal arteries. Somatic sensory innervation of the penis is from S3 and S4 via the ilioinguinal and genitofemoral nerves. Sympathetic vasomotor innervation derives from the hypogastric plexus, whereas the parasympathetic innervation originates from S2, S3, and S4 via the nervi erigentes. The nervi erigentes give rise to the cavernosal nerves that course on the posterior surface of the prostate en route to the corpora cavernosa of the penis. Injury to the cavernosal nerves during pelvic surgery can lead to impotence. The lymphatic drainage is to the superficial and deep inguinal nodes and then to the external iliac and hypogastric nodes.

163
Urologic Malignancy

Renal Cell Carcinoma

Renal cell carcinoma accounts for 2.3% of all adult cancers, has a peak incidence in the sixth decade of life, and has a male-to-female ratio of 2:1. Cigarette smoking is the only significant environmental risk factor that has been identified. Familial settings for renal cell carcinoma have been identified, but sporadic tumors are far more common. Renal cell carcinoma originates from the proximal tubule cells. Grossly, the tumor is yellow, at times pink, and often contains cystic areas of hemorrhage and necrosis. Microscopically, the dominant cells appear clear but are often mixed with granular cells. Various cell types and histologic patterns are observed. However, cell type and histologic pattern do not affect treatment.

Historically, 60% of patients present with gross or microscopic hematuria. Flank pain or an abdominal mass is detected in approximately 30% of cases. The triad of flank pain, hematuria, and mass are found in only 10% to 15% of patients and is often a sign of advanced disease. Symptoms of metastatic disease (cough, bone pain) occur in 20% to 30% of patients at presentation. Because of the current widespread use of ultrasound and computed tomographic (CT) scanning for diverse indications, renal tumors are sometimes detected incidentally in patients with no urologic symptoms. Paraneoplastic syndromes are not uncommon in renal cell carcinoma. Erythrocytosis from increased erythropoietin production occurs in 5%, although anemia is far more common. Stauffer's syndrome is a reversible syndrome of hepatic dysfunction in the absence of metastatic disease.

Over the past decade, CT has replaced intravenous pyelography and ultrasound as the radiologic modality of choice to evaluate renal masses. Characteristic features of renal cell carcinoma visible on CT include enhancement of lesion after injection of intravenous contrast medium, thickened irregular walls, thickened or enhanced septa within the mass, or multilocular mass. Computed tomography scanning is the most valuable imaging test for renal cell carcinoma. It confirms the character of the mass and further stages the lesion with respect to regional lymph nodes, renal vein, or hepatic involvement. It also gives valuable information on the contralateral kidney (function, bilaterality of neoplasm).

Chest radiographs exclude pulmonary metastases, and bone scans should be performed for large tumors and in patients with bone pain or elevated alkaline phosphatase levels. Magnetic resonance imaging (MRI) can be used for defining poorly characterized renal masses seen on CT or when CT is contraindicated in cases of allergy to intravenously administered contrast agent or poor renal function. In addition, MRI is an excellent method of assessing the presence and extent of tumor thrombus in the renal vein or vena cava.

Renal cancer is not responsive to irradiation and chemotherapy; therefore, radical nephrectomy remains the cornerstone of treatment of localized renal cancer. Radical nephrectomy with removal of the ipsilateral adrenal and evaluation of the hilar nodes is the standard operation for unilateral renal neoplasms. In this operation, the kidney is removed with the surrounding Gerota's fascia and perinephric fat. Early ligation and division of the pedicle minimize blood loss from the usually present, extensive collaterals. Removal of the primary tumor is occasionally followed by regression of metastases. Resection of isolated metastases in the lungs or extremities may prolong survival. Patients with a single kidney, bilateral lesions, or significant medical renal disease should be considered for partial nephrectomy. Patients with a normal contralateral kidney and good renal function but a small cancer (less than 4 cm) may be good candidates for partial nephrectomy as well.

There is a tendency for the tumor to invade its own venous system, extending into the vena cava and even into the right side of the heart. Resection of tumors with this marked intravascular extension is feasible, and cures have resulted. Tumors confined to the renal capsule (T1 to T2) demonstrate 5-year disease-free survivals of 90%

to 100%. Tumors extending beyond the renal capsule (T3 or T4) and node-positive tumors have 50% to 60% and 0% to 15% 5-year disease-free survival rates, respectively. No effective chemotherapy is available for metastatic renal cell carcinoma. Biologic response modifiers have received much attention. These include α-interferon and interleukin-2. Responders tend to have smaller tumor burdens and metastatic disease confined to the lung.

Testicular Cancer

Testicular cancer is the most common neoplasm in men aged 20 to 35 years. The typical presentation is a patient-identified painless nodule, and orchiectomy is necessary for diagnosis. From 90% to 95% of all primary testicular tumors are germ cell tumors. From a treatment standpoint, testicular carcinomas are divided into two major categories: (1) nonseminomas, which include embryonal cell carcinomas, teratomas, choriocarcinomas, and mixed cell types, and (2) seminomas. Testicular cancer is slightly more common on the right than on the left, which parallels the increased incidence of cryptorchism on the right side. From 1% to 2% of primary testicular tumors are bilateral, and up to 50% of these men have a history of unilateral or bilateral cryptorchism. The relative risk of developing malignancy is greatest for the intra-abdominal testis (1:20) and less for the inguinal testis (1:80). Placement of the cryptorchid testis into the scrotum (orchiopexy) does not alter the malignant potential of the cryptorchid testis; however, it facilitates examination and tumor detection.

The most common symptom of testicular cancer is painless enlargement of the testis. Patients are usually the first to recognize an abnormality, yet the typical delay in seeking medical attention ranges from 3 to 6 months, and an incorrect diagnosis is made at the initial examination in up to 25% of patients. Acute testicular pain resulting from intratesticular hemorrhage occurs in approximately 10% of cases. Ten percent manifest symptoms relating to metastatic disease, such as back pain (retroperitoneal metastases), cough (pulmonary metastases), or lower extremity edema (vena cava obstruction). A testicular mass or diffuse enlargement of the testis is found in most cases during physical examination. The examiner needs to differentiate between intraparenchymal testicular masses, which are often malignant, and extraparenchymal testicular masses, which are often benign.

On examination, the lesion is firm, nontender, and solid and does not transilluminate. Occasionally tumors are misdiagnosed as simple hydroceles because of the formation of a secondary hydrocele. The diagnosis of epididymitis may also be made erroneously in some situations. Examination should include a detailed evaluation of the neck, chest, and abdominal contents. In advanced disease, supraclavicular adenopathy may be detected, and abdominal examination may palpate a retroperitoneal mass. Gynecomastia is seen in 5% of germ cell tumors.

Several biochemical markers are important in the diagnosis and treatment of testicular carcinoma, including human chorionic gonadotropin (hCG), α-fetoprotein (AFP), and lactate dehydrogenase (LDH). α-Fetoprotein is not elevated in pure seminomas. Although hCG level is occasionally elevated in seminomas, levels tend to be lower than in nonseminomas. Lactate dehydrogenase level may be elevated in either type of tumor. It is a less sensitive and less specific marker than β-hCG or AFP for nonseminomatous germ cell tumors, but it may be the only marker that is elevated in seminomas. In addition, a significantly elevated serum LDH level has independent prognostic value for men with advanced seminoma.

Most intratesticular masses are malignant. If the lesion is confined to the testis on physical examination, inguinal exploration with early vascular control of the spermatic cord structures is the initial intervention to exclude neoplasm. Scrotal ultrasonography should be performed if uncertainty exists with respect to the diagnosis. Scrotal ultrasound can accurately distinguish intrinsic from extrinsic testicular lesions and can detect intratesticular lesions as small as 1 to 2 mm in diameter. Measurement of serum markers should be done prior to surgery, but surgical treatment should not be delayed for the results. Through an inguinal incision, the spermatic vessels are occluded before the testis is exteriorized for inspection to prevent the spread of tumor. Palpation of induration in the testis is an indication for radical orchiectomy, and there is little place for biopsy, because more than 90% of solid lesions of the testis in this age group are malignant. Scrotal violation through a scrotal incision or an attempt to "biopsy" the testis should be avoided because of concern for changing the lymphatic channels available to the testis tumor and potential for a poorer outcome. Further therapy depends on two pieces of information provided by histologic examination. The first is differentiation between a seminoma and a nonseminomatous tumor, and the second is a clear statement on the presence or absence of lymphovascular invasion. Patients are classified into groups with high risk or low risk of recurrence by presence of vascular invasion.

Once the diagnosis of testicular cancer has been established by inguinal orchiectomy, clinical staging of the disease is accomplished by chest, abdominal, and pelvic CT scanning. Conventional imaging involves CT of the chest, abdomen, and pelvis, which is prone to false-negative results. Magnetic resonance imaging offers equivalent (if not better) accuracy in imaging the abdomen and pelvis and is indicated when a patient is unable to have intravenous contrast. Magnetic resonance imaging also avoids exposure to radiation, but it is not always accessible. In many U.S. medical centers, patients are then definitively staged pathologically with lymph node dissection of the retroperitoneum, which is the first site of spread.

Retroperitoneal lymph node dissection (RPLND) is the only reliable method to identify nodal micrometastases and is the gold standard for providing accurate pathologic staging of the retroperitoneum. This extra step clearly minimizes clinical staging errors but at the expense of additional surgery. Stage I lesions are confined to the testis and cord. Stage II lesions have positive retroperitoneal nodes and are subdivided according to the extent of nodal involvement. Stage III designates nonregional metastases, involvement of visceral organs, or significant elevation of serum markers. Once surgery has been completed, it is important to follow the rate of marker decline. The predicted half lives of AFP and hCG are 5 to 7 days and 1 to 2 days, respectively. Any significant deviation from these numbers is predictive for metastatic disease, even in the absence of radiologically defined abnormalities. Such patients should be treated as if they have metastatic disease.

Testicular cancer is often curable, whether discovered in its early stage or as metastatic disease. Patients with disease confined to the testis have an overall survival rate of almost 100%. However, even many patients with disseminated disease can be treated with curative chemotherapy. For patients diagnosed with early-stage testicular cancer, radical orchidectomy is the primary therapeutic intervention. After orchiectomy, most patients with seminoma receive adjuvant radiotherapy as standard care, because seminomas are very radiosensitive. Most patients who relapse can be cured with cytotoxic chemotherapy. Retroperitoneal lymph node dissection is not generally used to treat seminoma.

For patients with nonseminomatous tumors, there are three therapeutic options; surveillance, adjuvant chemotherapy with cisplatinum-containing regimens, or retroperitoneal lymph node dissection. There is no consensus about the treatment of early nonseminomatous testicular cancer, because survival rate is almost 100% regardless of the initial treatment decision. Surveillance of patients with low-risk disease is acceptable, because testicular cancer is still curable if metastasis occurs. Pathologic analysis of the orchiectomy specimen enables definition of patients at high and low risk of relapse. Several studies have examined surveillance as a management strategy for patients with stage I nonseminoma. About 30% of patients relapse, but overall survival rate is 97% to 99%, because these patients can be cured with chemotherapy at relapse. Surveillance protocols involve a rigorous enforcement of regular examinations, chest x-rays, and tumor marker analysis. Computed tomography of the chest and abdomen is also required during the first 2 years. The major advantage of a surveillance protocol is that treatment is reserved for individuals who require it. Thus, for the 70% of patients with stage I disease who do not relapse after their primary orchiectomy, unnecessary surgery or chemotherapy is avoidable. Surveillance is suitable only for patients who lack vascular invasion in their orchiectomy specimen.

Retroperitoneal lymph node dissection after orchiectomy has been a therapeutic option for stage I nonseminomatous tumors for several years in the United Sates. The main supporting argument for this approach is that current radiologic techniques inadequately evaluate patients, so about 30% of patients diagnosed with stage I disease on the basis of a CT scan are subsequently found to have involved retroperitoneal lymph nodes at surgery. For patients with positive lymph nodes classified as having pathologic stage II disease, 60% to 90% can be cured by RPLND. Recurrence within the retroperitoneum is extremely rare after RPLND, so subsequent follow-up should not require routine abdominal CT. Historically, RPLND caused substantial morbidity, but this has been reduced recently because of better knowledge of the neuroanatomy and lymphovascular drainage. With nerve-sparing surgery, postoperative ejaculatory dysfunction associated with RPLND can now largely be avoided. Therefore, current clinical practice for nonseminomatous tumors recommends adjuvant treatment for patients with high-risk stage I disease.

164
Urologic Injuries

The most reliable sign of injury to the kidney is hematuria. However, the degree of hematuria is not correlated with the severity of injury. In blunt trauma, adults with microscopic hematuria and systolic blood pressure ≥90 mm Hg do not require imaging. All pediatric trauma patients, patients with gross hematuria, and patients with microscopic hematuria and systolic blood pressure <90 mm Hg require radiographic evaluation. Computed tomography (CT) is the first-line imaging modality for all suspected blunt renal traumas. A second CT scan, 10 minutes after initial imaging, is recommended to detect urinary extravasation or injury to the collecting system.

Grade I renal injury includes renal contusion, with or without subcapsular hematoma, and an intact renal capsule and collecting system. Grade II injuries include minor cortical lacerations without injury to the collecting system. Grade III injuries include deep parenchymal lacerations not involving the collecting system. Grade IV injuries involve deep parenchymal lacerations with extension into the collecting system or contained injury to the main renal artery or vein. Grade V injuries include shattered kidneys or renal artery or vein avulsion.

Historically, penetrating injury to the kidney mandated renal exploration. Current thought, however, is that accurate preoperative radiographic staging, usually with CT, can distinguish injuries that require exploration and repair from injuries that can be safely treated nonoperatively. Absolute preoperative indications for renal exploration include hemodynamic instability due to renal hemorrhage and grade V renal injury. In this instance, laparotomy is usually required before the injury is evaluated radiographically. Intraoperatively, a pulsatile or expanding retroperitoneal hematoma mandates renal exploration. In these cases, an on-table one-shot intravenous urogram should be performed to document contralateral renal function prior to exploration. If the injured kidney is imaged adequately and found to be normal, exploration can be omitted.

All grade I and II renal injuries, regardless of the mechanism of injury, can be managed without operation. In stable patients, grade III and nonvascular grade IV injuries can also be observed. Shattered kidneys (grade V) and vascular injuries (grades IV and V) require immediate renal exploration. The initial step is isolation of the renal vasculature before opening Gerota's fascia. This technique permits rapid control of bleeding. Isolation of the renal vessels is best performed by opening the peritoneum overlying the aorta. In the presence of large hematomas, the inferior mesenteric vein serves as a landmark for the aorta. Working cephalad along the aorta, the left renal vein is first encountered and subsequently both renal arteries. The best way to find the right renal artery is to dissect between the aorta and the vena cava. Isolation of the right renal vein may be easier after reflection of the right colon and duodenum. Vessel loops are applied around the renal artery and vein. Gerota's fascia is then opened. If release of the tamponade effect causes bleeding, clamping of the renal artery alone usually controls the hemorrhage, unless the renal vein is also injured. Clamp time should be limited to less than 30 minutes, if possible. Total exposure of the kidney by means of sharp and blunt dissection is performed. Renal repair includes debridement of all devitalized tissue, hemostasis, closure of the collecting system, and drainage. With these techniques, renal salvage should be possible in nearly 90% of kidney explorations. Nephrectomy should be reserved for destroyed kidneys that cannot be reconstructed or for serious renal injury associated with other life-threatening injuries. At the end of the procedure, drainage of the renal region is recommended.

Retroperitoneal drains should be removed within 48 hours unless the output is substantial. A comparison of the creatinine level in the fluid with the creatinine level in serum can distinguish urinary leakage from serous fluid. Persistent urinary leakage is evaluated with CT. Urinomas without infection usually resolve without intervention. Percutaneous drainage is required for infected urinomas and abscesses. Hypertension is a rare late complication of renal reconstruction. It is usually renin mediated from an ischemic segment of renal parenchyma. Excision of the nonperfused segment or nephrectomy may be required.

Renal artery thrombosis is usually associated with deceleration injury and is difficult to diagnose and treat. Successful revascularization occurs in less than 30% of cases, and delayed hypertension occurs even with successful revascularization. Therefore, revascularization is reserved for patients with bilateral renal injury or injury to a solitary kidney.

Injuries to the Ureters

Ureteral injury accounts for less than 1% of urologic injuries. The absence of physical signs of injury makes diagnosis difficult. A penetrating wound is the predominant cause of ureteral injury. Up to 50% of ureteral injuries caused by blunt trauma are not recognized immediately. Gross or microscopic hematuria occurs in only 30% to 70% of ureteral injuries. Computed tomography with delayed cuts should be performed when ureteral injury is suspected. However, ureteral injury may not be suspected until the time of laparotomy, when a hematoma is found near the kidney or ureter. If on-table intravenous urography is not diagnostic, direct inspection of the ureter is essential. Injection of indigo carmine directly into the collecting system may identify extravasation. All injuries to the ureter should be repaired, unless a delay in diagnosis results in an abscess or urinoma. In this case, drainage by percutaneous nephrostomy and ureteral stenting may allow the inflamed ureter to heal.

The repair techniques for ureteral injury include debridement of devitalized tissue, a spatulated tension-free anastomosis, watertight mucosal approximation, ureteral stenting, and drainage. Injuries to the ureter between the renal pelvis and the pelvic brim are repaired by ureteroureterostomy. After debridement, the ends are spatulated, and an interrupted repair is completed over a double J stent. Large defects in the ureter may require transureteroureterostomy, in which the injured ureter is passed behind the mesocolon to the contralateral side. Anastomosis of the injured ureter to a 1 to 2 cm opening in the medial normal ureter can be achieved without tension. With transureteroureterostomy, a stent crosses the anastomosis and is brought out through the bladder. Ureteral injuries below the pelvic brim should be debrided and reimplanted into the bladder. The distal stump is ligated, and, after the anterior bladder wall is opened, the proximal end of the ureter is brought through a new opening in the back wall of the bladder. The ureter is then spatulated and approximated to the bladder mucosa with interrupted chromic sutures. Large

defects can be bridged by performing a vesico-psoas hitch, in which the bladder dome is mobilized to bridge the ureteral defect and sewn to the central tendon of the psoas muscle. A retroperitoneal drain is essential in all ureteral repairs. Cystoscopic removal of the double J stent is usually performed 4 to 6 weeks after operation.

The same principles of repair apply to iatrogenic ureteral injury. Recognition of these injuries is often delayed until the patient develops a urinoma, abscess, ureterocutaneous fistula, or hydronephrosis. Injury diagnosed within a week of presentation can be repaired surgically at that time if there is no infection. Beyond this time, it is best to treat the injury with percutaneous nephrostomy drainage and an antegrade ureteral stent. An abscess or urinoma should be drained percutaneously. In some cases, 4 to 6 weeks of urinary diversion and stenting may allow resolution of the injury.

Injuries to the Bladder

Bladder rupture is most often caused by blunt trauma and is associated with gross hematuria in 95% of cases. Bladder rupture can be accurately diagnosed with CT cystography or plain-film cystography. Standard CT is inadequate for the diagnosis of bladder rupture, because the bladder is not sufficiently distended in most patients. Computed tomography cystography involves three sets of images: (1) initial fill images obtained after retrograde instillation of 100 mL of contrast material, (2) complete fill images obtained after instillation of 350 mL, and (3) images obtained after drainage. A plain-film cystogram is obtained after an initial scout film by instilling 300 to 400 mL of contrast through a urethral catheter. An anteroposterior view should be taken with the bladder full and after evacuation. In cases of intraperitoneal bladder injury, extravasation of contrast outlines the bowel loops and may track along the lateral gutters. Extraperitoneal injuries demonstrate flame-shaped extravasation in the pelvis.

Extraperitoneal bladder injuries caused by blunt trauma can be treated with catheter drainage for 10 days. After 10 days, plain-film cystography should be used to document healing. If extravasation persists, cystography should be repeated weekly until healing occurs. Contraindications to nonoperative management include urinary infection and the presence of bony fragments in the bladder. All penetrating injuries and all intraperitoneal ruptures of the bladder are treated with bladder exploration and repair. Bladder exploration can be performed via an intraperitoneal approach. Penetrating injuries and extraperitoneal ruptures are approached by opening the bladder with the electrocautery vertically at the dome and identifying the sites of rupture intravesically. These lacerations are then debrided and closed with interrupted 3-0 chromic catgut or Vicryl sutures, which approximate detrusor muscle and mucosa in one layer. The cystotomy is then closed with two layers of continuous 2-0 or 3-0 Vicryl sutures, the first layer consisting of mucosa and detrusor muscle and the second consisting of detrusor and serosa. Adequate urinary drainage is essential to successful healing of the repaired bladder. Large Foley catheter drainage is sufficient if bladder injuries are not extensive and hemostasis is successful. Extensive injuries and coagulopathy warrant additional drainage with a suprapubic tube, which allows irrigation of clots and proper decompression of the bladder. In addition, a closed-suction or a Penrose drain is placed near the bladder closure. For most patients with a bladder repair, 7 days of catheter drainage is sufficient to allow healing. Cystography may be indicated in cases of severe bladder injury or persistent output from drains. An infected pelvic hematoma can have disastrous consequences. Therefore, nonoperative treatment of extraperitoneal rupture must be undertaken with caution.

Injuries to the Urethra

Almost all injuries to the male urethra are caused by blunt trauma. Posterior urethral injuries in males occur in 5% of pelvic fractures, which is the most common cause of posterior urethral injury. The female urethra is seldom injured. It is almost always associated with bladder injury and pelvic fracture. Blood at the urethral meatus is the classic sign of injury to the male urethra. This is an indication for immediate urethrography. Attempt at catheter placement can convert incomplete injuries to complete disruptions and is contraindicated with suspected urethral injury. Traumatic urethral injuries are usually managed by suprapubic cystostomy, with reconstruction delayed for 3 to 6 months. Suprapubic cystostomy allows urinary diversion until all associated injuries and bony fractures have healed.

165
Neurogenic Bladder

The bladder is controlled by the autonomic nervous system. The bladder body is innervated by the parasympathetic nervous system. The bladder neck, proximal urethra, and, to a lesser extent, the bladder body are innervated by the sympathetic nervous system. The external or striated muscle sphincter of the proximal urethra is controlled by the somatic nervous system and is essential for continence. The innervation of the bladder includes sympathetic (hypogastric nerves), parasympathetic (pelvic nerves), and somatic innervation to the external sphincter (pudendal nerves). The primary motor nerve supply to the bladder is carried through the pelvic nerve. Sensation of bladder distension stimulates afferent fibers that are also carried in the pelvic nerve. This parasympathetic supply originates in the sacral portion of the spinal cord (S2, S3, and S4). The neurotransmitter is acetylcholine (cholinergic). Cholinergic stimulation promotes bladder contraction and emptying. The sympathetic innervation originates from the thoracolumbar spinal cord (T10 to L2). It travels through the presacral plexus and innervates the bladder via the hypogastric nerves. β-Adrenergic receptors predominate in the body of the bladder, while α-receptors densely populate the bladder neck. Stimulation of the β-receptors leads to relaxation of the body of the bladder, and α-stimulation closes the bladder neck. These actions lead to urine storage and maintain continence during bladder filling.

The bladder has two physiologic functions, the storage and emptying of urine. Normal bladder function requires (1) a compliant bladder that fills without concomitant rise in pressure at low volumes, (2) a competent bladder neck, (3) a sensation of desire to void when capacity is reached, (4) inhibition of micturition by cortical activity until an appropriate time, (5) facilitation of emptying by cortical pathways when voiding is desired, and (6) coordination between detrusor contraction and bladder neck relaxation. Classification of neurogenic bladder disorders categorizes patients as having neurologic disease that affects (1) sensory nerves to the bladder, (2) motor nerves to the

bladder, (3) both sensory and motor nerves, (4) descending and ascending spinal cord tracts, or (5) the cerebral cortex.

Sensory neurogenic bladder results from interruption of the peripheral sensory nerves from the bladder or the sensory components of the ascending spinal tracts. The patient is not aware of bladder filling and may initially have painless urinary retention and overflow incontinence. Typically, the patient with sensory neurogenic bladder disease voids infrequently and with time develops a large bladder capacity. With overdistention, the bladder loses its ability to effectively contract and empty. The cystometrogram demonstrates a large residual urine volume, absent sensation, and no uninhibited bladder contractions. The most common cause of sensory neurogenic bladder disease is diabetes mellitus. Any diabetic patient with voiding symptoms or recurrent urinary tract infection should be evaluated for sensory neurogenic bladder disease. Motor neurogenic bladder is an uncommon disorder that occurs with isolated damage to the parasympathetic motor supply to the bladder. As both motor and sensory nerves to the bladder are carried in the pelvic nerve, injury to the pelvic nerves by surgery or trauma does not result in pure motor neurogenic bladder. Patients typically have acute painful urinary retention. Motor neurogenic bladder is occasionally seen with herniated disc or viral illnesses. Another cause of acute painful urinary retention is psychogenic retention seen in young females.

Autonomous neurogenic bladder results from disruption of both the motor and sensory components of the parasympathetic bladder innervation. In this case the bladder is effectively denervated. Patients usually have urinary retention, and overflow incontinence may occur. A cystometrogram typically demonstrates a high residual urine volume, large bladder capacity, a lack of sensation, and no uninhibited or voluntary detrusor contractions. Any lesion affecting the sacral spinal cord, cauda equina, or pelvic nerves can produce this disorder. Trauma to the sacral portion of the spinal cord or cauda equina and congenital lesions such as myelomeningocele result in autonomous neurogenic bladders. In addition, patients who have undergone extensive pelvic surgery such as abdominoperineal resection for rectal cancer are at significant risk to develop this problem. Voiding dysfunction following radical pelvic surgery (e.g., abdominoperineal resection, proctocolectomy, radical hysterectomy, and low anterior resection) is common and usually results from direct injury to the innervation of the lower urinary tract. Most patients recover function within 4 to 6 months, and conservative management is warranted. Intermittent self-catheterization at periodic intervals should be instituted early to prevent bladder overdistention, recurrent infection, and overflow incontinence. Long-term antimicrobial therapy is not recommended because of the potential development of resistant organisms. The goals of treatment are preservation of renal function and establishment of urinary continence.

Reflex neurogenic bladder disease is seen in patients who have complete spinal cord lesions above the level of S2. When the ascending and descending spinal cord tracts are interrupted, the patient exhibits uncontrolled and uninhibited reflex-mediated bladder contractions secondary to bladder filling. Because reflex voiding cannot be inhibited by higher centers, patients with reflex neurogenic bladder disease usually have incontinence. A cystometrogram demonstrates a complete lack of sensation and uninhibited bladder contractions at low bladder volumes. Patients with reflex neurogenic bladder usually empty their bladders unless detrusor-striated sphincter dyssynergia is present. Patients with this syndrome exhibit contraction instead of relaxation of the striated pelvic floor muscles at the time of detrusor contraction.

Functional obstruction to urine flow may occur. This diagnosis should be considered for all patients with reflex neurogenic bladder who carry high residual urine volumes. Most patients with reflex neurogenic bladder disease are traumatic paraplegics. *Autonomic dysreflexia* is a serious medical condition that must be recognized and treated promptly in a patient with a spinal cord injury. Patients with injuries at T6 or higher are at risk for this autonomic reflex, which is usually triggered by visceral distention. Elevated blood pressure, sweating, pounding headache, and bradycardia occur with visceral autonomic nervous system activation (bladder distention, fecal impaction, bowel obstruction). Immediate treatment includes relief of the obstruction and the use of α-adrenergic blocking agents such as prazosin, terazosin, or nifedipine.

When a lesion develops in the cerebral cortex, the ability to suppress reflex bladder contractions is lost, resulting in uninhibited neurogenic bladder. During bladder filling, all is normal until the point of first sensation. At this point, a sudden desire to void occurs, the patient is unable to inhibit this, and micturition occurs. The bladder empties completely, and the stream is uninterrupted. Patients with uninhibited neurogenic bladder disease do not show detrusor-striated sphincter dysfunction. Patients usually have urgency and urgency incontinence. A cystometrogram shows a small residual urine volume, intact sensation, and uninhibited bladder contractions. These are similar to the observations in reflex neurogenic bladder; however, bladder sensation is absent in reflex neurogenic bladder and present in uninhibited neurogenic bladder. Uninhibited neurogenic bladder disease is common in elderly patients. Cerebrovascular disease and Parkinson's disease are common causes.

166
The Pediatric Surgical Patient

The perioperative care of infants and children presents many management problems that differ significantly from problems encountered with adults. This chapter is concerned with recognition and management of certain clinical problems that occur frequently in neonates, infants, and children, with special attention paid to five areas: (1) monitoring, (2) shock, (3) fluid and electrolyte management, (4) infection and antibiotics, and (5) nutritional support.

More emphasis is placed on the special needs of neonates (i.e., babies younger than 28 days) and infants (i.e., babies 28 days to 1 year of age), because treatment of very young children is quite different from treatment of adults or even older children. Several special conditions for which pediatric treatment differs substantially from adult treatment include intestinal obstruction, respiratory distress, and abdominal pain.

Temperature regulation is critical in neonates, because, compared with older children and adults, they have a large body surface area, little subcutaneous fat (and therefore poor thermal insulation), and reduced lean body mass (required for generating and retaining heat). Most of the heat loss from newborns occurs through radiation, convection, and evaporation. Very little heat is lost through conduction. Incubators are manufactured so as to minimize radiation and convection by decreasing airflow across the skin and by providing a tightly regulated, thermally neutral environment. Maintaining body temperature in neonates and young infants is critical both in the neonatal intensive care unit and in the operating room.

Measurement of body weight is especially helpful for evaluating neonates and young infants. Most acute changes in body weight result from changes in total body water. Serial measurements of body weight are therefore useful guides to fluid replacement. In general, a 1-g loss of body weight is equivalent to a 1-mL loss of total body water. Serial measurements should be made every 8 to 12 hours and possibly more frequently for neonates. It is important to keep in mind that, in their first day of life, newborns undergo significant diuresis that reduces extracellular fluid volume and total body water.

Urine flow is a very useful guide to fluid management in all age groups. Measurement of urine output requires accurate collections. An appropriate urine output is 1 to 2 mL/kg/hr with an osmolality of 250 to 300 mOsm/kg. In premature infants, the flow may need to be somewhat higher, and the osmolality may tend to be slightly lower.

Shock

The two most common types of shock occurring in infants, children, and adults are hypovolemic shock and septic shock. In infants and children, septic shock is the most common. How newborns and infants respond to the types of shock is substantially different from how older children and adults respond. For example, in a neonate affected by profound shock, bradycardia is a common response, rather than tachycardia, which is more common in adults. In addition, neonates, especially premature neonates, normally have a low blood pressure. Consequently, the shock insult often does not evoke a further significant reduction of blood pressure. Septic shock is usually caused by Gram-negative bacteria. Peritonitis caused by intestinal perforation is a common cause of septic shock in neonates and infants. Other causes are urinary tract infections, respiratory tract infections, and contaminated intravascular catheters.

The mainstay of treatment of hypovolemic shock is fluid and blood replacement. For neonates, the hematocrit should be maintained at 45% to ensure adequate oxygen delivery. For many infants, hypovolemic shock is caused not by hemorrhage but by dehydration (e.g., from severe gastroenteritis). The subsequent dehydration is usually hypertonic because of the loss of hypotonic fluid. As a rule, much more water is lost than electrolytes, which causes serum sodium levels to be as high as 150 mEq/L. The emergency treatment is infusion of hypotonic solutions of sodium chloride. Because septic shock, like hypovolemic shock, causes reduced circulating blood volume, initial therapy involves infusion of large volumes of colloid solutions. In addition, broad-spectrum antibiotics should always be administered.

Fluid and Electrolytes

Fluid and electrolyte management of neonates and infants requires a thorough understanding of the body's fluid compartment changes, which occur before and after birth. During the first trimester, total body water comprises 95% of body weight. This percentage falls to 80% by 32 weeks' gestation, to 78% at term, and to 75% by the end of the first postnatal week. Body water then decreases slowly over the next 1 to 2 years to 60% of total body weight. Similarly, extracellular fluid volume decreases from 60% of body weight during the second trimester to 45% at birth and eventually to 20% during the next 2 years. This normal physiologic process is interrupted in premature neonates, who must diurese excess fetal and postnatal total body water in a relatively short period after birth. This interruption has a significant effect on the fluid and electrolyte requirements of premature infants undergoing major surgery. An expanded extracellular fluid volume in a premature infant is a potent stimulus for the release of prostaglandin E_2, which maintains the patency of a ductus arteriosus.

Renal function is related to two physiologic processes, glomerular filtration and tubular excretion and reabsorption. In newborns, glomerular filtration rates are 25% of adult values, which are reached by 2 years of age. Likewise, renal concentrating ability is substantially reduced in both premature and full-term infants. A full-term infant can maximally concentrate urine to only 500 to 600 mOsm/kg (compared with 1,200 mOsm/kg for an adult). A premature infant has even less concentrating ability (up to a maximum of 400 mOsm/kg). As a consequence, newborns tolerate dehydration poorly.

Insensible water loss is a result of continuous loss of water from the respiratory tract and the skin. In both full-term and premature infants, transepithelial water loss is the major component of insensible water loss. Premature infants have a less developed stratum corneum than full-term infants and therefore experience a greater diffusion of water through the epidermal surface and a greater insensible water loss through the skin. In full-term neonates, in an environment of thermal neutrality and a humidity of 50%, total insensible water loss is 12 mL/kg/24 hr, of which 7 mL is lost through the skin and 5 mL through the lungs. In full-term infants, overhead radiant heaters and phototherapy can increase insensible water loss from skin by 50%. In premature infants, radiant heaters and phototherapy can increase insensible water loss from skin by 50% to 100%.

Full-term babies sweat at birth if body temperature exceeds 37.5°C (99.5°F); however, the amount of water they lose by this mechanism is quite small. Respiratory water loss accounts for about one-third of total insensible water loss in full-term infants and is related to the volume of inspired air, respiratory rate, body temperature, and the humidity of the expired air. Insensible water loss from the skin is minimized by the use of incubators in the neonatal ICU and extremity coverings in the operating room. Water loss from the lungs can be decreased by humidifying the inspired gases.

The sodium requirements of full-term infants average 2 mEq/kg/24 hr; preterm infants older than 32 weeks in gestational age require 3 mEq/kg/24 hr; and babies who are of younger gestational age or who are critically ill require 4 to 5 mEq/kg/24 hr. Conditions such as intestinal obstruction and peritonitis increase sodium loss and therefore increase the sodium requirements. Although full-term infants can retain sodium as well as adults do in the case of sodium deficit, they are unable to excrete excess sodium as effectively as adults. As a result, excessive infusion of intravenous sodium can rapidly cause hypernatremia.

Potassium requirements of infants are not well documented. The generally accepted requirements are 2 mEq/kg/24 hr after the first 2 to 3 days of life. Potassium requirements are important in the first few days of life, especially after a major operation, because, in the catabolic state, protein breakdown leads to nitrogen loss in the urine and a concomitant potassium loss. Thus, potassium should be administered in the first 1 or 2 days after an operation once urine output is established. Given all the considerations described, the initial fluid used for surgical management of the neonate and infant, both preoperatively and postoperatively, should be 5% or 10% dextrose in 0.2% saline at a dosage of approximately 100 to 150 mL/kg/24 hr.

Metabolic alkalosis caused by electrolyte loss, specifically chloride, can occur with prolonged gastric suction or vomiting and is usually easily corrected by replacement of the appropriate electrolytes (e.g., with potassium chloride). Metabolic acidosis, on the other hand, is usually the result of poor tissue perfusion and lactic acidosis. It is best corrected by treating the underlying cause of the poor perfusion.

Infection

Immediately after birth, bacterial colonization of the newborn begins. This process begins with the skin and shortly thereafter involves the gastrointestinal (GI) tract.

By 10 days of age, normal newborns have the common aerobic and anaerobic bacteria in their GI tract. Neonates in ICUs undergo delayed colonization with a small number of pathogenic bacteria. Normal barriers to invasive infection, especially the skin and GI tract, are underdeveloped in newborns. The normal mucosal barrier to bacterial invasion in the neonatal ileum is defective, which may explain the etiology of neonatal sepsis (see later) and possibly of necrotizing enterocolitis as well. Normal host defense mechanisms are also incompletely developed at birth; full immunocompetence develops during the first few months of life. In premature infants, antibody levels are not high enough for adequate response to invasive sepsis. Normal full-term infants have adequate levels of immunoglobulin (Ig)G antibodies from their mothers but a lack of IgM antibodies, which include many opsonins, making newborns susceptible to infection with Gram-negative bacteria. Secretory IgA antibodies from the intestine do not reach effective levels until 3 weeks of age. They are passively acquired from colostrum in the first few days of life. Phagocytes in breast milk are another source of passive protection for the neonate. Usually, the first sign of a postoperative infection is fever, except in neonates, who rarely manifest temperature elevation. The usual sites of postoperative infection are the lungs, the surgical wound, the urinary tract, and intravenous catheter sites.

Nutrition

The nutritional requirements of children and teenagers do not differ significantly from those of adults; however, the requirements of infants do. Sick infants in need of nutritional support pose therapeutic problems that are different from and frequently more complex than the needs of their adult counterparts. Not only must the metabolic demands of a major illness or operation be taken into account, but, additionally, special consideration must be given to the unique characteristics of pediatric patients, such as smaller body size, rapid growth, highly variable fluid requirements, and, in newborns, the immaturity of certain organ systems. Even a relatively short period of inadequate nutrition can lead to decreased host resistance, increased infection, and poor wound healing, which contribute appreciably to morbidity and mortality in infants and children with surgical disease. An infant's body contains more water than an adult's body (70% to 75% compared with 60% to 65%); therefore, infants require more water per unit of body weight. Healthy infants consume water at a daily rate of 10% to 15% of body weight, in contrast to a rate of only 2% to 4% for adults. They retain only 0.5% to 3% of their fluid intake: about 50% is excreted through the kidneys, 3% to 10% is lost through the GI tract, and 40% to 50% is insensible loss.

Infants also have much higher caloric requirements than older children and adults, and these requirements are further increased by periods of active growth and extreme physical activity. Most of an infant's caloric requirements are supplied by carbohydrates. Much less glycogen can be stored in an infant's liver than in an adult's liver. For this reason, fats are the other major nonprotein calorie source for infants. Protein needs of infants are based on the combined requirements for maintenance and growth. Protein constitutes 13% of an infant's body weight compared with 20% of an adult's. Most of the increase in body protein occurs during the first year of life, which explains why protein requirements are highest in infancy and decrease with age. In general, infants require more vitamins and minerals than adults. Increased amounts of calcium and phosphorus are particularly important because of the rapid growth rate of the infant's bones.

167
Pyloric Stenosis

Hypertrophic pyloric stenosis is the most common cause of nonbilious vomiting in infants. Gastric outlet obstruction results from hypertrophy of the circular muscle of the pylorus. It occurs in approximately 3:1,000 infants. The male-to-female ratio is 4:1; many being the firstborn male. The incidence of the disease is greater in offspring of mothers with a history of pyloric stenosis. It is also associated with other congenital defects such as Turner's syndrome, tracheoesophageal fistula, esophageal atresia, and trisomy 18. The primary etiology is unknown. Possible etiologic factors include abnormal muscle innervation, elevated prostaglandin levels, reduced levels of pyloric nitric oxide synthase, and hypergastrinemia. Erythromycin administration in neonates has also been implicated.

The most common symptom is nonbilious vomiting, which may be projectile in nature and can occur intermittently or immediately after feeding. The condition presents most commonly between ages 2 and 8 weeks. There is often a history of multiple changes in feeding formula before medical attention is sought. Infants generally become dehydrated because of frequent vomiting. The frequent vomiting leads to fluid loss as well as hydrogen and chloride ion losses, which result in a hypochloremic metabolic alkalosis. With volume depletion, the renal preservation of sodium can be achieved only in exchange with hydrogen ions, because potassium is already severely depleted. This will result in the classic "paradoxical aciduria" that further compounds the metabolic alkalosis. Sodium replacement therefore is crucial in correcting the problem.

Diagnosis can be made by palpation of a pyloric mass in 60% to 80% of cases. It is characterized as a firm, olive-shaped, mobile mass, approximately 2 cm in size. It is generally located in the midepigastrium to the right of the umbilicus beneath the liver's edge. A peristaltic wave may be visible that progresses from the left upper quadrant to the epigastrium with feeding. These classic findings on physical examination may be detected by the physician who is observing the infant while feeding. The diagnosis can be confirmed with ultrasound evaluation of the abdomen. A pyloric thickness of 3 to 4 mm or length greater than 15 to 18 mm secures the diagnosis. Contrasted studies with barium may demonstrate an elongated pyloric channel; however, these are infrequently required. The differential diagnosis includes gastroesophageal reflux, duodenal stenosis, pyloric duplication, adrenal insufficiency, and inborn errors of metabolism. These can be differentiated via radiographic evaluation as well as electrolyte panels.

Initially, treatment is focused on correcting acid–base and electrolyte abnormalities. Therefore, surgery should not be performed on an emergency basis in cases of pyloric stenosis. Fluid resuscitation is with an infusion of 0.45% to 0.9% saline plus 5% to 10% dextrose; 30 to 50 mEq/L is the preferred rate. Infants are kept non per os during this time with a nasogastric tube in place. The goal of fluid replacement is to achieve a serum bicarbonate level of less than 30 mEq/L. This is indicative of correction of alkalosis. Without correction, metabolic alkalosis can lead to postoperative apnea as a compensatory mechanism. The Ramstedt pyloromyotomy is the procedure of choice. The procedure can be conducted through a small transverse incision in the right upper quadrant, a periumbilical incision, or, more recently, laparoscopically. The pyloric muscle is split, leaving the mucosa intact. Vomiting may occur in about 50% of postoperative patients. This is thought to be due to edema at the pyloric incision site. Feeding can be resumed 12 to 24 hours postoperatively.

168
Pediatric Solid Tumors

The three most common solid tumors in infants and children are neuroblastoma, Wilms' tumor, and rhabdomyosarcoma, in decreasing order of incidence. Neuroblastoma is a tumor arising from neural crest cells and can be located anywhere along the sympathetic ganglia or adrenal medulla. Three-fourths of neuroblastomas originate in the abdomen, with half of these located in the adrenal medulla. The tumors that do not arise from an abdominal source tend to be in the posterior mediastinum. A very small number originate in the neck.

The incidence of neuroblastoma is approximately 1 in 10,000 persons, and it comprises 5% to 10% of all pediatric cancers. The median age at which neuroblastoma is diagnosed is 2 years, and approximately 95% of cases occur before age 10 years. Neuroblastoma has a variable course. Some tumors advance rapidly, and others regress spontaneously. Spontaneous resolution occurs most often in children with neuroblastoma before 1 year of age. The overall survival rate with neuroblastoma is less than 30%. Neuroblastoma comprises approximately 15% of childhood cancer deaths. Children with an early solitary mass have a surgical cure rate of 25%; however, many children have extensive local or metastatic disease at presentation and thus have a very poor prognosis.

Neuroblastoma most commonly appears as a fixed, lobular abdominal mass extending from the flank toward the midline. Children often have abdominal pain, distention, weight loss, and loss of appetite. Other presenting symptoms depend on the size and location of the primary tumor. Abdominal masses can compress the bowel and/or bladder, causing constipation or urinary bladder dysfunction. Children with masses arising in the posterior mediastium often present with Horner's syndrome, pneumonia, or dyspnea, and the mass is discovered on chest x-ray films. Cervical masses may be palpable or visible and can cause dysphagia or stridor. Presenting symptoms can also be due to metastatic lesions. Neuroblastoma most frequently metastasizes to cortical bones, resulting in localized swelling and tenderness. The tumor can also metastasize to the periorbital bones, causing proptosis and ecchymosis. Bone marrow is another common site of metastasis, which can lead to anemia and weakness. Metastasis to the liver can cause massive hepatomegaly, and in infants this can lead to respiratory distress and to the need for surgical decompression or mechanical ventilation. Less common is metastatic lesions to the skin, causing multiple dark spots. Because neuroblastomas are often functional, they have associated paraneoplastic syndromes, such as hypertension caused by increased catecholamine production or unremitting watery diarrhea due to high vasoactive intestinal polypeptide production. There is also cerebellar ataxia, involuntary movement, and nystagmus associated with some cases of neuroblastoma.

Generally, the diagnosis is made based on history, physical observations, and imaging studies; however, a definitive diagnosis requires histologic evaluation of the tissue. Imaging studies such as computed tomography (CT) or magnetic resonance imaging (MRI) are useful in evaluating the location, extent of metastasis, and resectability of the tumor. Masses that extend beyond the midline are usually considered unresectable. The initial laboratory studies should include complete blood count, kidney and liver function tests, and urine homovanillic and vanillymandelic acid levels. Elevated lactate dehydrogenase, serum ferritin, and neuron-specific enolase levels correlate with advanced disease and are poor prognostic indicators. Other prognostic indicators include the amplification of the N-*myc* oncogene, which tends to be associated with rapid progression of the tumor.

Staging is based on localization of the tumor, completeness of gross tumor excision, lymph node status, and presence of metastasis. Long-term survival rates range from 10% to 90% and depend on a combination of factors, including stage of the tumor, age of the patient (with children less than 1 year of age having markedly improved survival rate), level of N-*myc* amplification, and histology of the tumor. Unfortunately, most patients have less favorable combinations of risk factors.

Treatment for neuroblastoma is multidisciplinary, using surgery, chemotherapy, radiation, and immunotherapy. Surgical resection of the primary tumor and adjacent lymph nodes is the main objective and can be curative in early-stage disease. In cases in which the tumor is determined to be unresectable, incisional biopsy should be performed to allow for tumor histology studies. The tumor can be re-evaluated for resection after a course of adjuvant therapy.

Wilms' tumor is the most common primary malignant kidney tumor and the second most common solid tumor of childhood. The tumor usually occurs between the ages of 1 and 5 years, with the peak age being between 3 and 4 years. Bilateral Wilms' tumors occur in 13% of cases. A germline mutation on the short arm of chromosome 11 is responsible for the development of this tumor. Many other genes associated with genitourinary abnormalities and aniridia are located close to the Wilms' tumor gene, which explains these conditions frequently occurring with Wilms' tumor.

Wilms' tumor presents with a palpable abdominal mass in 60% of cases. There are usually no associated symptoms; however, one-fourth of the patients have hypertension, and about 15% have hematuria. Three syndromes are associated with Wilms' tumor. Denys-Drash syndrome consists of Wilms' tumor, intersex disorder, and progressive nephropathy. WAGR syndrome is an acronym for Wilms' tumor, aniridia, genitourinary anomalies, and mental retardation. Approximately 20% of patents with Beckwith-Wiedemann syndrome (omphalocele, visceromegaly, macroglossia, and hypoglycemia) develop Wilms' tumor. Because of these close associations, children with these syndromes should be closely screened for the development of Wilms' tumor.

Initial evaluation of a childhood abdominal mass should consist of ultrasonography to determine if the mass is solid or cystic and the origin of the mass. Because it can be difficult to distinguish Wilms' tumor from neuroblastoma, a CT scan or MRI is often useful to determine the origin of the mass. Another test to help distinguish the two solid tumors is measurement of urine catecholamines, because, unlike neuroblastoma, the levels should be normal in Wilms' tumor. A CT scan or MRI is also needed for preoperative evaluation to determine treatment options. If the tumor is bilateral, if it is present in a single horseshoe kidney, if there is tumor thrombus in the inferior vena cava extending beyond the hepatic veins, or if there is extensive metastatic disease, preoperative chemotherapy is indicated to attempt to shrink the tumor, to facilitate a complete resection of the tumor at a later time.

Surgical resection is important for both treatment and staging of the tumor. Removal of the entire tumor en bloc with surrounding organs that show invasion should be performed, with careful measures taken to avoid rupturing the tumor. Staging is based on completeness of gross tumor resection, extent of invasion into neighboring organs, whether the renal capsule remains intact, and lymphatic and hematogenous metastasis. Prognosis and postoperative treatment with chemotherapy and/or radiation are determined by the stage and histology of the tumor. Wilms' tumor was once lethal; however, with the current multidisciplinary approach to treatment, the overall survival rate exceeds 85%.

Rhabdomyosarcoma is a malignant tumor originating from skeletal muscle that typically presents before the age of 14 years. The most common primary sites are the head and neck, genitourinary tract, and extremities. However, they can occur in the trunk, gastrointestinal tract, the thorax, or perineal region. Most cases are sporadic, although some conditions pose an increased risk, including Li-Fraumeni, neurofibromatosis-1, and Beckwith-Wiedemann syndrome. Rhabdomyosarcoma largely presents as a palpable mass, with other symptoms being secondary to mass effect depending on the location of the tumor.

The overall prognosis is quite good for rhabdomyosarcoma, with a 5-year survival rate more than 60%. The prognosis is based on the patient's age, site of origin, tumor size and extent at the time of resection, and tumor histology. Children younger than 10 years have a more favorable prognosis. Tumors in the orbit, nonparameningeal head and neck, and biliary and genitourinary tracts tend to have a better prognosis. Children with tumors smaller than 5 cm have better outcomes than those with larger tumors. The ability to completely resect the gross tumor and the absence of metastatic disease also improve the prognosis. Histologically, botryoid and spindle cell types have better outcomes than embryonal, pleomorphic, alveolar, or undifferentiated subtypes.

All rhabdomyosarcomas need preoperative imaging with CT or MRI to determine the anatomy of the tumor and to evaluate for metastatic disease. Diagnosis requires a tissue sample, because there are no know tumor markers. Treatment involves surgical resection with wide local excision when possible and sampling of adjacent lymph nodes. Postoperatively, all rhabdomyosarcomas are followed by chemotherapy. Depending on the histology and extent of the tumor resection, radiation therapy may also be required. When complete resection of all gross tumor is impossible at the initial operation, a second operation should follow chemotherapy and/or radiation.

169
Pediatric Abdominal Wall Defects

Abdominal wall defects are the result of failure of the midgut to return to the abdominal cavity during embryonic development. During normal growth and development of the human embryo, the midgut herniates out of the abdominal cavity through the umbilical ring due to lack of space in the relatively small abdominal cavity for the enlarging midgut viscera. The midgut returns into the abdominal cavity, usually by the eleventh week of gestation, where it completes its rotation and becomes fixed in place, and the umbilical ring closes. There are two major abdominal wall defects that occur when there is failure of the normal reduction of the midgut herniation and closure of the umbilical ring. These are an omphalocele and a gastroschisis. Although the two types of defects have similar pathogenesis, there are important distinctions in the anatomy and prognosis associated with each abdominal wall anomaly.

An omphalocele is a herniation of some portion of the midgut through the umbilical ring into the umbilical cord. Depending on the size of the umbilical ring defect, the hernia sac can contain only a small portion of the small intestine, or it can be large with the entire small bowel, portions of the colon, and liver all in the sac. Either way, the bowel is covered by a membrane consisting of peritoneum and amnion, which separates the abdominal cavity contents from the amniotic fluid.

Many newborns with omphaloceles have associated anomalies. More than 50% of infants have other malformations that affect the cardiac, musculoskeletal, gastrointestinal, and genitourinary systems, with cardiac being the most common. Approximately one-third of infants have karyotype abnormalities such as trisomies 13, 18, and 21. Omphalocele is also one of the components in Beckwith-Wiedemann syndrome, along with hyperinsulinemia and macroglossia. Because of the association with additional congenital anomalies, a thorough evaluation of the infant prior to surgical repair is important. This should include a physical examination, chest radiograph, renal ultrasound, and possibly echocardiogram.

The options for surgical repair of omphaloceles depend primarily on the size of the defect. With small defects, the hernia contents are reduced back into the abdomen, the sac is excised completely, and the fascia and skin are closed. Large defects often require staged reductions over several days or weeks, with special attention to the monitoring of intra-abdominal pressures to avoid the development of abdominal compartment syndrome. Once the viscera are in the abdominal cavity, the fascia and skin can be closed. Again, these may require staged closures. Also in some very large defects, skin or fascia closure may not be possible, and the infant may have a large hernia until it can be closed a few years later.

In gastroschisis, the abdominal wall defect is always located to the right of the umbilical ring, and the umbilical cord is intact. The herniated viscera are not covered by a sac, which also helps distinguish gastroschisis from an omphalocele.

The cause of gastroschisis is unknown; however, the current theory is that the defect is caused by a normal involution of the second umbilical vein. Some risk factors have been identified, such as maternal cigarette, alcohol, and drug use, as well as use of aspirin, ibuprofen, and pseudoephedrine during the first trimester of pregnancy. The strongest risk factor is maternal age of less than 20 years, which leads to an 11-fold increase in occurrence.

Unlike omphalocele, there are rarely associated anomalies in infants with gastroschisis. The one exception is intestinal atresias of either small or large bowel, which occurs in up to 15% of children with gastroschisis. Infants with gastroschisis are prone to short gut syndrome due to the bowel being thickened, edematous, and matted together due to exposure to amniotic fluid or ischemia from the constricting abdominal wall defect. Although there may be adequate length of the small bowel, the damage to the bowel impairs the motility and the absorptive and digestive capacities, leaving the infant with short gut syndrome. Another consideration with gastroschisis is the large third-space fluid losses and increased risk for infection due to the exposed intestine.

Surgical repair of gastroschisis can be accomplished by (1) placing the bowel back in the intestine and surgically closuring the defect a few weeks later or (2) creating a proximal diverting stoma. A primary anastomosis is not recommended because of the relatively high risk of other atresias and the edematous condition of the bowel. Postoperatively, children tend to have a prolonged ileus and require parenteral nutrition.

170
Intussusception

Intussusception is the telescoping of a proximal portion of the intestine (intussusceptum) into an adjacent distal segment (intussuscipiens). The invaginated intestine is propelled further along by peristalsis. This condition is the most common cause of obstruction in children between 3 months and 6 years of age. The most common location is at the ileocecal junction. Other locations include ileo-ileocolic and, to a lesser extent, cecocolic. Intussusception occurs in adults also. The disease process is completely different in patients in these two age groups.

In children, there is rarely an associated pathologic lesion that provides a lead point for prolapse. A lead point is present in only 12% of pediatric patients and increases in incidence with age. Common lead points include Meckel's diverticula, polyps, the appendix, intestinal neoplasm, neurofibroma, hemangioma, and a foreign body. Often swelling of lymphoid tissue is found at the ileocecal valve. It is suspected that gastrointestinal infections may cause swelling of the Peyer's patches in the terminal ileum. The enlarged mounds of tissue lead to mucosal prolapse of the ileum into the colon.

Children with intussusception present acutely. Common symptoms include severe paroxysmal abdominal cramping, pain, and vomiting. In some cases, an abdominal sausage-shaped mass is palpated. As the obstruction progresses, the mesentery becomes constricted, causing bowel ischemia. Bleeding from the mucosa leads to passage of blood clots and mucus intermixed with the stool (currant jelly). Children often are seen with their legs drawn toward their abdomen during these episodes of pain. In between these episodes, the child may be completely asymptomatic.

The diagnosis can be made through clinical history and physical findings. Abdominal plain films may reveal a density in the area of the intussusception. Definitive diagnosis is provided by barium enema, which can be therapeutic as well as diagnostic. Typical findings include a filling defect where the advance of the barium is obstructed. A linear column of barium may be seen within the compressed lumen of the intussusceptum. Air enemas have been shown to be associated with fewer complications and have proved to be as effective. Ultrasound findings include a tubular mass on longitudinal images and a target appearance on transverse images.

Adults make up 5% of intussusception cases. In contrast to children, intussusception in adults is associated with an underlying pathologic process in 90% of cases. The most common lesions include neoplasms, inflammatory lesions, and Meckel's diverticula. Adult patients present with symptoms of intestinal obstruction (abdominal cramping and vomiting). Patients may also experience rectal bleeding. Also, in contrast to pediatric cases of intussusception, adult patients more often present with subacute or chronic symptoms and relapsing course.

In children, radiological reduction with hydrostatic or pneumatic pressure is successful in 70% to 90% if performed within 48 hours. The success rate decreases to 50% when symptoms are present greater than 48 hours. Surgical reduction is required when radiographic means fail. Resection is not required for children if the bowel appears viable. For adults, the presence of a pathologic lesion mandates surgical resection. There is no place for hydrostatic reduction in cases of adult intussusception. For children, the recurrence rate approaches 10% for radiographic methods and 2% to 5% for surgical reduction. Recurrence can most often be reduced radiologically.

171
Pediatric Hernias

Inguinal hernias occur in 1% to 5% of newborns, with about 30% occurring in premature infants. Males are affected six times more often than females. Right-side hernias are the most common, comprising 60% of hernias; 30% are left side, and 10% are bilateral. Inguinal hernias in children are due to the failure of the processus vaginalis to close after the testicle has descended into the scrotum. The processus vaginalis can persist to varying degrees and result in a hernia and communicating hydrocele or a hydrocele of the spermatic cord. The difference between rates of right- and left-side hernias is due to the later descent and obliteration of the of processus vaginalis of the right testis.

Inguinal hernias are identified by physical examination. They are detected as a bulge in the region of the inguinal ligament over the area of the external inguinal ring. The bulge can extend a variable distance into the scrotum or labia. Although the hernias are usually found on routine examinations, parents may also notice inguinal pain or inguinal bulges in the children during their crying episodes. The hernias can become incarcerated and strangulated and, for this reason, should be repaired surgically. The risk of incarceration and strangulation is higher for preterm infants.

Surgical repair of inguinal hernias in children usually requires high ligation of the hernia sac at the level of the internal inguinal ring. Generally, no further repair of the inguinal canal floor is necessary. The timing of surgical repair for premature infants is more complicated. Early repair has a greater incidence of recurrence, risk of damage to cord structures, and risk of anesthesia-related apnea. These risks must be weighed against the risks of incarceration and strangulation and the possibility of developing a larger hernia with loss of abdominal domain. The general consensus of pediatric surgeons is to wait until the neonate is ready to be discharged home. For infants born close to term and discharged home shortly after birth, most surgeons wait until the infant is more than 60 weeks postconception at which time the risk of anesthesia-related apnea is greatly reduced.

With an incarcerated hernia, the repair becomes more urgent. For males, the hernia usually contains incarcerated bowel. If the hernia can be reduced, the child should be observed for 24 to 48 hours and then the hernia repaired to allow tissue edema to decrease. If reduction is not possible, the child should undergo surgery emergently. With females, the ovary is the most common structure incarcerated in the hernia sac. Because the ovary is at a high risk for torsion, surgical repair should be undertaken within 24 hours. Another consideration in the correction of inguinal hernias is the practice of bilateral exploration in a child with a unilateral hernia. Contralateral patent processus vaginalis is common in children with inguinal hernias, especially in the first year of life. For this reason, surgeons generally do bilateral exploration in all children less than 1 year old. Many pediatric surgeons believe all females with unilateral inguinal hernias should have bilateral exploration due the risk of injury to reproductive structures. Bilateral exploration can be done using an open technique or with laparoscopic evaluation of the contralateral groin through the opened hernia sac.

Umbilical hernias are also common in the pediatric population. They are caused by the failure of the umbilical ring to completely close. Many do not require surgical repair, because 80% of umbilical hernias close spontaneously by age 4 to 6 years. In addition, umbilical hernias are far less likely than inguinal hernias to incarcerate or strangulate. Umbilical hernias that remain open after age 6 years require surgical closure. Indications for repair before age 6 years are a large defect (>2 cm, because these have a low probability of spontaneous closure), a history of incarceration, a large skin proboscis, and a child with a ventriculoperitoneal shunt. Surgical repair of umbilical hernias involves an infraumbilical semicircular incision, dissection of the hernia sac from the overlying umbilical skin, transaction of the sac, and primary repair of the fascial defect. For cosmetic reasons, the base of the umbilical skin is pexied to the underlying fascia.

Epigastric hernias are the least common of the abdominal wall hernias discussed in this chapter. The small, midline fascial defects occur between the umbilicus and the xiphoid process. The hernias tend to be small, allowing only preperitoneal fat through the defect. These are repaired surgically when discovered, because they can enlarge over time. When the preperitoneal fat is strangulated, it causes significant pain. Surgical repair involves making a small transverse incision over the mass, excision of the herniated fat, and primary repair of the fascial defect.

172
Surgery in the Elderly Patient

Advanced age is no longer considered a contraindication to surgery. An increasing number of surgical procedures of variable degrees of complexity are performed on older patients. However, in most instances, the elderly surgical patient is at a physiologic disadvantage compared with the younger patient. Understanding the unique physiology of aging is crucial to the surgeon's ability to provide adequate care to the elderly.

Several morphologic changes in the cardiovascular system take place with advancing age. The number of myocytes declines as the collagen and elastin content increases, resulting in fibrotic areas throughout the myocardium and a decline in ventricular compliance. Nearly 90% of the autonomic tissue in the sinus node is replaced by fat and connective tissue. Fibrosis in the conducting system contributes to the high incidence of sick sinus syndrome, atrial arrhythmias, and bundle branch blocks. Calcification of the aortic valve is common, but this is usually of no functional significance. Dilation of all four valvular rings may be responsible for the multivalvular incompetence in older persons. Finally, there is a progressive increase in rigidity and decrease in distensibility in the peripheral circulation. Changes in the peripheral vasculature lead to increased systolic blood pressure, increased resistance to ventricular emptying, and compensatory ventricular hypertrophy. Systolic function is well preserved with increasing age. Cardiac output and ejection fraction are maintained despite the increase in afterload.

The mechanism by which cardiac output is maintained during exercise, however, is somewhat different. In younger persons, output is maintained by increasing heart rate in response to β-adrenergic stimulation. With aging there is a "hyposympathetic state," and the heart becomes less responsive to catecholamines, possibly because of declining receptor function. The aging heart, therefore, maintains cardiac output not by increasing rate but by increasing ventricular filling (preload). Because of this dependence on preload, even minor hypovolemia can cause significant compromise in cardiac function. In contrast to the systolic function, diastolic function is affected by aging. Myocardial relaxation is more energy dependent and therefore requires more oxygen than contraction. With aging there is a progressive decrease in the partial pressure of oxygen. As a result, even mild hypoxemia can result in prolonged relaxation, higher diastolic pressures, and pulmonary congestion. Because early diastolic filling is impaired, maintenance of preload becomes even more reliant on the atrial kick. Loss of the atrial contribution to preload can result in further impairment of cardiac function. It is also important to remember that the manifestation of cardiac diseases in the elderly may be nonspecific and atypical. Although chest pain is still the most common symptom of myocardial infarction, as many as 40% of older patients have a nonclassic presentation with symptoms such as shortness of breath, syncope, acute confusion, or stroke.

Congestive heart failure (CHF) is the leading cause of postoperative morbidity and mortality after surgical procedures. Preoperative recognition of impaired cardiac function and reserve is essential to maintain proper fluid balance and limit myocardial stress. Patients with known CHF should have their fluid balance and hypertension well controlled before undergoing an elective procedure. Estimation of cardiac reserve can be difficult, because most elderly patients with cardiac dysfunction have compensated and only show signs of disease when stressed. Provocative testing with thallium scans or dobutamine stress test is helpful to identify patients with reversible ischemic heart disease. Patients with coronary artery disease are at particular risk for perioperative myocardial ischemia. Tachycardia and hypertension during the operation can increase cardiac work and decrease coronary blood flow, causing ischemia. Implementation of β-adrenergic blocking agents should begin before a planned procedure and continue throughout the perioperative period. Intraoperative intravenous nitroglycerin dilates the coronary circulation and reduces cardiac stress to prevent myocardial ischemia. The use of preoperative β-adrenergic blockade has been shown to decrease the incidence of postoperative cardiac complications and death in patients considered at increased cardiac risk. Present recommendations are that β-blockers should be started preoperatively and continued through the hospitalization.

Pulmonary changes associated with aging are evident by a loss of elastic recoil of the lung and impaired chest wall movement from muscle atrophy resulting in decreased intrathoracic volume displacement. Impaired elasticity also causes air trapping and ventilation–perfusion mismatching, leading to decreased oxygen transfer reflected by an increased alveolar–arterial oxygen gradient. Oxygenation is additionally impaired by an increased closure volume of small airways and decreased surface area for gas exchange as lung parenchyma is destroyed. Vital capacity decreases with age, reflecting an increase in dead space ventilation. Loss of parenchymal elasticity, joint stiffening, weakening of inspiratory muscles, and early small airway collapse also change gas flow characteristics. The forced expiratory volume in 1 second (FEV_1) progressively declines with aging, resulting in an FEV_1:VC (vital capacity) ratio <70. Uneven alveolar ventilation leads to ventilation–perfusion mismatches and a decline in arterial oxygen tension. The PCO_2 does not change despite an increase in dead space. This may be due to the decline in the production of CO_2 that accompanies the falling basal metabolic rates. Air trapping is also responsible for an increase in the residual volume. The overall effect of loss of elastic inward recoil of the lung is balanced somewhat by the decline in chest wall outward force. Total lung capacity therefore remains unchanged, and there is only a mild increase in resting lung volume or functional residual capacity.

The control of ventilation is also affected by aging. Ventilatory responses to hypoxia and hypercapnia fall by 50% and 40%, respectively. This may be the result of declining chemoreceptor function at either the peripheral or central nervous system level. In addition, pulmonary function is affected by alterations in the ability of the respiratory system to protect against infection. There is a decline in mucociliary clearance and a decrease in several components of the swallowing function. The loss of the cough reflex due to neurologic disorders combined with swallowing dysfunction may predispose an elderly patient to aspiration. The increased frequency and severity of pneumonia in older persons has been attributed to these factors and to an increased incidence of oropharyngeal colonization with Gram-negative organisms.

Several physiologic changes in renal function and fluid–electrolyte balance are associated with aging. Overall, these changes include decrease in total body water, decrease in glomerular filtration rate, decrease in urinary concentrating ability, increase in antidiuretic hormone (ADH), increase in atrial natriuretic peptide (ANP), decrease in aldosterone, decrease in thirst mechanism, and decrease in free-water clearance. Age-related changes in the renal system are characterized by a progressive reduction in renal mass caused by glomerulosclerosis, leading to decreased creatinine clearance in most aged patients. Glomerulosclerosis results in a decline in renal plasma flow and in glomerular filtration rate. Additionally, the age-related decline in cardiac output also negatively impacts renal plasma flow and glomerular filtration rate. Patients with an impaired glomerular filtration rate are more susceptible to volume overload in the perioperative period and to accumulation of metabolic substances and drugs. Slowed drug elimination can lead to prolonged sedative effects of anesthetic and narcotic medications and a propensity to drug-induced acute renal failure after administration of nonsteroidal anti-inflammatory medications, diuretics, and antibiotics. The plasma level of creatinine may measure low in elderly patients because of reductions in skeletal muscle mass, and calculated creatinine clearance remains the most sensitive marker of renal function.

Renal tubular function also declines with advancing age. The ability to conserve sodium and excrete hydrogen ion falls, resulting in a diminished capacity to regulate fluid and acid–base balance. Dehydration becomes a particular problem because losses of sodium and water from nonrenal causes are not compensated for by the usual mechanisms of increased renal sodium retention, increased urinary concentration, and increased thirst. The inability to retain sodium is believed to be due to a decline in the activity of the renin–angiotensin system. The increasing inability to concentrate the urine is related to a decline in end-organ responsiveness to ADH. The marked decline in the subjective feeling of thirst is also well documented but not well understood. Alterations of osmoreceptor function in the hypothalamus may be responsible for the failure to recognize thirst despite significant elevations in serum osmolality.

Maintaining appropriate intravascular volume is essential. Fluid overload or depletion can impair hemodynamic stability. Because of the increased afterload and the decreased inotropic and chronotropic responses caused by decreased sensitivity to catecholamines, the aging heart depends more on adequate preload. Dehydration from illness, hospitalization, invasive testing, diuretics, and fasting occurs easily in the elderly and may be underappreciated, because the thirst response is also less. Allowing oral intake of clear liquids up to 2 to 3 hours preoperatively, starting maintenance intravenous fluids early, and holding diuretics are helpful. Overhydration in a compromised heart, however, must also be avoided. For these reasons, intraoperative monitoring of intravascular volume by central venous catheters to measure central venous pressure or pulmonary artery catheters to measure pulmonary artery occlusion pressure is even more important for older patients, particularly those in whom large blood losses or large volume fluid shifts are expected. Because cardiac output in the elderly is maintained by increased stroke volume rather than increased heart rate, end-diastolic volumes must be higher. Optimum performance, therefore, occurs at a higher point on the Starling curve.

Sodium is the principal cation of the extracellular fluid. The age-related alterations in hormonal control of salt and water homeostasis predispose the aged to hyponatremia and hypernatremia. The most common manifestation of sodium imbalance is neurologic and ranges from mild confusion to seizures and coma. These alterations in neurologic function are due to changes in cell volume, with hyponatremia and hypernatremia resulting in brain swelling and brain shrinkage, respectively. For the older patient, improvement in the neurologic dysfunction may lag days behind correction of the electrolyte abnormality.

The most significant correlate of altered hepatobiliary function in the aged is the increased incidence of gallstones and gallstone-related complications. Gallstone prevalence rises steadily with age. Biliary tract disease is the single most common indication for abdominal surgery in the elderly population. Gallstones are associated with complications in more than 50% of cases in elderly patients. Overall, cholecystitis tends to be more severe in the elderly, and outcome is further worsened by the higher incidence of comorbidity such as atherosclerosis and diabetes. Delays in diagnosis and treatment because of the frequent absence of typical biliary symptoms may also be responsible for the bad outcome in the elderly. The typical presentation of right upper quadrant abdominal pain, tenderness, fever, leukocytosis, and peritoneal signs should not be expected in older patients. Awareness of this atypical presentation is the only means of improving the outcome of cholecystitis in the elderly.

Immune competence declines with advancing age. This is associated with an increased susceptibility to infections, an increase in autoantibodies, and an increase in tumorigenesis. This decline may not be apparent in the non-challenged state. For example, there is no decline in neutrophil count with age, but the ability of the bone marrow to increase neutrophil production in response to infection may be impaired. Elderly patients with major infections frequently have normal white blood cell counts, but the differential count will show a profound shift to the left, with a large proportion of immature forms.

Two perioperative factors may be related to the increased surgical morbidity in the elderly, pain and hypothermia. There are several misconceptions related to the physician's understanding of the elderly patient's analgesic requirements. There is a common misconception that a higher incidence of respiratory compromise follows administration of pain medicine in older patients and that they require less pain medication than younger patients. These misconceptions have caused untreated pain to be the most frequent complaint in hospitalized elderly patients. Special attention to the adequacy of analgesia in the postoperative period is required to minimize the level of physiologic stress and other pain-related complications in the elderly. Surgery can cause hypothermia in all patients because of environmental factors and the anesthetic-induced inhibition of normal thermoregulatory mechanisms. Elderly patients are at an even higher risk because of the changes in central and peripheral mechanisms of body temperature regulation that accompany aging. Intraoperative hypothermia in elderly patients with cardiac risk factors has been shown to be an independent predictor of postoperative cardiac events. Every effort should be made to prevent heat losses. Preoperative skin warmers should be used to prevent cooling before induction. Room temperature should be high while the patient is undraped, upper and lower forced air heating blankets should be applied, and all intravenous solutions should be warmed.

173
Surgical Problems of the Pregnant Patient

Breast Cancer in Pregnancy

Pregnancy-associated breast cancer is defined as breast cancer that is diagnosed during pregnancy or within 1 year following pregnancy. It is the most common non-gynecologic malignancy associated with pregnancy. It usually presents as a painless palpable mass with or without nipple discharge. Benign breast lesions account for 80% of breast masses that occur during pregnancy or during lactation. However, any palpable mass that persists for 4 weeks or longer should be evaluated. As in nonpregnant patients, ductal carcinoma is the most common pathologic type of tumor. Physiologic changes of breast engorgement, rapid cellular proliferation, and increased vascularity make a reliable physical examination difficult. Delays in diagnosis and treatment are common, and recent data show a mean delay of 1 to 2 months. When compared with age-matched nonpregnant controls, women with pregnancy-associated breast cancer present with a larger primary tumor and a higher risk of positive axillary lymph nodes. However, women with pregnancy-associated breast cancer have a similar stage-related prognosis compared with nonpregnant controls. Overall, these women have a poorer prognosis because of the more advanced disease at presentation. Pregnancy is a hyperestrogenic state and may correlate with rapid tumor proliferation and axillary lymph node metastases. In addition, diagnosis of pregnancy-associated breast cancer is often delayed because of the reluctance of surgeons to perform biopsies during pregnancy.

Because of the changes in the breast tissue with pregnancy, imaging modalities may be difficult to interpret. If used with appropriate shielding, mammography carries a limited risk to the fetus. Mammography has a high false-negative rate due to the increased density of the breast tissue, so it has limited usefulness in the evaluation of the pregnant patient. Ultrasonography can safely be performed as an initial evaluation or in conjunction with mammography. Ultrasound is able to distinguish solid from cystic lesions in 97% of patients and is helpful in guiding fine-needle aspiration or biopsy. Magnetic resonance imaging (MRI) of the breast is being used more frequently for the nonpregnant patient. Gadolinium crosses the placenta and has been associated with fetal abnormalities in rats, and MRI is not currently recommended for breast imaging in the pregnant patient.

Tissue diagnosis is essential. Core-needle biopsy with or without ultrasound guidance is a safe and reliable method for obtaining tissue. The risk of milk fistula may be reduced by stopping lactation for several days before biopsy and by emptying the breast of milk just before the procedure. If the biopsy is done postpartum, a 1-week course of bromocriptine may also be given before biopsy. Fine-needle aspiration may be a reliable alternative to core-needle or open biopsy. It can be performed safely with ultrasound guidance under local anesthesia, but its accuracy is dependent on the pathologist's experience.

The mainstay of therapy for pregnancy-associated breast cancer is surgical resection. Once the diagnosis of breast cancer is made, modified radical mastectomy should be done expeditiously; it should not be delayed because of the pregnancy. Modified radical mastectomy has long been considered the appropriate choice for local control. It eliminates the need for adjuvant radiation and its risk to the fetus. Axillary dissection is necessary because of the aggressive nature of pregnancy-associated breast cancer and the higher incidence of nodal metastasis. Sentinel node biopsy poses an unknown risk to the fetus and should be avoided until the safety of the radioisotope is determined. For patients diagnosed during the late second trimester or later, immediate breast-conserving lumpectomy and axillary dissection followed with radiation postpartum is a treatment option.

Chemotherapy is indicated for node-positive cancers or node-negative tumors greater than 1 cm. Current chemotherapeutic regimens are relatively safe after the first trimester, when the teratogenic risk is greatest. Antimetabolites such as methotrexate should be avoided because of the high risk of spontaneous abortion even after the first trimester. Chemotherapeutic regimens during the second and third trimesters that include fluorouracil, cyclophosphamide, and doxorubicin are not associated with congenital malformations. Cyclophosphamide and doxorubicin can enter breast milk. Therefore, breast-feeding is contraindicated during chemotherapy. Radiation is typically not offered during pregnancy because of its teratogenic risk and its risk of induction of childhood malignancies. Accordingly, lumpectomy with radiation therapy is an option only if radiation therapy can commence after delivery. Elective termination of the pregnancy to receive appropriate therapy without the risk of fetal malformation is no longer routinely recommended because no improvement in survival has been demonstrated.

Abdominal Pain in Pregnant Patients

The surgeon's natural inclination, when faced with a pregnant patient experiencing abdominal pain, is to temporize. This tendency, which arises from the misconception that surgical intervention may injure the fetus, is responsible for delays in diagnosis and ultimately for unfavorable outcomes. Acute abdominal surgical problems must be dealt with immediately. Management of less acute problems, however, must take into account the stage of the pregnancy. The risk of spontaneous abortion at operation is highest during the first trimester. The optimal time for elective surgery is during the second trimester, because the uterus is smaller at that time than it is in the third trimester and because the fetus can be maintained in a relatively stable condition during the administration of general anesthesia.

Appendicitis

Appendicitis is the most common surgical problem in pregnancy, but it occurs no more often in pregnant women than in nonpregnant women. The incidence is approximately the same in all three trimesters. Of all surgical problems during pregnancy, appendicitis causes the most fetal loss. The particular dangers of appendicitis in pregnancy lie in the varied presentation of symptoms and the higher chance of delayed diagnosis. The symptoms of appendicitis mimic symptoms of normal pregnancy—namely, anorexia, nausea, vomiting, and abdominal discomfort.

The most reliable symptom of appendicitis during pregnancy is periumbilical or diffuse abdominal pain that later localizes to the right lower quadrant. Although as the gravid uterus grows it pushes the appendix cephalad and posteriorly, right lower quadrant pain remains the most consistent symptom of appendicitis in any trimester.

It can be differentiated from adnexal or uterine pain with the help of the Adler sign: if the point of maximal tenderness shifts medially with repositioning on the left lateral side, the etiology is generally adnexal or uterine. Abdominal guarding and rebound tenderness are less common during the third trimester because of the laxity of the abdominal wall muscles.

Fever is not a consistent finding in pregnant patients with appendicitis. Laboratory values can be misleading, in that pregnancy can cause a leukocytosis as high as 15,000 leukocytes/mm^3 in the absence of a source of infection. The white cell differential is more useful than the absolute count; increased levels of band cells or immature forms suggest that the leukocytosis may be secondary to an infectious process. A urinalysis is necessary to rule out a urinary tract infection, which occurs in 10% to 20% of pregnant women.

Diagnostic radiology should be employed deliberately and judiciously. Ultrasonography of the lower abdomen or transvaginal ultrasonography can often visualize an inflamed appendix without risk to the fetus. It can also distinguish other causes of abdominal pain, such as an ovarian cyst. The clinical presentation and an ultrasonogram are often sufficient to establish the diagnosis of appendicitis. In very rare cases, a computed tomography (CT) study of the pelvis should be done as well to elucidate a complicated presentation. For both pelvic CT and directed spiral CT, the total radiation doses are well below the threshold of safety, which is 100 mGy.

The condition most often confused with appendicitis is pyelonephritis, which occurs in 1% to 2% of pregnant women. Because of the mechanical effects of the gravid uterus on the ureter, pyelonephritis is more common in pregnant women than in nonpregnant ones. Furthermore, urinalysis yields abnormal results, either pyuria or hematuria, in as many as 20% of patients with appendicitis as a result of extraluminal irritation of the ureter by the inflamed appendix.

Right lower quadrant pain during early pregnancy may also be a presentation of ectopic implantation. Typically, a patient misses a period and then experiences some degree of vaginal bleeding or spotting. Abdominal or pelvic pain and cervical motion tenderness are present, and a mass is often appreciated on pelvic examination. When ectopic pregnancy is suspected, a serum human chorionic gonadotropin (hCG) assay should be performed along with transvaginal ultrasonography. If the serum hCG level is higher than 2,000 IU/L and an intrauterine gestational sac is not visualized by transvaginal ultrasonography, laparotomy or laparoscopy is indicated.

When there is evidence of appendicitis and no alternative diagnosis seems likely, operative intervention is warranted no matter what stage the pregnancy has reached. The risk of the procedure to mother and child is minimal compared with the risks posed by delayed diagnosis, perforation, and abscess formation. With routine surgical management, maternal mortality rate is negligible, and fetal mortality rate is 2% to 8%. For a ruptured appendix, maternal mortality rate is 1%, and fetal mortality rate is as high as 35%. Negative laparotomy rates of 15% or lower are considered acceptable for the nonpregnant population, but negative laparotomy rates as high as 35% are considered acceptable for pregnant patients in light of the grave consequences of delayed diagnosis.

For appendectomy in the pregnant patient, a right lower quadrant muscle-splitting approach should be employed over the point of maximal tenderness. With late trimester pregnancies, this point of maximal tenderness may be higher than the traditional McBurney's point. If there is doubt about the diagnosis, a low midline incision or a right paramedian incision should be made, especially if the patient has diffuse peritonitis. If appendicitis is not found, the surgeon should thoroughly examine the peritoneal contents on the right side of the abdomen, taking care to avoid exerting traction on the uterus, which might lead to preterm labor. Appendectomy is advisable to avoid later confusion. If perforation occurs, the abdomen should be irrigated and drained. Skin closure should be avoided if abscess, advanced perforation, or gangrene is encountered. When the diagnosis of appendicitis is uncertain, a laparoscopic approach can help rule out salpingitis or ectopic pregnancy. In laparoscopic appendectomy, the first trocar for the camera is placed in the subxiphoid area under direct vision via an open technique. This step allows visualization of all pelvic structures and the appendix. The right upper quadrant and right lower quadrant trocars are then placed under direct vision.

Hepatobiliary Diseases

Hepatic adenomas are uncommon, benign lesions that are usually associated with oral contraceptive use in young women. They are usually solitary lesions, and they have a low potential for malignant transformation. The major risk of a hepatic adenoma during pregnancy is spontaneous rupture, which carries a mortality rate up to 60% for both mother and fetus even with surgical treatment. Spontaneous rupture presents with right upper quadrant pain with shock. Immediate laparotomy should be performed with cesarean section, control of hemorrhage, and resection of the adenoma if possible. Because of the high mortality rate associated with rupture of a hepatic adenoma, elective resection may be performed. Resection during the second trimester minimizes operative risk to the mother and fetus. Because of the unknown recurrence risk, subsequent pregnancy and oral contraceptive use may be discouraged in these patients.

Cholecystectomy for symptomatic cholelithiasis is second to appendectomy as the most common nonob-stetric surgical procedure performed during pregnancy. Pregnancy is associated with an increased incidence of cholelithiasis due to cholesterol supersaturation and biliary stasis promoted by pregnancy. Elevated estrogen levels increase cholesterol secretion by the liver, whereas elevated progesterone levels lead to bile stasis and decreased gallbladder contraction. The incidence of gallstone disease in pregnant women ranges from 3% to 12%; however, only 30% to 40% of patients with gallstones are symptomatic. Initial management of cholecystitis is conservative, comprising intravenous hydration, bowel rest, administration of meperidine and antibiotics, and fetal monitoring. This regimen is successful in 84% of patients. Operative intervention is indicated for failure of conservative management, recurrent disease, intractable nausea, maternal weight loss, fetal growth retardation, obstructive jaundice, gallstone pancreatitis, or peritonitis. Symptomatic gallstone disease is also a reasonable indication for surgical management. Half of patients with symptomatic gallstone disease require repeated hospitalizations. Of patients managed nonoperatively, 35% to 58% developed biliary colic refractory to medical management, requiring multiple hospitalizations.

Nonoperative management of gallstone disease results in increased maternal and fetal mortality rates. With gallstone pancreatitis during pregnancy, a maternal mortality rate of 15% and a fetal mortality rate of 60% have been reported. Because the adverse maternal and fetal outcomes are related more to the disease process rather than to the surgical treatment, surgical intervention should be considered as primary management of gallstones in pregnancy.

The timing of cholecystectomy for biliary colic depends on the gestational age and the severity of symptoms. A spontaneous abortion rate of 12% with open cholecystectomy during the first trimester falls to 5.6% and 0% during the second and third trimesters, respectively. The risk of preterm labor is nearly 0% during the second trimester and 40% during the third trimester. Therefore, the optimum time for cholecystectomy is the second trimester, when the risk of spontaneous abortion and preterm labor are the least, unless the patient develops a complication of cholelithiasis. Laparoscopic cholecystectomy is relatively safe during the second trimester. The gravid uterus is not usually large enough to interfere with visualization and also is less likely to be injured. The open technique is recommended for obtaining access to the abdomen. If intraoperative cholangiography is indicated, the uterus should be protected with appropriate shielding. If the severity of symptoms prevents delaying surgical intervention until after delivery, laparoscopic cholecystectomy can be safely performed during the third trimester, although the risk of preterm labor is substantially increased.

Splenic Artery Aneurysm

Splenic artery aneurysms are four times more common in women than in men, and 25% of all splenic artery ruptures occur during pregnancy. Several factors contribute to the relatively high incidence of such rupture in pregnant women. Splenic arterial pressure is unusually high during pregnancy as a result of the increased cardiac output, the increased blood volume, and the pressure placed on the abdominal aorta and the iliac arteries by the gravid uterus. Pregnancy is also believed to break down the connective tissue component of the arterial wall. Multiparous women in the third trimester are at highest risk for a ruptured splenic artery aneurysm. In the nonpregnant population, splenic artery rupture is associated with a 25% mortality rate; however, in pregnant women, it is associated with maternal and fetal mortality rates ranging from 75% to 95%, mainly as a consequence of erroneous diagnosis. Upon diagnosis of rupture, immediate operative repair is necessary. If a splenic artery aneurysm larger than 2 cm is found in a woman of childbearing age, elective resection is indicated.

Trauma in Pregnancy

Trauma is the leading nonobstetric cause of maternal mortality. The most common mechanisms of injury are falls and motor vehicle crashes. However, homicide is the most common cause of traumatic maternal death. The mother is the first priority: stabilization of the mother improves both maternal and fetal survival. When the mother survives, fetal death is most commonly related to abruptio placentae the earliest sign of which may be deceleration of the fetal heart rate. Early involvement of an obstetrician is important to evaluate both maternal and fetal well-being.

In the management of the pregnant trauma patient, the critical point is that resuscitation of the fetus is accomplished by resuscitation of the mother. Rapid assessment of the maternal airway, breathing, and circulation and ensuring an adequate airway avoids maternal and fetal hypoxia. In the later stages of pregnancy, uterine compression of the vena cava may result in hypotension from diminished venous return, so the pregnant trauma patient should be placed in a left lateral decubitus position. The increased blood volume associated with pregnancy has important implications for the trauma patient. Signs of blood loss such as tachycardia and hypotension may be delayed until the patient loses nearly 30% of her blood volume. As a result, the fetus may be experiencing hypoperfusion long before the mother manifests any signs. Early and rapid fluid resuscitation should be administered even in the pregnant patient who is normotensive. The expansion of intravascular fluid volume that occurs in pregnancy affects the amount of replacement fluid

needed. In the third trimester, patients should receive 1.5 times the amount of fluid that would ordinarily be given to compensate for this effect. Vasoconstrictive agents should never be used for hemodynamic stabilization until hypovolemia has first been treated. Epinephrine and norepinephrine lead to uteroplacental vasoconstriction and fetal compromise; ephedrine and phenylephrine may be used during pregnancy.

Special attention should be given to the abdominal examination. A pelvic examination should be performed, by an obstetrician if possible, to evaluate for vaginal bleeding, ruptured membranes, or a bulging perineum. Vaginal bleeding may indicate abruptio placentae, placenta previa, or preterm labor. Rupture of the amniotic fluid may result in umbilical cord prolapse, which compresses the umbilical vessels and compromises fetal blood flow. This requires immediate cesarean section. The Kleihauer-Betke (K-B) test for the assessment of fetomaternal transfusion is useful after maternal trauma and should be ordered with the initial laboratory studies that include a type and crossmatch. Because of the sensitivity of the K-B test, a small amount of fetomaternal transfusion may be undetected. Therefore, all Rh-negative pregnant trauma patients should be considered for Rh immunoglobulin (RhoGAM) therapy.

Radiographic investigation should be performed whenever necessary if the results are expected to affect management. It is usually possible to keep the total absorbed radiation dose below the level that is thought to increase teratogenic risk (i.e., 50 to 100 milligray [mGy]). Computed tomographic scanning of the abdomen with contrast may offer the greatest amount of information on injuries to the retroperitoneum, the peritoneum, and the pelvis. Ultrasonography is now being used for acute trauma assessment of both pregnant and nonpregnant patients. Peritoneal lavage done in an open fashion through a supraumbilical incision may facilitate rapid assessment of intra-abdominal hemorrhage in cases of blunt trauma. Early determination of gestational age by means of ultrasonography is a critical guide to further management decisions. Ultrasonography can also be used to monitor fetal heart tones, fetal activity, and amniotic volume. After the 20th week of gestation, cardiotocographic monitoring is an important adjunct for determining fetal status after trauma. Such monitoring should also be employed in the event of preterm contractions. As many as 40% of women experience preterm contractions, but only 3% progress to premature delivery. Placental abruption usually occurs within 4 hours of injury. Ultrasonography is not sensitive enough to detect this condition; therefore, cardiotocographic monitoring should be continued for 4 to 6 hours after stabilization and longer if any irregularity in the mother or fetus is noted.

In the event of acute maternal decompensation that does not respond to standard resuscitative measures, a cesarean section may be appropriate. Timing is critical. If anoxia is limited to 4 to 6 minutes, the fetus generally will not be harmed. Therefore, any attempt to deliver the fetus should begin within 4 to 6 minutes after maternal cardiac arrest. If the fetus appears to be viable after this period has passed, cesarean section should be performed. Fetal survival after delivery is dependent on its having reached a gestational age greater than 28 weeks. It is important to remember that (1) cesarean section should not be performed in an unstable patient because of an anticipated cardiac arrest, and (2) if cardiopulmonary resuscitation is successful before surgical delivery is attempted, cesarean section should not be performed, because in utero resuscitation is likely.

Deep Vein Thrombosis

Pregnancy is associated with increased risk of deep vein thrombosis (DVT) because of alterations in the coagulation system, such as increased levels of clotting factors and decreased fibrinolytic activity. The risk is exacerbated by the venous stasis and increased blood viscosity as well as compression of the iliac veins by the growing uterus. Leg swelling and prominent superficial veins are common in pregnancy and may delay the diagnosis of DVT. Real-time B-mode ultrasonography is an extremely sensitive examination that is useful in detecting DVT.

When the diagnosis is made, therapy with a low-molecular-weight heparin (LMWH) should be instituted for the duration of pregnancy. Postpartum anticoagulation with LMWH or warfarin is continued for 6 weeks. Unfractionated heparin can also be used during pregnancy. However, LMWHs have certain advantages over unfractionated heparin: once-daily or twice-daily subcutaneous administration, a predictable dose response, reduced passage across the placenta, and lower incidences of heparin-induced thrombocytopenia. Warfarin should not ordinarily be given for maintenance anticoagulation, because it has teratogenic potential during the first trimester and may induce bleeding during the later part of pregnancy. Prophylaxis of DVT is recommended for subsequent pregnancies.

Part XVI
Surgery Review Questions and Answers

1. Regarding contrast study for intestinal obstruction:
   (a) Gastrografin is preferred to barium for studying distal small bowel
   (b) Gastrografin has no therapeutic potential
   (c) Gastrografin is less hazardous than barium if aspiration occurs
   (d) Gastrografin can cause serious fluid shift
   (e) barium can convert partial small bowel obstruction into complete obstruction

2. An absolute contraindication to breast-conserving surgery for breast cancer is:
   (a) large tumor
   (b) tumor of high grade
   (c) early pregnancy
   (d) retroareolar tumor
   (e) clinical axillary nodes

3. The most common indication for surgery in chronic pancreatitis is:
   (a) jaundice
   (b) pain
   (c) pseudocyst
   (d) gastric outlet obstruction
   (e) endocrine deficiency

4. The most common cause of spontaneous intestinal fistula is:
   (a) radiation injury
   (b) malignancy
   (c) Crohn's disease
   (d) ulcerative colitis
   (e) diverticular disease

5. Gastrointestinal stromal tumors (GIST):
   (a) occur most commonly in the duodenum
   (b) are almost always malignant
   (c) can be treated adequately with enucleation
   (d) are often radioresistant
   (e) spread mainly via the lymphatics

6. Rightward shift of oxyhemoglobin dissociation curve occurs with:
   (a) hypothermia
   (b) acidosis
   (c) decrease in 2,3-diphosphoglycerate
   (d) hypocapnia
   (e) methemoglobinemia

7. The most common site of gastrointestinal lymphoma is:
   (a) small intestine
   (b) stomach
   (c) colon
   (d) duodenum
   (e) appendix

8. Meckel's diverticulum:
   (a) is a false diverticulum
   (b) is asymptomatic in most cases
   (c) commonly presents as gastrointestinal bleeding in adults
   (d) commonly presents with intestinal obstruction in children
   (e) is found in approximately 5% to 10% of people

9. Biliary-enteric fistula most commonly connects:
   (a) gallbladder and ileum
   (b) gallbladder and duodenum
   (c) common bile duct and jejunum
   (d) gallbladder and jejunum
   (e) common bile duct and ileum

10. Spontaneous closure is least likely in fistulae originating from:
    (a) colon
    (b) esophagus
    (c) pancreas
    (d) stomach
    (e) small intestine

11. Gastrointestinal diverticula do not occur in:
    (a) cecum
    (b) duodenum
    (c) rectum
    (d) jejunum
    (e) ileum

12. The hepatic caudate lobe:
    (a) drains directly into the inferior vena cava
    (b) represents segment IV
    (c) is supplied by the left portal vein only
    (d) is supplied by the right portal vein only
    (e) lies to the right of the inferior vena cava

13. von Willebrand's disease:
    (a) is an autosomal dominant disorder
    (b) results in prolonged prothrombin time
    (c) is associated with normal bleeding time
    (d) is due to decreased hepatic synthesis of von Willebrand's factor
    (e) is typically associated with joint bleeding

14. Which of the following is consistent with syndrome of inappropriate antidiuretic hormone (SIADH)?
    (a) hypovolemia
    (b) increased urine sodium
    (c) hypernatremia
    (d) plasma hyperosmolarity
    (e) excessive diuresis

15. Normal anion gap acidosis is associated with:
    (a) ketoacidosis
    (b) lactic acidosis
    (c) salicylate poisoning
    (d) severe diarrhea
    (e) uremic acidosis

16. Benign small bowel tumors most commonly present as:
    (a) small bowel obstruction
    (b) gastrointestinal bleeding
    (c) weight loss
    (d) incidental finding on laparotomy
    (e) intestinal perforation

17. The diagnostic test of choice for suspected acute sigmoid diverticulitis is:
    (a) barium enema
    (b) Gastrografin enema
    (c) computed tomography scan of the abdomen and pelvis
    (d) abdominal ultrasound
    (e) colonoscopy

18. Malignant small bowel neoplasms most commonly present with:
    (a) weight loss
    (b) abdominal pain
    (c) gastrointestinal bleeding
    (d) jaundice
    (e) intestinal perforation

19. Small bowel obstruction in an elderly female without external hernia or previous surgery is most likely caused by:
    (a) small bowel neoplasm
    (b) volvulus
    (c) gallstone ileus
    (d) abdominal abscess
    (e) obturator hernia

20. During cell cycle, DNA replication occurs in:
    (a) G_1 phase
    (b) G_2 phase
    (c) S phase
    (d) M phase

21. Li-Fraumeni syndrome shows increased incidence of:
    (a) colon cancer
    (b) ovarian cancer
    (c) lung cancer
    (d) breast cancer
    (e) pancreatic cancer

22. The best operative approach to choledochal cyst is:
    (a) cystoduodenostomy
    (b) cystojejunostomy
    (c) Roux-en-Y cystojejunostomy
    (d) Cyst excision and hepaticojejunostomy

23. Leiomyoma of the esophagus:
    (a) commonly presents with dysphagia
    (b) is more common in females
    (c) is usually multiple
    (d) is usually diagnosed with endoscopic biopsy
    (e) is usually located in the lower one-third of the esophagus

24. Hemangioma of the liver:
    (a) is the most common benign hepatic tumor
    (b) is diagnosed with percutaneous needle biopsy
    (c) is associated with α-fetoprotein level
    (d) should be resected as soon as diagnosed

25. Phosphorus:
    (a) is a major extracellular anion
    (b) is passively absorbed from the gastrointestinal tract
    (c) deficiency may result in insulin resistance
    (d) deficiency is rare in hospitalized patients

26. Hypermagnesemia is a complication of:
    (a) extensive burns
    (b) acute pancreatitis
    (c) oliguric renal failure
    (d) resection of the terminal ileum
    (e) diuretic therapy

27. The optimal management of traumatic duodenal hematoma is:
    (a) angiography and embolization
    (b) laparotomy and evacuation
    (c) laparotomy and gastrojejunostomy
    (d) observation

28. Hairy cell leukemia:
    (a) can be cured with splenectomy
    (b) is an aggressive form of leukemia
    (c) death is usually related to infectious complications
    (d) is a T cell leukemia

29. Overwhelming postsplenectomy sepsis:
    (a) commonly occurs after splenectomy for trauma
    (b) does not occur if accessory spleens are present
    (c) can be fatal within hours of onset
    (d) is most common in elderly patients
    (e) most fatal cases occur 10 to 15 years after splenectomy

30. The development of thrombocytopenia and arterial thrombosis with heparin requires:
    (a) continuation of heparin and platelet transfusion
    (b) continuation of heparin and thrombolysis
    (c) doubling the heparin dosage
    (d) changing the route of heparin administration
    (e) discontinuation of heparin

31. A trauma patient has a Glasgow Coma Scale score of 13, blood pressure 80/40; widened mediastinum on chest x-ray, and bloody peritoneal tap. The next step in management is:
    (a) obtain head computed tomography scan
    (b) perform thoracotomy
    (c) perform arch angiography
    (d) monitor intracranial pressure
    (e) perform laparotomy

32. Insulinomas:
    (a) are often multiple
    (b) are mostly benign
    (c) are a common component of multiple endocrine neoplasia type 1 (MEN 1)
    (d) are commonly located in the head of the pancreas

33. Intussusception in adults:
    (a) is idiopathic in most cases
    (b) usually requires resection
    (c) is often successfully treated with hydrostatic reduction
    (d) is seldom recurrent

34. Optimal treatment for an ileosigmoid fistula in Crohn's disease is:
    (a) closure of the fistula
    (b) proximal ileostomy
    (c) proximal ileostomy and closure of fistula
    (d) ileocecectomy and sigmoid colectomy
    (e) ileocecectomy and closure of the sigmoid defect

35. Obturator hernia:
    (a) is most common in older women with cachexia
    (b) is associated with pain in the sciatic nerve distribution
    (c) is repaired through a transverse incision in the upper medial thigh
    (d) is rarely strangulated

36. Gastrointestinal bleeding in Mallory-Weiss syndrome:
    (a) is occult in the vast majority of cases
    (b) can be controlled with balloon tamponade
    (c) stops with nonoperative management in most cases
    (d) is caused by mucosal tear in the lower one-third of the esophagus

37. The risk of overwhelming postsplenectomy sepsis is highest for patients requiring splenectomy for:
    (a) thalassemia
    (b) trauma
    (c) immune thrombocytopenic purpura
    (d) hereditary spherocytosis
    (e) acquired hemolytic anemia

38. After mastectomy, winging of the scapula results from injury to:
    (a) the medial pectoral nerve
    (b) the lateral pectoral nerve
    (c) the long thoracic nerve
    (d) the thoracodorsal nerve
    (e) the intercostal-brachial nerve

39. von Willebrand's disease:
    (a) is the most common congenital bleeding disorder
    (b) commonly results in hemarthrosis
    (c) affects males only
    (d) results in prolonged prothrombin time

40. Disc lesion between L4 and L5 will lead to:
    (a) reduced knee jerk
    (b) reduced ankle jerk
    (c) weakness of foot dorsiflexion
    (d) reduced sensation on the small toe

41. Kidney transplant recipients are at increased risk for:
    (a) epidermoid skin cancer
    (b) lung cancer
    (c) colon cancer
    (d) breast cancer
    (e) uterine cancer

42. The optimum management of medullary thyroid carcinoma in multiple endocrine neoplasia type 2 (MEN 2) is:
    (a) thyroid lobectomy
    (b) thyroid lobectomy and cervical lymphadenectomy
    (c) radioactive iodine
    (d) radiotherapy
    (e) total thyroidectomy ± radical neck dissection

43. Optimum management for a 2-cm mass in the head of the pancreas with hypoglycemia and high insulin levels is:
    (a) total pancreatectomy
    (b) Whipple resection
    (c) local excision
    (d) streptozotocin administration

44. Which of the following is not a risk factor for wound infection?
    (a) prolonged operative time
    (b) prolonged preoperative hospitalization
    (c) shaving the skin the night before surgery
    (d) patient's having upper respiratory tract infection
    (e) surgeon's hand scrub for 5 instead of 10 minutes

45. On the second day after abdominal aortic aneurysm repair, the patient passes grossly bloody stool. The next step is:
    (a) immediate exploratory laparotomy
    (b) sigmoidoscopy
    (c) computed tomography scan of the abdomen with intravenous contrast
    (d) barium enema
    (e) aortogram

46. Spontaneous pneumothorax:
    (a) is more common in young females
    (b) is typically postexertional
    (c) is recurrent in at least 30% of cases
    (d) often requires thoracotomy in the first episode
    (e) is often associated with severe persistent pain

47. The most common cause of hypercalcemic crisis is:
    (a) sarcoidosis
    (b) primary hyperparathyroidism
    (c) secondary hyperparathyroidism
    (d) malignancy
    (e) renal failure

48. A sudden onset of glucose intolerance in patients receiving total parenteral nutrition often indicates:
    (a) diabetes mellitus
    (b) sepsis
    (c) hypophosphatemia
    (d) adrenal insufficiency
    (e) zinc insufficiency

49. Pectus excavatum:
    (a) is usually associated with respiratory dysfunction
    (b) is usually associated with dysphagia
    (c) is often associated with cardiac dysfunction
    (d) cosmesis is usually the indication for surgery

50. Sacrococcygeal teratoma:
    (a) is usually malignant
    (b) is more common in males
    (c) requires complete excision of the coccyx
    (d) diagnosis is ruled out if calcification is absent on radiography

51. Dry, scaly, pruritic rash on the trunk and extremities of a patient receiving total parenteral nutrition is caused by:
    (a) zinc deficiency
    (b) vitamin A deficiency
    (c) vitamin C deficiency
    (d) free fatty acid deficiency

52. The main cause of postoperative death in children with chronic diaphragmatic hernia is:
    (a) increased intra-abdominal pressure
    (b) persistent lung collapse
    (c) patent ductus arteriosus
    (d) abnormal pulmonary microvasculature

53. A neonate has bilious vomiting and a double-bubble sign on plain x-ray. The most appropriate operation is:
    (a) division of annular pancreas
    (b) gastroenterostomy
    (c) duodenoduodenostomy
    (d) duodenal resection

54. The most common source of bacteria in wound infection after groin hernia repair is:
    (a) the patient's skin
    (b) the patient's nasopharynx
    (c) operating room air
    (d) surgical instruments
    (e) operating room staff

55. Enterocytes' energy requirements are provided by:
    (a) arginine
    (b) alanine
    (c) glutamine
    (d) glycine

56. In critical illness, immune function can be enhanced by:
    (a) arginine
    (b) glutamine
    (c) alanine
    (d) glycine

57. Intra-aortic balloon pump:
    (a) increases pulmonary wedge pressure
    (b) increases afterload
    (c) increases diastolic pressure
    (d) increases duration of systole
    (e) decreases duration of diastole

58. Popliteal artery aneurysms:
    (a) are less common than femoral aneurysm
    (b) are often bilateral
    (c) are more common in females
    (d) seldom result in limb ischemia

59. The most common cause of pneumaturia is:
    (a) Crohn's disease
    (b) ulcerative colitis
    (c) malignancy
    (d) radiation enteritis
    (e) diverticular disease

60. The most common benign hepatic lesion is:
    (a) hemangioma
    (b) adenoma
    (c) focal nodular hyperplasia
    (d) hamartoma

61. The most common etiologic factor for hepatocellular carcinoma worldwide is:
    (a) hepatitis C virus
    (b) hepatitis B virus
    (c) alcoholic cirrhosis
    (d) aflatoxin ingestion
    (e) schistosomiasis

62. Pulmonary hilar adenopathy with noncaseating granuloma is consistent with:
    (a) Hodgkin's disease
    (b) lymphoma
    (c) sarcoid
    (d) tuberculosis
    (e) metastatic carcinoma

63. A solitary lung nodule with a popcorn pattern of calcification is most likely:
    (a) a primary lung cancer
    (b) a metastatic lesion
    (c) an old tuberculosis lesion
    (d) histoplasmosis
    (e) a hamartoma

64. The most common presentation of gastric lymphoma is:
    (a) abdominal pain
    (b) weight loss
    (c) upper gastrointestinal bleeding
    (d) gastric perforation
    (e) nausea and vomiting

65. The protective immune function of immunoglobulin A is mediated through:
    (a) inhibition of bacterial adherence to epithelial cells
    (b) activation of complement
    (c) opsonization
    (d) direct destruction of microorganisms

66. The most potent stimulus for antidiuretic hormone secretion is:
    (a) hypovolemia
    (b) hyponatremia
    (c) hyperkalemia
    (d) raised serum osmolarity

67. Which of the following distinguishes adrenal insufficiency from sepsis?
    (a) hypotension
    (b) fever
    (c) tachycardia
    (d) altered mental status
    (e) hypoglycemia

68. For penetrating chest injury, thoracotomy is indicated if:
    (a) initial chest tube output is 500 cc
    (b) initial chest tube output is 1,000 cc
    (c) initial chest tube output is 1,500 cc
    (d) initial chest tube output is 2,000 cc
    (e) persistent chest tube output of 100 cc/hr

69. Which cell type is essential for wound healing?
    (a) neutrophil
    (b) macrophage
    (c) fibroblast
    (d) lymphocyte
    (e) endothelial

70. The treatment for osteosarcoma of the distal femur is:
    (a) above-knee amputation
    (b) chemotherapy followed by above-knee amputation
    (c) chemoradiation
    (d) chemotherapy alone
    (e) chemotherapy and limb-sparing surgery

71. Abnormal bleeding with normal prothrombin time occurs with:
    (a) heparin overdose
    (b) cirrhosis
    (c) hemophilia
    (d) von Willebrand's disease

72. The most significant prognostic factor for soft tissue sarcoma is:
    (a) site
    (b) size
    (c) grade
    (d) cell type

73. After reduction of posterior knee dislocation, the patient should undergo:
    (a) observation
    (b) discharge
    (c) splinting
    (d) angiogram
    (e) internal fixation

74. Metabolic acidosis is a complication of topical application of:
    (a) sodium mafenide
    (b) silver nitrate
    (c) silver sulfadiazine
    (d) Betadine
    (e) bacitracin

75. Stored blood is deficient in:
    (a) factor II
    (b) factor VII
    (c) factor VIII
    (d) factor IX
    (e) factor XI

76. Post-transplant lymphoproliferative disorders are related to:
    (a) cytomegalovirus
    (b) Epstein-Barr virus
    (c) human immunodeficiency virus (HIV)
    (d) herpesvirus
    (e) hepatitis B virus

77. Which of the following requires surgical drainage?
    (a) amebic liver abscess
    (b) peridiverticular abscess
    (c) appendiceal abscess
    (d) pancreatic abscess
    (e) subphrenic abscess

78. The main complication of topical silver nitrate is:
    (a) metabolic acidosis
    (b) metabolic alkalosis
    (c) hyperkalemia
    (d) hypocalcemia
    (e) hyponatremia

79. The adverse effects of steroids on wound healing can be reversed with:
    (a) vitamin C
    (b) vitamin A
    (c) copper
    (d) vitamin D
    (e) vitamin E

80. The most common source of infection in burn patients is:
    (a) burn wound
    (b) urinary tract infection
    (c) pneumonia
    (d) thrombophlebitis
    (e) endocarditis

81. The most common cause of death after kidney transplantation is:
    (a) operative technical complications
    (b) atherosclerotic complications
    (c) infection
    (d) cancer
    (e) graft rejection

82. Which of the following is least appropriate when evaluating a 14-year-old girl with a breast lump?
    (a) ultrasound
    (b) clinical follow-up
    (c) mammography
    (d) fine-needle aspiration
    (e) excisional biopsy

83. An absolute contraindication to renal transplantation is:
    (a) chronic osteomyelitis
    (b) diabetes mellitus
    (c) age >55 years
    (d) lung cancer treated 10 years ago
    (e) exertional angina

84. Changes occurring in stored blood include:
    (a) increased H^+
    (b) increased 2,3-diphosphoglycerate
    (c) decreased red cell fragility
    (d) decreased K^+
    (e) increased Ca^{2+}

85. The most effective method of treating hyperkalemia is:
    (a) intravenous calcium gluconate
    (b) intravenous sodium bicarbonate
    (c) hemodialysis
    (d) cation-exchange resin
    (e) intravenous glucose-insulin

86. The most common cause of hypercalcemia in hospitalized patients is:
    (a) primary hyperparathyroidism
    (b) metastatic carcinoma
    (c) sarcoidosis
    (d) immobility
    (e) milk alkali syndrome

87. Smoke inhalation is most reliably excluded by:
    (a) absence of carbonaceous sputum
    (b) normal carboxyhemoglobin level
    (c) normal xenon-133 inhalation scan
    (d) normal chest x-ray
    (e) normal flexible bronchoscopy

88. Which of the following ligands bind to cell surface receptors?
    (a) steroids
    (b) catecholamines
    (c) retinoids
    (d) thyroid hormones
    (e) vitamin D

89. von Willebrand's disease:
    (a) is autosomal dominant
    (b) results in prolonged prothrombin time
    (c) results in thrombocytopenia
    (d) is associated with normal bleeding time
    (e) is corrected by factor VIII therapy

90. Coumadin-induced skin necrosis is due to:
    (a) protein S deficiency
    (b) protein C deficiency
    (c) antithrombin III deficiency
    (d) disseminated intravascular coagulation

91. A patient receiving 1,800 cal/day in total parenteral nutrition will require:
    (a) 125 g protein/day
    (b) 150 g protein/day
    (c) 200 g protein/day
    (d) 250 g protein/day
    (e) 300 g protein/day

92. Apoptosis:
    (a) is an energy-dependent cell death
    (b) results in cell swelling
    (c) is associated with an inflammatory response
    (d) is usually toxin induced
    (e) is indistinguishable from necrosis

93. Splenic artery aneurysm:
    (a) is usually asymptomatic
    (b) is usually a pseudoaneurysm
    (c) is more common in young males
    (d) rupture is seldom fatal

94. The site of action of aldosterone is:
    (a) proximal renal tubules
    (b) distal renal tubules
    (c) collecting ducts
    (d) glomeruli
    (e) loop of Henle

95. The site of action of antidiuretic hormone is:
    (a) collecting ducts
    (b) glomeruli
    (c) proximal tubules
    (d) distal tubules
    (e) loop of Henle

96. The common bile duct:
    (a) lies to the right of the hepatic artery
    (b) is posterior to the hepatic artery
    (c) lies to the right of the portal vein
    (d) is posterior to the portal vein
    (e) lies to the left of the hepatic artery

97. A respiratory quotient (RQ) of 1 indicates that the main source of fuel is:
    (a) fatty acid
    (b) protein
    (c) carbohydrate
    (d) ketone
    (e) glycerol

98. Magnesium:
    (a) deficiency can be accurately diagnosed with serum level measurement
    (b) hypomagnesemia is associated with hyperkalemia
    (c) hypomagnesemia is associated with neuromuscular excitability
    (d) hypomagnesemia is a complication of renal failure
    (e) is a major extracellular cation

99. The management of pancreatic pleural fistula is:
    (a) distal pancreatectomy
    (b) pancreaticojejunostomy
    (c) cystogastrostomy
    (d) tube thoracostomy
    (e) thoracotomy and decortication

100. 48 hours after coronary artery bypass grafting, nausea with epigastric pain and tenderness are most likely due to:
    (a) perforated peptic ulcer
    (b) acute cholecystitis
    (c) acute pancreatitis
    (d) acute myocardial infarction
    (e) mesenteric ischemia

101. Hypotension develops after pneumoperitoneum and trocar placement for laparoscopic cholecystectomy. The next action is to:
    (a) convert to open cholecystectomy
    (b) deflate the abdomen
    (c) give intravenous fluids
    (d) place the patient in head down position
    (e) check for bowel injury

102. Delayed primary wound closure:
    (a) results in increased angiogenesis
    (b) results in decreased wound strength
    (c) results in lower collagen content
    (d) results in a wider scar

103. The most common cause of esophageal perforation is:
    (a) penetrating neck injury
    (b) iatrogenic
    (c) spontaneous
    (d) foreign body
    (e) malignancy

104. Multicentricity is characteristic of:
    (a) squamous cell carcinoma of the lung
    (b) small cell lung cancer
    (c) bronchoalveolar carcinoma
    (d) bronchial adenocarcinoma
    (e) bronchial carcinoid

105. DNA alkylation is the chemotherapeutic action of:
    (a) cyclophosphamide
    (b) vincristine
    (c) methotrexate
    (d) doxorubicin

106. Spontaneous perforation of the esophagus:
    (a) is usually seen in elderly females
    (b) is the most common cause of esophageal perforation
    (c) is usually located in the midesophagus
    (d) is usually preceded by history of dysphagia
    (e) typically presents with sudden onset

107. Fentanyl:
    (a) is normally found in the body
    (b) is 100 times more potent than morphine
    (c) has twice as long a duration of action as morphine
    (d) results in hypotension because of histamine release

108. Popliteal artery aneurysms:
    (a) are commonly complicated by rupture
    (b) occur equally in both sexes
    (c) are not surgically treated unless size is >4 cm
    (d) are bilateral in more than 50% of cases

109. The lower esophageal sphincter (LES) tone:
    (a) is increased by gastrin
    (b) is decreased by metoclopramide
    (c) is increased by nicotine
    (d) is increased by chocolate

110. Tachycardia is the main side effect of:
    (a) fentanyl
    (b) succinylcholine
    (c) morphine
    (d) pancuronium

111. Intralobar pulmonary sequestration often presents with:
    (a) chest pain
    (b) dyspnea
    (c) recurrent pneumonia
    (d) hemoptysis

112. Doxorubicin:
    (a) is an alkylating agent
    (b) is an antimetabolite
    (c) is an alkaloid
    (d) is an anthracycline antibiotic

113. A 45-year-old man has an 8×4 cm soft tissue mass in his right thigh. The most appropriate method to confirm the diagnosis of sarcoma is:
    (a) fine-needle aspiration
    (b) core biopsy
    (c) local excision
    (d) incisional biopsy
    (e) enucleation

114. Appropriate treatment of malignant hypothermia is intravenous:
    (a) morphine sulfate
    (b) dantrolene
    (c) benzodiazepines
    (d) KCl
    (e) calcium gluconate

115. Volkmann's contracture is a complication of:
    (a) humeral head fracture
    (b) femoral neck fracture
    (c) posterior dislocation of the knee
    (d) supracondylar humeral fracture
    (e) Colles' fracture

116. Decreasing glucose and increasing fat in total parenteral nutrition will:
    (a) increase respiratory quotient
    (b) increase CO_2 production
    (c) decrease minute ventilation
    (d) delay weaning from mechanical ventilation

117. Acute appendicitis in pregnancy:
    (a) has a higher incidence of wound infection
    (b) is least common in the third trimester
    (c) leukocytosis is important in making the diagnosis
    (d) initial observation is recommended when diagnosis is suspected

118. Eight hours after esophagogastroduodenoscopy (EGD), a patient complains of severe substernal pain. Chest x-ray film shows left pleural effusion. The next test is:
    (a) repeated EGD
    (b) celiotomy
    (c) computed tomography scan of the chest
    (d) water-soluble esophagogram
    (e) thoracotomy

119. The initial site of distant metastasis in breast cancer is:
    (a) lungs
    (b) liver
    (c) bones
    (d) brain

120. Arrest of cell cycle in the metaphase is the action of:
    (a) cyclophosphamide
    (b) methotrexate
    (c) doxorubicin
    (d) vincristine

121. After an acute myocardial infarction, elective operation should be postponed for at least:
    (a) 1 month
    (b) 3 months
    (c) 6 months
    (d) 1 year
    (e) 2 years

122. Succinylcholine is contraindicated for:
    (a) patients with hepatitis
    (b) emergency intubation of burn victims
    (c) celiotomy 2 weeks after spinal cord injury
    (d) parotidectomy
    (e) thyroidectomy

123. Splenic artery aneurysm:
    (a) can present with double-rupture phenomenon
    (b) is more common in males
    (c) is seldom multiple
    (d) will continue to enlarge if left untreated

124. One week after Coumadin therapy, a patient develops severe pain in the right leg with areas of skin necrosis. Appropriate action is:
    (a) transfusion of fresh-frozen plasma
    (b) intravenous vitamin K therapy
    (c) wound debridement and antibiotics
    (d) stopping Coumadin and starting heparin
    (e) lumbar sympathectomy

125. Mixed venous saturation is increased in:
    (a) hypovolemic shock
    (b) septic shock
    (c) cardiogenic shock
    (d) neurogenic shock
    (e) anaphylactic shock

126. Paraneoplastic syndrome is most commonly associated with:
    (a) bronchial adenocarcinoma
    (b) small cell lung cancer
    (c) bronchoalveolar carcinoma
    (d) bronchial carcinoid

127. The endothelial cells are the source of:
    (a) factor II
    (b) factor V
    (c) factor VII
    (d) factor VIII
    (e) factor X

128. Which of the following is likely to be multiple?
    (a) gastrinoma
    (b) insulinoma
    (c) somatostatinoma
    (d) vasoactive intestinal peptide–producing tumor
    (e) gluconoma

129. The mechanism of action of heparin is:
    (a) direct inhibition of thrombin
    (b) prevention of factor II synthesis
    (c) inhibition of cyclo-oxygenase
    (d) potentiation of antithrombin III action

130. Which of the following is an aminoester?
    (a) tetracaine
    (b) lidocaine
    (c) bupivacaine
    (d) mepivacaine
    (e) etidocaine

131. Vitamin K:
    (a) is required for factor VIII synthesis
    (b) is water soluble
    (c) is absorbed in the proximal small bowel
    (d) requires bile salts for absorption

132. Hyponatremia is a complication of topical application of:
    (a) bacitracin
    (b) povidone-iodine
    (c) silver sulfadiazine
    (d) Sulfamylon
    (e) silver nitrate

133. Which of the following is an etiologic factor in occlusive vascular diseases?
    (a) arginine
    (b) glutamine
    (c) methionine
    (d) homocystine
    (e) xanthine

134. Cardiomyopathy is a complication of:
    (a) methotrexate
    (b) tamoxifen
    (c) doxorubicin
    (d) cyclophosphamide
    (e) vincristine

135. Spontaneous antitumor activity is a function of:
    (a) macrophages
    (b) B lymphocytes
    (c) cytotoxic T cells
    (d) helper T cells
    (e) natural killer cells

136. Pulmonary fibrosis is a complication of:
    (a) bleomycin
    (b) cyclophosphamide
    (c) tamoxifen
    (d) vincristine
    (e) methotrexate

137. The best indicator of adequate resuscitation in shock is:
    (a) normal blood pressure
    (b) normal pulse
    (c) adequate urine output
    (e) improved mental status
    (f) decreased lactate level

138. Adrenal incidentalomas:
    (a) are commonly malignant
    (b) require endocrine evaluation
    (c) are commonly associated with hyperaldosteronism
    (d) are not resected unless they are >6 cm

139. Peaked T-wave on electrocardiogram is a feature of:
    (a) hypernatremia
    (b) hypermagnesemia
    (c) hyperkalemia
    (d) hypocalcemia
    (e) hyponatremia

140. Distinction between prerenal and renal azotemia is best made by:
    (a) urine sodium level
    (b) serum sodium level
    (c) urine creatinine level
    (d) serum creatinine level
    (e) urine microscopy

141. During prolonged starvation, the brain's main fuel is:
    (a) glucose
    (b) amino acids
    (c) ketones
    (d) short-chain fatty acids

142. Dobutamine:
    (a) has a major chronotropic action
    (b) decreases cardiac filling pressure
    (c) increases systemic vascular resistance
    (d) directly increases renal blood flow

143. Epidermal growth factor stimulates:
    (a) angiogenesis
    (b) wound contraction
    (c) fibroblast proliferation
    (d) epithelialization

144. Magnesium:
    (a) is an intracellular ion
    (b) deficiency leads to hyporeflexia
    (c) depletion is common in shock states
    (d) is excreted mostly in stool

145. The most commonly injured organ in a patient with seatbelt sign is:
    (a) the liver
    (b) the spleen
    (c) the colon
    (d) the pancreas
    (e) the small intestine

146. The development of necrolytic erythematous rash in a diabetic patient requires assessment of the serum level of:
    (a) insulin
    (b) somatostatin
    (c) cortisol
    (d) gastrin
    (e) glucagon

147. Appearance of a U-wave on electrocardiogram occurs in:
    (a) hyperkalemia
    (b) hypokalemia
    (c) hypermagnesemia
    (d) hypomagnesemia
    (e) hypercalcemia

148. Seizures can be associated with the use of:
    (a) aztreonam
    (b) Flagyl
    (c) clindamycin
    (d) ciprofloxacillin
    (e) imipenem-cilastatin

149. Nasotracheal intubation:
    (a) is contraindicated for suspected cervical spine injury
    (b) is contraindicated for apneic patients
    (c) is usually successful on the first attempt
    (d) is less tolerated by patients than is endotracheal intubation

150. The most important initial management of suspected blunt myocardial injury is:
    (a) electroencephalographic monitoring
    (b) chest computed tomography scan
    (c) assessment of cardiac enzymes
    (d) insertion of pulmonary artery catheter
    (e) echocardiogram

151. Headache, vomiting, and seizure may develop with rapid correction of:
    (a) hyponatremia
    (b) hypernatremia
    (c) hypokalemia
    (d) hyperkalemia
    (e) hypercalcemia

152. The most common microbial agent transmitted by blood transfusion is:
    (a) Cytomegalovirus
    (b) human immunodeficiency virus
    (c) hepatitis C virus
    (d) hepatitis B virus

153. The most frequent major complication of blood transfusion is:
    (a) volume overload
    (b) hemolytic reaction
    (c) human immunodeficiency virus infection
    (d) hepatitis C
    (e) hepatitis B

154. adenosine diphosphate–induced platelet aggregation is inhibited by:
    (a) aspirin
    (b) heparin
    (c) dipyridamole
    (d) Coumadin

155. Malignant hyperthermia
    (a) is rare in children
    (b) is an autosomal dominant disorder
    (c) results in respiratory alkalosis
    (d) is prevented by intravenous calcium gluconate

156. Colonic perforation in a patient with acquired immunodeficiency syndrome is most likely due to:
    (a) Clostridium difficile
    (b) Cytomegalovirus
    (c) Bacteroides
    (d) Salmonella typhi
    (e) Escherichia coli

157. Which of the following results of thyroid fine-needle aspiration indicates surgical treatment?
    (a) a nodule that disappeared on aspiration
    (b) clumps of follicular cells
    (c) anaplastic thyroid cells
    (d) lymphoma

158. Somatostatin:
    (a) is produced by antral G cells
    (b) has a half-life of 30 minutes
    (c) inhibits gastric motility
    (d) increases portal blood flow

159. The most common site for accessory splenic tissue is:
    (a) gastrosplenic ligament
    (b) gastrocolic ligament
    (c) splenic hilum
    (d) splenocolic ligament
    (e) the pelvis

160. The most sensitive indicator of increased hemolysis with hypersplenism is:
    (a) reticulocyte count
    (b) splenic enlargement
    (c) bilirubin level
    (d) hemoglobin level
    (e) haptoglobin level

161. Howship-Romberg sign is characteristic of:
    (a) femoral hernia
    (b) Spigelian hernia
    (c) obturator hernia
    (d) lumbar hernia
    (e) epigastric hernia

162. Which of the following is least indicated for evaluating adrenal incidentaloma?
    (a) magnetic resonance imaging
    (b) 24-hour urinary catecholamine testing
    (c) 24-hour urinary cortisol testing
    (d) low dexamethasone suppression test
    (e) fine-needle aspiration

163. Lobular carcinoma in situ:
    (a) is mostly found in premenopausal women
    (b) usually presents as a breast lump
    (c) has characteristic calcification pattern on mammography
    (d) is precancerous
    (e) associated cancer is lobular in nature

164. Sequence of return of gastrointestinal motility after surgery is:
    (a) intestine, stomach, colon
    (b) stomach, intestine, colon
    (c) colon, intestine, stomach
    (d) colon, stomach, intestine
    (e) stomach, colon, intestine

165. The treatment of choice for Barrett's esophagus with severe dysplasia is:
    (a) follow-up endoscopy and biopsy
    (b) esophagectomy
    (c) Nissen fundoplication
    (d) Proton pump inhibitors

166. Esophageal diverticula:
    (a) traction diverticula are false diverticula
    (b) pulsion diverticula are common in the midesophagus
    (c) pulsion diverticula are usually associated with enlarged lymph nodes
    (d) myotomy is always indicated for pulsion diverticula

167. The primary fuel source for enterocytes is:
    (a) short-chain fatty acids
    (b) glucose
    (c) triglycerides
    (d) lactulose
    (e) glutamine

168. Infection caused by dog and cat bites is due to:
    (a) *Pasteurella* species
    (b) *Mycobacterium*
    (c) *Staphylococcus aureus*
    (d) *Actinomyces*
    (e) *Candida*

169. Which of the following is preserved in radical neck dissection?
    (a) internal jugular vein
    (b) sternomastoid muscle
    (c) spinal accessory nerve
    (d) submandibular salivary gland
    (e) posterior belly of the digastric muscle

170. The organ most commonly involved in graft-versus-host reaction is:
    (a) lungs
    (b) kidneys
    (c) heart
    (d) skin

171. The most characteristic of malignancy in a cystic pancreatic neoplasm is:
    (a) size >6 cm
    (b) wall calcification
    (c) multiple loculations
    (d) dense vascularity

172. Which of the following is contraindicated for a paraplegic undergoing laparotomy?
    (a) benzodiazepines
    (b) sodium thiopental
    (c) succinylcholine
    (d) propofol
    (e) fentanyl

173. Which of the following is consistent with pleural transudate?
    (a) red blood cells count of 1,000/mm³
    (b) white blood cells count of 1,500/mm³
    (c) specific gravity of 1.120
    (d) protein concentration of 3.5 g/dL

174. Appropriate management of renal cell carcinoma extending into the inferior vena cava is:
    (a) radiotherapy
    (b) chemotherapy
    (c) chemoradiation
    (d) radical nephrectomy and caval tumor extraction
    (e) radical nephrectomy, caval resection, and graft interposition

175. The gastroduodenal artery is a branch of the:
    (a) celiac axis
    (b) right gastric artery
    (c) common hepatic artery
    (d) right hepatic artery
    (e) left hepatic artery

176. Inflammatory aortic aneurysm:
    (a) repair is associated with a higher incidence of graft infection
    (b) is more likely to rupture than is a noninflammatory aneurysm
    (c) leads to circumferential thickening of the aorta
    (d) may present with abdominal pain in the absence of rupture

177. The initial management of a diabetic patient with fever, plantar ulcer, and foot edema is:
    (a) antibiotics and elevation
    (b) hyperbaric oxygen
    (c) exploration and ulcer debridement
    (d) midtarsal amputation
    (e) femoropopliteal arterial bypass

178. Male breast cancer is associated with:
    (a) BRCA-1 gene
    (b) BRCA-2 gene
    (c) APC gene
    (d) p53 gene

179. The diagnosis of inflammatory breast cancer is confirmed by:
    (a) mammography
    (b) fine-needle aspiration
    (c) ultrasound
    (d) skin biopsy

180. The most common retroperitoneal sarcoma is:
    (a) liposarcoma
    (b) fibrosarcoma
    (c) leiomyosarcoma
    (d) neurosarcoma

181. Platelet dysfunction in uremia can be corrected with:
    (a) fresh-frozen plasma
    (b) cryoprecipitate
    (c) desmopressin (DDAVP)
    (d) factor VIII concentrate
    (e) vitamin K

182. Gynecomastia is a side effect of:
    (a) ketoconazole
    (b) amphotericin B
    (c) fluconazole
    (d) miconazole

183. Optimum approach to inflammatory breast carcinoma is:
    (a) total mastectomy
    (b) modified radical mastectomy
    (c) lumpectomy and radiotherapy
    (d) chemotherapy
    (e) chemotherapy, modified radical mastectomy, and radiotherapy

184. A potent inhibitor of T cell proliferation is:
    (a) transforming growth factor-β
    (b) platelet-derived growth factor
    (c) epidermal growth factor
    (d) basic fibroblast growth factor

185. The most reliable indicator of successful endotracheal intubation is:
    (a) chest x-ray
    (b) end-tidal CO_2
    (c) cord visualization
    (d) chest auscultation
    (e) pulse oximetry

186. The layer responsible for the strength of an intestinal anastomosis is the:
    (a) mucosa
    (b) submucosa
    (c) muscularis propria
    (d) serosa

187. Healing of the donor site for a split thickness skin graft is accelerated by:
    (a) transforming growth factor-β
    (b) recombinant human growth hormone
    (c) epidermal growth factor
    (d) platelet-derived growth factor

188. Prevention of empyema in a patient with residual hemothorax and a chest tube in place is best achieved by:
    (a) intravenous third-generation cephalosporins
    (b) placement of a second chest tube
    (c) needle thoracentesis
    (d) intravenous vancomycin

189. Popliteal artery entrapment:
    (a) is more common in females than males
    (b) is diagnosed by passive dorsiflexion of the foot
    (c) results from compression by the medial head of the gastrocnemius
    (d) requires bilateral exploration in most cases

190. Cervical anastomosis after esophagectomy for cancer:
    (a) has a lower leak rate than thoracic anastomosis
    (b) leak is likely to heal spontaneously
    (c) has a higher long-term mortality rate than thoracic anastomosis
    (d) has a lower operative mortality rate than thoracic anastomosis

191. Appropriate management of 3-cm squamous cell carcinoma of the anal canal is:
    (a) chemotherapy
    (b) abdominoperineal resection
    (c) local excision
    (d) radiotherapy + local excision
    (e) chemotherapy + radiation

192. Idiopathic thrombocytopenic purpura:
    (a) is caused by antiplatelet immunoglobulin G originating in the spleen
    (b) is associated with splenomegaly
    (c) is associated with prolonged prothrombin time
    (d) splenectomy is required for most pediatric cases
    (e) occurs with a male to female ratio of 3:1

193. The most common cause of death related to a central venous catheter is:
    (a) air embolism
    (b) central vein perforation
    (c) tension pneumothorax
    (d) catheter embolism
    (e) catheter-related sepsis

194. Postoperative morbidity after splenectomy for hematologic diseases is highest for:
    (a) idiopathic thrombocytopenic purpura
    (b) hereditary spherocytosis
    (c) myeloid dysplasia
    (d) sickle cell anemia
    (e) thalassemia

195. The respiratory quotient in prolonged starvation is:
    (a) 1.0
    (b) 1.2
    (c) 0.8
    (d) 0.7

196. The most abundant amino acid in the body is:
    (a) alanine
    (b) valine
    (c) leucine
    (d) glutamine
    (e) arginine

197. Maximum efficiency of glucose use in total parenteral nutrition occurs at the infusion rate of:
    (a) 4 mg/kg/min
    (b) 5 mg/kg/min
    (c) 6 mg/kg/min
    (d) 7 mg/kg/min

198. Refeeding syndrome is most commonly related to:
    (a) hyponatremia
    (b) hypocalcemia
    (c) hypophosphatemia
    (d) hypokalemia

199. Eczematoid rash at intertriginous areas with prolonged total parenteral nutrition is caused by:
    (a) zinc deficiency
    (b) fatty acid deficiency
    (c) copper deficiency
    (d) magnesium deficiency
    (e) niacin deficiency

200. The volume of air moved with maximum exhalation after deep inhalation measures:
    (a) vital capacity
    (b) inspiratory reserve volume
    (c) tidal volume
    (d) residual volume
    (e) total lung volume

201. Bleeding after adequate heparin reversal with protamine is usually caused by:
    (a) protamine toxicity
    (b) heparin rebound
    (c) hypothermia
    (d) thrombocytopenia
    (e) factor VIII depletion

202. Ileocolic intussusception in children:
    (a) presents with rectal bleeding in 90% of cases
    (b) is commonly caused by an underlying pathology
    (c) is ideally treated by operative reduction
    (d) is the most common cause of intestinal obstruction before the age of 3 years

203. Alopecia with prolonged total parenteral nutrition may be caused by:
    (a) zinc deficiency
    (b) magnesium deficiency
    (c) vitamin A intoxication
    (d) essential fatty acids deficiency
    (e) selenium deficiency

204. A 1-cm carcinoid found in the midappendix after appendectomy requires:
    (a) octreotide therapy
    (b) right hemicolectomy
    (c) streptozotocin therapy
    (d) no further action

205. The most common complication of heparin reversal with protamine is:
    (a) bradycardia
    (b) hypotension
    (c) thrombotic crisis
    (d) thrombocytopenia
    (e) leukopenia

206. The most common side effect of pancuronium is:
    (a) tachycardia
    (b) hypotension
    (c) hyperkalemia
    (d) hyperthermia
    (e) renal insufficiency

207. The most common cause of massive lower gastrointestinal bleeding in children is:
    (a) anal fissure
    (b) intussusception
    (c) Meckel's diverticulum
    (e) angiodysplasia

208. Fine-needle aspiration of bilateral upper cervical lymphadenopathy shows squamous cell carcinoma. No primary lesion is found on clinical examination. The most likely source is:
    (a) lungs
    (b) esophagus
    (c) tongue
    (d) tonsils
    (e) nasopharynx

209. Analysis of pleural effusion shows red blood cell count of $500/mm^3$, white blood cell count of $600/mm^3$, protein level of $1.5 g/dL$, and specific gravity of 1.010. The most likely diagnosis is:
    (a) congestive heart failure
    (b) parapneumonic effusion
    (c) hemothorax
    (d) bronchogenic carcinoma

210. Pulmonary sequestration:
    (a) commonly occurs on the right side
    (b) intralobar sequestration is supplied by the pulmonary artery
    (c) extralobar sequestration is supplied by the aorta
    (d) intralobar sequestration drains into systemic veins
    (e) extralobar sequestration drains into pulmonary veins

211. The most important diagnostic test for a thyroid nodule is:
    (a) ultrasound
    (b) radioactive isotope scan
    (c) thyroid function test
    (d) fine-needle aspiration
    (e) computed tomography scan

212. Pleomorphic parotid adenoma:
    (a) requires core biopsy before resection
    (b) is adequately treated with enucleation
    (c) commonly undergoes malignant transformation
    (d) commonly results in facial palsy
    (e) is the most common parotid neoplasm

213. The mean arterial pressure is:
    (a) diastolic pressure + 1/2 pulse pressure
    (b) systolic pressure + pulse pressure
    (c) systolic pressure + 1/3 pulse pressure
    (d) diastolic pressure + 1/3 pulse pressure

214. A contraindication to breast-conserving therapy is:
    (a) age more than 70 years
    (b) coronary artery disease
    (c) family history of breast cancer
    (d) collagen vascular disease

215. Death from tension pneumothorax is caused by:
    (a) decreased venous return
    (b) cardiac arrhythmia
    (c) acute hypoxia
    (d) acute hypercapnia

216. The most important element in the history of an infant with vomiting is:
    (a) the frequency of vomiting
    (b) the amount of vomiting
    (c) the presence of fever
    (d) if vomiting is projectile
    (e) if vomiting is bile stained

217. The substrate for nitric oxide synthetase is:
    (a) glutamine
    (b) alanine
    (c) L-arginine
    (d) valine

218. The most frequent complication of giant gastric ulcer is:
    (a) gastric outlet obstruction
    (b) perforation
    (c) upper gastrointestinal bleeding
    (d) gastroenteric fistula

219. Mucosal defense is provided by immunoglobulin:
    (a) A
    (b) G
    (c) M
    (d) D
    (e) E

220. The most common cause of nipple discharge is:
    (a) duct ectasia
    (b) breast cancer
    (c) intraductal papilloma
    (d) pituitary adenoma
    (e) fibrocystic disease

221. The most common agent transmitted by blood transfusion is:
    (a) human immunodeficiency virus
    (b) hepatitis B virus
    (c) hepatitis C virus
    (d) *Cytomegalovirus*

222. Advantage of full thickness over split thickness skin graft is:
    (a) less wound contraction
    (b) better take
    (c) more resistance to infection
    (d) better sensory function

223. Cyclosporin A inhibits the production of:
    (a) interleukin–1
    (b) interleukin–2
    (c) interleukin–6
    (d) tumor necrosis factor-α

224. The main component of urinary stones complicating resection of terminal ileum is:
    (a) urate
    (b) oxalate
    (c) phosphate
    (d) ammonium

225. A characteristic feature of toxic shock syndrome in children with burns is:
    (a) purulent wound drainage
    (b) leukopenia
    (c) hypothermia
    (d) bradycardia

226. The rate of axonal regeneration after nerve injury is:
    (a) 1 cm/month
    (b) 1 mm/day
    (c) 1 mm/week
    (d) 1 cm/week

227. The optimal treatment for bleeding gastric varices in chronic pancreatitis is:
    (a) distal pancreatectomy
    (b) splenorenal shunt
    (c) portocaval shunt
    (d) splenectomy
    (e) transjugular intrahepatic portosystemic shunt procedure

228. Electrical burn injury:
    (a) can be estimated by the extent of skin damage
    (b) typically affects the trunk more than the extremities
    (c) requires close cardiac monitoring
    (d) is inversely related to tissue resistance

229. The highest rate of metastasis occurs in carcinoid arising from:
    (a) appendix
    (b) bronchus
    (c) ileum
    (d) stomach

230. The most common presentation of ductal carcinoma *in situ* is:
    (a) breast pain
    (b) breast lump
    (c) nipple discharge
    (d) microcalcification

231. The main source of fuel in sepsis is:
    (a) glucose
    (b) fatty acids
    (c) ketones
    (d) amino acids

232. A patient with electrical burn of the leg complains of pain on passive movement of the foot. The pedal pulses are diminished. The next step is:
    (a) escharotomy
    (b) femoral angiogram
    (c) leg elevation and intravenous heparin
    (d) fasciotomy

233. The most common complication of blood transfusion is:
    (a) hemolytic reaction
    (b) human immunodeficiency virus transmission
    (c) allergic reaction
    (d) volume overload
    (e) coagulopathy

234. The highest concentration of immunoglobulin A–producing cells is in:
    (a) bloodstream
    (b) oral cavity
    (c) bronchial tree
    (d) small intestine
    (e) urogenital tract

235. In the treatment of coagulopathy:
    (a) calcium should be routinely infused with massive transfusion
    (b) desmopressin (DDAVP) stimulates the release of factor VIII
    (c) von Willebrand's disease can be treated with factor VIII concentrate
    (d) the effect of aspirin can be reversed by fresh-frozen plasma

236. The most common source of metastatic small bowel tumor is:
    (a) lungs
    (b) melanoma
    (c) breast
    (d) soft tissue sarcoma

237. Myeloid metaplasia:
    (a) is a disease of young females
    (b) is rarely associated with splenomegaly
    (c) results in extramedullary hematopoiesis
    (d) results in increased bone marrow megakaryocytes

238. Which of the following is contraindicated in managing corrosive esophagitis?
    (a) gastric lavage
    (b) esophagogastroduodenoscopy
    (c) corticosteroids
    (d) tracheostomy

239. Which of the following is effective in treating refractory Crohn's fistula?
    (a) total parenteral nutrition
    (b) prednisone
    (c) infliximab
    (d) azathioprine

240. Hypothermic coagulopathy:
    (a) is associated with clotting factor depletion
    (b) can be corrected with fresh-frozen plasma transfusion
    (c) is associated with prolonged prothrombin time and partial thromboplastin time
    (d) is a complication of massive transfusion

241. Secretin:
    (a) stimulates gastrin secretion
    (b) stimulates pancreatic enzyme secretion
    (c) inhibits intestinal motility
    (d) stimulates gastric acid secretion

242. The use of inverse ratio ventilation will:
    (a) decrease auto-positive end-expiratory pressure
    (b) improve alveolar ventilation
    (c) increase incidence of pneumonia
    (d) decrease mean airway pressure

243. The optimal management of esophageal leiomyoma is:
    (a) Ivor-Lewis esophageal resection
    (b) transhiatal esophageal resection
    (c) segmental esophageal resection
    (d) esophagomyotomy and enucleation
    (e) endoscopic resection

244. Hand infection caused by a human bite is due to:
    (a) *Staphylococcus aureus*
    (b) *Clostridium difficile*
    (c) *Herpes simplex*
    (d) *Eikenella corrodens*
    (e) *Candida* species

245. Gastric intrinsic factor is secreted from:
    (a) parietal cells
    (b) chief cells
    (c) antral G cells
    (d) D cells

246. 246 Which of the following directly induces coagulation?
    (a) superglue
    (b) oxidized cellulose
    (c) absorbable gelatin sponge
    (d) microfibrillar collagen (Avitene)

247. Which of the following inhibits gastric bicarbonate secretion?
    (a) prostaglandins
    (b) vagal stimulation
    (c) aspirin
    (d) gastrin

248. A characteristic of prerenal azotemia is:
     (a) abnormal urine sediment
     (b) fractional excretion of sodium value <1%
     (c) urine sodium level <40 mEq/L
     (d) blood urea nitrogen/serum creatinine level >10

249. At an operation for small bowel obstruction, cecal volvulus is diagnosed. The cecum is viable. The procedure of choice is:
     (a) cecopexy
     (b) tube cecostomy
     (c) right hemicolectomy
     (d) resection, ileostomy, and mucous fistula

250. For a patient with a serum potassium level of 7 mEq/dL and an absent P-wave on electrocardiogram, the initial management is:
     (a) intravenous Lasix
     (b) intravenous glucose/insulin
     (c) Kayexalate enema
     (d) intravenous sodium bicarbonate
     (e) intravenous calcium gluconate

251. Optimal management of mucosa-associated lymphoid tissue (MALT) lymphoma is:
     (a) chemotherapy
     (b) total gastrectomy
     (c) chemoradiation
     (d) antibiotics

252. Positive end-expiratory pressure therapy will result in:
     (a) decrease in extravascular lung water
     (b) increase in cardiac preload
     (c) decrease in atrial natriuretic peptide
     (d) decrease in functional residual capacity

253. At the initiation of swallowing, the pressure at the lower esophageal sphincter:
     (a) remains unchanged
     (b) decreases and then increases
     (c) increases and then decreases
     (d) increases and then returns to baseline

254. The serum sodium level in a 60-year-old man who weighs 70 kg is 125 mEq/L. His sodium deficit is:
     (a) 130 mEq
     (b) 210 mEq
     (c) 360 mEq
     (d) 520 mEq
     (e) 850 mEq

255. A colorectal tumor that invades through the muscularis propria into the subserosa is a:
     (a) T1 lesion
     (b) T2 lesion
     (c) T3 lesion
     (d) T4 lesion

256. Glutamine:
     (a) is supplied in total parenteral nutrition
     (b) increases intestinal cellularity
     (c) is an essential amino acid
     (d) is a substrate for gluconeogenesis

257. Which of the following is a defect in the hemoglobin chain that responds to splenectomy?
     (a) idiopathic thrombocytopenic purpura
     (b) hereditary spherocytosis
     (c) thalassemia
     (d) glucose-6-phosphate deficiency

258. A central scar in a hepatic lesion is characteristic of:
     (a) focal nodular hyperplasia
     (b) hepatic adenoma
     (c) hemangioma
     (d) hamartoma
     (e) hepatocellular carcinoma

259. The initial step in management of a hypercalcemic crisis is intravenous:
     (a) steroids
     (b) calcitonin
     (c) saline
     (d) furosemide
     (e) mithramycin

260. Hepatic focal nodular hyperplasia:
     (a) usually occurs in women of reproductive age
     (b) is related to oral contraceptive use
     (c) presents with abdominal pain in most cases
     (d) carries the risk of spontaneous rupture

261. The most accurate measure of adequacy of nutritional support is:
     (a) serum albumin level
     (b) body weight
     (c) triceps skinfold measurement
     (d) serum prealbumin level

262. Refractory hypokalemia can be caused by:
     (a) hypocalcemia
     (b) hyponatremia
     (c) hypophosphatemia
     (d) hypomagnesemia

263. A respiratory quotient of 1.2 indicates:
    (a) lipogenesis
    (b) ketogenesis
    (c) pure fat utilization
    (d) carbohydrates are the source of fuel
    (e) proteins are the source of fuel

264. Mallory-Weiss tear is located:
    (a) in the distal esophagus
    (b) anteriorly across the gastroesophageal junction
    (c) posteriorly across the gastroesophageal junction
    (d) on the lesser curve of the cardia
    (e) on the greater curve of the cardia

265. The blood supply of the thoracic stomach used for esophageal replacement depends on:
    (a) the left gastric artery
    (b) the short gastric vessels
    (c) the right gastroepiploic artery
    (d) the left gastroepiploic artery

266. The most serious complication of gastric bypass procedure is:
    (a) hepatic failure
    (b) anastomotic leak
    (c) urolithiasis
    (d) intestinal obstruction
    (e) hypocalcemia

267. *Helicobacter pylori:*
    (a) colonization is highest in childhood
    (b) eradication does not influence ulcer recurrence
    (c) is isolated in up to 90% of duodenal ulcer cases
    (d) metronidazole achieves eradication as a single agent

268. L5–S1 disc lesion will result in:
    (a) weak plantar flexion
    (b) weak dorsiflexion
    (c) absent knee jerk
    (d) lost sensation in the big toe

269. A patient with head injury opens his eyes and withdraws his arm to pain. He is making incomprehensible sounds. His Glasgow Coma Scale score is:
    (a) 12
    (b) 10
    (c) 8
    (d) 6

270. Perianal Crohn's disease:
    (a) typically occurs late in the course of the disease
    (b) fistulas are usually multiple
    (c) fecal diversion is usually curative
    (d) lesions are typically located posteriorly
    (e) granulomas are seldom found on biopsy

271. Appropriate management of chronic pancreatitis with pancreatic duct ectasia is:
    (a) pancreaticoduodenectomy
    (b) distal pancreaticojejunostomy
    (c) longitudinal pancreaticojejunostomy
    (d) near total pancreatectomy
    (e) sphincteroplasty

272. The most common cause of massive bleeding in chronic pancreatitis is:
    (a) pseudoaneurysm
    (b) arteriovenous fistula
    (c) mycotic aneurysm
    (d) fibromuscular dysplasia

273. Colonic distension in toxic megacolon is most prominent in the:
    (a) cecum
    (b) ascending colon
    (c) transverse colon
    (d) descending colon
    (e) sigmoid colon

274. At the lung functional residual capacity:
    (a) chest wall exerts inward elastic recoil
    (b) lungs exert outward elastic recoil
    (c) alveolar pressure equals pleural pressure
    (d) lungs and chest wall exert equal and opposing recoil

275. Which of the following inhibits intestinal motility?
    (a) gastrin
    (b) cholecystokinin
    (c) epinephrine
    (d) motilin
    (e) serotonin

276. The most common site of ectopic pheochromocytoma is:
    (a) lower pole of the kidney
    (b) para-aortic tissue
    (c) mediastinum
    (d) pelvis

277. Which of the following is poorly absorbed in achlorhydria?
    (a) proteins
    (b) fats
    (c) bile salts
    (d) vitamin D
    (e) vitamin B_{12}

278. The most common cause of hypophosphatemia in hospitalized patients is:
    (a) renal failure
    (b) sepsis
    (c) glucose overload
    (d) diarrhea

279. The main fuel for colonocytes is:
    (a) glutamine
    (b) short-chain fatty acids
    (c) alanine
    (d) glucose
    (e) ketones

280. Pulmonary fibrosis is a complication of:
    (a) doxorubicin
    (b) methotrexate
    (c) bleomycin
    (d) cyclophosphamide
    (e) vincristine

281. The most useful serum marker for cancer screening is:
    (a) prostate-specific antigen
    (b) CA 19.9
    (c) α-fetoprotein
    (d) carcinoembryonic antigen

282. The inferior parathyroid gland originates from the:
    (a) first pharyngeal pouch
    (b) second pharyngeal pouch
    (c) third pharyngeal pouch
    (d) fourth pharyngeal pouch

283. Hypotension and decreased end-tidal CO_2 during laparoscopy are likely due to:
    (a) tension pneumothorax
    (b) inferior vena cava compression
    (c) CO_2 embolism
    (d) anesthetic overdose

284. The main fuel for most cancer cells is:
    (a) butyrate
    (b) glutamine
    (c) L-arginine
    (d) glucose
    (e) ketones

285. Which of the following is an inhibitor of wound contraction?
    (a) glucocorticoids
    (b) d-penicillamine
    (c) colchicine
    (d) aspirin

286. Fetal wound healing is characterized by:
    (a) increased angiogenesis
    (b) increased hyaluronic acid synthesis
    (c) increased inflammatory response
    (d) decreased collagen

287. Death from postoperative renal failure is most commonly due to:
    (a) myocardial infarction
    (b) bleeding
    (c) sepsis
    (d) liver failure

288. Regarding graft rejection:
    (a) hyperacute rejection is antibody mediated
    (b) hyperacute rejection is reversed with steroids
    (c) acute rejection is B cell mediated
    (d) acute rejection occurs over month

289. The most important prognostic variable for melanoma is:
    (a) gender
    (b) age
    (c) Clark's level
    (d) Breslow's thickness
    (e) complexion

290. Follicular thyroid carcinoma:
    (a) is the most common thyroid cancer
    (b) is readily diagnosed with fine-needle aspiration
    (c) spreads via hematogenous route
    (d) is commonly multifocal

291. Multiple endocrine neoplasia is associated with germline mutation in:
    (a) *p53* gene
    (b) *RET* proto-oncogene
    (c) *N-myc* gene
    (d) *APC* gene

292. Optimal treatment of cloacogenic carcinoma of anal canal is:
    (a) local excision
    (b) abdominoperineal resection
    (c) chemotherapy alone
    (d) radiotherapy alone
    (e) chemoradiation

293. The most common hernia in women is:
    (a) femoral hernia
    (b) obturator hernia
    (c) inguinal hernia
    (d) umbilical hernia
    (e) spigelian hernia

294. Gastroschisis:
    (a) is usually associated with other anomalies
    (b) is usually associated with chromosomal disorders
    (c) is located on the left of the umbilical cord
    (d) repair is followed by prolonged ileus

295. The most common visceral aneurysm is:
    (a) celiac
    (b) superior mesenteric artery
    (c) splenic
    (d) hepatic

296. Gastroschisis is associated with an increased risk of:
    (a) hepatomegaly
    (b) intestinal atresia
    (c) microcephaly
    (d) cardiac anomalies

297. The cremaster muscle is derived from:
    (a) the external oblique muscle
    (b) the internal oblique muscle
    (c) the transversus abdominis muscle
    (d) the transversalis fascia

298. The time for platelet transfusion during splenectomy for idiopathic thrombocytopenic purpura is:
    (a) on making the incision
    (b) after ligation of the splenic artery
    (c) on induction of anesthesia
    (d) after removal of the spleen

299. The most common congenital cardiac defect is:
    (a) atrial septal defect
    (b) ventricular septal defect
    (c) transposition of great vessels
    (d) aortic coarticulation

300. The most appropriate method to diagnose small bowel injury in a conscious trauma patient with seatbelt injury is:
    (a) diagnostic peritoneal lavage
    (b) ultrasound
    (c) computed tomography scan
    (d) serial abdominal examination
    (e) plain abdominal film

301. On postoperative day 1, a patient develops a temperature of 104°F and foul-smelling wound drainage. The most likely isolate is:
    (a) Gram-negative rods
    (b) Gram-positive rods
    (c) Gram-negative cocci
    (d) Gram-positive cocci

302. A hemodynamic consequence of carbon dioxide pneumoperitoneum is:
    (a) decrease in cardiac index
    (b) decrease in systemic vascular resistance
    (c) decrease in mean arterial pressure
    (d) increase in cardiac preload

303. In the diabetic foot:
    (a) atherosclerosis often involves the pedal arteries
    (b) foot sepsis is often polymicrobial
    (c) ankle–brachial index accurately measures the degree of ischemia
    (d) diabetic neuropathy involves only sensory nerves

304. Decreased hemoglobin affinity to oxygen at the tissue level is caused by:
    (a) increased body temperature
    (b) decreased 2,3-diphosphoglycerate
    (c) decreased pCO_2
    (d) increased pH

305. A patient with pelvic fracture is hypotensive and has grossly positive diagnostic peritoneal lavage. The next step is:
    (a) angiography and embolization
    (b) computed tomography of the abdomen and pelvis
    (c) celiotomy
    (d) application of C-clamp
    (e) application of pneumatic antishock garment

306. Heparin:
    (a) prevents platelet aggregation
    (b) prevents factor VII synthesis
    (c) is a cyclo-oxygenase inhibitor
    (d) potentiates the action of antithrombin III

307. Cholecystokinin:
    (a) stimulates the sphincter of Oddi
    (b) is secreted by the antral mucosa
    (c) stimulates pancreatic enzyme secretion
    (d) stimulates gastric emptying

308. The earliest and most specific sign of malignant hyperthermia is:
   (a) high fever
   (b) hypotension
   (c) increase in end tidal CO_2
   (d) tachycardia
   (e) hypoxia

309. The most frequent manifestation of blunt myocardial contusion is:
   (a) atrioventricular block
   (b) atrial flutter
   (c) premature ventricular contractions
   (d) premature atrial contractions
   (e) atrial fibrillation

310. The most commonly injured nerve under general anesthesia is:
   (a) radial nerve
   (b) ulnar nerve
   (c) median nerve
   (d) brachial plexus
   (e) common peroneal nerve

311. Respiratory distress associated with goiter is most commonly caused by:
   (a) recurrent laryngeal nerve palsy
   (b) malignant tracheal invasion
   (c) retrosternal goitrous extension
   (d) hemorrhage in large goiter

312. Malignant hyperthermia:
   (a) can be induced by local anesthetics
   (b) can be induced by nondepolarizing muscle relaxants
   (c) can be induced by nitrous oxide
   (d) is related to disordered K^+ metabolism
   (e) is more common in children than adults

313. The most common cardiac anomaly found in adults is:
   (a) atrial septal defect
   (b) ventricular septal defect
   (c) transposition of great vessels
   (d) coarctation of the aorta

314. The most common complication of epidural analgesia is:
   (a) hypotension
   (d) nausea
   (c) respiratory depression
   (d) deep vein thrombosis

315. The lateral boundary of a femoral hernia is:
   (a) the femoral nerve
   (b) the femoral artery
   (c) the femoral vein
   (d) the lacunar ligament

316. A characteristic of primary hyperaldosteronism is:
   (a) hyperkalemia
   (b) hyper-reninism
   (c) hypertension
   (d) hyperplasia of zona reticularis
   (e) hyperplasia of zona fasciculata

317. Regarding the adrenal gland:
   (a) the adrenal cortex does not have nerve supply
   (b) the adrenal medulla is supplied by postganglionic adrenergic fibers
   (c) the right adrenal vein drains into the renal vein
   (d) the left adrenal vein drains into the inferior vena cava

318. At an operation for appendicitis, the appendix is found to be normal and the fallopian tube is found to be thickened with surrounding purulent exudate. The operative management should be:
   (a) appendectomy
   (b) appendectomy and salpingectomy
   (c) salpingectomy
   (d) no operative intervention

319. In the preoperative preparation of pheochromocytoma, medications are given in the following order:
   (a) diuretics and then α-blockers
   (b) α-blockers and then β-blockers
   (c) β-blockers and then α-blockers
   (d) diuretics and then β-blockers

320. Hyperinsulinism in a newborn is most likely caused by:
   (a) nesidioblastosis
   (b) glycogen storage disease
   (c) benign insulinoma
   (d) malignant insulinoma

321. A patient with abdominal wall desmoid tumor should be screened for:
   (a) lung cancer
   (b) colon polyps
   (c) breast cancer
   (d) medullary thyroid carcinoma
   (e) pancreatic cancer

322. Which of the following is a vasoconstrictor?
    (a) procaine
    (b) bupivacaine
    (c) lidocaine
    (d) cocaine

323. Paralytic ileus is a complication of:
    (a) cyclophosphamide
    (b) vinca alkaloids
    (c) methotrexate
    (d) cisplatin
    (e) doxorubicin

324. Neutropenic enterocolitis is a complication of:
    (a) cytarabine
    (b) cyclophosphamide
    (c) doxorubicin
    (d) cisplatin

325. Severe peripheral neuropathy is a complication of:
    (a) vinca alkaloids
    (b) cyclophosphamide
    (c) cytarabine
    (d) cisplatin

326. Watery diarrhea, hypokalemia, hypochloremia, and acidosis are features of:
    (a) insulinoma
    (b) gastrinoma
    (c) vasoactive intestinal peptide–producing tumor
    (d) glucagonoma

327. Characteristics of somatostatinoma are:
    (a) mild diabetes, skin rash, glossitis
    (b) ulcer diathesis, diarrhea
    (c) mild diabetes, diarrhea, gallstones
    (d) diarrhea, hypokalemia, hypochloremia

328. An inhibitor of platelet aggregation is:
    (a) prostacyclin I
    (b) thromboxane A_2
    (c) adenosine diphosphate
    (d) serotonin
    (e) von Willebrand's factor

329. Regarding gastrointestinal bleeding in children:
    (a) anal fissure is the leading cause
    (b) clear nasogastric aspirate rules out upper gastrointestinal bleeding
    (c) Meckel's diverticulum is seldom the cause of massive bleeding
    (d) bleeding is the most common presentation of intussusception

330. The colon secretes:
    (a) water
    (b) sodium
    (c) chloride
    (d) potassium

331. Mild diabetes, skin rash, and glossitis are features of:
    (a) somatostatinoma
    (b) gastrinoma
    (c) glucagonoma
    (d) insulinoma

332. The most common intra-abdominal solid tumor in children is:
    (a) nephroblastoma
    (b) neuroblastoma
    (c) rhabdomyosarcoma
    (d) fibrosarcoma

333. Distinction between toxic epidermal necrolysis and staphylococcal scalding skin syndrome is based on:
    (a) degree of erythema
    (b) bullae formation
    (c) level of exfoliation
    (d) response to steroids

334. An indication for laparotomy in neonatal necrotizing enterocolitis is:
    (a) distended bowel loops
    (b) thickened bowel wall
    (c) abdominal wall erythema
    (d) pneumatosis intestinalis

335. Regarding congenital diaphragmatic hernia:
    (a) requires emergency operation if respiratory distress is present
    (b) foramen of Bochdalek hernia is the most common type
    (c) foramen of Morgagni hernia presents with respiratory distress
    (d) is rarely associated with underlying lung pathology

336. Regarding neonatal Hirschsprung's disease:
    (a) diagnosis is confirmed by barium enema
    (b) enterocolitis is the leading cause of death
    (c) mainly affects females
    (d) shows absent nerve trunks in the aganglionic segments

337. Prosthetic graft infection is most commonly due to:
    (a) *Staphylococcus epidermidis*
    (b) *Staphylococcus aureus*
    (c) *Escherichia coli*
    (d) *Streptococcus faecalis*

338. Sinistral portal hypertension is most commonly due
     to:
     (a) hypercoagulable states
     (b) schistosomiasis
     (c) alcoholism
     (d) chronic pancreatitis

339. Cervical sympathectomy is least likely to improve:
     (a) hyperhidrosis
     (b) scleroderma
     (c) causalgia
     (d) frostbite

340. Management of deep vein thrombosis during
     pregnancy is:
     (a) 10-day intravenous heparin and then Coumadin
         until term
     (b) 10-day intravenous heparin and then Coumadin
         for 6 months
     (c) 10-day intravenous heparin and then prophy-
         lactic subcutaneous heparin until term
     (d) 10-day intravenous heparin and then therapeu-
         tic subcutaneous heparin until term

341. A pleural fluid pH >6.5:
     (a) is normal
     (b) indicates esophageal perforation
     (c) indicates pleural transudate
     (d) indicates bacterial infection

342. The most accurate method to diagnose traumatic
     aortic arch injury is:
     (a) upright chest x-ray
     (b) chest computed tomography
     (c) magnetic resonance imaging
     (d) transesophageal echocardiogram

343. Lung resection is contraindicated if:
     (a) preoperative PO_2 is 60
     (b) preoperative PCO_2 is 50
     (c) $FEV_1 = 1$ liter
     (d) FEV_1/VC is 75%
     (e) MBC is 60%

344. Immediately after intravenous (IV) injection of
     5,000 U of heparin, the effect can be reversed with
     IV:
     (a) 10 mg protamine sulfate
     (b) 20 mg protamine sulfate
     (c) 30 mg protamine sulfate
     (d) 40 mg protamine sulfate
     (e) 50 mg protamine sulfate

345. The most common cause of small bowel obstruction
     during pregnancy is:
     (a) incarcerated groin hernia
     (b) adhesions
     (c) gallstone ileus
     (d) intestinal volvulus
     (e) intussusception

346. Which of the following is an analgesic?
     (a) sodium thiopental
     (b) ketamine
     (c) etomidate
     (d) propofol

347. A contraindication to the use of ketamine is:
     (a) hypotension
     (b) head injury
     (c) asthma
     (d) hypoventilation

348. The cytokine directly responsible for hepatic acute
     phase response is:
     (a) interleukin-1
     (b) interleukin-2
     (c) interleukin-6
     (d) tumor necrosis factor-α

349. In multiple endocrine neoplasia type 1:
     (a) almost all patients have parathyroid hyper-
         plasia
     (b) almost all patients have pancreatic endocrine
         tumor
     (c) almost all patients have pituitary adenoma
     (d) all patients have hyperparathyroidism, pancre-
         atic, and pituitary lesions

350. Postoperative cardiac events are most likely if pre-
     operative electrocardiogram shows:
     (a) ST-T wave changes
     (b) bundle branch block
     (c) left ventricular hypertrophy
     (d) Q-wave

351. An indication for preoperative angiography for
     elective abdominal aortic aneurysm surgery is:
     (a) suspected contained rupture
     (b) suspected inflammatory aneurysm
     (c) aneurysm larger than 7 cm
     (d) history of claudication

352. An early feature of lidocaine toxicity is:
     (a) arrhythmia
     (b) muscle twitching
     (c) respiratory depression
     (d) hypotension

353. The superior pancreaticoduodenal artery is a branch of:
    (a) the celiac axis
    (b) the superior mesenteric artery
    (c) the hepatic artery
    (d) the right gastric artery
    (e) the gastroduodenal artery

354. Which of the following pancreatic enzymes is secreted in an active form?
    (a) lipase
    (b) phospholipase A
    (c) trypsin
    (d) elastase

355. A tracheostomy-related tracheoinnominate fistula is best managed by:
    (a) division of innominate artery and ligation of both ends
    (b) division of innominate artery and vein graft
    (c) division of innominate artery and polytetrafluoroethylene graft
    (d) primary repair of the innominate artery

356. Optimum calorie/nitrogen ratio for protein synthesis is:
    (a) 25–50:1
    (b) 50–75:1
    (c) 75–100:1
    (d) 100–150:1

357. Aldosterone:
    (a) stimulates sodium resorption in proximal renal tubules
    (b) stimulates sodium resorption in distal renal tubules
    (c) stimulates potassium resorption in proximal renal tubules
    (d) stimulates potassium resorption in distal renal tubules

358. Hypertension in cases of extra-adrenal pheochromocytoma is caused by:
    (a) combined epinephrine and norepinephrine
    (b) pure epinephrine
    (c) pure norepinephrine
    (d) rennin, epinephrine, and norepinephrine

359. The highest bicarbonate concentration is found in:
    (a) saliva
    (b) gastric secretions
    (c) biliary secretion
    (d) pancreatic secretion
    (e) small intestine

360. A 70-kg male with 50% body surface area second-degree burn requires:358
    (a) 7,000 mL of lactated Ringer's solution over the first 6 hours
    (b) 7,000 mL of lactated Ringer's solution over the first 8 hours
    (c) 8,000 mL of lactated Ringer's solution over the first 8 hours
    (d) 10,000 mL of lactated Ringer's solution over the first 8 hours

361. A complication that enteral and parenteral feeding have in common is:
    (a) increased incidence of sepsis
    (b) intestinal villous atrophy
    (c) elevated liver transaminases
    (d) hyperosmolar nonketotic coma
    (e) diarrhea

362. The most common organism isolated from bile is:
    (a) *Escherichia coli*
    (b) *Klebsiella*
    (c) *Staphylococcus aureus*
    (d) *Bacteroides*
    (e) *Proteus*

363. The protein loss equivalent to 100g of negative nitrogen balance is:
    (a) 75 g
    (b) 150 g
    (c) 375 g
    (d) 525 g
    (e) 625 g

364. The most common cause of cancer-related death in females is:
    (a) breast cancer
    (b) colon cancer
    (c) ovarian cancer
    (d) pancreatic cancer
    (e) lung cancer

365. The highest potassium concentration is found in:
    (a) saliva
    (b) gastric secretion
    (c) bile
    (d) small intestine
    (e) pancreatic secretion

366. The risk of regional node metastases in 0.70 mm thick melanoma is:
    (a) <5%
    (b) 10%
    (c) 20%
    (d) 30%
    (e) 50%

367. The initial fluid bolus for an injured child is:
     (a) 10 mL/kg of lactated Ringer's solution
     (b) 20 mL/kg of lactated Ringer's solution
     (c) 30 mL/kg of lactated Ringer's solution
     (d) 40 mL/kg of lactated Ringer's solution

368. Elevation of urinary 5-hydroxyindole acetic acid is diagnostic of:
     (a) pheochromocytoma
     (b) Cushing's disease
     (c) carcinoid syndrome
     (d) aldosteronoma

369. Regarding hypertrophic pyloric stenosis:
     (a) more common in males
     (b) most commonly presents in the first week of life
     (c) vomit is typically bile stained
     (d) diagnosis should be confirmed with upper gastrointestinal contrast study

370. A colon polyp with the highest malignant potential is:
     (a) 1 cm tubular adenoma
     (b) 4 cm hyperplastic polyp
     (c) 2 cm villous adenoma
     (d) 2 cm tubulovillous adenoma
     (e) 3 cm juvenile polyp

371. Gastric smooth muscle tumors present most commonly as:
     (a) upper gastrointestinal hemorrhage
     (b) incidental finding on esophagogastroduodenoscopy
     (c) gastric outlet obstruction
     (d) intermittent epigastric pain
     (e) weight loss

372. The desired minimum distal margin of resected rectal cancer is:
     (a) 1 cm
     (b) 2 cm
     (c) 3 cm
     (d) 4 cm
     (e) 5 cm

373. Regarding gastric adenocarcinoma:
     (a) the intestinal type is more common in younger patients
     (b) the intestinal type is often associated with peritoneal spread
     (c) the intestinal type has worse prognosis than diffuse type
     (d) the intestinal type is often distal in location

374. In the TNM staging, stage II colorectal cancer is:
     (a) T1, N1, M0
     (b) T2, N0, M0
     (c) T3, N1, M0
     (d) T4, N0, M0
     (e) T3, N1, M1

375. Postoperative radiation without chemotherapy:
     (a) improves survival in stage II colon cancer
     (b) improves local recurrence in stage II colon cancer
     (c) improves local recurrence in stage III rectal cancer
     (d) improves local recurrence and survival in stage III rectal cancer

376. Risk of irreversible tissue damage in pressure sores is highest with:
     (a) constant pressure of 50 mm Hg for 2 hours
     (b) constant pressure of 70 mm Hg for 2 hours
     (c) constant pressure of 100 mm Hg for 30 minutes
     (d) constant pressure of 150 mm Hg for 20 minutes

377. In caustic esophageal injury:
     (a) upper endoscopy is contraindicated in the acute phase
     (b) early induced emesis is helpful in minimizing the period of mucosal contact
     (c) alkalis cause coagulative tissue necrosis
     (d) acids cause severe gastric rather than esophageal injury

378. Toxic epidermal necrolysis in children is most commonly related to:
     (a) *Pseudomonas aeruginosa*
     (b) *Escherichia coli*
     (c) *Staphylococcus aureus*
     (d) *Streptococcus pneumoniae*

379. The most essential step in management of esophageal reflux and Barrett's change is:
     (a) Nissen fundoplication
     (b) close endoscopic surveillance
     (c) esophageal resection
     (d) medical management of reflux disease

380. A prominent "v" wave in the right atrial venous waveform indicates:
     (a) tricuspid valve regurgitation
     (b) atrial fibrillation
     (c) pulmonary embolism
     (d) atrial septal defect
     (e) atrial flutter

381. The mainstay of treatment of blunt carotid artery injuries is:
    (a) surgical exploration and vein patch graft
    (b) endoluminal stenting
    (c) catheter thrombolysis
    (d) anticoagulation

382. Regarding the anatomy of the esophagus:
    (a) the cervical esophagus lies to the right of the midline
    (b) the thoracic esophagus is anterior to the aortic arch
    (c) the left vagus nerve passes posterior to the esophagus
    (d) the cervical esophagus is supplied by the inferior thyroid artery
    (e) the abdominal esophagus is supplied by the right gastric artery

383. The most common cause of early postoperative death in elective abdominal aortic aneurysm repair is:
    (a) acute renal tubular necrosis
    (b) ischemic stroke
    (c) acute myocardial infarction
    (d) respiratory failure
    (e) exsanguination from anastomotic disruption

384. The initial test in cases of suspected gastroesophageal reflux should be:
    (a) Barium swallow
    (b) upper endoscopy
    (c) gastric pH monitoring
    (d) esophageal manometry

385. Which of the following organisms is slime-producing?
    (a) *Candida albicans*
    (b) *Staphylococcus aureus*
    (c) *Staphylococcus epidermidis*
    (d) *Klebsiella pneumoniae*
    (e) *Enterobacter aerogenes*

386. An increased incidence of adenocarcinoma of the esophagus is associated with:
    (a) achalasia
    (b) lye ingestion
    (c) Barrett's esophagus
    (d) Plummer-Vinson syndrome

387. Insulinomas:
    (a) are usually benign
    (b) are usually multiple
    (c) are commonly located in the tail of the pancreas
    (d) are less common than gastrinoma

388. The initial step in management of a 25-year-old male with a painless scrotal mass is:
    (a) fine-needle aspiration and cytology
    (b) abdominal computed tomography scan
    (c) observation and repeat examination in 2 weeks
    (d) scrotal ultrasound
    (e) orchiectomy

389. The most common anterior mediastinal tumor is:
    (a) thymoma
    (b) retrosternal goiter
    (c) lymphoma
    (d) teratoma

390. The hallmark of multiple endocrine neoplasia type 2 syndromes is:
    (a) hyperparathyroidism
    (b) pheochromocytoma
    (c) medullary thyroid carcinoma
    (d) pituitary adenoma
    (e) neural gangliomas

391. The cranial nerve most commonly injured during carotid endarterectomy is:
    (a) IX
    (b) X
    (c) XI
    (d) XII

392. Inadvertent tissue extravasation of intravenous dopamine is best managed with:
    (a) topical steroids and elevation
    (b) local ice packs and elevation
    (c) local infiltration of nitroglycerin
    (d) local infiltration of phentolamine
    (e) local infiltration of 1% lidocaine

393. Hürthle cell thyroid carcinoma:
    (a) is adequately treated with thyroid lobectomy
    (b) is seldom bilateral
    (c) often metastasizes to the cervical lymph nodes
    (d) is often related to previous neck radiation

394. Which of the following contributes to the arterial supply of the thoracic esophagus?
    (a) right gastric artery
    (b) bronchial artery
    (c) pulmonary artery
    (d) innominate artery

395. Regarding postoperative myocardial infarction:
    (a) it is often associated with chest pain
    (b) ischemic injury is more common postoperatively rather than intraoperatively
    (c) T-wave changes are the most specific finding for acute myocardial infarction
    (d) it occurs most commonly within the first 48 hours after surgery

396. The least appropriate test in the initial evaluation of adrenal incidentaloma is:
    (a) magnetic resonance imaging of the abdomen
    (b) fine-needle aspiration biopsy
    (c) follow-up computed tomography of the abdomen in 6 months
    (d) 24-hour urinary vanillylmandelic acid (VMA) level
    (e) serum potassium level

397. A 58-year-old female with a tubo-ovarian abscess should be treated with:
    (a) antibiotics and laparoscopic drainage
    (b) antibiotics with hysterectomy and bilateral salpingo-oophorectomy
    (c) antibiotics and unilateral salpingo-oophorectomy
    (d) antibiotics and computed tomography–guided drainage
    (e) antibiotics and observation

398. Cannon "a" waves on a right atrial waveform tracing indicate:
    (a) atrial flutter
    (b) atrial fibrillation
    (c) tricuspid regurgitation
    (d) pulmonary embolism
    (e) atrioventricular block

399. Intralobar pulmonary sequestration:
    (a) is supplied by the aorta
    (b) is drained by the azygos venous system
    (c) is commonly associated with diaphragmatic defect
    (d) has a separate pleural covering

400. Specific therapy for heparin-induced thrombocytopenia is:
    (a) low-molecular-weight heparin
    (b) Coumadin
    (c) dextran-60
    (d) aspirin
    (e) lepirudin

401. Hürthle cell thyroid carcinoma:
    (a) can be readily diagnosed with fine-needle aspiration
    (b) is often associated with previous neck radiation
    (c) is more aggressive than follicular thyroid carcinoma
    (d) typically shows avid ^{131}I uptake

402. Burn-associated inhalation injury can be excluded if:
    (a) the chest x-ray on admission is normal
    (b) there is no abnormal finding on flexible bronchoscopy
    (c) the arterial oxygen saturation is over 90%
    (d) the FEV_1/FVC is normal

403. The lateral boundary of a left paraduodenal hernia is:
    (a) the splenic artery
    (b) the left renal vein
    (c) the superior mesenteric vein
    (d) the inferior mesenteric artery
    (e) the inferior mesenteric vein

404. The carotid body:
    (a) is a pressure receptor
    (b) is an osmoreceptor
    (c) is a subintimal structure
    (d) is located in the adventia
    (e) is located in the media

405. Barrett's esophagus:
    (a) is commonly congenital in origin
    (b) is associated with epidermoid carcinoma of the esophagus
    (c) is reversed by a successful antireflux surgery
    (d) is an indication for life-long endoscopic surveillance

406. The most common causative agent in nosocomial sinusitis in the ICU is:
    (a) Pseudomonas aeruginosa
    (b) Staphylococcus aureus
    (c) Staphylococcus epidermidis
    (d) Streptococcus pneumoniae

407. The treatment of hyperacute kidney transplant rejection is:
    (a) administration of OKT-3
    (b) administration of massive doses of steroids
    (c) immediate transplant nephrectomy
    (d) observation and dialysis

408. Blunt cardiac injury:
    (a) most commonly affects the left ventricle
    (b) most commonly results in ventricular arrhythmias
    (c) can be reliably excluded if cardiac enzymes are normal
    (d) should be suspected if admission electrocardiogram is abnormal

409. A characteristic of Buerger's disease is:
    (a) superficial migratory thrombophlebitis
    (b) female predominance
    (c) severe involvement of the aortoiliac segment
    (d) the disease is restricted to the lower extremities

410. Recurrence of thyroid carcinoma after definitive treatment is best detected by:
    (a) ultrasound of the neck
    (b) thyroid-stimulating hormone level measurement
    (c) thyroglobin serum measurement
    (d) computed tomography scan of the neck
    (e) triiodothyronine/thyroxine measurement

411. The primary regulator of aldosterone secretion is:
    (a) angiotensin II
    (b) serum K level
    (c) adrenocorticotropic hormone
    (d) prostaglandins

412. The optimum management of a T4 breast cancer is:
    (a) modified radical mastectomy and radiation
    (b) chemoradiation only
    (c) simple mastectomy and radiation
    (d) chemotherapy followed by mastectomy and radiation
    (e) radiation therapy only

413. The diagnosis of esophageal achalasia is confirmed by:
    (a) bird's beak appearance on barium swallow
    (b) subatmospheric intraluminal esophageal pressure on manometry
    (c) endoscopic evidence of distal esophagitis
    (d) failure of lower esophageal sphincter relaxation on manometry
    (e) hyperperistalsis of the body of the esophagus

414. Factor VIII–related antigen is a marker of:
    (a) Kaposi's sarcoma
    (b) melanoma
    (c) postmastectomy angiosarcoma
    (d) desmoid tumors
    (e) Merkel cell carcinoma

415. The indication for fine-needle aspiration biopsy of an adrenal incidentaloma is:
    (a) suspected pheochromocytoma
    (b) suspected aldosteronoma
    (c) suspected adrenal carcinoma
    (d) suspected adrenal metastases

416. Male breast cancer:
    (a) has a peak incidence at the age of 40 years
    (b) is typically hormonally dependent
    (c) typically presents with bloody nipple discharge
    (d) is seldom an indication for tamoxifen therapy

417. A non-anion gap metabolic acidosis is associated with:
    (a) diabetic ketoacidosis
    (b) hemorrhagic shock
    (c) excessive sodium chloride administration
    (d) uremia
    (e) ingestion of ethylene glycol

418. Inverse ratio ventilation:
    (a) decreases mean airway pressure and increases intrathoracic pressure
    (b) decreases mean airway pressure and decreases intrathoracic pressure
    (c) increases mean airway pressure and increases intrathoracic pressure
    (d) increases mean airway pressure and decreases intrathoracic pressure

419. Duodenal atresia:
    (a) is caused by intrauterine mesenteric vascular accident
    (b) commonly exhibits normal muscular wall with a mucosal web
    (c) is seldom associated with normal passage of meconium at birth
    (d) is rarely associated with other congenital anomalies

420. Angiotensin-converting enzyme is produced by:
    (a) type I pneumocytes
    (b) type II pneumocytes
    (c) hepatocytes
    (d) juxtaglomcrular cells
    (e) vascular endothelial cells

421. Hereditary nonpolyposis colorectal cancer:
    (a) is an autosomal recessive disorder
    (b) is associated with higher incidence of ovarian cancer
    (c) is associated with higher incidence of endometrial cancer
    (d) is mostly left-side colon cancer

422. Auto-positive end-expiratory pressure in mechanical ventilation is most likely to develop with:
    (a) high rates and prolonged I:E ratio
    (b) high rates and decreased I:E ratio
    (c) decreased rate and decreased I:E ratio
    (d) decreased rate and prolonged I:E ratio

423. Initial management of T4 invasive lobular breast carcinoma is:
    (a) tamoxifen therapy
    (b) modified radical mastectomy
    (c) radiation therapy to the breast and ipsilateral axilla
    (d) neoadjuvant chemotherapy

424. The fluid of chylothorax is composed of:
    (a) pure fat
    (b) fat and neutrophils
    (c) fat and lymphocytes
    (d) fat and macrophages

425. The most common cause of renovascular hypertension is:
    (a) aneurysm of the renal artery
    (b) fibromuscular hyperplasia
    (c) renal artery calcinosis
    (d) renal artery atheroma

426. Merkel cell carcinoma:
    (a) is highly radiosensitive
    (b) has the best prognosis when it occurs on the trunk
    (c) seldom spreads to regional lymph nodes
    (d) is less likely than melanoma to recur after local excision

427. A complication of tacrolimus therapy is:
    (a) new-onset diabetes
    (b) upper gastrointestinal bleeding
    (c) thrombocytopenia
    (d) cardiac arrhythmia
    (e) bronchospasm

428. Extralobar pulmonary sequestration:
    (a) typical presents with repeated pulmonary infections
    (b) is drained by the pulmonary veins
    (c) is supplied by the aorta
    (d) is more common on the right side
    (e) is commonly connected with the bronchial tree

429. Appropriate management of radiation mastitis is:
    (a) local heat application
    (b) danazol therapy
    (c) therapeutic breast massage
    (d) simple mastectomy
    (e) pentoxifylline therapy

430. Optimum therapy for effort thrombosis of the axillary vein is:
    (a) therapeutic heparin followed by Coumadin for 3 months
    (b) therapeutic heparin followed by Coumadin for 6 months
    (c) thrombolysis, anticoagulation, and possible first rib resection
    (d) thrombolysis, anticoagulation, and balloon angioplasty
    (e) thrombectomy, anticoagulation, and stent placement

431. Drooling from the corner of the mouth after submandibular gland excision is due to:
    (a) injury of the lingual nerve
    (b) injury of the ansa cervicalis
    (c) injury of the hypoglossal nerve
    (d) injury of the marginal mandibular nerve

432. The component of blood transfusion responsible for immunosuppression is:
    (a) red cells
    (b) immunoglobulins
    (c) white blood cells
    (d) platelets

433. In therapeutic immunosuppression, rapamycin:
    (a) blocks interleukin-1 production
    (b) blocks interleukin-1 action
    (c) blocks interleukin-2 production
    (d) blocks interleukin-2 action

434. Gallstones diagnosed during pregnancy:
    (a) may resolve spontaneously after delivery
    (b) are the most common cause of jaundice during pregnancy
    (c) are seldom the cause of recurrent acute cholecystitis during the same pregnancy
    (d) are most commonly pigment stones

435. Trauma cesarean section is indicated if the fetus is viable and:
    (a) the mother is unstable and cardiac arrest is anticipated
    (b) 5 minutes of cardiopulmonary resuscitation were successful
    (c) 5 minutes of cardiopulmonary resuscitation were unsuccessful
    (d) cardiopulmonary resuscitation has just been initiated

436. The single most common abdominal operation for the elderly is:
   (a) adhesiolysis for small bowel obstruction
   (b) closure of perforated duodenal ulcer
   (c) resection of colon cancer
   (d) cholecystectomy
   (e) appendectomy

437. An age-related change in respiratory functions is:
   (a) increased total lung capacity (TLC)
   (b) decreased total lung capacity (TLC)
   (c) decreased functional residual capacity (FRC)
   (d) increased residual volume (RV)
   (e) increased vital capacity (VC)

438. Fetal death during pregnancy is most commonly due to:
   (a) abruptio placentae
   (b) subarachnoid hemorrhage
   (c) penetrating fetal injury
   (d) maternal demise

439. A physiologic change of aging is:
   (a) increased total body water
   (b) decreased antidiuretic hormone secretion (ADH)
   (c) decreased aldosterone secretion
   (d) exaggerated thirst response
   (e) decreased atrial natriuretic peptide (ANP)

440. Which of the following is contraindicated during pregnancy for treating breast cancer?
   (a) methotrexate
   (b) 5-fluorouracil
   (c) doxorubicin
   (d) cyclophosphamide

441. In the elderly:
   (a) there is decreased insensible water loss
   (b) there is increased antidiuretic hormone response
   (c) there is increased volume of distribution of water-soluble medications
   (d) there is decreased volume of distribution of lipid-soluble medications

442. During pregnancy:
   (a) acute appendicitis is more common than in the nonpregnant state
   (b) intestinal obstruction is most commonly caused by adhesions
   (c) laparoscopic cholecystectomy is contraindicated
   (d) leukocytosis is often indicative of a surgical abdominal pathology

443. An 80-year-old male is confused, lethargic, and has tonic spasms. He has been receiving intravenous 5% dextrose in water in one-half normal saline for 3 days after right hemicolectomy. The most likely cause is:
   (a) hypokalemia
   (b) hyperkalemia
   (c) hypocalcemia
   (d) hypernatremia
   (e) hyponatremia

444. A physiologic change in pregnancy is:
   (a) increased gallbladder contractility
   (b) elevated alkaline phosphatase
   (c) elevated alanine aminotransferase (AST)/ aspartate aminotransferase (ALT)
   (d) direct hyperbilirubinemia
   (e) indirect hyperbilirubinemia

445. In the elderly:
   (a) the myocardium is oversensitive to the effect of catecholamines
   (b) systolic function is more impaired than diastolic function
   (c) diastolic function is more impaired than systolic function
   (d) systolic and diastolic functions are equally impaired

446. A Crohn's disease–related internal fistula:
   (a) most commonly presents with florid sepsis
   (b) most commonly presents with Crohn's disease flare–up
   (c) requires excision of both organs involved for surgical treatment
   (d) most commonly involves small bowel to small bowel fistulation
   (e) requires surgical intervention as soon as the diagnosis is made

447. In inflammation, early "rolling" of neutrophils on endothelium is a function of:
   (a) selectins
   (b) N-cahedrins
   (c) immunoglobulin superfamily
   (d) integrins
   (e) complement activation

448. A paraesophageal hernia:
   (a) is a type I hiatal hernia
   (b) is most common in men <50 years of age
   (c) may present with chronic anemia
   (d) is often associated with reflux
   (e) requires surgery only if symptomatic

449. The most common cause of large bowel obstruction is:
     (a) colorectal cancer
     (b) Crohn's colitis
     (c) diverticulitis
     (d) adhesions
     (e) volvulus

450. Hypophosphatemia is associated with:
     (a) increased hemoglobin p50, respiratory failure, and encephalopathy
     (b) decreased hemoglobin p50, hemolysis, and respiratory failure
     (c) respiratory failure, hypothyroidism, and hemolysis
     (d) ataxia, cardiomyopathy, and hypothyroidism

451. Preoperative radiotherapy for rectal adenocarcinoma:
     (a) improves survival
     (b) increases postoperative morbidity
     (c) down-stages tumor in up to 50% of cases
     (d) is less effective than postoperative radiation

452. The principal side effect of ganciclovir therapy is:
     (a) bone marrow suppression
     (b) elevated liver enzymes
     (c) acute pancreatitis
     (d) acute renal failure
     (e) prolonged ileus

453. In contrast to ulcerative colitis, Crohn's disease:
     (a) is not associated with increased cancer risk
     (b) may spare the rectum
     (c) is more commonly associated with sclerosing cholangitis
     (d) is more commonly associated with toxic megacolon

454. The negative predictive value of a test is:
     (a) the proportion of patients with the disease who have a positive test
     (b) the proportion of patients without the disease who have a negative test
     (c) the proportion of patients without the disease who have a positive test
     (d) the proportion of patients with a positive test who have the disease
     (e) the proportion of patients with negative test who do not have the disease

455. Radiation enteritis of the large bowel most commonly affects:
     (a) the cecum
     (b) the splenic flexure
     (c) the sigmoid
     (d) the rectum

456. Eight hours after treatment for a scald injury, an infant has a temperature of 40°C and a white blood count of 5,000/mm³. The burn wound is clean. The most likely diagnosis is:
     (a) *Cytomegalovirus* infection
     (b) clostridial wound infection
     (c) toxic shock syndrome
     (d) *Pseudomonas* wound infection
     (e) *Pneumocystis pneumoniae*

457. The medial boundary of the femoral canal is:
     (a) the femoral vein
     (b) the femoral artery
     (c) the lacunar ligament
     (d) the inguinal ligament
     (e) the femoral nerve

458. Hemorrhagic dermal bullae are characteristic of wound infection caused by:
     (a) coagulase-negative *Staphylococcus*
     (b) *Streptococcus pyogenes*
     (c) *Clostridium perfringens*
     (d) *Clostridium tetani*
     (e) *Eikenella*

459. A marker with prognostic significance in cases of seminoma is:
     (a) α-fetoprotein
     (b) human chorionic gonadotropin-β
     (c) alkaline phosphatase of hepatic origin
     (d) testosterone level
     (e) serum lactate dehydrogenase

460. Collagen synthesis in the actively healing wound is best assessed by:
     (a) glutamine content
     (b) arginine content
     (c) hydroxyproline content
     (d) alanine content

461. The main motor nerve supply to the urinary bladder is:
     (a) the pelvic nerve
     (b) the hypogastric nerve
     (c) the pudendal nerve
     (d) the presacral nerve

462. Compared with hepatitis B virus, hepatitis C virus:
     (a) is an RNA virus
     (b) less commonly results in persistent viremia
     (c) can be prevented with effective vaccination
     (d) can be transmitted via the fecal-oral route

463. The positive predictive value of a test is:
    (a) the proportion of patients with the disease who have a positive test
    (b) the proportion of persons without the disease who have a negative test
    (c) the proportion of persons with a positive test who have the disease
    (d) the proportion of persons with a negative test who do not have the disease

464. The circulating level of which cytokine can be used as prognostic marker in sepsis?
    (a) interleukin-1
    (b) interleukin-2
    (c) interleukin-6
    (d) interleukin-8
    (e) tumor necrosis factor-α

465. Nitric oxide:
    (a) is a potent vasoconstrictor
    (b) prevents platelets aggregation
    (c) requires cyclic adenosine monophosphate for its actions
    (d) is normally stored in endothelial cells

466. The most common cause of facial nerve paralysis is:
    (a) parotid surgery
    (b) faciomaxillary injury
    (c) Bells' palsy
    (d) pleomorphic adenoma of the parotid gland
    (e) carcinoma of the parotid gland

467. Most renal absorption of sodium takes place in:
    (a) the proximal tubules
    (b) the loop of Henle
    (c) the distal tubules
    (d) the collecting ducts

468. Distinction between hemorrhagic and cardiogenic shock can be based on:
    (a) level of urinary sodium
    (b) ventricular filling pressures
    (c) system vascular resistance
    (d) serum lactate level
    (e) mixed venous oxygen saturation

469. Renin–angiotensin system is activated by:
    (a) hyponatremia
    (b) hypernatremia
    (c) hypokalemia
    (d) hypocalcemia
    (e) hypercalcemia

470. The thoracodorsal nerve:
    (a) is purely motor
    (b) supplies motor innervation to the serratus anterior muscle
    (c) injury during axillary dissection will lead to winged scapula
    (d) injury will result in loss of sensation on the medial surface of the upper arm

471. Hypocalcemia is a complication of chemotherapy with:
    (a) cyclophosphamide
    (b) vincristine
    (c) methotrexate
    (d) mithramycin
    (e) Adriamycin

472. Male breast cancer most commonly presents with:
    (a) mastodynia
    (b) bleeding per nipple
    (c) breast mass only
    (d) breast mass and bleeding per nipple
    (e) breast mass with ulceration

473. Which of the following is a clear indication of surgery for necrotizing enterocolitis?
    (a) generalized gas distension of the intestine
    (b) bleeding rectum
    (c) pneumatosis intestinalis
    (d) gas in the portal vein
    (e) pneumoperitoneum

474. An infected dog bite is most readily treated with:
    (a) gentamicin
    (b) ampicillin
    (c) vancomycin
    (d) clindamycin

475. During CO_2 pneumoperitoneum:
    (a) the mean arterial pressure increases
    (b) the mean arterial pressure decreases
    (c) the systemic vascular resistance increases
    (d) the systemic vascular resistance decreases
    (e) the cardiac output increases

476. In diabetic foot ulcers:
    (a) neuropathy is restricted to somatic nerves
    (b) the heel is the most common location
    (c) motor neuropathy mostly affects toe flexors
    (d) cold, dry foot is a classic finding
    (e) the ankle–brachial index is an accurate measure of the degree of ischemia

477. A sign of early sepsis is:
    (a) metabolic alkalosis
    (b) metabolic acidosis
    (c) respiratory alkalosis
    (d) respiratory acidosis

478. In contrast to a keloid, a hypertrophic scar:
    (a) is more likely to be familial
    (b) may subside spontaneously
    (c) may develop in delayed fashion years after initial injury
    (d) often extends beyond the limits of the original wound

479. In transplant recipients, there is an increased incidence of:
    (a) colon cancer
    (b) anal cancer
    (c) lung cancer
    (d) breast cancer
    (e) prostate cancer

480. The most common cause of small bowel bleeding in adults is:
    (a) Crohn's disease
    (b) arteriovenous malformation
    (c) leiomyosarcoma
    (d) Meckel's diverticulum
    (e) carcinoid neoplasms

481. A type IV hiatal hernia:
    (a) is a sliding hiatus hernia
    (b) is a traumatic diaphragmatic hernia
    (c) is a hernia that contains the stomach
    (d) is a hernia that contains parts of the intestine and colon

482. Isosulfan blue injection for sentinel node biopsy may result in:
    (a) cardiac arrhythmia
    (b) inaccurate pulse oximetry
    (c) malignant hyperthermia
    (d) hypercapnia
    (e) skin sloughing

483. The most common complication of gastric ulcer is:
    (a) malignant transformation
    (b) perforation
    (c) upper gastrointestinal bleeding
    (d) gastric outlet obstruction

484. The preferred neuromuscular-blocking agent in a liver failure patient is:
    (a) vecuronium
    (b) atracurium
    (c) pancuronium
    (d) pipecuronium

485. The most common fatal infection in burn victims is:
    (a) pneumonia
    (b) venous line–related sepsis
    (c) burn wounds sepsis
    (d) urinary tract infection

486. The cardiac ejection fraction:
    (a) is normally 45%
    (b) is an accurate indicator of cardiac dysfunction in the elderly
    (c) is increased in mitral stenosis
    (d) is decreased in mitral incompetence
    (e) is increased in ventricular septal defect

487. After 3 years, vein graft failure in the lower extremities is mostly caused by:
    (a) technical complications
    (b) anastomotic aneurysm
    (c) atherosclerosis of the graft
    (d) intimal thickening

488. The predominant parathyroid pathology in multiple endocrine neoplasia is:
    (a) a single parathyroid adenoma
    (b) multiple parathyroid adenomas
    (c) parathyroid hyperplasia
    (d) parathyroid carcinoma

489. In renal artery stenosis, angiotensin-converting enzyme inhibitors will:
    (a) decrease glomerular filtration rate
    (b) increase glomerular filtration rate
    (c) result in dilation of the afferent arterioles
    (d) result in constriction of the afferent arterioles
    (e) result in constriction of the efferent arterioles

490. The appropriate agent for prophylaxis in elective colectomy is:
    (a) Flagyl
    (b) imipenem
    (c) vancomycin
    (d) cefotetan
    (e) cefazolin

491. Which of the following is a dopamine antagonist?
    (a) phentolamine
    (b) propofol
    (c) haloperidol
    (d) clonidine

492. Peripheral neuropathy is the main side effect of:
    (a) cyclophosphamide
    (b) vincristine
    (c) methotrexate
    (d) mithramycin
    (e) Adriamycin

493. In liver transplantation, biliary complications are most commonly related to:
    (a) adequacy of hepatic venous outflow
    (b) adequacy of portal venous flow
    (c) adequacy of hepatic arterial flow
    (d) length of the donor's common bile duct

494. The optimum management of aspiration pneumonitis is:
    (a) endotracheal intubation and mechanical ventilation
    (b) endotracheal intubation, mechanical ventilation, and bronchial lavage
    (c) endotracheal intubation, ventilation, bronchial lavage, and steroids
    (d) endotracheal intubation, ventilation, bronchial lavage, and antibiotics

495. Malignant hyperthermia:
    (a) is triggered by the stress of surgery or anesthesia only
    (b) is a contraindication to future general anesthesia
    (c) can be prevented by perioperative calcium channel blockers
    (d) is associated with intraoperative rise of end tidal CO_2

496. The long thoracic nerve:
    (a) is purely motor
    (b) provides sensation to the medial wall of the axilla
    (c) provides sensation to the medial aspect of the upper arm
    (d) supplies motor innervation to the latissimus dorsi muscle
    (e) its injury results in weakness of arm abduction

497. The likelihood of malignancy in cystic pancreatic neoplasm is related to:
    (a) high glycogen content
    (b) mucin content
    (c) sunburst appearance on computed tomography scan
    (d) previous history of pancreatitis

498. Colovesical fistula:
    (a) is most commonly caused by colon cancer
    (b) is more common in females than in males
    (c) is readily diagnosed with barium enema in most cases
    (d) requires segmental colectomy and partial cystectomy for treatment
    (e) most commonly presents with pneumaturia

499. The optimum management for stage II thyroid lymphoma is:
    (a) total thyroidectomy
    (b) total thyroidectomy and radical neck dissection
    (c) total thyroidectomy and chemotherapy
    (d) chemoradiation
    (e) cervical radiation

500. The most reliable indicator of successful ventilatory weaning is:
    (a) PO_2 >100 with FiO_2 of 40%
    (b) PCO_2 <40 mm Hg
    (c) negative inspiratory force less (more negative) than −30 cm HO_2
    (d) f/Vt <100

501. Chronic allograft rejection:
    (a) can be prevented with adequate immunosuppression
    (b) is the main cause of death after liver transplantation
    (c) is more common with liver than heart transplantation
    (d) is more common with kidney than liver transplantation

502. The most accurate test to determine the need for neoadjuvant therapy in esophageal carcinoma is:
    (a) endoluminal ultrasound
    (b) chest computed tomography scan
    (c) bronchoscopy
    (d) barium swallow
    (e) esophagogastroduodenoscopy

503. The most characteristic metabolic abnormality in glucagonoma is:
    (a) hypoglycemia
    (b) hypoaminoacidemia
    (c) hypocholesterolemia
    (d) hypercholesterolemia

504. A local anesthetic that can be safely administered with tetracaine allergy is:
    (a) lidocaine
    (b) cocaine
    (c) procaine
    (d) chloroprocaine

505. Clonidine is:
    (a) an α_1-agonist
    (b) an α_1-antagonist
    (c) an α_2-agonist
    (d) a β_1-agonist
    (e) a β_2-agonist

506. A definitive diagnosis of inflammatory breast cancer is provided by:
    (a) unique mammographic appearance
    (b) finding tumor emboli in dermal lymphatics
    (c) finding extensive inflammatory cell infiltration of the tumor
    (d) elevated white cell count, fever, axillary lymphadenopathy
    (e) ultrasound appearance of cavitation

507. Tissue loss almost always results from ligation of the:
    (a) popliteal artery
    (b) common femoral artery
    (c) superficial femoral artery
    (d) brachial artery
    (e) portal vein

508. Male breast cancer:
    (a) is associated with the *BRCA-1* gene mutation
    (b) can only be of ductal origin
    (c) is seldom hormone receptor positive
    (d) develops at a much younger age than female breast cancer

509. Keloid formation has been associated with an increased amount of:
    (a) transforming growth factor-β
    (b) platelet-derived growth factor
    (c) epidermal growth factor
    (d) basic fibroblast growth factor
    (e) tumor necrosis factor-α

510. The anteroposterior anatomic relationship at the renal hilum is:
    (a) vein—artery—ureter
    (b) artery—vein—ureter
    (c) ureter—artery—vein
    (d) ureter—vein—artery

511. Endophthalmitis is characteristic of:
    (a) *Escherichia coli* sepsis
    (b) toxic shock syndrome
    (c) systemic candidiasis
    (d) facial necrotizing fasciitis

512. The most important determinant of survival of retroperitoneal sarcoma is:
    (a) the use of adjuvant chemotherapy
    (b) the size of the primary tumor
    (c) the histologic type of the primary
    (d) the use of intraoperative radiotherapy
    (e) complete surgical resection

513. A pulmonary embolus is associated with:
    (a) decrease in pulmonary capillary wedge pressure
    (b) decrease in mean pulmonary artery pressure
    (c) decrease in central venous pressure
    (d) decrease in dead space/tidal volume ratio

514. Pyoderma gangrenosum is typically associated with:
    (a) advanced colonic adenocarcinoma
    (b) rectal carcinoid
    (c) ulcerative colitis
    (d) villous adenoma of the colon

515. Popliteal artery aneurysms:
    (a) commonly present with rupture
    (b) seldom result in limb ischemia
    (c) are the most common peripheral arterial aneurysms
    (d) require operation only if they result in embolization
    (e) are most commonly false aneurysms

516. After vigorous exercise, an athlete develops pain on dorsiflexion of the foot and decreased sensation in the first web space. Appropriate action should be:
    (a) color duplex scan and immediate heparinization
    (b) leg elevation, ice packs, and nonsteroidal anti-inflammatory medications
    (c) immediate fasciotomy
    (d) immediate femoral arteriogram

517. The most common presentation of testicular cancer is:
    (a) a painless scrotal mass
    (b) acute testicular pain
    (c) a secondary hydrocele
    (d) gynecomastia
    (e) retroperitoneal lymphadenopathy

518. Which of the following is most likely to cause a false-positive fecal occult blood test?
    (a) oral iron therapy
    (b) Coumadin therapy
    (c) aspirin therapy
    (d) nonsteroidal anti-inflammatory medications
    (e) dietary peroxidases

519. Aldosteronoma is associated with:
    (a) hypertension, hypokalemia, high aldosterone and high renin levels
    (b) hypertension, hyperkalemia, high aldosterone and low renin levels
    (c) hypertension, hyperkalemia, high aldosterone and high renin levels
    (d) hypertension, hypokalemia, high aldosterone and low renin levels

520. A PO_2 of 90 torr, PCO_2 of 28 torr, and pH of 7.16 on room air are indicative of:
  (a) hypovolemic shock
  (b) alveolar hypoventilation
  (c) prolonged nasogastric suctioning
  (d) hyperventilation

521. Idiopathic thrombocytopenic purpura is most likely to respond to splenectomy if:
  (a) the spleen is enlarged
  (b) the patient is a female
  (c) the disease is chronic
  (d) the disease responded to steroids

522. A marker that would distinguish nonseminoma from seminoma is:
  (a) lactate dehydrogenase
  (b) alkaline phosphatases
  (c) human chorionic gonadotropin
  (d) α-fetoprotein

523. Positive end-expiratory pressure:
  (a) increases cardiac output
  (b) decreases functional residual capacity
  (c) increases right to left shunting
  (d) lowers PCO_2
  (e) decreases alveolar–arterial oxygen gradient

524. Estrogen therapy for postmenopausal women is associated with:
  (a) increased incidence of thrombophlebitis
  (b) increased incidence of hepatic adenoma
  (c) increased incidence of endometrial cancer
  (d) increased incidence of breast cancer

525. A 10-year-old boy comes from a family of "bleeders." His coagulation profile shows: prolonged bleeding time, normal prothrombin time, and prolonged partial thromboplastin time. His platelet count is 150,000/mm³. The most likely diagnosis is:
  (a) idiopathic thrombocytopenic purpura
  (b) thrombotic thrombocytopenic purpura
  (c) hemophilia
  (d) Christmas disease
  (e) von Willebrand's disease

526. A single organism is usually the causative agent in:
  (a) pelvic inflammatory disease
  (b) perforated diverticulitis
  (c) acute cholecystitis
  (d) primary peritonitis
  (e) diabetic foot infections

527. Neurogenic bladder dysfunction with intact bladder sensation is associated with:
  (a) nerve injury with abdominoperineal resection
  (b) cauda equina lesion
  (c) myelomeningocele
  (d) paraplegia
  (e) cerebrovascular accident

528. Tumor necrosis factor-α antagonist is useful in treating:
  (a) disseminated intravascular coagulopathy
  (b) septic shock
  (c) Crohn's disease
  (d) metastatic melanoma

529. An 83-year-old female presents with vomiting and abdominal distension. She complains of pain in the medial aspect of the right thigh, and a palpable lump can be felt on the right side on rectal examination. The appropriate action is:
  (a) nasogastric tube, intravenous fluids, and observation
  (b) flexible sigmoidoscopy and drainage of the rectal mass
  (c) urgent laparotomy
  (d) Gastrografin study with small bowel follow-through
  (e) right groin exploration and hernia repair

530. A normal-sized spleen is found in:
  (a) idiopathic thrombocytopenic purpura
  (b) myelodysplasia
  (c) Gaucher's disease
  (d) thalassemia
  (e) schistosomiasis

531. Neurogenic bladder after extensive pelvic surgery is characterized by:
  (a) painful urine retention
  (b) large bladder capacity with overflow incontinence
  (c) small residual volume and uninhibited bladder contractions
  (d) autonomic dysreflexia

532. Regarding cytokines:
  (a) serum level is not related to the severity of illness
  (b) are stored intracellularly as preformed molecules
  (c) are produced by a limited number of specific cells
  (d) most commonly function in an endocrine fashion
  (e) low serum levels are normally detected in healthy individuals

533. Hypothermic coagulopathy is characterized by:
    (a) normal prothrombin time and normal partial thromboplastin time
    (b) normal prothrombin time and prolonged partial thromboplastin time
    (c) prolonged prothrombin time and normal partial thromboplastin time
    (d) depletion of factor VII
    (e) depletion of factor VIII

534. A patient with diagnosed pseudomembranous colitis is developing a worsening clinical picture and is taken for urgent laparotomy. The appropriate surgical procedure should include:
    (a) segmental colectomy and exteriorization of the ends
    (b) total abdominal colectomy
    (c) diverting proximal colostomy
    (d) segmental colectomy and primary anastomosis
    (e) segmental colectomy, primary anastomosis, and diverting colostomy

535. The specificity of a test is:
    (a) the proportion of patients with the disease who have a positive test
    (b) the proportion of patients without the disease who have a negative test
    (c) the proportion of patients with a positive test who have the disease
    (d) the proportion of patients with a negative test who do not have the disease

536. A 45-year-old-male complains of severe chest pain after a diagnostic upper endoscopy. He has crepitus on palpation of his neck. The next step in management should be:
    (a) repeated upper endoscopy
    (b) immediate endotracheal intubation
    (c) Gastrografin swallow
    (d) administration of aspirin and sublingual nitrite
    (e) admission to ICU, administration of intravenous narcotics, and observation

537. Familial adenomatous polyposis:
    (a) is caused by inactivation of a tumor suppressor gene
    (b) has normal life expectancy after prophylactic colectomy
    (c) is associated with increased risk of right-side colon cancer
    (d) is inherited as an autosomal recessive trait

538. The most common posterior mediastinal mass in children is:
    (a) neuroblastoma
    (b) teratoma
    (c) lymphoma
    (d) pheochromocytoma

539. In the absence of sepsis, glucose intolerance with total parenteral nutrition may indicate:
    (a) copper deficiency
    (b) zinc deficiency
    (c) magnesium deficiency
    (d) chromium deficiency

540. The most common presentation of gastric cancer is:
    (a) hematemesis and melena
    (b) acute abdominal pain due to perforation
    (c) vague abdominal pain and weight loss
    (d) an epigastric mass

541. In burn victims, the finding most indicative of inhalation injury is:
    (a) singed nasal hair
    (b) soot around the mouth
    (c) dyspnea
    (d) carbonaceous sputum

542. A child with anaphylactoid purpura develops an acute colicky abdominal pain and bleeding per rectum. The most likely diagnosis is:
    (a) perforated duodenal ulcer
    (b) bleeding Meckel's diverticulum
    (c) enterocolitis with perforation
    (d) intussusception

543. The most reliable means of preoperative nutritional assessment is:
    (a) clinical history of weight loss
    (b) serum albumin level
    (c) impaired cell-mediated immunity
    (d) triceps skinfold measurement

544. In contrast to adults, fetal wound healing:
    (a) has a higher content of type III collagen
    (b) has a higher level of transforming growth factor-β
    (c) has an exaggerated inflammatory phase
    (d) has much less hyaluronic acid content

545. The greatest amount of maintenance intravenous fluids is required for:
    (a) 21-year-old male athlete
    (b) 55-year-old obese male office worker
    (c) 21-year-old housewife
    (d) 75-year-old female with recent weight loss

546. The most accurate test to detect subclinical hypothyroidism is:
    (a) radioactive iodine uptake
    (b) thyroid-stimulating hormone level
    (c) total thyroxine level
    (d) free thyroxine level

547. A 28-year-old male has a closed head injury, pulmonary contusion, grade III splenic injury, and closed femoral shaft fracture. The ideal management of his fracture is:
    (a) external fixation
    (b) skeletal traction
    (c) intramedullary nailing within 24 hours of injury
    (d) intramedullary nailing 1 week after the injury
    (e) use of metal plates and screws

548. Accessory spleens are most commonly found in:
    (a) idiopathic thrombocytopenic purpura
    (b) thrombotic thrombocytopenic purpura
    (c) schistosomiasis
    (d) hereditary spherocytosis

549. The effectiveness of prophylactic antibiotics in surgery is mostly related to the:
    (a) use of broad-spectrum agents
    (b) continuation of antibiotics for 24 hours after surgery
    (c) timing of initial administration
    (d) use of two synergistic agents
    (e) use of bactericidal agents

550. A 6-year-old boy has a right undescended testicle. His parents should be advised that:
    (a) right orchiectomy should be performed
    (b) a course of endocrine treatment is advisable
    (c) orchiopexy is performed to improve spermatogenesis and prevent cancer
    (d) orchiopexy is performed but with no effect on spermatogenesis or cancer prevention
    (e) the right testicle is probably atrophic and can be left undisturbed

551. The sensitivity of the test is:
    (a) the proportion of patients with the disease who have a positive test
    (b) the proportion of patients without the disease who have a negative test
    (c) the proportion of patients with a positive test who have the disease
    (d) the proportion of patients with a negative test who do not have the disease

552. Regarding an amebic liver abscess:
    (a) surgical drainage is usually required
    (b) negative stool testing for amebiasis rules out the disease
    (c) it should be drained percutaneously under computed tomography guidance
    (d) it is treated with metronidazole

553. An infant has been having episodic coughing for 48 hours. On examination, he is wheezing with decreased aeration of the left chest. A chest x-ray shows an overinflated left lung. The next step in management should be:
    (a) insertion of left-side chest tube
    (b) insertion of right-side chest tube
    (c) endotracheal intubation
    (d) administration of steroid inhaler and observation
    (e) rigid bronchoscopy

554. A 40-year-old female has a 4-cm hemangioma in the right lobe of the liver on computed tomography scan. She is asymptomatic. Appropriate action should be:
    (a) fine-needle biopsy
    (b) arrangement for elective resection
    (c) no further action
    (d) angiographic embolization

555. A non-anion gap metabolic acidosis is associated with:
    (a) methane intoxication
    (b) large amount of saline resuscitation
    (c) diabetic ketoacidosis
    (d) cardiogenic shock
    (e) hemorrhagic shock

556. The gold standard for the diagnosis of pelvic inflammatory disease is:
    (a) vaginal microbiology swab
    (b) pelvic ultrasound
    (c) laparoscopy
    (d) pelvic computed tomography scan
    (e) endometrial biopsy

557. A 60-year-old alcoholic male presents with severe
     chest pain after repeated vomiting. A chest x-ray
     shows a small left pleural effusion. The next step in
     management is:
     (a) obtain cardiac enzymes and admit to coronary
         care unit
     (b) insert nasogastric tube, administer intravenous
         fluids, and observe
     (c) insert nasogastric and left-side chest tube and
         antibiotics
     (d) administer Gastrografin swallow test
     (e) perform upper endoscopy

558. Mediastinal granulomas may be associated with:
     (a) epiphrenic esophageal diverticulum
     (b) Zenker's diverticulum
     (c) esophageal traction diverticulum
     (d) achalasia

175
Surgery Review Answers

1. d	40. c	79. b	118. e	157. b	196. d
2. c	41. a	80. c	119. c	158. c	197. d
3. b	42. e	81. c	120. d	159. c	198. c
4. c	43. c	82. c	121. c	160. a	199. a
5. d	44. e	83. a	122. c	161. c	200. a
6. b	45. b	84. a	123. a	162. e	201. b
7. b	46. c	85. c	124. d	163. a	202. d
8. b	47. d	86. b	125. b	164. a	203. d
9. b	48. b	87. e	126. b	165. b	204. d
10. d	49. d	88. b	127. d	166. d	205. b
11. c	50. c	89. a	128. a	167. e	206. a
12. a	51. d	90. b	129. d	168. a	207. c
13. a	52. d	91. a	130. a	169. c	208. e
14. b	53. c	92. a	131. d	170. d	209. a
15. d	54. a	93. a	132. e	171. b	210. c
16. a	55. c	94. b	133. d	172. c	211. d
17. c	56. a	95. a	134. c	173. a	212. e
18. a	57. c	96. a	135. e	174. d	213. d
19. c	58. b	97. c	136. a	175. c	214. d
20. c	59. e	98. c	137. e	176. d	215. a
21. d	60. a	99. d	138. b	177. c	216. e
22. d	61. b	100. c	139. c	178. b	217. c
23. e	62. c	101. b	140. a	179. d	218. b
24. a	63. e	102. a	141. c	180. a	219. a
25. c	64. a	103. b	142. b	181. c	220. c
26. c	65. a	104. c	143. d	182. a	221. d
27. d	66. a	105. a	144. a	183. e	222. a
28. c	67. e	106. e	145. e	184. a	223. b
29. c	68. c	107. b	146. e	185. b	224. b
30. e	69. b	108. d	147. b	186. b	225. b
31. e	70. e	109. a	148. e	187. c	226. b
32. b	71. b	110. d	149. b	188. b	227. d
33. b	72. c	111. c	150. a	189. c	228. c
34. e	73. d	112. d	151. a	190. b	229. c
35. a	74. a	113. d	152. a	191. e	230. d
36. c	75. c	114. b	153. d	192. a	231. d
37. a	76. b	115. d	154. c	193. b	232. d
38. c	77. d	116. c	155. b	194. c	233. c
39. a	78. e	117. b	156. b	195. d	234. d

235. b	289. d	343. b	397. b	451. b	505. c
236. b	290. c	344. e	398. e	452. a	506. c
237. c	291. b	345. b	399. a	453. b	507. a
238. a	292. e	346. b	400. e	454. e	508. b
239. c	293. c	347. b	401. c	455. d	509. a
240. d	294. d	348. c	402. b	456. c	510. a
241. c	295. c	349. a	403. e	457. c	511. c
242. b	296. b	350. d	404. d	458. b	512. e
243. d	297. b	351. d	405. d	459. e	513. a
244. d	298. b	352. b	406. a	460. c	514. c
245. a	299. b	353. e	407. c	461. a	515. c
246. d	300. d	354. a	408. d	462. a	516. c
247. c	301. b	355. a	409. a	463. c	517. a
248. b	302. a	356. d	410. c	464. c	518. e
249. c	303. b	357. b	411. a	465. b	519. d
250. e	304. a	358. c	412. d	466. c	520. a
251. d	305. c	359. d	413. d	467. a	521. d
252. c	306. d	360. b	414. c	468. b	522. d
253. b	307. c	361. d	415. d	469. a	523. e
254. b	308. c	362. a	416. b	470. a	524. c
255. c	309. c	363. e	417. c	471. d	525. e
256. b	310. b	364. e	418. c	472. c	526. d
257. c	311. c	365. a	419. b	473. e	527. e
258. a	312. e	366. a	420. e	474. b	528. c
259. c	313. a	367. b	421. c	475. c	529. c
260. a	314. c	368. c	422. a	476. c	530. a
261. d	315. c	369. a	423. d	477. d	531. b
262. d	316. c	370. c	424. c	478. b	532. a
263. a	317. a	371. b	425. d	479. b	533. a
264. d	318. a	372. b	426. a	480. b	534. b
265. c	319. b	373. d	427. a	481. d	535. b
266. b	320. a	374. d	428. c	482. b	536. c
267. c	321. b	375. c	429. e	483. b	537. a
268. a	322. d	376. b	430. c	484. b	538. a
269. c	323. b	377. d	431. d	485. a	539. d
270. b	324. a	378. c	432. c	486. e	540. c
271. c	325. d	379. b	433. d	487. c	541. d
272. a	326. c	380. a	434. a	488. c	542. d
273. c	327. c	381. d	435. c	489. a	543. a
274. d	328. a	382. d	436. d	490. d	544. a
275. c	329. a	383. c	437. d	491. c	545. a
276. b	330. d	384. b	438. d	492. b	546. b
277. e	331. c	385. c	439. c	493. c	547. c
278. c	332. b	386. c	440. a	494. a	548. d
279. b	333. c	387. a	441. b	495. d	549. c
280. c	334. c	388. d	442. b	496. a	550. d
281. a	335. b	389. a	443. e	497. b	551. a
282. c	336. b	390. c	444. b	498. e	552. d
283. c	337. a	391. b	445. c	499. e	553. e
284. b	338. d	392. d	446. d	500. d	554. c
285. c	339. b	393. c	447. a	501. d	555. b
286. b	340. d	394. b	448. c	502. a	556. c
287. c	341. b	395. b	449. a	503. b	557. d
288. a	342. d	396. b	450. b	504. a	558. c

Bibliography

Books

ACS Surgery: Principles and Practice 2004. Wilmore DW et al. (eds.) New York: WebMD Professional Publishing, 2004.

ACS Surgery: Principles and Practice 2005. Wilmore DW (ed). Electronic book. New York: WebMD Professional Publishing, 2005. Available at http://online.statref.com.

Anesthesia, 5th edition. Miller RD (ed). New York: Churchill Livingstone, 2000.

Anesthesia, 6th edition. Miller RD (ed). New York: Churchill Livingstone, 2004.

Anesthesia Secrets, 2nd edition. Duke J. Philadelphia: Hanley & Belfus, 2000.

APC Medicine 2005. Dale DC (ed). Electronic book. New York: WebMD Professional Publishing, 2005. Available at http://online.statref.com.

Basic Science Review for Surgeons. Simmons RL, Steed DL (eds). Philadelphia: W.B. Saunders Company, 1992.

Brenner & Rector's The Kidney, 7th edition. Brenner BM, Livine SA (eds). Philadelphia: W.B. Saunders Company, 2004.

Campbell's Operative Orthopaedics, 10th edition. Canale ST (ed). Philadelphia: Mosby Publishers, 2002.

Cecil Textbook of Medicine, 21st edition. Goldman L, Bennett C (eds). Philadelphia: W.B. Saunders Company, 2000.

Cecil Textbook of Medicine, 22nd edition. Goldman L, Ausicllo D (eds). Philadelphia: W.B. Saunders Company, 2004.

Clinical Oncology, 2nd edition. Abeloff MD, Armitage JO, Lichter AS, Niederhuber JE. New York: Churchill Livingstone, 2000.

Clinical Oncology, 3rd edition. Abeloff MD, Armitage JO, Niederhuber JE, Kastan MB, McKenna WG. New York: Churchill Livingstone, 2004.

Current Critical Care Diagnosis & Treatment, 2nd edition. Bongard FS. Stamford, CT: Appleton & Lange, 2003.

Current Surgical Diagnosis & Treatment, 11th edition. Way LL, Doherty GM (eds). New York: McGraw-Hill, 2002.

Current Surgical Therapy, 7th edition. Cameron JL (ed). Philadelphia: Mosby Year Book, Inc., 2001.

Current Surgical Therapy, 8th edition. Cameron JL (ed). Philadelphia: Mosby Year Book, Inc., 2004.

Essentials of Basic Science of Surgery. Savage EB, Fishma S, Miller LD (eds). Philadelphia: Lippincott Williams & Wilkins, 1993.

Evaluation of the patient with established venous thrombosis. Bauer KA, Lip GYH. Available at http://patients.uptodate.com/topic.asp?file=coagulat/7266.

Grainger & Allison's Diagnostic Radiology, 4th edition. Grainger RG, Allison DJ, Adam A, Dixon AK (eds). New York: Churchill Livingstone, 2001.

The ICU Book, 2nd edition. Marino PL. Philadelphia: Lippincott Williams & Wilkins, 1998.

Internal Medicine, 5th edition. Stein JH (ed). St. Louis: Mosby Year Book, Inc., 1998.

Management of inherited thrombophilia. Bauer KA. Available at http://patients.uptodate.com/topic.asp?file=coagulat/7802.

Mastery of Surgery, 4th edition. Baker RJ, Fischer JE (eds). Philadelphia: Lippincott Williams & Wilkins, 2001.

The Merck Manual of Diagnosis and Therapy, 17th edition. Beers MH, Berkow R (eds). New York: John Wiley and Sons, Inc., 1999.

Nelson Textbook of Pediatrics, 17th edition. Behrman RE (ed). Philadelphia: W.B. Saunders Company, 2003.

Obstetrics: Normal and Problem Pregnancies, 4th edition. Gabbe SG, Neibyl JR, Simpson JL (eds). Philadelphia: W.B. Saunders Company, 2002.

Physiologic Basis of Modern Surgical Care. Miller T, Rowlands BJ (eds). St. Louis: C. V. Mosby Company, 1988.

Physiologic Basis of Modern Surgical Care, 2nd edition. Miller T (ed). St. Louis: Quality Medical Publications, 1996.

The Physiologic Basis of Surgery, 3rd edition. O'Leary JP (ed). Philadelphia: Lippincott Williams & Wilkins, 2002.

Principles and Practices of Surgery for the Colon, Rectum and Anus, 2nd edition. Gordon PH, Nivatvongs S. St. Louis: Quality Medical Publishers, 1999.

Principles of Surgery, 6th edition. Schwartz SI, Shires GT, Spencer FC, Husser WC (eds). New York: McGraw-Hill, Inc., 1994.

Review for Surgery: Scientific Principles and Practice, 3rd edition. Greenfield LJ, Lillemoe KD, Mulholland MW, Oldham KT, Zelenock GB (eds). Philadelphia: Lippincott Williams & Wilkins, 2002.

Review of Medical Physiology, 21st edition. Ganong WF. New York: McGraw Hill. 2003.

Robbins and Cotran: Pathologic Basis of Disease, 7th edition. Kumar V, Abbas AK, Fausto N (eds). Philadelphia: W.B. Saunders Company, 2005.

Sabiston Textbook of Surgery: The Biological Basis of Modern Surgical Practice, 16th edition. Townsend CM, Beauchamp RD, Evers BM, Mattox K (eds). Philadelphia: W.B. Saunders Company, 2000.

Sabiston Textbook of Surgery: The Biological Basis of Modern Surgical Practice, 17th edition. Townsend CM, Beauchamp RD, Evers BM (eds). Philadelphia: W.B. Saunders Company, 2004.

Schwartz's Principles of Surgery: A Modern Approach, 7th edition. Schwartz SI, Shires GT, Spencer FC, Daly JM, Fischer JE, Galloway AC (eds). New York: McGraw-Hill, 1999.

Schwartz's Principles of Surgery: A Modern Approach, 8th edition. Brunicardi FC, Anderson DK, Billiar TR, Dunn DL, Hunter JG, Andersen DK, Pollock RE (eds). New York: McGraw-Hill, 2004.

Shackelford's Surgery of the Alimentary Tract, 5th edition. Zuidema GD, Yeo CJ (eds). Philadelphia: W.B. Saunders Company, 2001.

Sleisenger & Fordtrans's Gastrointestinal and Liver Disease, 7th edition. Feldman M, Friedman L, Sleisenger MH. Philadelphia: W.B. Saunders Company, 2002.

Textbook of Critical Care, 4th edition. Shoemaker WC, Ayres SM, Grenvik A, Holbrook PR (eds). Philadelphia: W.B. Saunders Company, 2000.

Textbook of Medical Physiology, 9th edition. Guyton AC, Hall JE (eds). Philadelphia: W.B. Saunders Company, 1996.

Vascular Surgery, 5th edition. Rutherford RB (ed). Philadelphia: W.B. Saunders, Company, 2000.

Williams Textbook of Endocrinology, 10th edition. Larsen PR, Kronenburg HM, Melmed S (eds). Philadelphia: W.B. Saunders Company, 2003.

Scientific Journal Articles

Baillie JM. Tumors of the gallbladder and bile ducts. J Clin Gastroenterol 1999; 29(1):14–21.

Baylis TB, Norris BL. Pelvic fractures and the general surgeon. Curr Surg 2004; 61:30–35.

Beigi RH, Wiesenfeld HC. Pelvic inflammatory disease. New diagnostic criteria for treatment. Obstet Gynecol Clin North Am 2003; 30:777–793.

Berger A. Magnetic resonance imaging. BMJ 2002; 324:35.

Biffl WL, Smith WR, Moore EE, et al. Evolution of multidisciplinary clinical pathway for the management of unstable patients with pelvic fractures. Ann Surg 2001; 233: 843–850.

Brem H, Sheehan P, Boulton AJ. Protocol for the treatment of diabetic foot ulcers. Am J Surg 2004; 187(5A):1S–10S.

Buchwald H, Avidor Y, Braunwald E, Jensen MD, Pories W, Fahrbach K, Scholelles K. Bariatric surgery: A systematic review and meta-analysis. JAMA 2004; 292(14):1724–1737.

Cannistra SA. Cancer of the ovary. N Engl J Med 2004; 351: 2519–2529.

Colditz GA. Economic costs of obesity. Am J Clin Nutr 1992; 55(Suppl 2):503S–507S.

Davies MG, Fulton GJ, Hagen PO. Clinical biology of nitric oxide. Br J Surg 1995; 82:1598–1610.

Deitel M. Overweight and obesity worldwide now estimated to involve 1.7 billion people. Obes Surg 2003; 13:329–330.

Loran DB, Zwischenberger JB. Thoracic surgery in the elderly. J Am Coll Surg 2004; 199:773–784.

Lowry SF. Cytokine mediators of immunity and inflammation. Arch Surg 1993; 128:1235–1241.

Luckey AE, Parsa CJ. Fluid and electrolytes in the elderly. Arch Surg 2003; 138:1055–1060.

Nieweg OE, Tanis PJ, Kroon BB. The definition of a sentinel node. Ann Surg Oncol 2001; 8:538–541.

Patti MG, Gantert W, Way LW. Surgery of the esophagus. Surg Clin North Am 1997; 77:959–970.

Raeburn CD, Sheppard F, Barsness KA, Arya J, Harken AH. Cytokines for surgeons. Am J Surg 2002; 183:268–273.

Snyder HS. Blunt pelvic trauma. Am J Emerg Med 1988; 6:618–627.

Wolf AM, Colditz GA. The current estimates of the economic costs of obesity in the United States. Obes Res 1998; 6:97–106.

Other Sources

National Center for Health Statistics. Available at http://www.cdc.gov/nchs/data/nhis/earlyrelease/200406_06.pdf. Accessed January 25, 2005.

National Comprehensive Cancer Network. Clinical Practice Guidelines in Oncology. Colon Cancer v.2.2005. Available at http://www.nccn.org.

Index